ADAPTABILITY
OF VASCULAR WALL

Adaptability
of Vascular Wall

PROCEEDINGS OF THE XIth INTERNATIONAL

CONGRESS OF ANGIOLOGY-PRAGUE 1978

Editors:

Z. REINIŠ, J. POKORNÝ, J. LINHART,

R. HILD and A. SCHIRGER

With 486 Figures and 205 Tables

1980

AVICENUM CZECHOSLOVAK MEDICAL PRESS PRAGUE

SPRINGER-VERLAG BERLIN HEIDELBERG NEW YORK

ISBN-13: 978-3-540-09907-9   e-ISBN-13: 978-3-642-67582-9
DOI: 10.1007/ 978-3-642-67582-9

Publishers:

AVICENUM — Czechoslovak Medical Press, Prague

SPRINGER-VERLAG — Berlin—Heidelberg—New York

XIth INTERNATIONAL CONGRESS OF ANGIOLOGY
ADAPTABILITY OF VASCULAR WALL

Prague, Czechoslovakia July 2.–8. 1978

Organizing Committee

(on behalf of International Union of Angiology and of Czechoslovak Medical Society
J. E. Purkyně)

President

Z. REINIŠ

Secretary General

J. POKORNÝ

Scientific Secretary

J. LINHART

International Scientific Committee

E. Betz (Tübingen), M. Degni (Sao Paolo), R. Hild (Heidelberg),
N. Klüken (Essen), J. F. Merlen (Lille), A. N. Klimov (Leningrad),
K. Seki (Tokyo), A. Schirger (Rochester), G. Martorell (Barcelona),
F. Pratesi (Firenze) and J. Rannie (Newcastle upon Tyne)

PREFACE

The International Congresses of Angiology have had a 25-year tradition. Let us remember the 10 previous International Congresses, the first of which took place in Paris in 1952. On this occasion a stimulus for the foundation of the International Union, "Union Internationale d' Angéiologie" came into existence.

The period of 25 years is long enough to evaluate the scientific progress which has been made in diagnosis, therapy and prevention of vascular diseases. Proceedings of the previous International Congresses of Angiology became attractive resources for scientific information in libraries all over the world. They represent really historic documents of remarkable development of angiology and wittness successful international cooperation in the settlement of serious medical problems of the twentieth century.

The Proceedings of the XI. International Congress of Angiology held in Prague 1978 under the stimulating title "Adaptability of Vascular Wall" contains 284 original papers dealing with scientific and clinical research in arterial, venous and lymphatic circulation. The papers are incorporated into 12 chapters according to the main topics.

In the first sections the questions of atherogenesis and thrombogenesis are discussed with regard to the adaptability of vascular wall in various metabolic, immunobiologic, and hemodynamic disorders. In the further sections attention is paid to new procedures in investigation, treatment, and prevention of arterial, venous, and lymphatic diseases. Peripheral microangiopathies, renovascular hypertension, and coronary circulation represent another part.

Many histochemical studies have shown that vascular tissue is of high biologic activity and is protected against pathologic processes by specific enzymatic systems. Regression of atherosclerosis was confirmed not only in experimental animals but it was also predicted in human beings when exogenous risk factors were eliminated. The adaptation of venous grafts into the arterial circulation revealed a remarkable ability of vascular tissue to be „arterialized" and to function in aorto-coronary or in femoro-tibial bypass as well.

New diagnostic methods in vascular diseases were presented and the findings were compared with radioisotopic, ultrasonic, and angiographic procedures. Pharmacotherapy was enriched by new drugs with anticoagulant and thrombolytic effect or with hypolipemic and vasodilation efficiency. Reconstructive surgery of arterial occlusions achieved unexpected progress. Recent epidemiologic studies confirmed the validity of the risk factor theory and several multifactorial preventive programmes are being conducted at present in different parts of the world.

The goal of the scientific program of the Congress was to bring together experts in the multiple disciplines that have a bearing on blood vessels. Participation of pathologists, histochemists, biochemists, radiologists, dermatologists, internists, and surgeons in the experimental and clinical research in the vascular diseases has shown that angiology is a modern interdisciplinary branch of medicine.

Presenting the Proceedings on „Adaptability of Vascular Wall" to medical people all over the world, we are convinced it will be fruitful for every medical doctor who is interested in new diagnostic, therapeutic and preventive procedures of vascular diseases.

Z. REINIŠ

CONTENTS

ATHEROGENESIS

THROMBOGENESIS

IMMUNOLOGICAL ASPECTS OF VASCULAR DISEASES

ADAPTABILITY OF VASCULAR TISSUE SURGERY

EPIDEMIOLOGY AND PREVENTION OF VASCULAR DISEASES

INVESTIGATION OF ARTERIAL AND VENOUS DISORDERS

PERIPHERAL MICROANGIOPATHIES

VENOUS AND LYMPHATIC CIRCULATION

PHARMACOLOGY AND THERAPY OF VASCULAR DISEASES

Pharmacology and pharmakokinetics of Trimepranol (Symposium)

RENOVASCULAR HYPERTENSION

CORONARY CIRCULATION

ATHEROGENESIS

EXPERIMENTAL ATHEROSCLEROSIS
REGRESSION OF ATHEROSCLEROSIS
LONG-TERM COURSE OF OBLITERATIVE ATHEROSCLEROSIS

1

PHYSIOLOGICAL, MORPHOLOGICAL AND ANGIOCHEMICAL CHANGES IN AORTA AND LOWER EXTREMITY ARTERIES IN MACACA FASCICULARIS MONKEYS FED AN ATHEROGENIC DIET FOR 3 YEARS

H. D. GREEN, D. J. FARRAR, M. G. BOND, W. D. WAGNER
AND R. A. GOBBEE

*Departments of Physiology and Comparative Medicine, Bowman Gray School
of Medicine, Winston-Salem, N.C., U.S.A.*

Seven *M. fascicularis* monkeys (test) were fed an atherogenic diet (45% of calories from lard with 1 mg. of cholesterol per KCal) for 36 months. Six control monkeys were fed the same diet but without added cholesterol (0.05 mg. of cholesterol per KCal) for 36 months. These 13 monkeys of uniform size were studied at sacrifice at completion of the diet period at which time total serum cholesterol concentrations were: test 647 ± 81 mg/dl (mean $\pm$ SEM) and control 180 ± 15 mg/dl. Four types of studies were done: (a) physiological measurement (invasive and non-invasive) of simultaneously detected pulse contours in the subclavian and femoral arteries and the toe volume pulses (Fig. 1 A and B) plus measurements of the distances between detection sites, (b) measurements of static circumferential distensibility of excised strips of the aorta, (c) macroscopic evaluation of atherosclerosis, and (d) chemical analyses of arterial wall composition. Pulse wave velocities were calculated as 1/transit time (sec^{-1}) or as distance divided by transit time (M/sec).

Results

The velocity of the foot of the pulse wave increased linearly with increase of arteria diastolic pressure in both the aortic segment (Fig. 2) (subclavian artery to femoral artery) and the leg segment (Fig. 3) (femoral artery to toe); the average velocity was less in the latter.

The velocity of the foot of the pulse wave in the aortic segment was faster in the test monkeys than in the controls at all levels of arterial diastolic pressure (Fig. 2), however, consistent changes were not observed in the velocity of the wave peak. Increases in pulse wave velocities of the leg segment were not seen in the test monkeys (Fig. 3).

Fourier harmonic analysis of the pulse waves revealed that the apparent phase velocities of the second through seventh harmonics were comparable to the veloci-

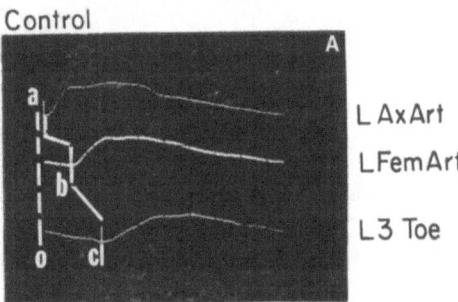

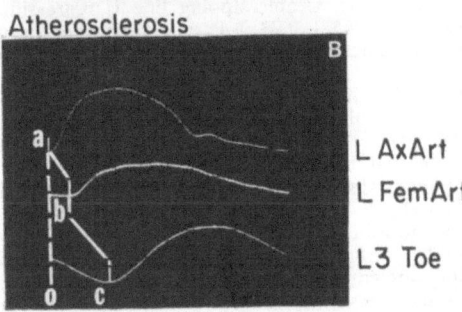

Fig. 1. Simultaneously recorded pulses: (a) subclavian artery, (b) femoral artery, and (c) toe pulses in (A) control, and (B) test (atherosclerotic) M. fascicularis monkeys. Note shorter foot-to-foot time in aortic segment $(a - b = \Delta\alpha)$ in test compared with control monkey.

3

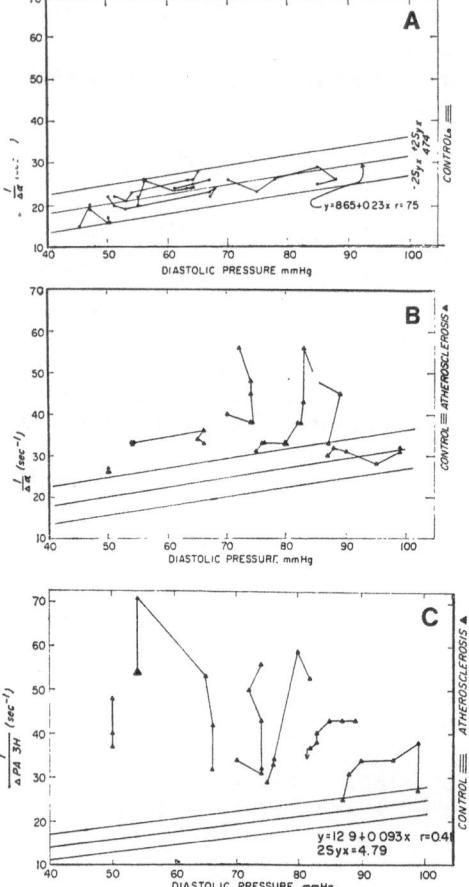

using the linear regression data in the controls, these velocities in the aortic segment of the test monkeys averaged approximately twice that of the control monkeys at 70 mm Hg (Fig. 2) but were not different from control in the leg segment (Fig. 3).

As a group the enhanced aortic pulse wave velocity correlated closely with the increased stiffness (decreased distensibility of circumferential segments of the aortic wall and with the increased thickness of the wall, i.e., both were approximately doubled. However, there was no significant change in Young's elastic modulus, i.e., in stiffness divided by thickness. Cholesterol

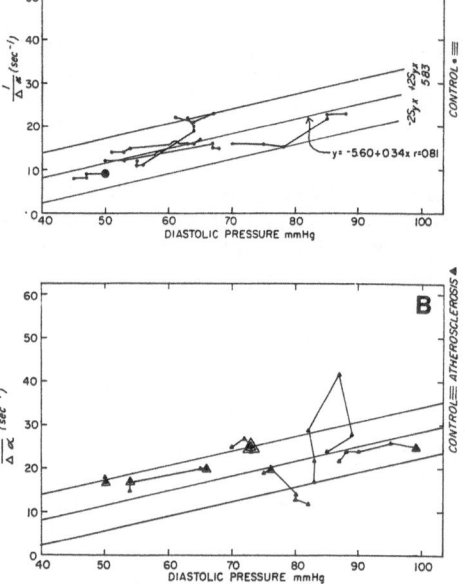

Fig. 2. A — Plot of reciprocal of control transit times $1/\varDelta\alpha$ (sec^{-1}) for foot-to-foot of pulses for aortic segment (subclavian to femoral detection sites). Center sloping line is regression line ($y = 8.65 + 0.23x$). Parallel lines above and below regression line represent ±2 sd of y on $x = \pm4.7$ sec^{-1}. Reciprocal times — ordinate scale — can be converted to approximate velocity by multiplying by 0.31 meters; this yields 7.67 M/sec at 70 mm Hg for control. Points connected by a line represent data from one animal. Abscissa — aortic diastolic pressure in mm Hg. B, C — Plots of aortic segment for (B) foot-to-foot and (C) — apparent phase velocity of 3rd harmonic of test animal (points). Parallel lines are control data (regression and confidence limits); lines in B are same as those in A.

Fig. 3. Plots, similar to Fig. 2 A and B, of leg segment (femoral artery to toe plethysmographic pulse) — both recorded non-invasively. A — points are for control monkeys; in B points are for test animals; parallel lines in both A and B are the same and represent control data regression line and confidence limits. Equation for control is $y = -5.60 + 0.34x$. Reciprocal time (sec^{-1}) can be converted to approximate velocity by multiplying reciprocal time by 0.35 meters, yielding a foot-to-foot control velocity of 6.37 M/sec at 70 mm Hg.

ties of the foot of pulse wave in aortic and femoral segments of both test and control monkeys (Fig. 2 C). When corrected to 70 mm Hg diastolic pressure,

and calcium content per unit of intimal surface area, and concentration per unit volume of wall substance were increased dramatically in the test group to approximately 10 times that of the control group. In contrast, in the test aortas, collagen and elastin content per unit area of intima increased more nearly in proportion to the wall thickness, wall rigidity and wave velocity and all five of these measurements were approximately twice that in the control aortas (*Farrar et al.*, 1978).

Conclusions

In *M. fascicularis* test monkeys a 36 month high cholesterol diet caused highly significant stiffening of the aortic wall (Wind Kessel) related to increased wall thickness and content of collagen and elastin, whereas no significant changes occurred in the control animals fed a diet low in cholesterol. This aortic stiffening is related to increase of the pulsepressure and can be detected by non-invasive registration of the pulse wave transit times between the carotid and femoral arteries.

Supported by National Institutes of Health, Grants HL 00487, SCOR-HL14164 and HL 05392.

REFERENCE

Farrar, D. J., Green, H. D., Bond, M. G., Wagner, W. D., and Gobbee, R. A. (1978): Aortic pulse wave velocity, elasticity, and composition in a non-human primate model of atherosclerosis. Circulation Res. 43: No. 1, July (in press).

H. G., Bowman Gray School of Med. Dept. of Physiology Winston-Salem, North Carolina, U.S.A.

THE PROLIFERATIVE ACTIVITY OF AORTIC ENDOTHELIUM AND ITS SIGNIFICANCE FOR ATHEROGENESIS

J. KUNZ

Institute of Pathology, Humboldt University, Berlin, G.D.R.

In recent years numerous studies have shown that mechanical (1, 2) and chemical (3, 4) injuries of the endothelial cells can exacerbate the formation of atherosclerotic lesions. The initial changes in this layer of cells are quite different. These are disturbances in the surface coat (5), increased cell turnover (6), occurrence of hexagonal or silver binding cells (3) and focal loss of foldings and bridges. It can also be shown by scanning electron microscopy that focal monocellular lesions occur after 3 days of cholesterol diet and crater-like changes after 6−7 weeks of this diet (4).

We assume that the physiologically existing regional differences in the proliferative activity of the endothelium are important for the development of atheromatous lesions. In investigations of autoradiograms of endothelial plane preparations of rabbit aorta after application of ^{3}H-thymidine, a nearly homogenous distribution of DNA − synthetizing cells is visible in areas without blood flow abnormalities. In previous studies we could demonstrate that aortic endothelial cells of adult animals in these areas are extremely long lived due to a small growth fraction and a generation time of about four months of the proliferating cells. With increasing age, there is a decrease in the labelling intensity as can be established by visual evaluation in accordance with the results of automatic image analysis (7, 8).

However, in comparison to this almost homogenous distribution, the proliferative behaviour of endothelium in the neighbourhood of branching sites is completely different. In these areas (ostia of the intercostal arteries), a higher labelling index can be found, especially in the ostium near endothelial cells (Fig. 1, Table I). These are the same sites where atheromatous lesions are manifested most distinctly (Fig. 2). The increased proliferative activity of these areas can be explained by 3 different mechanisms: 1. These regions may be growth centres comparable to the intestinal crypts; this is, however, not very probable. 2. These areas are still involved in growth and have not yet achieved a steady state.

However, most probable is the third possibility, that various flow − mechanical influences, such as locally increased pressure load, shearing forces and suction effects, are responsible for the increased proliferation at these sites. It has repeatedly been demonstrated electron-microscopically that here there is an increased rate of cell loss (9); Svendson and Jørgensen (10) found, by scanning electron microscopy, desquamations of cells from the basement membrane, breaks near the intercellular junctions, twisting of cells and platelet deposits on the denuded

Table 1. Mean labelling indices (= ^{3}H-thymidine labelled aortic endothelial cells per 1000 cells)

Animal	Zone I	Zone II	Zone III
1	10.2	5.0	5.9
2	7.3	6.9	4.7
3	15.6	10.7	8.1
4	5.8	3.3	3.6
5	2.2	0.7	3.6
6	24.0	10.0	5.9
Σ	65.1	36.6	31.8
Σ/6	10.9	6.1	5.3

Zone I   = ostium-near endothelial cells
Zone II = intermediary zone
Zone III = ostium-far endothelial cells
The breadth of every zone was 240 μm.

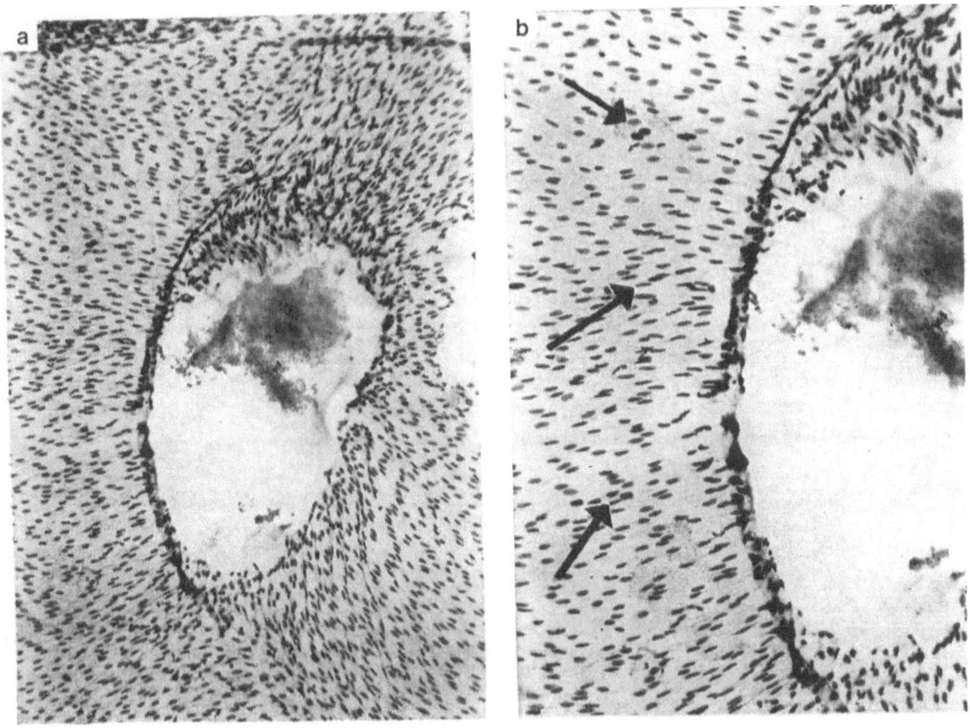

Fig. 1. Rabbit aortic endothelium. Plane preparation. Ostium of an intercostal artery. Autoradiogram after ^{3}H-thymidine-application. a 173×, b 277×. Numerous DNA-synthesizing cell in the zone near the ostium.

areas. Probably the proliferation triggering substances formed by the thrombocytes (12) start the cell division of media myocytes and in

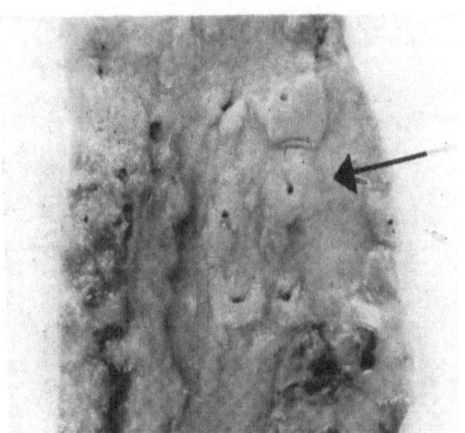

Fig. 2. Human aorta thoracica: Atheromatous changes in areas of the ostia of intercostal arteries. 1,7×.

this way stimulate the growth of atheromatous plaque. In areas with increased endothelial cell proliferation a higher permeability for Evans Blue (2, 11) and preferred deposits of lipoproteins in the subendothelium were also demonstrated. We feel that the above mentioned changes in the endothelial cells in certain areas — especially increased proliferation and permeability — can be aggravated by the known risk factors, so that functionally important lesions can be recognized microscopically. Further factors not associated with the endothelium, such as changes in the metabolism and structure of glycosaminoglycans of the media contribute decisively to this development.

However, it appears that some cases of atheromatosis, where no such atherogenic influences such as essential hypertension and hypercholesterolemia play a role, can be triggered off by flow mechanical factors alone.

7

REFERENCES

1. *Gertz, S. D. et al. (1976):* J. Neurosurg. 45 514—519.
2. *Stemerman, M. B. et al. (1977):* Amer. J. Pathol. 87, 125—142.
3. *Christensen, B. C. (1974):* Virchows Arch. A Pathol. Anat. and Histol. 363,33—46.
4. *De Bruijn, W. C. and W. van Mourik (1978):* Virchows Arch. A Pathol. Anat. and Histol. 365, 23—40.
5. *Weber, G. et al. (1973):* Virchows Arch. A Pathol. Anat. and Histol. 359, 299—307.
6. *Schwartz, St. M. and E. P. Benditt (1977):* Circul. Res. 41, 248—255.
7. *Kunz, J. and U. Keim (1975):* Mechanisms of Ageing and Development 4, 361—369.
8. *Kunz, J. et al. (1978):* Acta histochem. 61, 53—63.
9. *Gutstein, W. H. et al. (1973):* Labor. Invest 29, 134—149.
10. *Svendsen, E. and L. Jørgensen (1978):* Acta pathol. microbiol. scand. Sect. A 86, 1—13.
11. *Caplan, B. A. and C. J. Schwartz (1973):* Atherosclerosis 17, 401—417.
12. *Thorgeirsson, G. and A. L. Robertsen, Jr. (1978):* Atherosclerosis 30, 67—78.

J. K., Pathologisches Institut der Humboldt-Universität, Berlin, G.D.R.

ULTRASTRUCTURAL ASPECTS OF ATHEROGENESIS AND ATHEROREGRESSION

G. WEBER

Center of Research on Atherosclerosis, Institute of Pathological Anatomy, University of Siena, Italy

Transmission electron microscope observations have shown that atherosclerotic lesions chiefly consist of smooth muscle cell hyperplasia and that the matrix is produced by the proliferating cells. Smooth muscle cell proliferation (which occurs with necrosis and lipid accumulation) is promoted by atherogenic hyperlipoproteinemia, platelet factors, etc., acting through endothelial lesions.

Endothelial lesions are easily produced by many agents such as endotoxin or noradrenalin, hypoxia or exposure to CO; in various "immunologic" conditions, endothelial lesions, necrosis and extensive endothelial loss have been described (*Weber et al.*, 1977a).

In dietetic experimental atherogenic hyperlipemia, endothelial lesions have been described in rabbits (*Weber*, 1975) at the surface coat level together with the presence of vacuoles and sub-endothelial edema. Surface changes in dietary hyperlipemia may cause the endothelial surface to be more susceptible to mechanical disruption (*Imai et al.*, 1966). Increased numbers of mitoses, altered orientation of endothelial cells and changes in their argyrophilic properties have also been described (*Veress et al.*, 1970; *Somer et al.*, 1972). Detachment of endothelial cells has been observed experimentally under different conditions (*Gutstein and Parl*, 1973; *Gutstein et al.*, 1975; *Scott et al.*, 1967); a large number of detached endothelial cells circulating in the blood have been found in guinea pigs by Payling Wright (1973) in anyphylactic shock, in dogs after endotoxin injection by Gerrity et al. (1976), in rabbits on a short-term hypercholesterolemia (*Weber*, 1977). One of the most accepted opinions concerning etiology and pathogenesis of atherosclerosis proposes that the endothelial cells, once subtly or grossly injured, become susceptible to the sharing stress of blood flow and may desquamate (*Ross and Harker*, 1976; *Ross and Glomset*, 1976; *Bierman and Ross*, 1977), leading to a sequence of atherogenic events.

As clearly stated by Thomas et al. (1977), arterial cell births and deaths go hand in hand with atherogenesis: in the early stages, necrotic changes occur both in scattered individual smooth muscle cells and endothelial cells or in small foci; the cell debris rapidly disintegrates; the early lesions therefore consist largely of proliferating smooth muscle cells. Increased numbers of divisions of endothelial cells, not accompanied by piling up, necessarily reflects a loss of endothelial cells from the surface. (*Thomas et al.*, 1977). Degenerative lesions in the early stages of experimental cholesterol and immunological atherogenesis in rabbits have also been observed (*Weber*, 1978; *Weber et al.*, 1978) both in endothelial and in smooth muscle cells in areas still devoid of proliferative lesions, which seem to be more prone to be flattened in pressure fixed aortas after a very short period of cholesterol diet or after two heterologous serum injections at a fortnightly interval in SEM examination.

Regression of atherosclerosis has been observed in different animal species once the atherogenic diets have been withdrawn. Parietal lesions are strongly reduced in number and extent or almost disappear; the residual plaques are smaller, less protruding, more whitish. Their smooth muscle cells are reduced in number

(*Stary*, 1974) and are losed the accumulated lipids, while the endothelial layer is regenerated over the residual lesions. Arterial cell injury and cell deaths have been observed by Stary et al. (1976) and by Starý (1977), not only in hypercholesterolemia but also after its reduction: Starý et al. (1976) reported that the mode of foam cell disappearance is by cell death.

At present, we don't yet know which forces are active in remodeling the fibrous tissue and cells of the residual lesions or in enhancing endothelial regeneration and much is still to be learned on the properties of regenerated endothelial cells (*Weber et al.*, 1977c). Anti-atherosclerotic dietary and/or drug intervention, may help regression, as has repeatedly shown by Wissler's group in rabbits and also in monkeys in a collaborative study (*Weber et al.*, 1977b).

REFERENCES

Weber, G. (1975): Relationship of endothelium to smooth muscle. Polysaccharide endothelial coating. Adv. Exp. Med. Biol. 57, 231—237.

Weber, G. (1977): The regression of arterial lesions: facts and problems. Intern. Conf. on Atherosclerosis, Milan 9—11 nov (in press) Ref.

Weber, G. (1978): Ultrastructural aspects of experimental atherogenesis. Intern. Symp. "Immunità e Arteriosclerosi" Florence 16—18 march (in press) Ref.

Weber, G., Fabbrini, P., Resi, L. (1977a): Arterial intimal changes in the early phases of experimental atherogenesis. Atherosclerosis Reviews (in press) Ref.

Weber, G., Fabbrini, P., Resi, L., Jones, R., Vesşelinovitch, D., Wissler, R. W. (1977b): Regression of arteriosclerotic lesions in Rhesus monkey aortas after regression diet. Atherosclerosis 26, 535—547.

Weber, G., Fabbrini, P., Resi, L., Pierli, C., Tanganelli, P. (1977c): Regeneration of endothelial cells. Conf. on Atherosclerosis, Milan 9—11 nov (in press) Ref.

G. W., Inst. of Patholog. Anatomy, University of Siena,
Via Laterina 8, 53100 Siena, Italy

ATHEROSCLEROSIS OF THE CORONARY ARTERY IN NORMOLIPEMIC SWINE INDUCED BY WITHDRAWAL OF HYPERVITAMINOSIS D₃

S. TAURA, M. TAURA, F. A. KUMMEROW and H. IMAI

H. E. Moore Heart Research Foundation, Champaign, Illinois, U.S.A.

Introduction

The usual arterial lesions induced by hypervitaminosis D are fibromuscular intimal thickening and medial calcification. By a combination of hypervitaminosis D and hyperlipemia, coronary atherosclerosis has been produced in experimental animals. In our recent study (*Taura, in press*), similar coronary atherosclerosis was induced in normolipemic swine that were initially fed a basal ration supplemented with 250,000 IU of vitamin D_3/kg of diet for 4 months and subsequently the basal ration alone for 3 months. The current study was designed to correlate graded doses of vitamin D_3 with coronary atherosclerosis quantitatively, and to determine the minimum effective dose.

Materials and methods

Forty three Yorkshire swine (barrows and gilts), averaging 2 months of age, were used. The animals were divided into 3 groups. Group 1 was fed a corn and soybean meal ration containing a vitamin and mineral premix which contained 387 IU of vitamin D_3 and 580 mg of calcium per kg of diet. Group 2 comprised the vitamin D supplemented group and was fed the basal ration supplemented with 250,000 IU, 125.000 IU, 62.500 IU, 12.500 IU and 2.500 IU

of vitamin D_3/kg of diet for 3 months. Group 3 was the vitamin D_3 withdrawal group and was fed the same 5 doses of vitamin D_3 as group 2 for the same time period, after which time it received only the basal ration for the following 3 months. Groups 2 and 3 were sacrificed at the end of the experimental period. Blood samples were taken at the time of sacrifice. An average of 30 samples were taken from each heart, and 10 samples each from the 3 major branches. Tissues were processed for light and electron microscopy.

Results

Biochemical studies disclosed that the serum cholesterol levels were slightly depressed and serum calcium levels were abnormally high in the animals of group 2 receiving the highest doses of vitamin D; both levels were within normal limits in all the animals of group 3.

Histologically, the animals in group 1 had no abnormal areas of intimal thickening or calcific lesions in the coronary arteries. In group 2, calcified lesions were noted in the 3 subgroups receiving the higher doses of vitamin D. These calcified lesions were focally located in the internal elastica and were frequently accompanied by fibromuscular intimal thickening. In group 3, atherosclerotic lesions were

Table I.	Parameter studies	250.000 IU	125.000 IU	62.500 IU	12.500 IU	2.500 IU
	Animals	3	4	4	3	4
	Animals with atheroma	3	4	4	0	0
	Segments examined	105	108	93	98	115
	Segments with atheroma	36	22	10	0	0
	Incidence of atheroma (U)	34.3	20.4	10.7	0	0
	Distribution of atheroma					
	left descending branch	17	9	4	0	0
	left circumflex branch	7	6	2	0	0
	right coronary artery	12	7	4	0	0

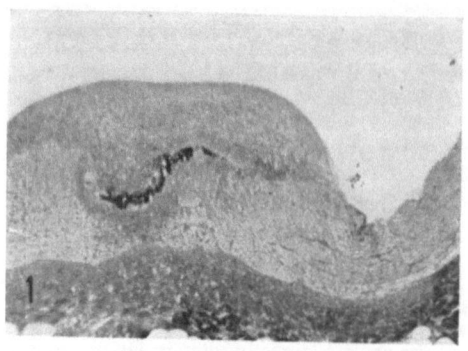

Fig. 1. 125.000 IU vitamin D_3 withdrawal (Von Kossa stain) Atherosclerotic lesion consists of intimal atheroma above the calcific internal elastica.

produced in 100% of the animals which received the 3 larger doses of vitamin D and in none which received the 2 lower

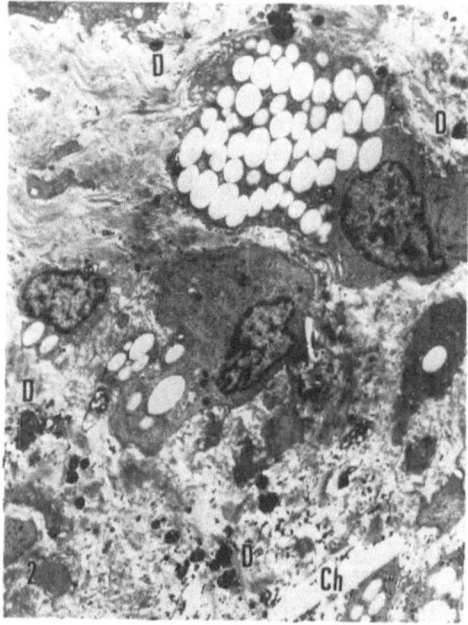

Fig. 2. 250.000 IU vitamin D_3 withdrawal (uranyl acetate and lead citrate stains). Atherosclerotic intima consists of many foam cells, dense particles (D) and cholesterol deposits (Ch).

doses. The incidence of atherosclerotic lesions was proportional to the dosage of vitamin D_3 fed and tended to involve the left descending branches more often than any other branches as shown in Table I. The largest atheroma was always located in the proximal portion of the left descending branches. Atherosclerotic lesions consisted of lipid rich intima, calcified internal elastica, and caused luminal narrowing (Fig. 1). Extracellular cholesterol crystals were noted in the deep intima. Calcified deposits in group 3 were lower than in group 2 under the same levels of vitamin D. Electron microscopically, atherosclerotic intima contained many foam cells and extremely dense particles in the stroma (Fig. 2). These dense particles contained calcium and phosphorus as determined by x-ray microanalysis.

In the present study hypervitaminosis D_3 resulted in calcified internal elastica and fibromuscular intimal thickening of the coronary artery in swine by the 3rd month. When the excessive vitamin D_3 was withdrawn, characteristic atherosclerosis developed in the following 3 months. These serial changes were observed in all animals which were fed over 62.500 IU vitamin D_3/kg of diet. Since atherosclerotic lesions were always associated with calcified internal elastica, atherosclerotic involvement must necessarily be preceeded by calcified lesions as observed in group 2. The present study also suggested atherosclerosis was related to the mural factor rather than the serum cholesterol factor. To date, no other investigators have produced coronary atherosclerosis in normolipemic animals. Recently, several investigators have produced aortic atherosclerosis by mechanical injury in normolipemic animals (*Moore*, 1973). The present authors believe the calcified lesions may act as another source of arterial injury. The current atherosclerotic lesions resembled morphological features of human coronary atherosclerosis (*Lansing*, 1948).

S. T., H. E. Moore Heart Res. Fd. 503 S. Sixth Str., Champaign, IL 61801, U.S.A.

THE EFFECT OF DIFFERENT CHOLESTEROL DIETS ON THE LOCALISATION OF SUDANOPHILIC LESIONS IN RABBITS

M. R. ROACH and J. FLETCHER

University of Western Ontario, London, Canada

There has been much debate in the literature about the reliability of rabbit models for studying atherosclerosis. One of the major criticisms has been that lesions which develop rapidly may be different from those which develop slowly. We (*Roach* 1977) have provided evidence that the shape and location of the lesions can be explained by the alterations in flow near a branch. Most lesions are distal to the orifices, but the coronary lesions surround the orifice, presumably because of the eddies created in the aortic sinus (*Cornhill and Roach* 1976). We (*Roach and Flectcher* 1976) also showed by nephrocto-mizing cholesterol-fed rabbits that the localization of the lesions was determined both by the nature of the flow into the branch, and also by the velocity profile of the blood approaching the branch.

In this paper, we will assess whether the shape and location of the lesions are different with different dietary regimes. We showed previously that the lesions were comparable in rabbits fed a diet with 2% cholesterol and 6% corn oil plus chow (*Roach, Fletcher and Cornhill* 1976) and in others fed a diet of 0.2% cholesterol and 6% corn oil plus chow (*Roach, Cornhill and Fletcher* 1978). Two other groups of animals were similarly studied (a) with one egg yolk added to the rabbit pellets each day and (b) with two egg yolks added to the diet each day. The analysis of the lesions was similar, and details will be published elsewhere. Figure 1 shows the differences in serum cholesterol with these four diets. Note that measurements in general were done only at the time of sacrifice with six rabbits in each group.

A detailed analysis of the lesions showed no differences in the shape of the lesions around any one orifice for all diets, i.e. all of the coronary lesions encircled the orifices, and the others were distal. However, as shown in Figure 2, there were marked differences in the rate at which lesions developed. Table I shows this for the combined data. The numbers shown are the percentage value for the orifices with lesions, and those in brackets show the numbers that were complex and surrounded more than one orifice. Detailed analysis of the data with linear regression analysis showed that in any one group the best correlation was with the time on the diet. If all the groups were lumped, then the best correlation (and it was not a significant one) was with the cholesterol-

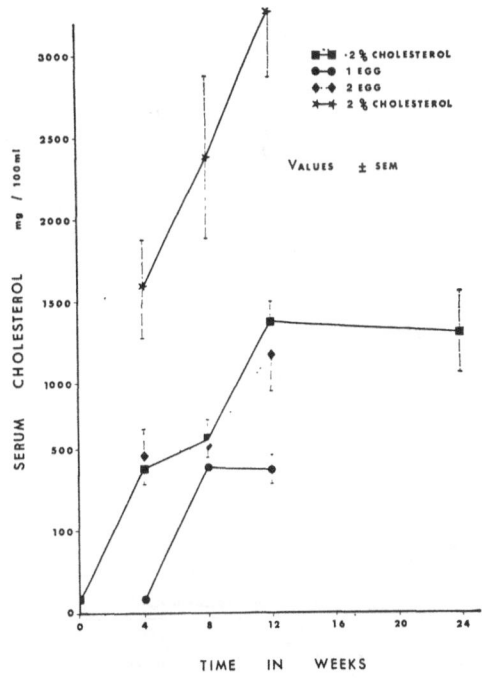

Table I. Effect on Different Diets on the Development of Lesions*

	2% cholesterol	2 eggs	0.2% cholesterol	1 egg
Right coronary	71.6 (11.7)	56.3 (0)	37.5 (0)	14.3 (0)
Left coronary	71.6 (11.7)	62.5 (0)	25.0 (0)	21.4 (0)
Intercostals 1—3R	69.8 (7.0)	2.6 (0)	9.1 (0)	7.1 (0)
1—3L	60.5 (7.0)	28.2 (7.2)	13.6 (0)	11.9 (0)
4—6R	51.0 (19.6)	29.4 (0)	25.0 (0)	6.7 (0)
4—6L	71.6 (19.6)	29.4 (0)	20.8 (0)	6.7 (0)
7—9R	65.2 (45.6)	23.5 (7.8)	11.8 (0)	4.4 (0)
7—9L	67.4 (45.6)	21.6 (0)	17.7 (0)	2.2 (0)
Coeliac	88.2 (11.8)	82.3 (0)	50.0 (0)	23.1 (0)

* All involvement is expressed as a percentage of the total number of orifices in the group for all periods up to twelve weeks. The numbers in the brackets show the percentage that involved more than one orifice.

time index. (i.e. cholesterol x time : 2). We believe that this correlation might be better if we measured the area under the cholesterol-time curve for each animal, but this would require serial measurements which we did not do. The marked differences in rate of rise of cholesterol with time in Figure 1 show why these serial measurements would be preferable.

We can conclude that any cholesterol diet produced comparable lesions in rabbits. Thus we could suggest that the high cholesterol diet for 4—6 weeks is the best one for hemodynamic studies.

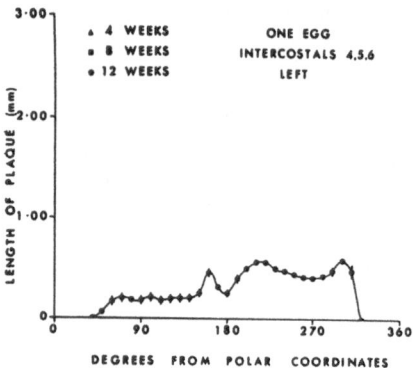

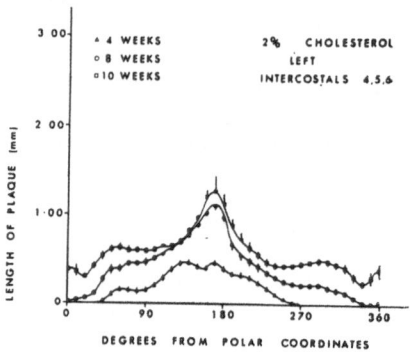

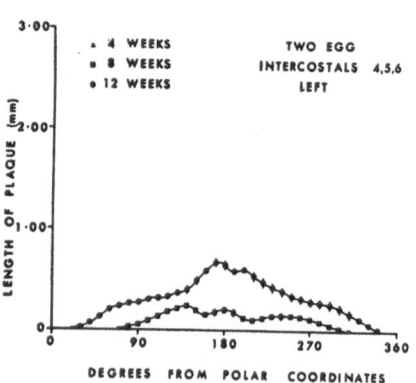

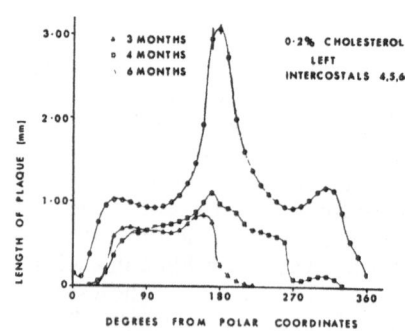

REFERENCES

Cornhill, J. F. and Roach, M. R. (1976): A quantitative study of the localisation of atherosclerotic lesions in the rabbit aorta. Athero- sclerosis 23: 489—501.

Roach, M. R. (1977): The Effects of Bifurcations and Stenoses on Arterial Disease in Hwang, N. H. C. and Normann, N. A. Cardiovascular Flow Dynamics and Measurements. University Park Press. Baltimore. pp. 489—539.

Roach, M. R. and Fletcher, J. (1976): Effect of unilaterial nephrectomy on the localisation of aortic sudanophilic lesions in cholesterol-fed rabbits. Atherosclerosis 24: 327—333.

Roach, M. R., Fletcher, J. and Cornhill, J. F. (1976): The effect of the duration of cholesterol feeding on the development of sudanophilic lesions in the rabbit aorta. Atherosclosis 25: 1—11.

Roach, M. R., Fletcher, J. and Cornhill, J. F. (1978): A quantitative study of the development of sudanophilic lesions in the aorta of rabbits fed a low-cholesterol diet for up to six months. Atherosclerosis 29: 259—264.

M.R.R. Department of Biophysics Health Sciences Centre University of Western Ontario London, Ontario, N6A5C1 Canada

LOCALIZATION OF SOME PEPTIDASES IN THE VASCULAR WALL

Z. LOJDA

*Laboratory of Histochemistry and Laboratory of Angiology,
Faculty of General Medicine, Charles University, Praha, Czechoslovakia*

Our knowledge on the activity and distribution of peptidases in the vascular wall is rather scanty (*Adams*, 1967; *Kirk*, 1969) although it would be highly desirable particularly from the viewpoint of atherogenesis and of the disputed problem of possible regression of atherosclerotic lesions. Therefore we have studied peptidases of the normal and atherosclerotic arterial wall of man and some animal species both with biochemical and improved histochemical methods (*Lojda et al.*, 1976; *Lojda*, 1977). In this communication data on aminopeptidase M and dipeptidylaminopeptidase IV are given.

Aminopeptidase M (membrane aminopeptidase 1, E.C. 3.4.11.2) is a zinc containing peptidase which can completely hydrolyze large peptides as long as the terminal aminoacid is not modified and is in the L-form. Its activity given in mM NA/1 g wet weight/1 hour at 37 °C in intima-media samples of macroscopically normal human aorta amounts to 0.0169 with Leu-2 NA and 0.0477 with Ala-2 NA. For mini-pig thoracic aorta the respective values are 0.0168 and 0.0369, for rat aorta 0.0128 and 0.0290 and for rabbit aorta 0.0148 (with Leu-2 NA). Values with Leu-2 NA calculated per 1 g of protein are 16.94 mM (human thoracic aorta), 13.7 mM (mini-pig thoracic aorta), and 12.6 mM (rabbit aorta). In the abdominal aorta the values were 1.45× (man, $p < 0.01$), 1.32× (mini-pig, $p < 0.01$), and in human coronary artery 1.24× ($p < 0.05$) higher than in the thoracic aorta. The activity is inhibited by about 70% by o-phenanthroline. Our data on human aorta are in agreement with *Kirk* (1969). The data on other species are new. Kirk did not mention the superiority of

the Ala-compound and designated the determined activity erroneously as leucine aminopeptidase.

The histochemical investigation confirmed the superiority of the Ala- over the Leu-MNA. In normal vessels the activity is very low. Only in connective tissue cells of the adventitia which penetrate with vasa vasorum also into the media a high activity is found. This may cause high biochemical values when the sample is not cleaned thoroughly from the adventitia. A strong reaction resides also in cells of the thickened intima, e.g. in the abdominal aorta of mini-pig (Fig. 1 A) and this might be the reason for a higher activity of the abdominal aorta as determined biochemically. In intima-media samples of atherosclerotic segments biochemical examination did not reveal significant differences in any animal species. However, histochemical examination demonstrated a relatively high activity in some cells of

Fig. 1: Activity of aminopeptidase M (Ala-MNA, Fast Blue B, chloroform-acetone pretreated cryostat sections adherent to semipermeable membranes) in A) thickned intima of abdominal aorta of a mini-pig; B) in cells of a fibrous plaque of human aorta; C) in the vicinity of a necrotic focus (arrow) of an atheromatous plaque of human aorta.
Activity of DAP IV (Gly-Pro-MNA, Fast Blue B, chloroform-acetone pretreated cryostat sections adherent to semipermeable membranes): D) Strong activity of the endothelium of a vas vasis penetrating into the media in mini-pig aorta; E) in endothelium of vasa vasorum (arrows) in the outer media of human aorta; F) in endothelium of capillaries of rat myocardium; G) in foam cells of cholesterol atheroma in the aorta of a cock; H) in foam cells of atheroma of a coronary artery of a cock; I) in endothelium of capillaries (arrows) at the bottom of an atheromatous plaque of human aorta.

Fig. 1

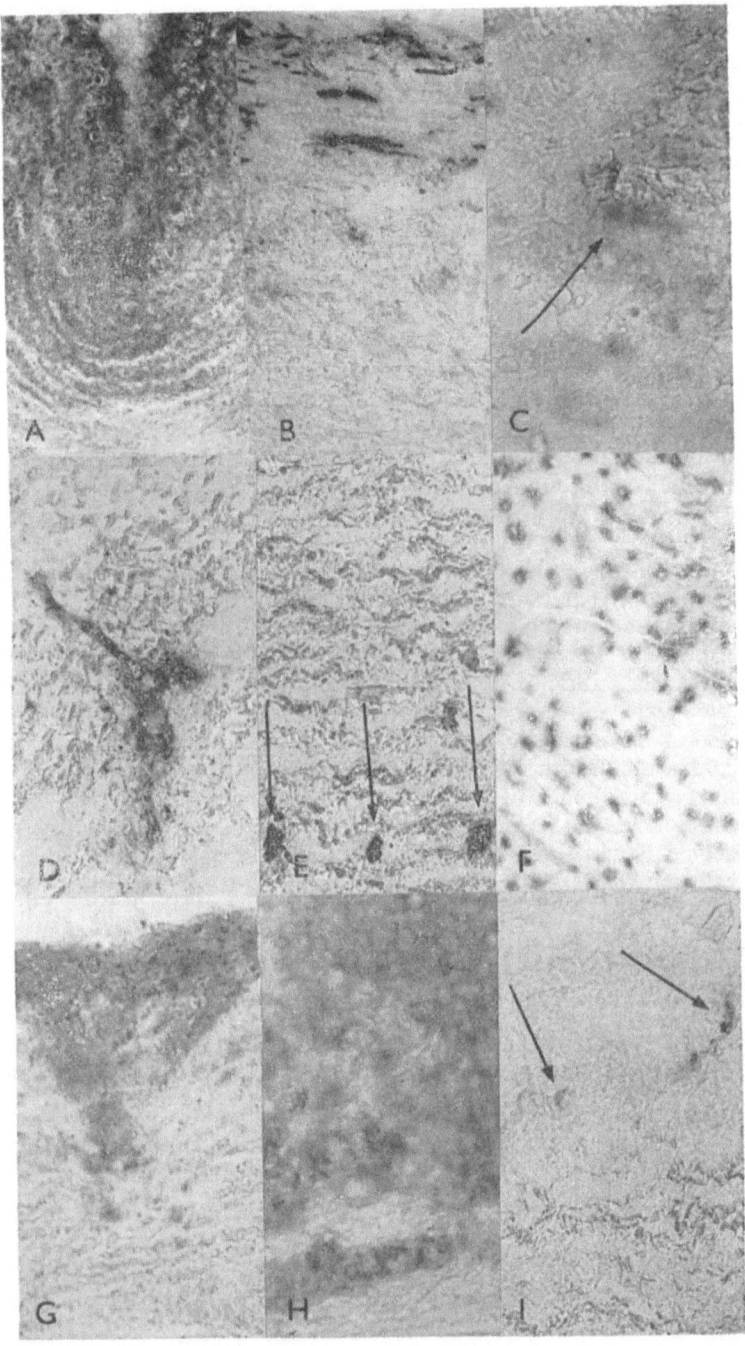

fibrous plaques (Fig. 1 B) and a diffuse extracellular staining in atheromatous plaques (Fig. 1 C) of human aorta. In fatty streaks and plaques of experimentally induced atherosclerosis in rabbit and cock only a very weak activity was found. No changes in the media were observed. Alanine aminopeptidase (E.C. 3.4.11.−) does not seem to be a great bias in the studies on the vascular wall performed with Ala-2 NA or Ala-MNA.

Our findings indicate that in fibrous and atheromatous plaques there is an activity which can participate in the degradation of proteins.

Dipeptidyl(amino)peptidase IV (DAP IV, glycyl-proline naphthyl-amidase, E.C. 3.4.14.4) is a serine peptidase which removes N-terminal dipeptides from polypeptides with proline in the penultimate position with only little regard for the N-terminal L-aminoacid. It may participate in the degradation of collagen (cf. Lojda, 1977). Its activity given in mM of 2 NA (MNA)/1 g wet weight/1 hour at 37 °C in intima-media samples of normal human thoracic aorta amounts to 0.0200 (0.0389), for mini-pig thoracic aorta 0.0183 (0.0250), for rabbit aorta 0.0159 (MNA) and for rat aorta 0.0134 (2 NA). There were no significant differences between thoracic, abdominal aorta and coronary arteries in man. In mini-pig the values for abdominal aorta were about 10% lower. No significant differences were found between normal segments and those affected with atherosclerosis. The activity was inhibited totally by DFP (10^{-3}M), by about 45% by E600 and by about 10% by phenanthroline, unaffected by EDTA and maleimide. Without the knowledge of the localization one can speculate about the participation of media muscle cells in the degradation of collagen. However, the histochemical examination shows that DAP IV activity is confined particularly to the endothelium of a portion of vasa vasorum which penetrate from the adventitia into the media in all animals (Fig. 1 D: mini-pig; 1 E: man) No reaction was observed in the arterial endothelium and a negligible (if any) reaction in muscle cells. DAP IV activity is confined to the endothelium of the venous part of the capillary bed of many organs (Fig. 1 F: rat myocardium). In atherosclerotic vessels an intense staining of foam cells resides in the cock arteries only (Fig. 1 G, H). In foam cells of other species it does not occur. In atheromatous plaques of human aortae the reaction is confined to capillaries only (Fig. 1 I).

These findings show that DAP IV does not participate in the catabolism of collagen in large arteries (with the exception of atherosclerotic plaques of the cock). Neither aminopeptidase M nor DAP IV belong to enzymes indicating early changes in atherogenesis. From the examples presented the importance of histochemical studies is clearly evident.

REFERENCES

Adams, C. W. M. (1967): Vascular Histochemistry. Lloyd-Luke, London.
Kirk, J. E. (1969): Enzymes of the arterial wall. Academio Press, N. Y.

Lojda, Z. (1977): Histochemistry 54, 299—309.
Lojda, Z., Gossrau, R., Schiebler, T. H. (1976): Enzymhistochemische Methoden. Springer, Berlin—Heidelberg—New York.

Z. L., Laboratory of Histochemistry, Studničkova 2, 12800 Praha 2, Czechoslovakia

SPONTANEOUS CALCIFYING MEDIAL SCLEROSIS OF RABBITS

F. SCHNEIDER

Department of Pathology, County Hospital, Kecskemét, Hungary

Calcifying medial sclerosis (CMS) refers macroscopically to a hard yellowish-white plaque-like thickening of the rabbit aorta, which is microscopically characterized by necrosis, calcification of degenerated elastic fibers, regeneration and chondroid metaplasia of aortic smooth-muscle cells. It can be observed in experimental sclerotic rabbits and sometimes in normal control animals. The purpose of this lecture is: 1. to study the histopathological process in the aortic wall during the disease and 2. to find some connection between experimental cholesterol-sclerosis and CMS in rabbits.

Material and methods

120 male LATI rabbits weighing 2—3 kg divided into 3 groups were investigated. Group I. — 28 animals-fed normal food. Group II. — 60 animals-fed 1 g cholesterol daily. Group III. — 32 animals-fed 3000 I.U. Vitamin-D$_3$ and 1 g cholesterol daily. The animals were sacrificed after the 1st, 2nd, 3d, 6th and 12th week of treatment.

The aortas were investigated. 3—4 mm wide part of the ascending aorta was fixed in Ca-formol over 24 hours. Slides were obtained by freezing-microtome stained with oil-red 0. Other 3—4 mm wide parts of the aortas were fixed in alcohol: formol 4 : 1 mixture over 24 hours and embedded in paraffin. Slides were then stained with 0.1% toluidine-blue solution at pH 1, 3 and 5. Slides were stained with toluidine-blue and different molar concentration of MgCl$_2$ to estimate "critical electrolyte concentration" — CEC-value of different metachromatic stained chromotrops. Other slides were digested with testicular hyaluronidase at 37 °C for 16 hours and stained with 0.1% toluidine-blue solution. Kossa silver-impregnation, fenol reaction according to Ebner and picrosyrius staining were also carried out. Preparations were investigated under the Zeiss-Amplival-polmicroscope in normal and in polarized light.

Results

CMS occurred with 20% frequency in the normal group. Occurrence of CMS in group II 40% and in group III 80%. The histological picture is summarized in Fig. 1. At the periphery of the small necrotic area smoothmuscle cells are regenerated. Calcified degenerated elastic fibers can also be observed. On the other side a great amount of collagen fiber can be seen, as a result of reparative tendency (Fig. 1. a, b, c.).

There were larger necrotic regions in the other parts of the aortas. At the border of the lesion was observed metachromatic staining at pH 3 and negative birefringence due to collagen and mucopolysaccharides. Around these chondroid-like cells, metachromatic stained material proved to be partly hyaluronidase—sensitive, partly hyaluronidase-resistant. The MgCl$_2$ CEC-value of the latter was 0.8 M. In the necrotic area between the degenerated elastic lamellas, mucopolysaccharide-secreting, modified smooth-muscle cells could be observed (Fig. 1. d, e, f.).

A foam-cell group in deep media was observed very rarely in the neighbourhood of a necrosis. (Fig. 2. a.). Medial smooth-muscle cells might be the source of these foam-cells. In the necrotic area massive lipid infiltration was visible and much more less lipid in regenerated areas. When CMS was localized under the intimal foam-cell plaque, the same phenomenon could be seen. There was also lipid under it. There was no lipid under the repaired CMS in the aortic wall (Fig. 2. b, c, d). In this latter stage increased Evans-blue detected permeability failed in the aorta (Fig. 2. e).

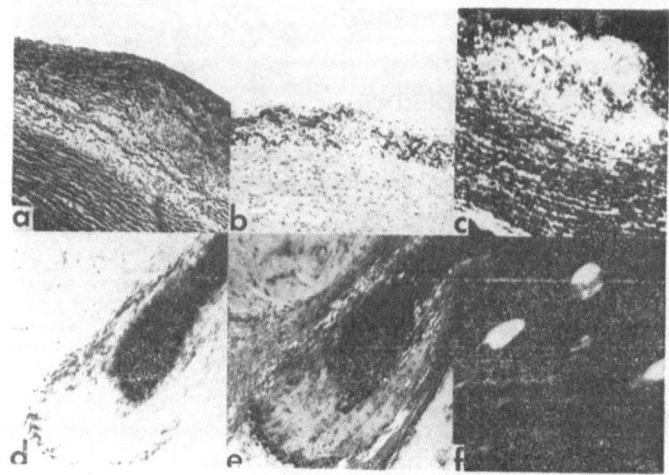

Fig. 1. a: Subintimally small necrotic area. In the periphery of lesion-regenerating groups of muscle-cells (toluidine-blue, pH 5) *b*: Calcified degenerated elastic fibers can be observed in this focus (Kossa silver-impregnation). *c*: A large amount of positive birefringent collagen fiber can be seen as a result of the reparative tendency (Picrosyrius staining, polarisation photomicrograph). *d, e*: In the middle of the orthochromatic stained necrotic area, on the border of the lesion metachromatic stained region, with crossed polars negative birefringence due to collagen and mucopolysaccharides. (toluidine-blue staining pH 3, d: normal light photomicrograph, e: polarization photomicrograph). *f*: In the necrotic area between degenerated elastic lamellas mucopolysaccharide secreting modified smooth-muscle cells. (toluidine-blue staining, pH 3. Polarization photomicrograph).

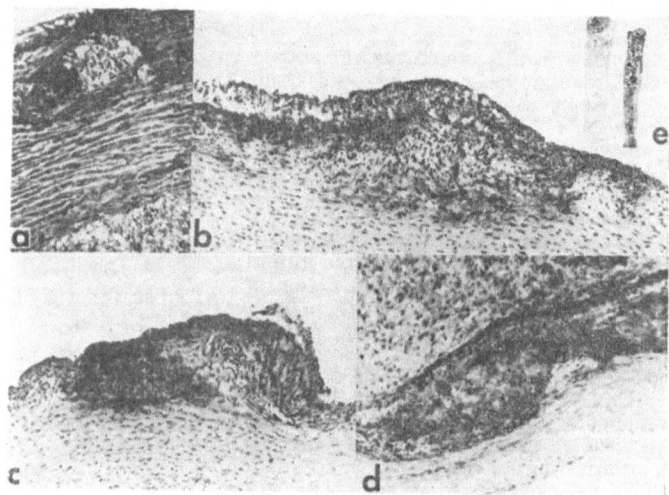

Fig. 2. a: Developed atheromatous plaque in the intima. In deep media there is a small necrosis and in the neighbourhood a small foam-cell group (toluidine-blue pH 5). *b*: Under a foam-cell plaque there is a necrotic regenerating area, under which lipid can also be observed in the media. *c*: Small initiating necrosis and lipid infiltration. *d*: Developed intimal foam-cell plaque. Under it chondroid metaplastic repaired necrosis. No lipid underneath (b, c, d: oil-red 0 staining). *e*: No Evans-blue imbibation can be seen in left side CMS aorta. Right side aorta has many atheromatous plaques, no CMS.

Discussion

CMS is a non-specific reaction of rabbit-aorta to different noxes, including known and unknown metabolic stresses such as cholesterol-feeding and Vitamin D_3-administration. These latter increased the frequency of CMS from 20% to 40–80%.

Massmann and Weidenbach demonstrated by electronmicroscopic examinations that cells in this area displaying chondroid metaplasia are modified smooth-muscle cells. In our experiment mucopolysaccharide-secretion of these cells was observed. Their material is thought to be partly chondroidsulphate (metachromatic staining at pH 1–3, hyaluronidase-sensitivity), partly keratosulphate around the elongated and rounded off chondroid-like cells (metachromatic staining, hyaluronidase-resistency, $MgCl_2$ 0.8 M CEC-value). Medial necrosis and cholesterol-induced atheromatosis are different pathogenetically. Their coincidence in time raises the question of now necrosis influences lipid deposition. In deep medial necrotic areas, smooth-muscle cells may develop into foam-cells. A necrotic area subintimally localized has no barrier effect against hyperlipidemic sera and lipid-can be trapped in the structurally altered aortic wall. The repaired aortic wall is the end-stage of the process and neither lipid-rich sera trapping nor increased Evans-blue permeability can then be observed.

F. S., Dept. of Pathology, County Hospital, Kecskemét, Hungary

EXPERIMENTAL PATHOLOGICAL STUDY ON ARTERIAL WALL INJURY GIVEN BY ELEVATED INTRAVASCULAR PRESSURE AND ITS REPAIR — BLOOD PRESSURE AND CIRCUMFERENTIAL TENSION —

T. JOSHITA, N. SAKATA, Y. YOSHIDA AND G. OONEDA

Department of Pathology, School of Medicine, Gunma University, Maebashi, Japan

It is a widely known fact that hypertension is responsible for the generation and development of arteriosclerosis and other arterial lesions. It is, however, scarcely known, what sort of lesion is produced solely by elevation in internal pressure. When the adult is standing straight, the internal pressure in the dorsalis pedis artery becomes higher than 200 mm Hg because of the addition of hydrostatic pressure. But despite this, no one has ever reported that this part is more susceptible to hypertensive arterial lesion than any other arteries. In the pulmonary artery, however serious arterial lesion is produced when the internal pressure is increased to $100 - 120$ mm Hg owing to ventricular septal defect or other lesion. These contradictory facts demonstrates that the elevation of internal pressure does not directly injure the arterial wall. We have devised a method for controlling intravascular pressure of the vessel, and by means of this, we have investigated the relationship between luminal pressure, arterial architecture and arterial lesion. Furthemore, we calculated circumferential tension by the Oka-Azuma's formula, and thus succeeded to clarify how intimately this circumferential tension was related with the production of the lesion observed after elevation of the internal pressure.

Method for controlling the interval pressure of the vessel (Joshita, 1970)

An experimental animal is fixed, the aimed vessel is exposed under anesthesia, and after blocking the blood flow with rubber-coated clips at the proximal and distal points, a manometer and an infusion apparatus, connected with a three-way cock, are inserted into the segment of vessel between the two clips (Fig. 1). By this means, the maximum and minimum intravascular pressures, their durations and the total length of the action can be freely altered in the segment. Also the liquid for controlling the pressure can be chosen freely. After the termination of the manometeric operation, the opening in the vascular segment is closed with Spongel, Aron alpha A and Tefron paper to prevent blood

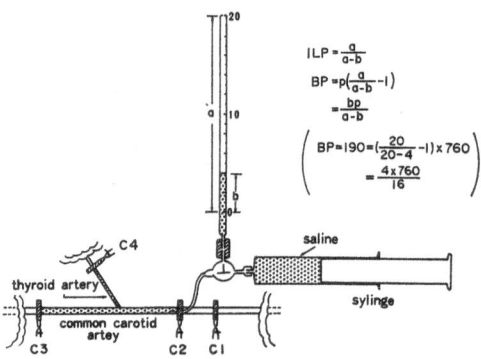

Fig. 1. Method for controlling the internal pressure of the vessel C_1, C_3, C_4: Heifetz's clips, C_2: rubber covered forceps.

leakage, and the clips are removed to reopen blood flow, and morphology and function of the segment are sequentially observed. In measuring the intravascular pressure, two methods are used: One utilizes a mercury column, and the other determines change in the air volume in the glass tube by the Biol's law. The former can determine the pressure below 200 mm Hg in a small scale, and when connected to a simple device, can record the sequential pressure change on paper. The latter can be performed with a very simple apparatus, and is able to determine the pressure as high as $500 - 1000$ mm Hg.

Circumferential tension

It has generally been accepted that law of Laplace ($T = PR$) is not applicable to the circumferential tension in thick-walled blood vessels. *Oka* and *Azuma* (1970) have obtained a formula for circumferential tension in a hollow cylindrical tube.

$$T = P_1 r'_2 - P_2 r'_2$$

Where P_1 and P_2 are the internal and external pressure, and r'_1 and r'_2 are the inner and outer radius of the tube, respectively. The circumferential tension due to the local control on intravascular pressure was computed by the Oka-Azuma's formula in order to pursue the relation between changes in the circumferential tension and arterial lesion.

Adaptation of arterial wall to elevated intravascular pressure and its failure

No injury was given to the artery when the intravascular pressure produced negative circumferential tension. The intravascular pressure which gave $T = 0$ was about 150 mm Hg for the common carotid artery and somewhat higher for the thyroid artery in the rabbit (Fig. 2) (*Joshita*, 1974). In the case of $T \geqq 0$, there developed medial hyperplasia; in $T \gg 0$, medial hyperplasia and intimal thickening; in $T \ggg 0$, medial thinning and intimal thickening; and in $T \ggg 0$, smooth muscle cell disappearance, fibrosis or

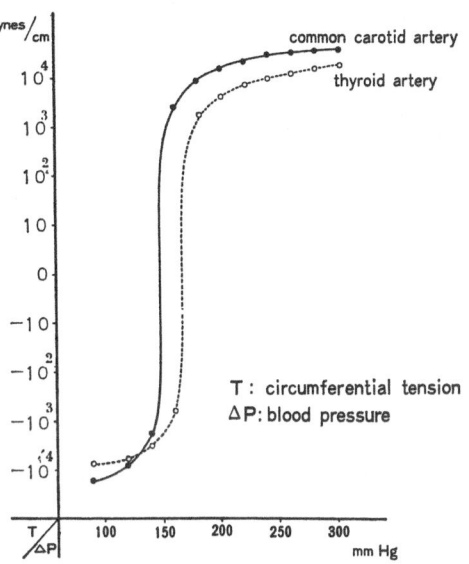

Fig. 2. Relation between circumferential tension and blood pressure. Circumferential tension changes with alteration in internal pressure of rabbit's common carotid artery and thyroid artery.

calcification in the media and reduction or abolishment of thickening ability of the intima. When the intraarterial pressure was controlled in various arteries of human autopsy materials and the subsequently induced change in the circumferential tension was calculated, it was found that the natural calibre and mural thickness of the human artery (except coronary artery) were very intimately related with intravascular pressure reigning in that part,

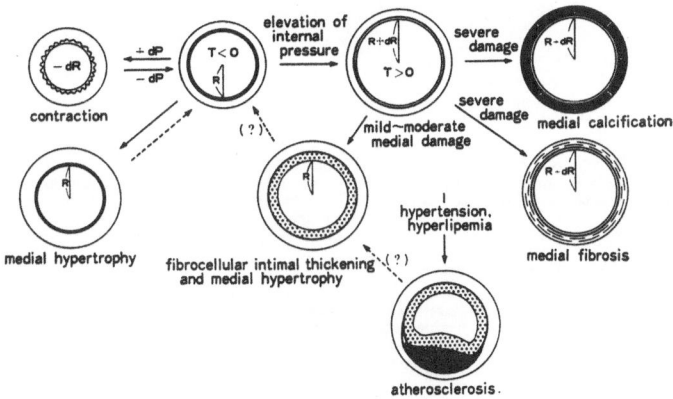

Fig. 3. Behaviour of arterial wall in response to elevation of arterial internal pressure. (Adaptation and its failure)

23

and that the hypertensive arterial lesion was apt to develop in the part (for example, cerebral arteries whose media is originally thinner than other arteries), where the condtition of $T > 0$ was easily induced. In the pulmonary artery, even the action of normotensive systemic circulation alone could induce $T \gg 0$, thus giving the clear genetic explanation of pulmonary arteriosclerosis. The immediate vascular adaptation is made by luminal reduction due to contraction of smooth muscle cells and delayed adaptation, by the medial hyperplasia and intimal thickening. And disorder in this adaptation causes the arterial lesion (Fig. 3).

REFERENCES

Joshita, T., Ooneda, G. (1970): Pathological Study on Arterial injury by A method for controlling the internal intravascular pressure of the vessel. J. Jap. Coll. Angiol. 10, 381. (In Japanese)

Joshita, T., Ooneda, G. (1974): Experimental pathological study on arterial wall injury given by elevated intravascular pressure, and its repair. Jap. J. Atheroscler. 2, 73—79. (In Japanese)

Oka, S., Azuma, T. (1970): Physical theory of tension in thick-walled blood vessel in equilibrium. Biorheology 7, 109.

Takashi Joshita Dept. of Pathology, School of Med. Gunma Univ.
3—39 Showamachi, Maebashi, 371 Japan

EFFECTS OF CERTAIN DRUGS ON EXPERIMENTAL ATHEROSCLEROSIS IN SWINE

K. T. LEE AND W. M. LEE

Dept. of Pathology, Albany Medical College, Albany, New York, U.S.A.

Studies in man and animal models reveal that the atherosclerotic lesion, in its early phases, is characterized by the accumulation of lipid and the proliferation of smooth muscle cells and the production of collagen, mucopolysaccharides and elastic tissue. In the more advanced stages, atheromatous lesions with foci of necrotic debris, with or without foci of calcification, appear.

There have been many studies employing various agents including anti-proliferative and anti-inflammatory drugs in animal models to learn if the course of experimental atherosclerosis can be modified by these therapeutic agents. In our previous studies, the effects of two anti-metabolites, mercaptopurine and hydroxyurea, and a platelet aggregation inhibitor, pyridinolcarbamate, have been studied on cholesterol induced atherosclerosis in rabbits.

In the current study, the effects of hydroxyurea and pyridinolcarbamate on retardation of progression of atherosclerosis was investigated in swine. For this study, 33 young, male Yorkshire swine weighing average 11 kg were used. The intimal cells of the abdominal aorta of all swine were partially denuded using a balloon catheter.

This balloon procedure has recently been devised by *Baumgarten and Spaet* (1970) for partially denuding an artery of the intimal cells with apparently minimal damage to the underlying tissue. The procedure involves pulling an inflated balloon through a portion of the artery of an experimental animal. The balloon is inflated through a catheter to the point where it fits snugly against the intimal lining. As the balloon is pulled along the artery, patches of endothelial cells become detached. When the procedure is combined with an atherogenic diet, the two procedures appear to act synergistically to produce lesions, the extent and thickness of which are far greater than those expected by summing up the effect when the two procedures are used separately. The lesions produced by this combined method have many of the characteristics of advanced human lesions (*Nam et al.,* 1973).

After the balloon procedure, all swine were given a hypercholesterolemic diet for six months. They were divided into three groups of 11 swine each at the outset, one group for control, and two groups for test drugs. The control group received the hypercholesterolemic diet (Table I)

Table I. Composition of Daily Diet Given Each Swine

Ingredients	Amount, gram
Peanut oil	15
Lard	185
Mash	330
Sodium Cholate	10
Cholesterol	15
Salt Mix	15
Vitamin Mix	10
Milk Powder	15
Total	630 grams
Total Calories	3200 Cal.

without drug treatment, and each of the other two groups received the diet plus either hydroxyurea (50 mg/kg/day) or pyridinolcarbamate (50 mg/kg/day) for six months.

At the end of six months, all swine were sacrificed. The cholesterol concentrations of the serum, aorta, and liver were measured and the extent of atherosclerosis in the abdominal aorta was measured by light microscopy using an eye piece micrometer.

Four to six segments of abdominal aorta were taken under rigidly standardized conditions. Those segments were cut into two portions: one for light microscopy and the remainder for chemical analysis for cholesterol content. On each light microscopy section the percent of surface involved by atherosclerotic lesions was determined. In addition, the wall areas occupied by lesions and normal areas were measured by using a micrometer. Since our sampling was extensive and rigidly standardized, we could assume that the composite results from many sections would give us the ratio of lesion to non-lesion tissue in the entire abdominal aorta.

The extent of the intimal surface and the medial wall involved by atherosclerotic lesions were significantly less in both

Table II. Extent and Size of Aortic Lesions in Swine After 6 Months of Progression Studies

Group	% of intimal surface involved by lesions	Lesion areas expressed as % of total medial area
Control	61.5 ± 2.6	40.5 ± 3.6
PC	45.0 ± 4.7*	22.1 ± 3.5**
U-OH	47.4 ± 4.4*	23.6 ± 2.5**

* P < 0.02 as compared to control group.
** P < 0.01 as compared to control group.

drug-treated groups than in the untreated control group (Table II). The cholesterol contents in the serum, aorta and liver among the three groups were not significantly different (Table III).

In conclusion, hydroxyurea and pyridinolcarbamate retarded progression of atherosclerotic lesions in the swine aorta produced by a combination of a hypercholesterolemic diet and the balloon injury.

Table III. Cholesterol Concentrations in Serum, Aorta and Liver in Swine after 6 Months of Progression Studies

Group	Serum* (mg/dl)	Thoracic Aorta (mg/g wet wt)	Abdominal Aorta (mg/g wet wt)	Liver (mg/g wet wt)
Control	623 ± 55	2.7 ± 0.4	5.1 ± 1.8	15.4 ± 1.0
PC	592 ± 40	3.8 ± 0.4	5.3 ± 0.8	15.7 ± 3.5
U-OH	538 ± 51	3.9 ± 0.5	3.4 ± 0.8	20.0 ± 2.3

* Calculated from monthly measurements
There are no significant differences among the three groups

REFERENCES

Baumgarten, H. R. and Spaet, T. H. (1970): Endothelial replacement in rabbit arteries. Fed Proc. 29: 710.
Nam, S. C., Lee, W. M., Jarmolych, J., Lee, K. T. and *Thomas, W. A.* (1973): Rapid production of advanced atherosclerosis in swine by a combination of endothelial injury and cholesterol feeding. Exp. Mol. Pathol. 18: 369—379.

K. T. L., Department of Pathology Albany Medical College Albany, New York 12208, U.S.A.

REGRESSION OF ATHEROSCLEROSIS: THE CELLULAR RESPONSE AND THE LOCAL ACTION OF HDL

C. W. M. ADAMS, Y. H. ABDULLA AND O. B. BAYLISS

Department of Pathology, Guy's Hospital Medical School, London University, U.K.

Atherosclerosis in the rhesus monkey regresses over a period of 1,5 — 2 years when the animals are returned to a low-lipid diet after the disease has been established by feeding a cholesterol-enriched diet (Vesselinovitch et al., 1976). By contrast, the rabbit represents a species that is resistant to regression and shows only slight, if any real reversal (review by Adams & Morgan, 1978). The possible reversibility of human lesions remains quite uncertain and is further complicated by the distinction between removal of lipid and resorption of fibrous material Even in "fast-regression" species, such as the rhesus monkey, the speed of the process is slow compared with the rate of resorption of lipids from experimental implants under the skin (Adams et al., 1975a) or from xanthomas (Adams et al., 1975b).

Some reasons for this relative metabolic inertia of atheroma lipids in situ include the following factors (Adams et al., 1975b): —
a) absence of cholesterol degradative enzymes in the arterial wall
b) absence or inadequacy of reticuloendothelial phagocytes in the centre of fibro-fatty human plaques.
c) physical inaccessibility of cholesterol crystals to metabolic processes and their relative resistance to cellular handling.

Cholesterol degradative enzymes. The liver is unique in its capacity to catabolize cholesterol to cholic acids and to excrete them plus free cholesterol into the bile. Apart from excretion into serum and metabolism by the endocrine system, other tissues lack any significant capacity to catabolize cholesterol. This metabolic deficiency would, thus, lead to the retention of cholesterol deposited within arterial tissue.

Reticuloendothelial cells. Histochemical and some electron microscopic evidence suggests that blood monocytes do not enter deeply into the typical human fibro-fatty plaque, hence in the centre of the lesion reticuloendothelial cells are not available for phagocytosis of lipid. Blood monocytes enter the subendothelial region of the human arterial wall and progress only a little deeper (Fig. 1; Adams et al., 1975b, 1976a; Gaton & Wolman, 1977). This resistance by monocytes to deep penetration is probably a reflection of hypoxia of the arterial wall and atheromatous lesions (Lehninger 1959; Adams 1967). By contrast most vascular smooth muscle is enzymically adapted to hypoxia (Adams & Bayliss, 1976b) and fluorishes within the lesions. Smooth muscle is probably at best only a weakly phagocytic cell and is relatively ineffective in transporting lipid out of the arterial wall.

Although the typical fibro-fatty plaque contains few deeply placed monocytes, the position alters when the plaque becomes capillarized following repair by organization of ulcerated, thrombosed or

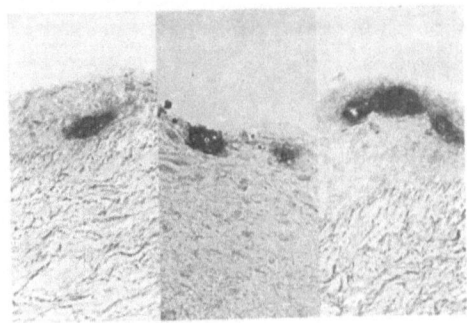

Fig. 1. Monocytes confined to subendothelial position in a non-capillarized human atherosclerotic lesion, modified cytochrome oxidase technique, × 210.

haemorrhagic lesions. Such complicated lesions show a number of monocytes in their depth, and this is associated with the appearance of capillaries within the plaque (Adams & Bayliss 1976 a & b). Such infiltration of monocytes is associated with focal giant cell formation (Adams & Bayliss, to be published), usually manifested as pallisades of macrophages around cholesterol clefts (Fig. 2). Pallisading or circumfusion of macrophages is the initial response in the formation of giant cells around experimental subcutaneous implants of cholesterol; subsequent interiorization of the crystal results in the characteristic appearance of lipid-phagocytosis by a giant cell (Bayliss, 1976).

In human autopsy material, it is difficult to be certain whether lipid resorption has occurred in advanced capillarized lesions which contain macrophages and occasional giant cells. However, we have gained the impression of a reduction in lipid content in the region of substantial infiltrations of monocytes. Likewise cholesterol clefts seem to be deficient in regions where giant cells have formed. The amount of lipid resorbed, however, seem at best to be quite modest in extent.

Physical accessibility of crystals The low surface area/volume ratio of cholesterol crystals had previously suggested to us that such crystals would be relatively inaccessible to metabolic

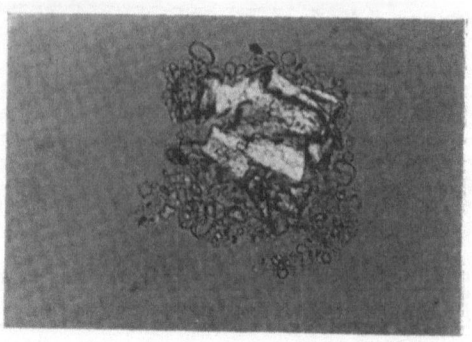

Fig. 3. Crystal of free cholesterol partly solubilized by HDL (3 mg/ml). Note corona of liposome (Ω myelin buds) at edge of crystal. Viewed in polarized light with half-crossed analyser, × 210.

processes and, therefore, difficult to resorb. This view was supported by autoradiographic evidence of poor in-vivo labelling of atheroma cholesterol crystals by exchange with radioactive plasma cholesterol in contrast to the marked labelling of dispersed atheroma lipids (Adams et al., 1975c).

In further investigations on the accessibility of cholesterol crystals, we were surprised to find that crystals of tritium-labelled cholesterol were solubilized in vitro by human highdensity lipoprotein (HDL) with a resulting marked increase in radioactivity in the supernatant. Examination of this reaction under the microscope showed that HDL caused the formation of liposomes (myelin buds or figures) at the surface of cholesterol crystals (Fig. 3). Cholesterol was used as reagent crystals or derived from human atheroma lipids. The rate of formation of these liposomes was much increased by adding a polyunsaturated soya lecithin (Lipostabil, Nattermann, Koln) to the incubating medium. A suspension of cholesterol crystals (20 mg/ml) was cleared and solubilized by 18 hr. incubation with HDL and such phospholipid. Low-density lipoprotein, very low-density lipoprotein and albumin were ineffective in solubilizing cholesterol crystals.

Biochemical studies on these liposomes showed that their "molecular weight" varied between $5 - 50 \times 10^6$ which clearly

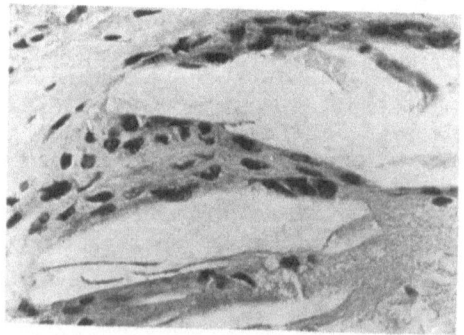

Fig. 2. Circumfusion of monocytes (early stage in giant cell formation) around a cholesterol crystal in an advanced capillarized human atherosclerotic plaque. Haematoxylin and eosin, × 210.

distinguished them from HDL. The liposomes contained more cholesterol, but less protein and phospholipid than HDL (Abdulla and Adams, 1979).

The solubilization of cholesterol crystals by HDL (with or without added phospholipid) clearly differs from the physiological removal of cholesterol from cell membrane and its carriage back to the liver on the HDL molecule, as proposed by Glomsett (1968). The accessibility of cholesterol crystals to this action of HDL might well prove to be important in the regression of atherosclerotic lesions. However, at present we do not know whether this process acts in vivo. It is perhaps particularly relevant that the HDL apoproteins are known to penetrate the arterial wall quite readily (Stein & Stein, 1973) and thus, the reaction could be physiologically feasible *in vivo*.

Table I. Biochemical comparison of HDL and liposomes derived by interaction between HDL and cholesterol crystals

composition dry weight	HDL	Large	Medium Liposome	Small
Protein	0.47	0.103	0.208	0.42
Cholesterol	0.021	0.59	0.48	0.206
Cholesterol-ester	0.18	0.26	0.22	0.157
Phospholipid	0.263	0.047	0.157	0.19
Size	10 nm	μm	200 nm	100 nm

REFERENCES

Abdulla, Y. H. and Adams, C. W. M. (1979): The action of high-density lipoprotein on cholesterol crystals. Part 2. Biochemical observations. In preparation.

Adams, C. W. M. 1967: Vascular Histochemistry, Lloyd-Luke, London, p. 86—93.

Adams, C. W. M. and Bayliss, O. B. (1976a): Detection of macrophages in atherosclerotic lesions with cytochrome oxidase. Brit. J. Exp. Path., 57, 30—36.

Adams, C. W. M. and Bayliss, O. B. (1976b): Succinic dehydrogenase and cytochrome oxidase in arterial, venous and other smooth muscle. Atherosclerosis, 23, 367—370.

Adams, C. W. M. and Morgan, R. S. (1978): Regression of atheroma in the rabbit, Atherosclerosis, 28, 399—404.

Adams, C. W. M., Knox, J. and Morgan, R. S. (1975a): The resorption rate of atheroma lipids in situ and implanted subcutaneously. Atherosclerosis, 22, 79—90.

Adams, C. W. M., Bayliss, O. B., and Turner, D. R. (1975b). Phagocytes, lipid-removal and regression of atheroma. J. Pathol., 116, 225—238.

Adams, C. W. M., Knox, J. and Morgan, R. S. (1975c). Exchange of plasma radioactive cholesterol with atheroma lipids in situ and implanted subcutaneously. Atherosclerosis, 22, 229—240.

Bayliss, O. B., (1976): The giant cell in cholesterol resorption Brit. J. Exp. Path. 57, 610—618.

Gaton E., and Wolman M. 1977: The role of smooth muscle & haematogenous macrophages in atheroma J. Pathol. 123, 123—128.

Glomsett, J. A. (1968): The plasma lecithin: cholesterol acyltransferase reaction. J. Lipid Res., 9, 155—167.

Lehninger, A. L. (1959): The metabolism of the arterial wall. In A. I. Lansing (Ed). The Arterial Wall, Williams & Wilkins, Baltimore, p. 220—246.

Stein, Y., and Stein, O. (1973): Lipid synthesis and degradation and lipoprotein transport in mammalian aorta. In Atherogenesis: Initiating Factors, Ciba Symposium, 12 (NS), 165—183.

Vesselinovitch, D., Wissler R. W., Hughes R., and Borensztajn, J. (1976): Reversal of advanced atherosclerosis in rhesus monkeys. Part 1. Light microscopic studies. Atherosclerosis 23, 155—176.

C. W. M. A., Department of Pathology, Guy's Hospital Medical School, St. Thomas' Street, London SE1 9 RT. U.K.

DRUGS AFFECTING ARTERIAL PERMEABILITY AND ATHEROGENESIS

F. NUMANO

Tokyo Medical and Dental University, Tokyo, Japan

Modern science has elucidated the important role of vascular injuries in initiation and acceleration of atherosclerosis and the function and metabolism of endothelial cells in the arterial wall has been extensively investigated in relation to the pathogenesis of the disease.

In 1960, Shimamoto and his group found that a single dose of cholesterol, epinephrine, angiotensin II, cigarette smoking or painful stimuli as applied to animals, all of which are considered to be risk factors for atherosclerosis, induced edematous changes in the aortic wall.[1,2] Later, using fluorescent techniques we found that such injury results in acute infiltration of lipids including VLDL and LDL into the aortic wall.[3] We observed contracted endothelial cells and increased phagocytic activity in the edematous changed aorta[4] and that large particles of lipoprotein passed through the open junction between contracted endothelial cells. This observation naturally led us to focus our attention on the metabolic changes of endothelial cells and possible measures to protect the vessel wall from vascular injury. A repetition of such challenges in animals promoted a thickening of the intima in the aortic wall and this was followed by atherosclerotic lesions.[5]

From this point of view, the changes of ATP and cAMP levels or the cAMP phosphodiesterase (cAMPPDE), phosphofructokinase (PFK), glucose-6-phosphate dehydrogenase activity were studied in intima of rabbits challenged with one dose of angiotensin II (10 µg/kg i.v.) or cholesterol (1 g/kg p.o.) and epinephrine (10 µg/kg i.v.) by using Lowry's micro assay method as modified by our group.[6,7]

There was a statistically significant decrease in cAMP and ATP levels and also a decrease in the PFK activity in the intima of edematous changed aorta as compared with findings in placebo control rabbits. On the contrary, the activity of cAMPPDE and G-6PDH exhibited an increase in these intima without a statistically significant difference. There were no striking changes of these enzymes or nucleotides in the media.[8] (Tables I, II)

Table I. Changes of ATP, Cyclic AMP and Cyclic AMP Phosphodiesterase in the Intima and Media of Aortic Wall of Rabbits Challenged by Epinephrine, Cholesterol and Angiotensin II

| | Aorta | | | | | |
| Treatment | Intima | | | Media | | |
	ATP	cAMP	cAMPPDE	ATP	cAMP	cAMPPDE
Placebo Control	14.3 ± 1.7	5.55 ± 0.3	12.8 ± 1.0	27.1 ± 2.3	1.73 ± 0.3	15.1 ± 1.6
Epinephrine (10 µg/kg) & Cholesterol (1 g/kg)	$10.6 \pm 1.3^{*}$	$4.01 \pm 0.2^{*}$	13.9 ± 0.8	$17.3 \pm 1.5^{*}$	$2.56 \pm 0.4^{*}$	13.6 ± 1.8
Angiotensin II (10 µg/kg)	$9.2 \pm 1.0^{**}$	$3.72 \pm 0.3^{**}$	15.1 ± 1.2	$18.3 \pm 1.1^{*}$	2.17 ± 0.5	12.5 ± 2.1

* <0.05, ** $P < 0.01$ Placebo control vs challenged group

Table II. Changes of Phosphofructokinase (PFK) and Glucose-6-Phosphate Dehydrogenase (G--6PDH) Activities in Intima and Media of Aorta of Rabbits Challenged by Angiotensin II or Cholesterol and Epinephrine

| Treatment | Enzyme Activity of Aorta | | | |
| | PFK | | G-6PDH | |
	Intima	Media	Intima	Media
Placebo Control	0.92 ± 0.07	1.48 ± 0.21	0.15 ± 0.20	0.20 ± 0.03
Cholesterol (1 g/kg p.o.) & Epinephrine (10 µg/kg)	$0.63 \pm 0.09*$	1.40 ± 0.15	0.18 ± 0.02	0.23 ± 0.01
Angiotensin II (10 µg/kg .v.)	$0.58 \pm 0.14*$	1.55 ± 0.29	0.17 ± 0.05	0.21 ± 0.02

The enzyme activity was expressed as moles of substrate converted per kg of dry weight of tissue per hour. * $P < 0.05$ Challenged group vs placebo control

Table III shows substances capable of preventing this injury to the vascular wall. Estrogen, glucocorticoid, aspirin, cyproheptadine, nialamide, all of which reportedly have preventive effects on experimentally induced atherosclerosis, were all confirmed to prevent acute vascular changes induced by the administration of cholesterol, epinephrine, or angiotensin II.

Table III. Substances capable of preventing acute vascular injury and their threshold values

Diethylstilbestrol	1.0 mg/kg p.o.
Estradiol Benzoate	2.0 mg/kg s.c.
Conjugated Estrogens	5.0 mg/kg i.v.
Estriol Succinate	5.0 mg/kg i.v.
Prednisolone	0.1 mg/kg p.o.
Dexamethasone	0.5 mg/kg p.o.
Cyproheptadine	5.0 mg/kg p.o.
Aspirin	50.0 mg/kg p.o.
Aminopyrine	50.0 mg/kg p.o.
Nialamide	50.0 mg/kg p.o.
Trasylol	300.0 U/kg i.v.
Soybean Trypsin Inhibitor	1.0 mg/kg/min (for 15 min)
Colchicine	1.0 mg/kg i.v.
Dibutyryl cAMP	15.0 mg/kg i.v.
ATP	5.0 mg/kg i.v.
Iproveratril	1.0 mg/kg i.v.
Vinblastine	1.0 mg/kg i.v.
Pyridinolcarbamate	1.0 mg/kg p.o.
Phthalazinol	1.0 mg/kg p.o.

CAMP, ATP or iproveratril, which inhibit calcium entry, also helped prevent vascular injury. Pyridinolcarbamate and phthalazinol, both of which were synthesized by Shimamoto and Ishikawa in 1965 & 1975 respectively, can protect the arterial wall of rabbits from vascular injury. Pyridinolcarbamate is a pyridine derivative and is reported to have a preventive effect against experimentally induced atherosclerosis.[2] Furthermore, this substance was confirmed to have an inhibitory effect on platelet aggregability induced by ADP, epinephrine, or thromboxane A_2. It was also found to increase in vitro the activity of PFK, malate dehydrogenase and ATP in the human aorta.[9] These metabolic effects of pyridinolcarbamate may explain its favorable effect in preventing vascular injury and the progression of atherosclerosis. Pyridinolcarbamate has been widely studied clinically and is being prescribed therapeutically in many countries.

Phthalazinol is a phthalazine derivative and reveals pharmacologically a potent inhibitory effect on cAMPPDE activity.[10] Experimentally, studies showed that this compound has an inhibitory effect on platelet aggregation and a preventive effect on experimentally induced atherosclerosis. These effects in turn suggest the important roles of cyclic nucleotide metabolism in the progression of atherosclerosis, platelet aggregation and/or vascular injury. Shimamoto also reported the antagonistic effect of phthalazinol on thromboxane A_2.[11] Since 1977, clinical studies of phthalazinol have been performed in neurological, angiological and cardiological fields and a considerable amount of positive data has been obtained.[12,13]

In our attempts to control experimentally induced vascular permeability, we have come to the conclusion that metabolism and/or functions of the endothelium and arterial wall may well be controlled by pharmacological agents.

REFERENCES

1. *Shimamoto, T., Yamazaki, H., Inoue, M., Fujita, T., Sagawa, N., Ishioka, T. and Sunaga, T. (1960):* Effect of adrenaline and noradrenaline on "silicone-like property" of blood vessels. Proc. Japan Acad. 36: 234—239.
2. *Shimamoto, T. (1963):* The relationship of edematous reaction in arteries to atherosclerosis and thrombosis. J. Atheroscler. Res. 3: 87—102.
3. *Shimamoto, T., Kobayashi, M. and Numano, F. (1975):* Immunofluorescent demonstration of plasma protein entry into arterial wall by cholesterol, epinephrine, norepinephrine and angiotensin II. Acta Path. Jap. 25: 51—67.
4. *Shimamoto, T., and Sunaga, T. (1972):* Contraction of endothelial cells as a key mechanism in atherogenesis. Proc. Japan Acad. 48: 633—638.
5. *Numano, F., Kobayashi, M., Moriya, K., Kuroiwa, T., Takahashi, T., Watanabe, Y., Takano, T., Takeno, K. and Shimamoto, T. (1975):* Histochemical and microbiochemical studies on the initial change of aortic wall to atherosclerosis. J. Jap. Atheroscler. Soc. 2: 257—266.
6. *Numano, F., Watanabe, Y., Takeno, K., Takano, T., Arita, M., Numano, F., Maezawa, H., Shimamoto, T. and Adachi, K. (1976):* Microassay of cyclic nucleotides in vessel wall. 1. Cyclic AMP. Exptl. Mol. Path. 25: 172—181.
7. *Numano, F. et al. (1978):* Microassay of cyclic nucleotides in vessel wall. II. Cyclic AMP phosphodiesterase activity. Microvasc. Res. 15: 229—238.
8. *Numano, F., Kuroiwa, T., Takeno, K., Takano, T., Watanabe, Y., Maezawa, H., Moriya, K. and Shimamoto, T. (1978):* Changes in phosphofructokinase, glucose-6-phosphate dehydrogenase activity and cyclic nucleotides in the aortic wall of rabbits with vascular injury induced by angiotensin II or cholesterol & epinephrine. Blood Vessels.
9. *Numano, F., Yamazawa, S., Takano, T. and Shimamoto, T. (1973):* On the mechanism of antiatheroscleotic agents. Microchemical studies on the in vitro effects of pyridinolcarbamate and estrogen (Premarin) on phosphofructokinase and malate dehydrogenase in the arterial wall. Mech. Ageing Develop. 2: 43—53.
10. *Adachi, K. and Numano, F. (1977):* Phosphodiesterase inhibitors: Their comparative effectiveness in vitro in various organs. Japan J. Pharmac. 27: 97—103.
11. *Shimamoto, T., Takashima, Y., Kobayashi, M., Moriya, K. and Takahashi, T. (1976):* A thromboxane A_2-antagonistic effect of pyridinolcarbamate and phathalazinol. Proc. Japan Acad. 52: 591—594.
12. *Shimamoto, T., Murase, H. and Numano, F. (1976):* Treatment of senile dementia and cerebellar disorders with phthalazinol. Cyclic AMP-increasing agent, phthalazinol, in therapeutic trials in hitherto incurable morbid conditions (1) Mech. Ageing Develop. 5: 241—250.

F. N., Dept. of Int. Med., Tokyo Med. and Dental Univ., Yushima-1, Bunkyoku, Tokyo 113, Japan

EXPERIMENTAL ATHEROSCLEROSIS: SURVIVAL AND SPONTANEOUS REGRESSION

C. A.-VILLAVERDE, J. C. MARTÍNEZ, L. MASSANET,
L. BADIMÓN AND F. G.-VALDECASAS.

Dept. Pharmacol. C.S.I.C. Barcelona. Spain

In the last International Congress on Angiology (Tokyo, 1976), we presented a method of rapid atherosclerosis production in rats with an induction period of 15 days. The procedure was: a first phase (4 days) of treatment with vitamin D and cholesterol in an olive oil suspension, and a second phase (11 days) of a hyperlipidemic diet with butter and thyroid function suppression by thiouracil.

Macroscopic results, already presented, showed aorta endothelial surface alteration and lipidic heaps strongly coloured by Herxeimers stain. Microscopically, we observed the existence of calcic infiltrations and elastic fiber dilaceration in arterial walls; myocardial infarction areas were also visible.

Compared to different experimental animal models (*Wissler*, 1974), this is a method that reveals lesions more similar to human atherosclerosis disease. However, the model had the inconvenience of a high mortality rate; only 33% survival. Although this is a good result compared to other proposed infarctal techniques, such as Howard's or Hartroff's that attained only 15 or 20% survival, we tried to improve the survival rate and this was obtained by changing the previous procedure in both time phases. The improved atherogenic method is depicted in Figure 1; 1.5 ml./K. of vit. D and cholesterol in olive oil were administered over 3 days and the hyperlipemic diet was administered ad libitum over 12 days. The total induction period of 15 days was not changed; the previous scheme was modified, giving one dosage less of vit. D suspension and increasing in one day the lipid diet ingestion, so that slight modification produced a great change in mortality as Fig. 3 shows; the first scheme had a mortality rate of 66% and the second one of 28%; this represents 71% survival.

The morphological characteristics of lesions have not changed, either in distribution nor quality. Histological study of aortas previously stained by Herxeimers confirms the lipidic deposits at different wall levels; staining, with Hematoxiline, calcic depositions, dilaceration and disruption of elastic fibers and endothelial proliferation can be seen.

The histological characteristics of the model were completed with study of plasma lipidic patterns. Figure 2 shows the results obtained (cholesterol, total lipids and triglycerids) in normal and atherosclerotic rats. The initial pattern of β-lipoprotein lower than α (normal in rats) is reversed after atherosclerosis induction; β-lipoproteins exhibited a great increase similar to human atheroclerostic disease in which the β/α coefficient increased considerably (normal rats: 0.3;

1st. Phase	Vitamine D$_2$ ..... (320.000, u.u.)	
	Cholesterol .... 40 mgr.	Days:
	Olive Oil .... c.s.p. 1.5 ml.	1—3
	(Daily Dosis: 1.5 ml./K.)	
2nd. Phase	Cholesterol .... 50 g	
	Thiouracil.............. 3 g	
	Cholic Acid 20	
	Butter 400	
	Sucrose 160	
	Casein.................. 200	Days:
	Choline Chloride........ 10	4—15
	Salts 40	
	Cellulose Powder 100	
	Magnesium Oxide 5	
	Inositol 2	
	B Vitamins 0.12	
	(Ad libitum)	

Fig. 1

33

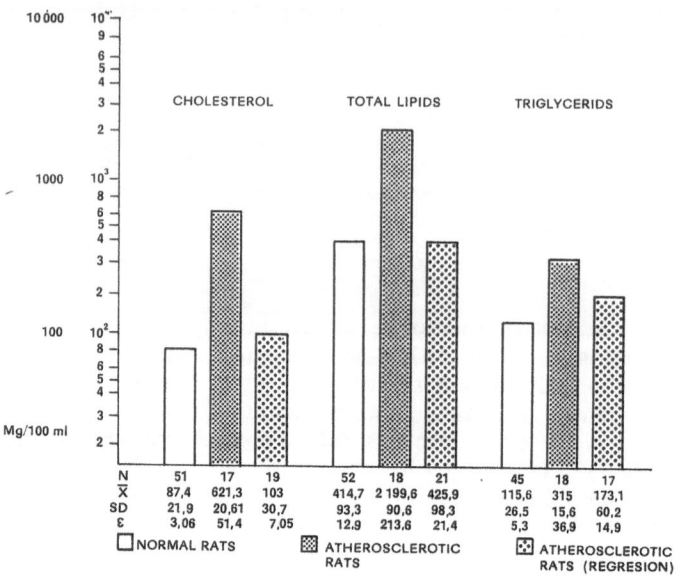

	CHOLESTEROL			TOTAL LIPIDS			TRIGLYCERIDS		
N	51	17	19	52	18	21	45	18	17
X̄	87,4	621,3	103	414,7	2 199,6	425,9	115,6	315	173,1
SD	21,9	20,61	30,7	93,3	90,6	98,3	26,5	15,6	60,2
ε	3,06	51,4	7,05	12,9	213,6	21,4	5,3	36,9	14,9

☐ NORMAL RATS   ▨ ATHEROSCLEROTIC RATS   ▧ ATHEROSCLEROTIC RATS (REGRESION)

Fig. 2

atherosclerotic rats: 1.5) and chylomicrons appear. Total proteins, measured by a refractometric method, exhibited a slight increase which is not significant in atherosclerotic rats (7.2 g%) compared to normal ones (6.9 g%). Protein electrophoretic patterns not change.

Studying rat atherosclerosis regression when rats were restored to normal diet for 75 days after the atherogenic diet, we found decreased Sudan-stained lesions (lipidic depots) but maintenance of fibrous streaks, rugosity and calcifications. Plasma lipidic patterns (figure 3) changed, cholesterol and total lipids decreased (showing no significant difference compared to normal values), while triglycerides remained significantly ($p < 0.0005$) increased. The lipoprotein ratio β/α returned to normal values (0.3) and chylomicrons disappeared. Total proteins and protein and protein electrophoretic patterns did not change compared to previous values.

In summary, a rapid (15 days) and inexpensive (71% rat-survival) atherosclerosis experimental model has been described. The method produces macro and microscopic lesions similar to human ones and an increased pattern of lipidic parameters, reversing the lipoprotein ratio β/α compared to normal rats.

Regression studies reveated disappearance of lipid accumulation and persistence of fibrous lesions in the arterial walls; plasmatic cholesterol and total lipids returned to normal values leaving increased triglycerides.

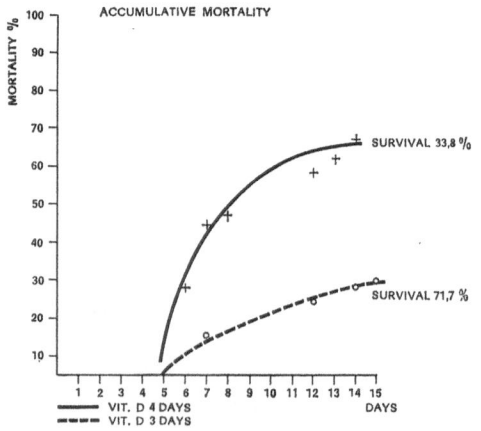

Fig. 3

34

REFERENCES

Altman R. F. A., (1972): A simple method for the rapid production of atherosclerosis in rats. Sperientia, 29, 2.

Gresham G. A., Howard A. N. (1960): The independent production of atherosclerosis and thrombosis in the rat. Brit. J. Exp. Path., 41, 395—402.

Villaverde C. A., Badimón L., Escolar G., Valdecasas F. G., (1976): The role of hyperlipemia and fibrinolysis in the experimental atherosclerosis and myocardial infarction. 7th. European Congress of Cardiology (Abstract book II, p. 185).

Villaverde C. A., Escolar G., Badimón L., Valdecasas F. G., (1976): Etiopathogenic aspects of atherosclerosis in rat. Proceedings X Internat. Congress of Angiology, p. 285.

Wissler R. V., Vesselinovitch, (1974): Differences between human and animal atherosclerosis. Atherosclerosis III, Edit. Schettler and Weizel, p. 319.

C. A. V., Dept. of Pharmacology C.S.I.C. C/Jorge Girona Salgado s/n. Barcelona-34. Spain

REGRESSION OF EXPERIMENTAL ATHEROSCLEROSIS

MAGDOLNA BIHARI-VARGA

2nd Department of Pathology, Semmelweis Medical University, Budapest, Hungary

Various trends in the prevention and therapy of atherosclerosis are intended to influence the humoral and vascular factors playing role in the pathogenesis of the disease. Nevertheless, interventions are mainly focused on the normalization of the blood cholesterol or blood lipid pattern and there are hardly any studies for the influence of the local biochemical processes involved in the formation of plaques. Our studies were carried out, to

continued for six weeks. The applied agents were: Anavar, Lipostabil, Miscleron and Chinoin-123, respectively. The fifth group was kept on a cholesterol diet and served as a control.

The effect of the treatment on the average serum lipid concentrations is demonstrated in Table I. In pre-established hyperlipidemia a significant decrease was observed in the concentration of total-, ester- and free cholesterol and triglycerides

Table I. The effect of antilipidemic agents on the serum lipid levels of cholesterol-fed rabbits (% change in concentration)

Drug	Total cholesterol	Tri-glycerides	Phospho-lipids	Cholest. ester	Free chol.
Miscleron	−74.0	−59.0	−38.0	−64.0	−83.0
Anavar	−16.0	−18.0	+58.0	−14.0	−15.0
Lipostabil	−28.0	−17.0	−41.0	−38.0	−6.0
Chinoin-123	−48.0	−39.0	+75.0	−45.0	−34.4

Table II. The effect of antilipidemic agents on the lipid content of the aorta of cholesterol-fed rabbits (% change in concentration)

Drug	Cholesterol	Triglycerides	Phospholipids
Miscleron	−29.0	−12.0	−7.0
Anavar	−35.0	−22.0	−9.0
Lipostabil	−32.0	−17.0	−2.0
Chinoin-123	−30.0	−13.0	+14.

perform comparative investigations on the effects of various antilipidemic agents on the tissue level.

Cholesterol atherosclerosis was produced in five groups of six month old rabbits. Each group consisted of fifteen animals. Three months after feeding the high cholesterol diet, treatment with antilipidaemic drugs started in four parallel groups of animals and was then

during the six-week course of treatment with the drugs; Miscleron and Chinoin-123 were found to be the most effective. The phospholipid content was decreased by Miscleron and Lipostabil, while Anavar and even more significantly Chinoin-123 administration resulted in a pronounced elevation of the latter lipid component.

A similar decrease could be demonstrated in the cholesterol and triglyceride

Table III. The effect of antilipidemic agents on the composition of the intimal ground substance of cholesterol-fed rabbits (% change in concentration)

Drug	Struct. water	Total GAG	HA + CS	CSA-4 + CSA-6	DS	He + HS
Miscleron	+14.5	+18.0	+10.0	+14.0	+4.0	+7.0
Anavar	−11.5	−5.0		not measured		
Lipostabil	+0.8	+10.0		not measured		
Chinoin-123	+17.2	+19.4	+13.0	+6.0	+7.0	−5.0

Abbreviations: GAG: glycosaminoglycan, HA: hyaluronic acid, CS: chondroitin, CSA-4: chondroitin-4-sulfate, CSA-6: chondroitin-6-sulfate, DS: dermatan sulfate, He: heparin, HS: heparan sulfate

content of the aorta intimas in all the four groups of experimental animals (Table II). Phospholipid concentrations were slightly reduced by Miscleron and Anavar, were not altered by lipostabil and showed a further increase of about 13% in the aortas of the animals receiving Chinoin-123.

The glycosaminoglycan (GAG) content and the amount of structural water bound to the proteoglycans of the ground substance was found to decrease in the aortas of rabbits receiving Anavar (Table III). At the same time, treatment with the three other compounds resulted in an increase of structural water and GAG concentrations, connected with the induction of an active repair process. With the two most effective drugs, Miscleron and Chinoin-123, alterations taking place in the intimal GAG-pattern of cholesterol-fed rabbits were also studied. There was a difference between the action of the two agents: the amount of nonsulfated acidic GAG-s increased in both experiments, as did the chondroitin-sulfates, but, while Miscleron enhanced mainly CSA-4 and CSA-6 synthesis, as a result of Chinoin-123 administration the increase in the dermatan-sulfate level was more significant. The heparin + heparan sulfate-containing fractions also behaved dissimilarly: their concentration increased during Miscleron administration and decreased in the aortas of Chinoin-123 treated animals.

Studies in the last fifteen years have indicated that focal accumulation of acidic GAG-s accompanies deposition of lipids within the arterial intimal region. The involvement of the lipoproteins and acidic GAG-s in atherosclerosis suggested an *in vivo* complexing process which might play an important role in arteriosclerosis pathogenesis (Gerö et al., 1960). Thus it seemed to be of interest to examine the effect of antilipidemic drugs on the intimal GAG-lipoprotein complexes, preestablished by cholesterol feeding. By application of a thermoanalytical method (*Bihari-Varga et al.*, 1968) it could be demonstrated that, in the arteries of rabbits with cholesterol-induced atherosclerosis, one part of the GAG-s became bound to lipoproteins. The amount of GAG-lipoprotein-containing lesions was definitely smaller in the aortas of the treated animals. From among the four drugs Miscleron and Chinoin-123 seemed to be the most effective.

A further alteration of significance could be demonstrated in the fibrillar protein components of the intimal tissue. Based on the results of thermal analysis (*Bihari-Varga*, 1971) in the aortas of cholesterol-fed rabbits, a pathological increase of protein stability, probably due to the deposition of some lipid compounds into the fibrillar protein molecules, took place. As a result of treatment with antilipidemic drugs, this cholesterol-induced increase in structural stability was found to be partly reversible.

M. B.-V., 2nd. Dept. of Pathology, 1450 Budapest, Üllöi út. 93, Hungary

THE REVERSIBILITY OF THE HUMAN ATHEROSCLEROTIC PLAQUE

K. T. LEE

Dept. of Pathology, Albany Medical College, Albany, New York, U.S.A.

Abundant evidence has been presented indicating that even advanced necrotic atherosclerotic lesions can be made to regress in experimental animals. Under appropriate conditions lipid can be removed; necrotic debris can disappear; collagen can be reabsorbed at least to some extent; and even calcium deposit can be reduced in size. Also, the excessive proliferative activity of the lesion smooth muscle cells that characterizes the active lesion can be reduced to the level of the smooth muscle cells in the normal media.

Since human lesions have similar components to those of the experimental animal lesions, it is natural to infer that they too can be made to regress. However, convincing evidence that substantial regression of advanced lesions can be induced in man is difficult to obtain.

In this presentation, I shall review some of the data from many centers on regression in man.

The earliest morphologic study that I have found is that of *Aschoff* in 1924. Aschoff reported that there was a diminution in the amount of aortic atherosclerosis observed at autopsy during the semi-starvation period in Germany at the end of World War I. *Veriainen and Kaniverain* (1947) reported a similar finding in the corresponding post World War II period. These studies, though suggestive, are largely impressionistic and untrolled and cannot be accepted as clearly established facts.

Wilens of New York in 1947 used a different approach that did permit some degree of control and statistical analysis. He studied aortas and coronaries from individuals dying of wasting diseases with terminal weight loss up to 45 kg. These were compared with corresponding arteries from autopsied individuals who had little or no terminal weight loss. The data showed convincingly that the group with the wasting diseases had less atherosclerosis.

However, Wilen's study must be viewed with some reservations because of the manner in which he selected his groups. The wasting disease group would consist largely of cancer patients. The control group would be heavily weighed with patients who died of complications of advanced atherosclerosis. The latter group would be expected to show more atherosclerosis regardless of other conditions.

Eilersen and Faber from Copenhagen in 1960 reported on a somewhat similar type of study using chemical data for comparison. They chose as their wasting disease tuberculosis. The controlled material-sisted of aortas from accidents or diseases of short duration. Patients with heart disease, hypertension, or diabetes were excluded. This seems to us to be an acceptable control group. Evaluations were made on the basis of chemical analysis for calcium and cholesterol in the intima and media. Comparisons were made on an age-related basis using two ages for the tuberculosis group L (1) age at death and (2) age at which weight loss began. In theory this device would permit them to detect either progression, regression, or no change. What they found in their study was progression of calcium accumulation and no change in cholesterol content, which suggests retardation of progression but not regression.

Zelis et al. of Bethesda in 1970 reported a study of plethysmographic changes in hyperlipidemic patients with peripheral vascular disease treated with a therapeutic diet and clofibrate. There was significant improvement in peak reactive hyperemia blood following ischemia suggesting the possibility of regression of the atherosclerotic process in certain patients.

More recently the most promising way of studying changes in atherosclerotic lesions appears to be by serial angiography. There seems to be solid angiographic evidence that changes in size of lesions can be seen in a relatively short period of time.

Blankenhorn and his associated in Los Angeles in 1977 assessed the effect of weight reducing diet, stopping smoking, and an exercise program in 38 patients who had at least one myocardial infarction by serial coronary arteriography. After an average of 15 months, 6 patients were improved, 16 unchanged, and 16 showed progression suggesting that regression and or stabilization of atherosclerotic lesions occur in certain patients.

Buchwald et al. of Minnesota in 1977 reported serial evaluation of coronary atherosclerotic plaque changes by arteriography for 1−2 years after partial ileal bypass. Data are inconclusive but evidence of plaque regression has been noted in 3 patients.

In conclusion, data presented thus far on the reversibility of atherosclerotic plaque in humans is not as conclusive as that seen in experimental atherosclerosis in animal models. However, encouraging data are being slowly accumulated and all available data suggest that human atherosclerosis can be made to regress in certain circumstances.

REFERENCES

Aschoff, L. (1924): Lectures in Pathology, Chapter 6, Atherosclerosis. Lane Lecture, Hoeber, N.Y.

Blankenhorn, D. (1977): Angiographic evidence of atherosclerosis regression in man. Proceedings of 4th International Symposium on Atherosclerosis, p. 414. Springer-Verlag, Heidelberg, New York.

Buchwald, H., Guzman, I. J., Moore, R. B. and Varco, R. L. (1977): Surgical management of hyperlipidemia. Proceedings of 4th International Symposium on Atherosclerosis. P. 528. Springer-Verlag, Heidelberg, New York.

Eilersen, P. and Faber, M. (1960): The human aorta. Arch. Path. 70: 103.

Veriainen, I. and Kaniverain, K. (1947): Arteriosclerosis and wartime. Ann. Med. Exp. Biolog. Fenniae 36: 748.

Wilens, S. L. (1947): Resorption of Arterial atheromatic deposits in wasting disease. Am. J. Path. 23: 793.

Zelis, R., Mason, D. T., Braunwald, E. and Levy, R. I. (1970): Effects of hyperlipoproteinemia and the treatment on the peripheral circulation. J. Clin. Invest. 49: 1007.

K. T. L. Department of Pathology Albany Medical College, Albany, New York 12208 U.S.A.

ELECTRON MICROSCOPY REMARKS ON THE POSSIBILITY OF REGRESSION OF HUMAN ATHEROSCLEROSIS

M. TESI, L. CARAMELLI and A. BORGIOLI

Department of Angiology, Main Regional Hospital of S. Maria Nuova, Florence, Italy

In atherosclerosis, a few main points have been raised. This disease is localized in certain zones of the arterial system corresponding to ramifications, bifurcations, curves, etc. The formation of a fibrous plaque is the most important manifestation of this disease, and it is linked to the proliferation of smooth muscle cells, variously stimulated. As long as the endothelium remains integral, the smooth muscle cells remain untouched; a focal damage of the endothelium is followed by a focal proliferation of these cells with formation of the

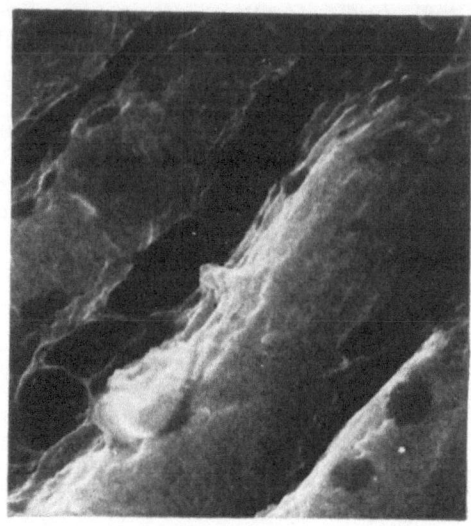

Fig. 2. Normal Left Gastric Artery ($\times$ 5000). At this enlargement the folds are still visible, and appear distinctly separated from one another by spaces of varying widths. In these, filaments of tissue which seem to connect one plica to the adjacent one, can be observed. These are the so-called "intercellular bridges" stretched between contiguous endothelial cells; not only their function, but even their existence is still under discussion.

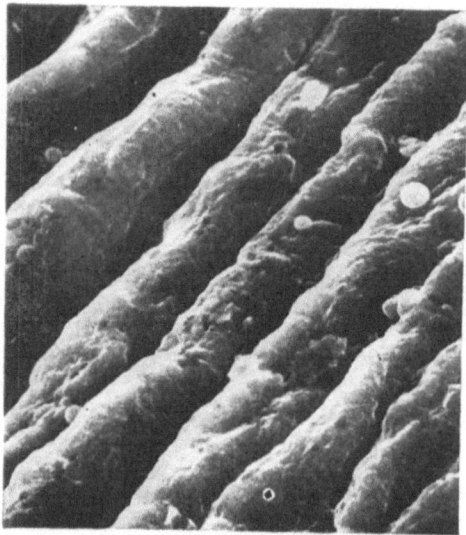

Fig. 1. Normal Left Gastric Artery ($\times$ 1200). The normal intima is formed of parallel endothelial folds which run down the wall like columns. Between the plicae are spaces which look like depressions or valleys. These intimal plicae seem to be formed by the endothelial cells aligned one with another, which lift the intima against the lumen of artery.

fibrous plaque. Therefore, research of arterial endothelium, both under experimental and clinical conditions, has become important. One of the methods used in studying endothelium is that of scanning electron microscopy (SEM), which allows us to observe the vascular intima from the front, i.e., "en face".

Experimental conditions

The problem of regression of atherosclerosis has been explored in experimental

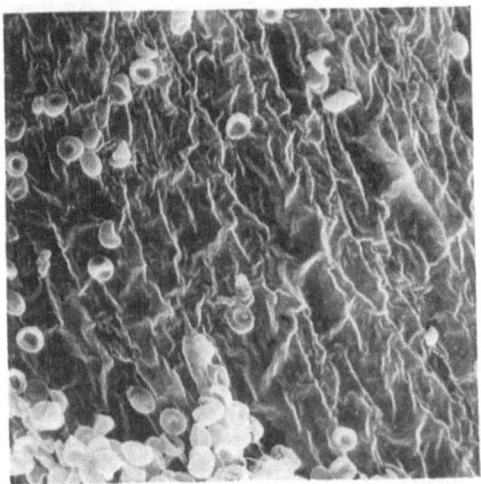

Fig. 3. Atherosclerotic Posterior Tibial Artery (×1000). This is a panoramic picture of the arterial intimal surface which only resembles that of the normal artery to a certain degree. An orientation toward folds can still be distinguished; however, the plicae project only slightly and are differentiated from one another as dry and wrinkled. At some points, a few endothelial folds conserve the intercellular bridges. Numerous red cells appear on the surface, some on the right agglutinated together.

animals. In rhesus monkey, in particular, certain high-lipid diets induce atherosclerotic lesions. With the abolition of these diets, in groups of animals previously fed this type of diet which should therefore show indications of atherosclerotic lesions, this type of alterations cannot be observed. Therefore elimination of the high-lipid diet seems to cause regression of certain manifestations of experimental atherosclerosis.

Human atherosclerosis

Using scanning electron microscopy, our group has made a series of observations of the human arterial intima in conditions both of normality and of atherosclerotic disease. These observations were the first of the published ones concerning the study by scanning of normal and pathological human material (*Tesi et al.*, 1973, 1975). Study of this type had been made in animals too by various authors.

(*Shimamoto et al.*, 1969, *Christensen and Garbarsch* 1972, Ready and Bowyer 1977, Weber et al., 1977).

All of the arteries that are to be described belong to human material. The samples were obtained in the operation room, where fixation was also carried out. The processes of dehydration, vaporization etc. up to final reading by the electronic microscope were performed successively.

The figures observed in the two groups of atherosclerotic patients, the first on a non-restricted diet and the second on a controlled diet as regards lipids and glycides, do not show significant differences. The figures of arterial endothelium observed are practically similar, and the morphological items described are characteristic of atherosclerotic disease in evolutive phase.

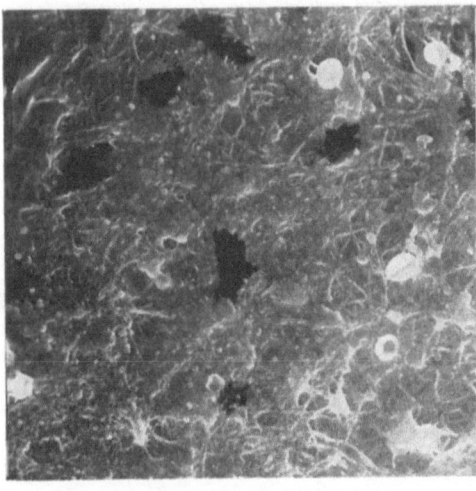

Fig. 4. Atherosclerotic Aorta, Proximal to the Thrombus (×1000). The intimal architecture appears hidden by an opaque veil which includes or recovers a reticulum, which is sometimes confused and other times arranged in small radiate structures. The meshwork winds around blood red cells and platelets. At the bottom and to the right, there appears a formation of soft material, constituted of small spherical granules, a part of the intimal plaque. In the velum disruptions can be observed giving origin to fenestrae which appear dark, with filamens of the reticulum running through them.

41

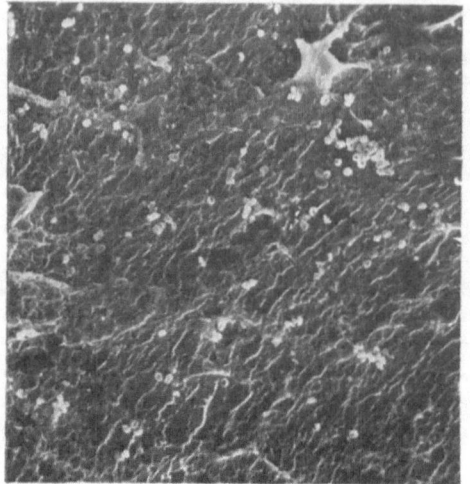 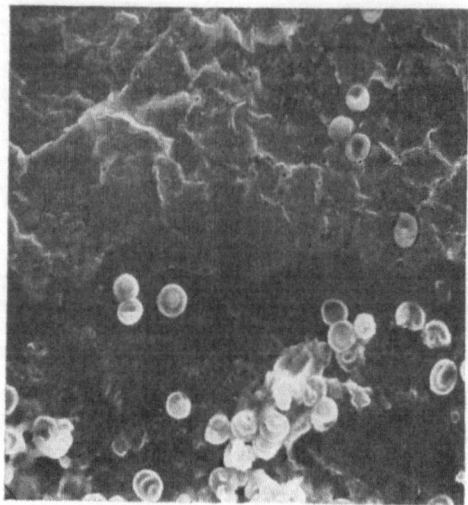

Fig. 5. Atherosclerotic Aorta, in patient on long term diet control as regards lipids and glycides (× 300). The arterial intima does not seem different from that observed during the preceding preparations. The organisation of the plicae appears disordered; slightly raised, indistint folds which give the endothelium on the whole a dry wrinkled aspect, can be observed. In the picture appears a grayish stratified substance which is lacking in the upper left-hand corner only. Dark points reveal falling of the endothelial lining. Blood red cells and a few platelets appear on the surface.

Fig. 6. Atherosclerotic Aorta, in patient on long term diet control as regards lipids and glycides (× 1000). The preparation shows two parts distinctly separated from each other. In the upper part a residuum of severaly altered plicae, can be seen on the left side; the disorder is even greater, on the right, and a gryish matter engulfs blood red cells and platelets. In the lower part the endothelium has fallen down, and in the background can be observed blood red cells altered in various ways. in one point conglutinated to a mass.

This conclusion is only apparently in contrast to the observations made by *Constantinides et al.,* (1960), *Wessler et al.,* (1965), *Vesselinovich et al.,* (1972), *Gresham* (1976), *Weber et al.,* (1977). This research was made in fact in animals and it was divided according to the description of regression regarding certain lesions of the atherogenetic phase.

Our study, instead, was done in man,

and the atherosclerotic disease in the patients observed, had gone far beyond the stage of atherogenesis. We have studied patients with atherosclerotic disease and arterial obliteration; where the atherosclerosis, from the phase of anatomical lesions, has become a clinical process with the consequent symptomology. At this stage, the alterations are probably definite and not susceptible to regression.

REFERENCES

Christensen B. C., Garbarsch C.: Scanning electron microscopic (SEM) on the ensothelium of the normal rabbit aorta. Angiologica 9, 15, 1972.
Constantinides P., Pooth J.,Carlson G.: Production of advanced cholesterol atherosclerosis in the rabbit. Arch. Path., 70, 712, 1960.
Gresham G. A.: Is atheroma a reversible lesion? Atherosclerosis 23, 379, 1976.

Redy M. A., Bowyer D. E.: The morphology of aortic endithelium in haemodynamic stressed areas associated with branches. Atherosclerosis 26, 181, 1977.
Shimamoto T., Yamashita Y., Sunaga T.: Scanning electron microscopic observation of endothelial surface of hear and blood vessels. Proc. Jap. Acad. 45, 707, 1969.

Tesi M., Caramelli L., Pollastri L., Tarantelli M.: Rilievi di microscopia elettronica a scansione nell'aterosclerosi umana. Convegno Sez. Tosco Umbra di Cardiologia, Pisa 17 Novembre 1973, e Boll. Soc. Ital. Card., 4, 383, 1774.

Tesi M., L. Caramelli, A. Borgioli, C. Tesi: L'intima artérielle dans la maladie diabétique. Etude en microscopie electronique de balayage. Expansion Scientifique Editeur, Paris 1975, pag. 224.

Vesselinovitch D., Getz G. S., Hughes R., Wissler R. W.: Coronary artery lesions in rhesus monkey fed with corn oil, outter fat, or peanut oil. Circulation 25, 46, 1972.

Weber G., Fabbrini P., Resi L., Jones D., Vesselinovitch D., Wissler R. W.: Regression of atherosclerosis lesions in rhesus monkey aortas after regression diet. Atherosclerosis 26, 635, 1977.

Wissler R. W., Hughes R. H., Frazier L. E., Getz G. S., Turner D.: Aortic lesions and blood lipids in rhesus monkey fed with "table prepared" human diets. Circulation 32, 220, 1965.

M. T., Department of Angiology, Main Regional Hospital of S. Maria Nuova, 50129 Firenze, Italy

SERUM LIPIDS AND VASOMOTORIC RESPONSE OF RATS DURING EXPERIMENTAL ATHEROSCLEROSIS

P. BRAVENÝ, L. VACEK, L. MÁCHOVÁ

Laboratory of Pathophysiology of Circulation, Faculty of Medicine, Purkyně University, Brno, Czechoslovakia

Female Wistar rats were kept for 20 weeks on an atherogenic dietary regimen which in a previous study had been shown to produce severe hyperlipemia and atheromatosis (*Vacek and Máchová*, 1974).

In parallel to the day by day serum lipids examination, the systemic blood pressure response of these animals to the standard stimuli of a broad spectrum of vasoactive agents was established (*Vacek and Bravený*, 1978).

A diet lasting 24 hours nearly doubled the total serum lipids, especially due to an increase in phospholipids and triglycerides. The spectrum of lipoproteins revealed a very early decrease in the alpha-fraction. The serum cholesterol level displayed a delayed but steady increase concomitant with the increase of triglycerides. Although the level of serum phospholipids doubled in 4 days, a further increment appeared extremely slowly.

Intravenously administered standard doses of adrenaline and acetylcholine

(0.4 µg/kg) were found to be most informative as an early sign of altered hemodynamic response. In comparison with control animals, the response to both vasoactive agents was significantly di-

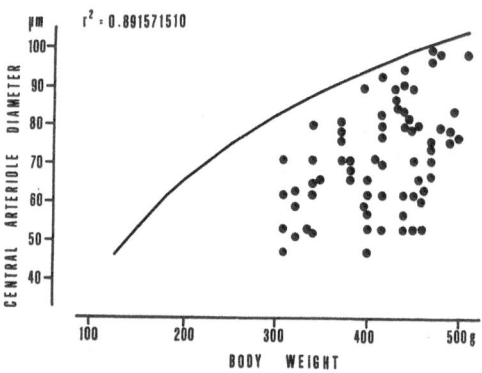

Fig. 2. The changes of mean arterial blood pressure response to a bolus administration of acetylcholine (0.4 µg/kg) after 3 (A 3) and 6 (A 6) weeks of atherogenic diet. Time in seconds.

minished after 6 weeks and stabilized after 12 weeks of the dietary regimen.

Approximately at the same time, i.e. 6 weeks, the first morphological changes were noticed in the liver, namely as a marked lipoid infiltration. Impairment of the other organs ensued with a distinct delay. Lipoid infiltration and enlargement of the media interfibrillar spaces in the aorta and in the main arteries, general lipid thesaurismosis, frequent pneumonias, and cholesterol granulomas in hypodermic and abdominal spaces were a late consequence of the deep metabolic deterioration.

The very early shift in serum lipoproteins as well as in serum lipids preceded

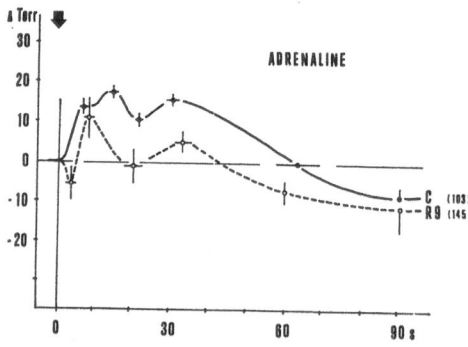

Fig. 1. Early changes of serum lipid components during the atherogenic dietary regimen. TSL = total serum lipids, CH = total cholesterol, PL = phospholipids, TG = triglycerides.

the first morphological changes in the liver. Significant deviation of vasomotoric response appeared in parallel to the change in the liver tissue but was recorded before any morphological alteration in the cardiovascular system proper. Thus the impairment of the liver metabolism seems to represent an important factor in early atherogenesis.

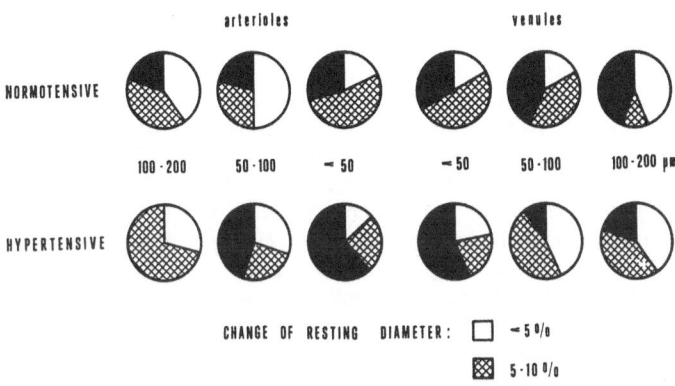

Fig. 3. The changes of mean arterial blood pressure response to a bolus administration of adrenaline (0.4 μg/kg) after twelve (A 12) weeks of atherogenic diet

REFERENCES

Vacek, L., Bravený, P. (1978): Blood pressure response to bolus administration of vasoactive drugs in the rat. Physiol. Bohemoslov. 27, 35—41.

Vacek, L., Máchová, L. (1974): Experimental hyperlipemia in the rat. Scripta med. (Brno) 47, 339—346.

L. V., Lab. Path. Circulation, Pekařská 53, 656 91 Brno, Czechoslovakia

DIFFUSIBLE CHOLESTEROL AND ATHEROGENESIS

S. I. CSÖGÖR

Institute for Arteriosclerosis Research at the Universtiy of Münster, Münster, F.R.G.

The solubility of cholesterol in water is only 0.18 mg/100 ml, most of the cholesterol is transported in blood by lipoproteins. Part of the cholesterol is found in plasma as a structural component of lipoproteins (*Fredrickson and al.*, 1967); the other part is only solubilized and is exchangeable between lipoproteins and cells. The biological activity of a substance is related to the plasma concentration of its unbound, diffusible form, because the distribution of protein-bound substances is limited by to the distribution of their carriers. To obtain data concerning the amount of plasma cholesterol physically supplied to tissues, solubilized, loosely bound or diffusible cholesterol must be determined.

If serum is mixed with decane, $CH_3 . . (CH_2)-CH_3$, some of the cholesterol diffuses into the decane while the lipoproteins remain in the serum. The cholesterol fraction remaining in serum is strongly bound by lipoproteins, while the amount of cholesterol diffusing into the decane is loosely bound or diffusible. The partition of cholesterol between serum and decane is determined by the lipid — protein interactions and the partition coefficient of cholesterol between water and decane. Under standardized experimental conditions, the amount of cholesterol diffusing into the decane is dependent on the loosely bound, diffusible fraction of serum cholesterol.

The separation of the solubilized fraction from structurally bound lipids is a difficult task, because the extraction of loosely bound lipids may alter the interactions of proteins with the residual lipids. In order to minimize the alteration of lipoproteins by the lipid solvent used for cholesterol extraction, in these experiments a chemically inert substance, decane, was used, which does not modify the ultraviolet absorption spectrum of serum proteins and their electrophoretic migration. The decane-treated lipoproteins have altered electrophoretic mobility due to their partial delipidation.

A mixture of 0.5 ml of serum and 4.0 ml of decane as well as 0.1 ml of stabilizer was incubated at 37 °C with a Cenco Test-Tube-Rotator moving in a vertical plane. After the incubation, the decane was separated from the serum by centrifugation and the cholesterol which had diffused into decane was determined with

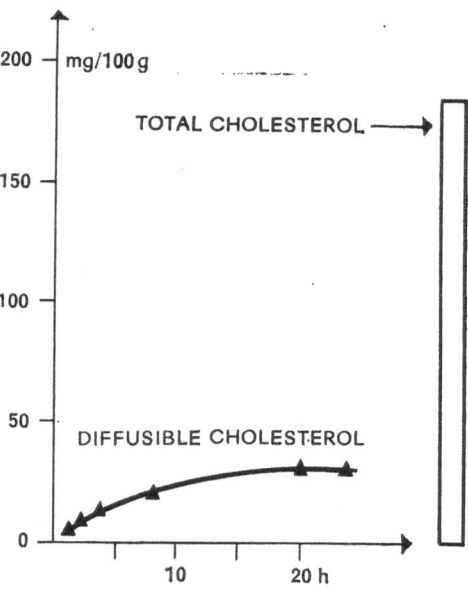

Fig. 1. Diffusion of serum cholesterol into decan. The curve represents the diffusible cholesterol entering the decan. The column indicates the total serum cholesterol.

the ferric chloride-method after evaporation of the solvent under nitrogen. Figure 1 shows the time course of diffusion of serum cholesterol into decane.

The serum-decane interface plays an important role in the kinetics of cholesterol exchange between the two phases and it is determined by the volume ratio of serum and decane, the length of incubation, the geometrical properties of the tube and the composition of the serum. This interface may be smooth or may be extended by emulsification. 10 mg Tween 20 and 20 mg Span 20/ml water stabilize the serum-decane interface as a water-in-oil emulsion and their use improves the reproducibility of the results. The esterification of free cholesterol during the incubation may be inhibited with dinitrodithiodibenzoic acid (2 mg/ml). These stabilizers do not alter the electrophoretic migration of lipoproteins.

Table I summarizes our data on the species-related difference in the diffusible fraction of serum cholesterol. The absolute amount of diffusible cholesterol is significantly lower in rats and rabbits than in man ($P < 0.001$). In rabbits fed a cholesterol-rich diet, there is an increase in diffusible cholesterol to values significantly higher than that determined in normal or hyperlipoproteinemic man ($P < 0.001$).

We could not find any close positive correlation between total cholesterol and its diffusible fraction in any of the species in normal condition.

The atherogenic activity is very low or lacking completely in normal rats and rabbits; it is present in "normal" man, high in hyperlipoproteinemic patients and extreme in cholesterol-fed rabbits. Consequently, there is an interesting correlation between the degree of atherogenic activity and the absolute values of diffusible cholesterol.

The passage of hydrophilic lipoproteins into the cells is impeded by the hydrophobic cell membrane, but the loosely bound lipids can leave their protein vehicles and can diffuse into the cellular wall (*Razin and Rottem*, 1978; *Csögör* 1972, 1975). Dissolution of plasma lipids in the lipid phase of endothelial cells followed by its transfer into deeper portions of the artery may be one of the mechanisms of cholesterol accumulation in the arterial wall, without endocytosis and degradation of lipoproteins (*Goldstein and Brown*, 1974). Thus the increase in the diffusible fraction of serum cholesterol, of the cholesterol physically available to the tissues, is particularly interesting with regard to the pathogenesis and treatment of atherosclerosis.

Table I. Total cholesterol and diffusible cholesterol in various species. No., number of examinations a.m., arithmetical mean; s.e.m., standard error of the mean

Groups	No	Total chol. mg/100 ml a.m. ± s.e.m.		Diffusible chol. mg/100 ml a.m. ± s.e.m.	
Normal man	18	191	5.1	35.4	1.9
Hyperlipemic patients	8	336	5.5	70.1	2.8
Normal rabbits	12	53	4.7	10.3	1.4
Cholesterol-fed rabbits (1% chol., after 2 month)	8	1504	134	244	13
Normal rats	19	90	0.9	12.0	0.9
Diabetic rats (streptozotocin, after 1 month)	7	76	5.4	17.0	1.5

S. I. C., Institut für Artherioskleroseforschung, Westring 3, 4400 Münster, F.R.G.

STUDIES ON VESSEL WALL CELLS OF NORMAL, HYPERTENSIVE AND STREPTOZOTOCIN DIABETIC ANIMALS
I. THE PROLIFERATIVE CAPACITY

R. DÉNES, R. LEHMANN, R. NIENHAUS, T. KERÉNYI,
J. MEY, and W. H. HAUSS

*Institute for Arteriosclerosis Research and Institute for Medical
Information and Biometry, University of Münster, Federal Republic
of Germany and 3rd Medical Clinic and 2nd Department of Pathology,
Semmelweis University Budapest, Hungary*

It is generally accepted that the accelerated proliferation of arterial smooth muscle cells is one of the most important events in the development of vascular disease. In our experiments the proliferation kinetics of aortic and venous smooth muscle cells and aortic fibroblasts were investigated using a new *in vivo-in vitro* model (Fig. 1). In this model Streptozotocin diabetes of different severity or renal hypertension was produced in male Wistar rats *in vivo*, the proliferation kinetics of the vascular cells prepared from these animals was followed in cell cultures *in vitro*.

The severity of diabetes was classified as latent, mild or serious according to the glucose elimination and insulin secretion observed. Renal hypertension was produced by artificial perinephritis. After two weeks of diabetes or hypertension explant cultures were prepared from the media

or adventitia of the thoracic aorta and the vena cava inferior. Aortic and venous smooth muscle cells and aortic fibroblasts isolated from the explants were subcultivated according to a precise time schedule (1) and the proliferation kinetics

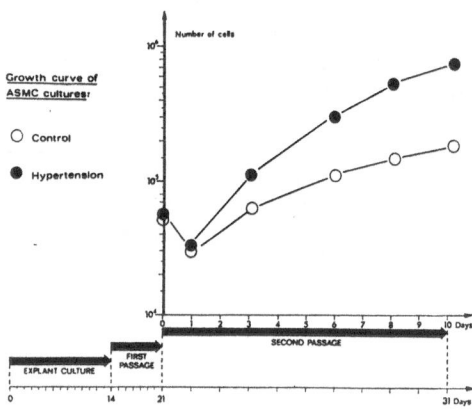

Fig. 2. Diagram of cell growth of the aortic smooth muscle cells (17 SMC) in the 2nd subculture after experimental diabetes.

was assessed in the second and sixth passage by cell counting. Using a function describing the growth we characterized the proliferative capacity of cells from each individual donor and the parameters of the growth function were evaluated statistically (2).

Aortic smooth muscle cell cultures from diabetic rats showed a significantly increased proliferation as related to the controls. The increase was independent of

IN VIVO — IN VITRO

RISK FACTORS:
Diabetes or Hypertension

CONTROL

Comparison of proliferative capacity in tissue culture

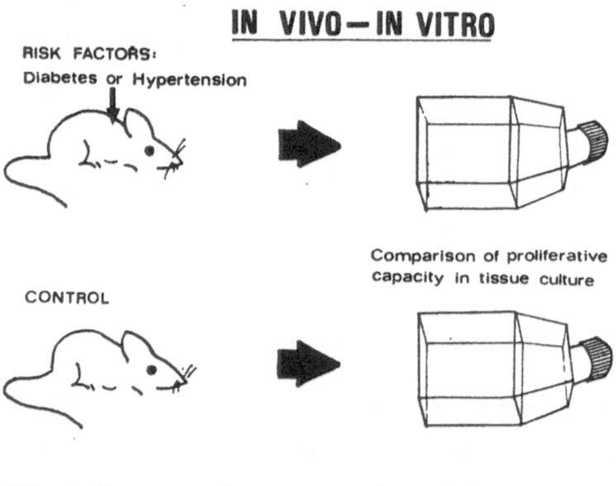

Fig. 1. Conceptual representation of the method.

48

the severity of diabetes (Fig. 2) and was maintained also in the sixth passage.

Cultures of venous smooth muscle cells proliferated significantly slower than those of aortic smooth muscle cells. No difference was detectable in the proliferative capacity of venous smooth muscle cells from control or treated animals. Venous smooth muscle cell cultures showed the same low proliferative capacity after two weeks or three months of serious diabetes. Present results may contribute to the understanding of the different reactions of the arterial and venous walls to the pathogenic factors of arteriosclerosis.

Since all cells were obtained and processed under identical conditions the difference in their proliferative capacity appeared to be genuine. Based on these results we assume that there exist in the vessel wall smooth muscle cells of different reactivity to proliferation enhancing stimuli.

Aortic smooth muscle cells obtained from rats with renal hypertension also showed significantly increased proliferative capacity proving that the phenomenon was not specific for diabetes (Fig. 3).

No difference was detectable between the proliferation of control fibroblast cultures and of those from diabetic or hypertensive rats. Thus apparently not all vascular cells were affected in the same way by experimental diabetes or hypertension.

We suggest that both diabetes and hypertension may induce in the aortic wall selection of smooth muscle cells of high proliferative capacity. Thus the reaction seems to be general and factor independent. The results correlate well with the pathologic concept of non specific mesenchymal reaction (3) and with findings of uniform alteration of DNA template activity of artery wall cells by different risk factors (4). The selective advantage of rapidly proliferating cells is readily detected in tissue cultures and subcultures. In the artery wall the same phenomenon may be involved in the pathologic smooth muscle cell proliferation in vascular disease. The induced selection of rapidly proliferating smooth muscle cells would be one of the possible mechanisms of smooth muscle cell population dynamics in arteriosclerosis.

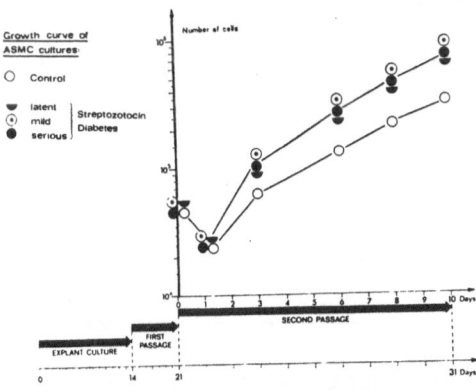

Fig. 3. Diagram of cell growth of the aortic smooth muscle cells (17 SMC) in the 2nd subculture after exprimental hypertension.

REFERENCES

1. *Dénes, R., Mey, J., Lehmann, R. and Hauss, W. H. (1978):* Vascular smooth muscle cells in culture after experimental diabetes. In: "State of Prevention and Therapy in Human Ateriosclerosis and in Animal Models" (Ed. by W. H. Hauss, R. W. Wissler and R. Lehmann), Westdeutscher Verlag, Köln, pp. 249—266.
2. *Nienhaus, R., Dénes, R. and Lehmann, R.:* Studies on vessel wall cells of normal, hypertensive and Streptozotocin diabetic animals. II. The biomathematical evaluation of proliferative capacity. (in this volume).
3. *Hauss, W. H., Junge-Hülsing, G. and Gerlach, U.:* Die unspezifische Mesenchymreaktion. Georg Thieme, Stuttgart 1968.
4. *Lehmann, R., Dénes, R., Kerényi, T. and Hauss, W. H. (1978):* Alteration of DNA template activity in artery wall cells induced by risk factors. In: "State of Prevention and Therapy in Human Arteriosclerosis and in Animal Models" (Ed. by W. H. Hauss, R. W. Wissler and R. Lehmann), Westdeutscher Verlag, Köln, pp. 267—283.

R. D., 2nd Department of Pathology, 1450 Budapest, Üllöi út 93, Hungary

STUDIES ON VESSEL WALL CELLS OF NORMAL, HYPERTENSIVE AND STREPTOZOTOCIN DIABETIC ANIMALS II. BIOMATHEMATICAL EVALUATION OF THE PROLIFERATIVE CAPACITY

RÓZSA NIENHAUS, R. DÉNES, and R. LEHMANN

Institute for Medical Information and Biometry and Institute for Arteriosclerosis Research, University of Münster, F.R.G. and 3rd Medical Clinic, Semmelweis University Budapest, Hungary

The proliferation of cultivated vessel wall cells was investigated. A new *in vivo in vitro* model (1) was used to detect changes in the proliferative capacity of these cells after experimental diabetes and hypertension. The increased proliferative capacity of cultivated aortic smooth muscle cells of treated, relative to that of control, animals suggests the role of a selection mechanism in the population dynamics of the pathologic aortic smooth muscle (2).

In these experiments, it was necessary to statistically compare the proliferation kinetics of different cell types (smooth muscle cells and fibroblasts), from different vessels (aorta and vein), from differently treated rats (Streptozotocin diabetes, renal hypertension and control) in different subcultures (2. and 6. passage).

The proliferation kinetics was followed by repeated assesment of the cell count from the first to the tenth day of sub-cultivation. At each point in time two tissue culture flasks, were prepared from each animal, from each flask two samples were taken and from each sample four counts.

The graphic presentation of the cell count versus time relationship for aortic and venous smooth muscle cell cultures from each induvidual animal showed "allometric" growth from the 1st to the 10th day (Fig. 1). The function yielding a curve with optimal fitting to the experimental values was:

$$y = a \cdot e_{bt}$$

a, b are parameters, b characterizes the rapidity of the growth. The parameters of the particular functions have been approximated by the least-squares method.

The graphic presentation of cell count

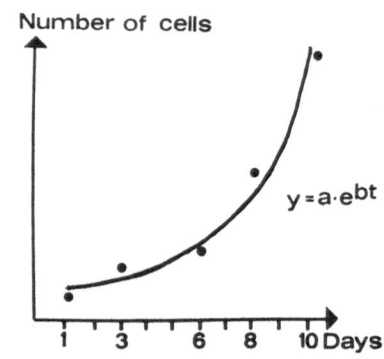

$$y = a \cdot e^{bt}$$

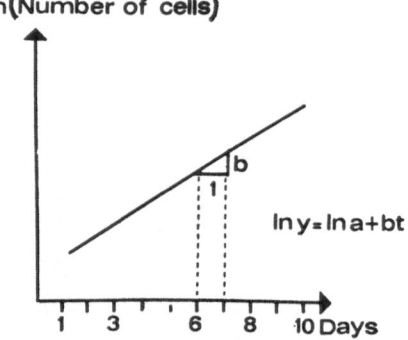

$$\ln y = \ln a + bt$$

The proliferative capacity is characterized by b

Fig. 1. Growth function of vascular smooth muscle cells in the subculture.

50

versus time relationship for aortic fibro-blast cultures derived from individual animals yielded an S-shaped curve in the 1th to 10th day period (Fig. 2). In the interpretation of the curve the logistic growth function was found to fit best:

$$y = \frac{P_1}{1 + e^{(P_2 t + P_3)}}$$

P_1, P_2, P_3 are parameters, the growth rate is characterized by P_3. The parameters have been approximated by an iterative proceeding using the least-square method (3).

The estimated parameters of the differently treated groups were compared by one-way variance analysis with the model:

$$y_{ij} = \mu + a_i + \varepsilon_{ij}$$

y_{ij} is the rapidity of the growth, b or P_3 of j-th animals in the i-th group and
μ is the mean of the random variables Y_{ij}
a_i is effect of i-th group
ε_{ij} is the error factor

In order to assess the sources of error in the final calculations, two animals per group were selected randomly and was the error of the induvidual readings per sample, the difference between the two samples per flask, the difference between the two flasks per animal and finally the biological difference between the two randomly selected animals (Fig. 3) were estimated. The model of the three level anova is:

$$y_{hijv} = \mu + a_h + b_{hi} + c_{hij} + \varepsilon_{hijv}$$

y_{hijv} is the number of cells at v-th counts of the j-th samples in the i-th flasks for the h-th animal
a_h is the animal effect
b_{hi} is the effect of flasks from the same animal
c_{hij} is the effect of samples per flask
ε_{hijv} is the error in the readings proper.
a_h, b_{hi}, c_{hij}, ε_{ijhv} are random variables with variance σ_v^2, σ_b^2, σ_c^2, σ_ε^2.

Number of cells

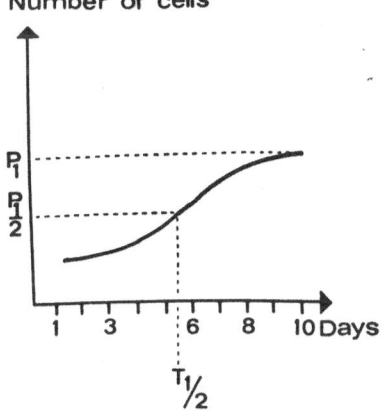

The proliferative capacity is characterized by P_3 (P_3 is proportional to rapidity of the growth.)

Fig. 2. Growth function of vascular fibroblasts in the subculture.

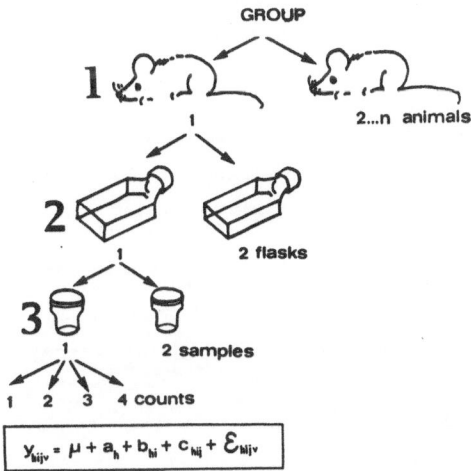

Fig. 3. The three-level nested anova for the data from the *in vivo — in vitro* model.

51

The interclass correlation coefficient was determined by means of the estimated variances. The results revealed strong correlation between the readings, samples and flasks from a single same animal. Thus any item of these data is highly informative in itself. In addition, the readings of the samples of the same flask and animal as well as the readings of the differential flasks of the same animal are strongly correlated. Thus the overwhelming majority of the variances originates from the individual animals themselves. Therefore, the results obtained *in vitro* reflect true biological differences rather than methodical errors. This fact justifies the comparison of animals on the tissue culture level.

REFERENCES

1. *Dénes, R., Mey, J., Lehmann, R. and Hauss, W. H. (1978):* Vascular smooth muscle cells in culture after experimental diabetes. In: "State of Prevention and Therapy in Human Arteriosclerosis and in Animal Models" (Ed. by W. H. Hauss, R. W. Wissler and R. Lehmann), Westdeutscher Verlag, Köln. pp. 249–266.
2. *Dénes, R., Lehmann, R., Nienhaus, R., Keré-nyi, T., Mey, J. and Hauss, W. H.:* Studies on vessel wall cells of normal, hypertensive and Streptozotocin diabetic animals. I. The proliferative capacity. (in this volume).
3. *Wingert, F.:* Eine Verallgemeinerung der logistischen Wachstumsfunction. Schriftenreihe des Deutschen Rechenzentrums. Heft S-9. Deutsches Rechenzentrum, Darmstadt 1969.

R. N. Institut für Medizinische Informatik and Biomathematik, 4400 Münster, Hüfferstr. 75, G.F.R.

MOLECULAR DISTRIBUTION OF PLASMA TRIGLYCERIDE IN ARTERIAL OCCLUSIVE DISEASE

J. SKOŘEPA, V. PUCHMAYER, S. VINOGRADOV and J. ZAPLETALOVÁ

IVth Medical Clinic, Faculty of Medicine, Charles University, Prague, Czechoslovakia

Hyperlipidaemia and especially hyper-triglyceridaemia are consideret to be important risk factors in atherosclerosis, even if the causal relations have not yet been proven to exist. There are many retrospective and prospective studies investigating the relationship between the plasma lipids level and coronary heart disease. On the other hand, the problem of plasma lipids in the ischemic diseases in the lower limbs, is less well know.

In our present paper we would like to report on a comparative study of the levels of cholesterol and triglycerides in a group of men with obliterating atherosclerosis and in a reference group.

Method

The determination of plasma lipids was studied by the gas chromatographic method proposed in 1967 by Kuksis and collaborators and modified in our own laboratory. The method permits the determination of free cholesterol, cholesterol esters, total cholesterol and composition of plasma triglycerides from a single analysis because this method separates triglycerides according to their molecular weight. Individual triglyceride fractions are marked with "carbon number". The carbon number is the sum of all carbon atoms of fatty acid chains bound to glycerol in individual molecules.

The reference values of cholesterol were determined in 197 persons and those of triglycerides in a group of 199 persons. All persons of this group were clinically healthy and free of all disorders which might influence lipid metabolism. The ponderal index was less then 1.1. Plasma fasting glycemia and uricemia were normal. The levels of plasma lipids in this group were adjusted according to sex and age. In this way we obtained normal lipid values in individual age groups in men as well as in women. The relationship of

Table I.

Number of men 30	Age range 35—65 years	Average range 51.6 years	Number of lower Extremities 42

Localisation of stenoses and occlusions					

Aorto-iliac prothesis with iliac occlusion	Abdominal aorta		Iliac artery		Femoral artery		Popliteal artery		Crural artery	
	Stenoses	Occlus.	S	O	S	O	S	O	S	O
	2	—	11	1	6	26	10	10	3	16
2	2		12		32		20		19	
	87 total									

plasma triglycerides to age on men has a distinct regression character and there is marked difference in this relationship between men and women.

On the other hand we observed no significant difference in the percent age molecular composition of plasma triglycerides in different age groups in men and women. The fraction of carbon number 56, which contains 2 fatty acids with 18 carbons and one with 20 carbons is present in an average of about one percent regardless of sex.

The group of persons suffering from ischemic disease of the lower limbs was composed of 30 men aged 35 to 65 years, with an average age of 51.6 years. We intentionally excluded all diabetics from this group. All men of this group suffered from obliterating arteriosclerosis in different parts of the arterial bed of the lower limbs (Table I).

All received complete clinical examination including x-ray examination of the chest and electrocardiogram. The biochemical examinations consisted of analysis of the plasma lipid profile plasma fasting glycemia and uricemia. The angiological investigation consisted of the palpation and auscultation of all accesible arteries, the position test, oscillogram at rest and after exercise, ultrasonic measurement of the systolic blood pressure on the radial, popliteal, posterior and arterior tibial arteries with determination of pressure gradient. Finally they underwent arteriographical investigation of the aorto-iliac segment as well as of the arteries of the lower extremities. The oscillographical and ultrasound investigationes were an available functional supplement to arteriography which is the decisive diagnostic method. The average diagnostic accordance of the noninvasive methods with arteriography was 86%.

Table II. Heterogenous triglyceridaemia in obliterative atherosclerosis in comparison with a reference group

Group	n	Augmented C_{56} Fraction
Obliterative Atherosclerosis	30	5
Reference	199	9

Fourfold table test $\chi^2 = 5.47$ P 0.05

Table II. shows a comparison of cholesterolaemia and triglyceridaemia in both groups. The values of total cholesterol are adjusted to sex and to the age of forty years. There is no significant difference between the two groups. Also the values of triglyceride are adjusted to sex and to an age of forty years. Between the reference group and the group of men with obliterating arteriosclerosis there is a significant difference in the mean level of plasma triglyceride. As regards the composition of plasma triglyceride there is also a significant difference between the two groups. (Table III).

Table III. Lipidemia in obliterative atherosclerosis in comparison with a reference group

Group	n	Cholesterol	Triglyceride
		Log values adjusted to sex and to age of 40 years	
Obliterative atherosclerosis	30	126.43 ± 9.64[a]	97.57 ± 17.43[c]
Reference	197	128.66 ± 8.74	95.38 ± 17.87[b,c]

[a] mean $\pm$ S.D.
[b] n = 199
[c] difference between means: t = 3.34, P 0.001

Results

In arterial occlusive disease we can much more frequently observe abnormal triglyceride fractions which consist of higher carbon number molecules. The fourfold table test is significant on the 5 percent level. The triglyceride fractions with carbon numbers of 56 and more generally contain 1 to 2 acyl chains with 20 or 22 carbons. It is of interest that these molecules are also found in patients with normal triglyceride levels.

Conclusion

From these results can be concluded that the arteriosclerotic process is not only in relationship to hypertriglyceridaemia but that there is also a significant association with abnormal compositions of triglyceride.

In other studies which are in progress we will try to find out more about abnormal triglyceride molecules and to study their composition. We feel that study of this question may contribute to more knowledge of the pathogenetic factors of the atheromatous infiltration of the arterial wall.

J. S., IVth Medical Clinic, Faculty of Medicine, Charles Univ., U nemocnice 2, 120 00 Prague 2, Czechoslovakia

LECITHIN CHOLESTEROL ACYLTRANSFERASE (LCAT) IN PROGNOSIS OF CARDIOVASCULAR COMPLICATIONS

MILADA DOBIÁŠOVÁ, K. VONDRA, J. STŘÍBRNÁ and J. VÁLEK

Isotope Laboratory, Biol. Inst., Czechoslovak Acad. Sci. and Institute of Clinical and Experimental Medicine, Prague, Czechoslovakia

Detailed knowledge of the internal dynamics of cholesterol metabolism is essential for understanding the role of cholesterol in aetiopathogenesis of cardiovascular diseases, especially of states without manifest hyperlipidemia. LCAT may be taken as an indicator of the rate of endogenous cholesterol turnover.

In view of the fact that the LCAT activity is influenced in a complex manner by the enzyme concentration and substrate capacity of plasma lipoproteins, the final value obtained from assays using an autologous substrate does not express the effect of the individual components. Hence, we attempted to eliminate the role of the individual lipoprotein spectrum and to determine the range of the normal values of basal LCAT activity in a large set of healthy individuals using the slightly modified method of *Glomset and Wright* (1964). On the basis of these values and their relationships we estimated the deviations in patients with so-called IHD risk diseases — obesity, hypertension, diabetes and hyperlipoproteinemia II — and in patients with an IHD — myocardial infarction.

While the differences in relative body weight, serum cholesterol and triglycerides between the groups of healthy men and women (Table I) were insignificant, there was a highly significant difference in the average value of LCAT activity. The higher values of LCAT in men give rise to a higher rate of fractional cholesterol turnover. The values of cholesterol ester production derived from plasma volume and from LCAT activity were very close to the values obtained *in vivo* (*Kudchodkar*, 1976, *Nestel*, 1970). Correlation analysis

detected and confirmed (*Akanuma*, 1973) a close dependence of LCAT on the relative body weight (Fig. 1). This dependence holds for both reference groups, the level of significance being greater in men than in women. This led us to introducing the LCAT/weight/length index which may serve as a more exact criterion for evaluating deviations than the mean LCAT value of the reference group. It followed that, in healthy individuals, there is a certain normal value of basal LCAT which is best expressed in relation to the body weight (LCAT/w/l) but is different for men and women. (Table I). Furthermore, the basal LCAT activity in healthy individuals is in equilibrium with the plasma cholesterol content. This internal balance between the rate of turnover of free cholesterol in plasma and the concentration of cholesterol is expressed by the fractional turnover value.

The results obtained in the reference group were compared with those from patients with diseases considered as risk factors for the IHD formation (Table I). In obese men, the basal LCAT activity increased proportionally up to 130% relative body weight. For higher excess weight the LCAT activity did not increase further. The rate of fractional turnover even at higher cholesterol levels remained the same as with men of the reference group. In obese women the fractional turnover was greater than in healthy women. In hypertension the relation of LCAT and relative body weight was preserved on an average in both men and women. The rate of fractional turnover in men decreased while in women it remained on the same level as the reference group,

Table I. Lipid concentration and basal LCAT activity in healthy individuals, patients with "risk" IHD and patients with myocardial infarction

Groups	weight[a]	TCH μmol/l	TG mg/100 ml	LCAT μmol/l/h	Fractional turnover %	LCAT w/l
REFERENCE						
men (n = 67)	95.8	5555	84.6	94.1	7.29	0.985
women (58)	94.8	5639	78.8	84.4	6.10	0.898
	N.S.	N.S.	N.S.			
OBESITY						
men (n = 18)	136.8	6505	156.5	115.5	7.33	0.875
women (13)	170.9	5837	128.5	104.3	7.10	0.617
					N.S.	
HYPERTENSION						
men (n = 23)	109.3	6706	195.5	106.2	6.15	0.984
women (15)	112.3	7453	102.8	135.1	5.85	0.928
					N.S.	N.S.
DIABETES						
men (n = 29)	108.2	7262	239.3	108.4	5.71	0.998
						N.S.
women (15)	119.1	7977	193.1	122.3	6.26	1.054
					N.S.	
HLP II.						
men (n = 12)	103.7	9890	250.0	104.4	4.10	1.009
						N.S.
I.M.						
men (n = 37)	111.0	7328	239.8	100.8	5.31	0.915
					N.S.	

a = weight/lenght index (kg/cm-100 . 100); TCH = total cholesterol; TG = triglycerides; LCAT = = lecithincholesterol acyltransfer rate; fractional turnover = per cent of free cholesterol esterified; LCAT/w/l = index of dependence LCAT rate on relative body weight; N.S. = nonsignificant differences between men and women in the reference group and between men of reference group and other groups and women of the reference group and other groups. All other differenes were statistically significant.

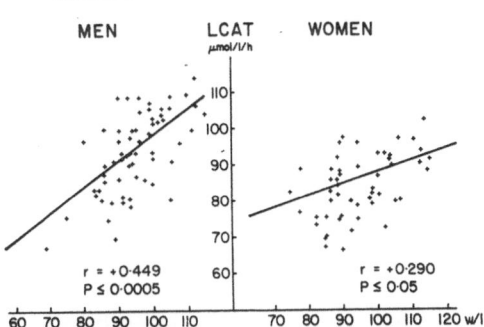

Correlation between LCAT rate and w/l index

MEN · LCAT μmol/l/h · WOMEN

r = +0·449 P ≤ 0·0005

$\dfrac{\text{LCAT}}{\text{w/l}} = 0·9845$ S.E. ±0·0145

r = +0·290 P ≤ 0·05

$\dfrac{\text{LCAT}}{\text{w/l}} = 0·8977$ S.E. ±0·0173

even if plasma cholesterol increased by 30%. In diabetes in men, the average ratio of LCAT to relative weight did not differ from the healthy group, but the rate of

fractionai turnover was lower. In women, although the content of plasma cholesterol increased by 40%, the rate of fractional turnover did not differ from healthy. In hyperlipoproteinemia II there was a relationship between LCAT and relative weight (on an average), just as in the preceding groups and the rate of fractional turnover decreased further. In IHD — myocardial infarction 16 of 37 male patients did not suffer from any of the risk diseases studied. The mean rate of fractional turnover was very low and there was no longer any relationship between LCAT and realtive body weight.

To assess the dependence between LCAT-dependent indicators and IHD we designed criteria for evaluating deviations in individuals in all the groups of men studied (Table II). The criteria included a deviation from the mean value of the

LCAT/w/l index of the reference group; further the values of the rate of fractional turnover were lower than 6% and the values of total cholesterol exceeded 7.500 μmol per liter. The number of individuals for whom deviations were found increased gradually from the reference group to obesity, hypertension, diabetes, HLP II, to myocardial infarction. Most deviations were found in patients with infarctions even if they did not suffer from a risk disease. The presence of a risk disease increased the number of deviations.

On the basis of the results presented here, we assume that there is a relationship between IHD and LCAT-dependent disturbances of endogenous regulations of cholesterol metabolism even if these disturbances are not manifested clinically by hypercholesterolemia. Presumably LCAT activity could also be used in clinical practice for testing these latent disturbances.

REFERENCES

Akanuma, Y. et al. (1973): Positive correlation of serum lecithin: cholesterol acyltransferase activity with relative body weight. Europ. J. Clin. Invest. 3, 136—141.

Glomset, J. A., Wright, J. L. (1964): Some properties of a cholesterol esterifying enzyme in human plasma. Biochim. Biophys. Acta 83, 266—276.

Kudchodkar, B. J., Sodhi, H. S. (1976): Plasma cholesteryl esters turnover in man: comparison in vivo and in vitro methods. Clin. Chim. Acta 68, 187—194.

Nestel, P. J. (1970): Cholesterol turnover in man. Advances in lipid research, R. Paoletti and D. Kritchevski (eds.) 8, 1. Academic Press Inc.

M. D., Isotope Laboratory, Biol. Inst., Czechoslovak Acad. Sci., Prague 4-Krč, Vídeňská 1083, Czechoslovakia.

THE EFFECT OF CHELATON III ON CALCIUM METABOLISM IN THE ARTERIAL WALL

(Clinical Observation with Experimental and Cytochemical Study)

OLGA BRÜCKNEROVÁ, A. ZECHMEISTER and E. HADAŠOVÁ

Introduction

Arteriosclerosis is the most frequent ethiopathogenetic factor of the occlusive arterial disease. The incidence of simultaneous damage to arteries of multiple organs increases with age which also is one of the risk factors of arteriosclerosis. The contraindications of vasodilating therapy or reconstructive surgery increase with age and therefore drugs without vasodilatory effect have been studied with which arteriosclerosis could be treated.

Clinical results

After the favourable results of *Lamar* (1964, 1966) Chelaton III ($Na_2EDTA = C_{10}H_{14}N_2Na_2O-.2H_2O$) which is disodium ethylendiaminotetraacetate was applied in the form of a slow intravenous infusion (in the dose of 3 g in 500 ml of the 5% fructose solution, the duration of an infusion 4 hours, decreasing gradually to 3 hours). One series of treatment consisted in 30 infusions given daily (for five days each week). All patients were put on anti-atherogenic, milk free diet during the treatment. In 48 patients (40 men, 8 women) with prevalence of the occlusion of large arteries (ileofemoral, or aortoiliac section) the results of treatment were estimated as good in 40 cases, in 8 cases as none. The average age at the beginning of the syndrome of claudication was 54.5 for men and 64.5 for women, at the beginning of the treatment with Chelaton III the average age was 60 for men and 66 for women.

The objective estimation of the therapeutical effect of Chelaton III, namely the regression of resting pain and trophic skin changes, further the prolongation of walking distance has been described in our previous reports (*Brücknerová et al.,* 1968, 1972, 1975).

The mechanism of the action of Chelaton III therapy is not yet elucidated. *Lamar* explained the effect of chelating therapy by direct disintegration of atherosclerotic plaques in the arterial wall and by elimination of metastatic calcium from the deposits. But the proof has been missing till now.

Experimental part

The decalcifying effect of Chelaton III has been followed in experimentally provoked calcification (with dihydrotachysterol, AT 10) in rabbits. In 21 white rabbits of the same breed, one year of age, average weight about 3.500 g, experimental calcification has been induced by a single administration of AT 10 in the dose of 8 mg per one rabbit. In 12 rabbits there has been administered Chelaton III intravenously in the dose of 120 mg per one rabbit. In six cases the dose was applied daily from the first till the 17th day of the experiment – the group in which the preventive effect of Chelaton III on the development of experimental calcification was followed. In other six rabbits Chelaton III was applied from the 3rd till the 17th day of the experiment – the group in which the therapeutical decalcifying effect of Chelaton III was tested. The 9 control animals were sacrificed on the 3rd, 11th and 18th day after AT 10 administration, the 12 animals with Chelaton III (both groups – with

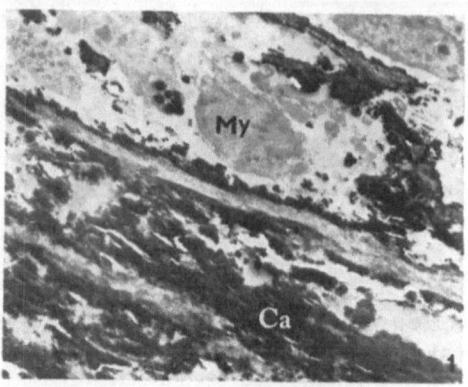

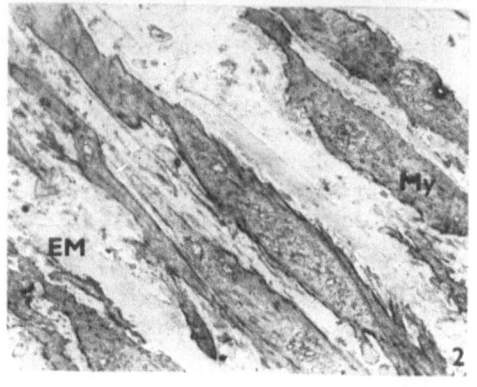

Fig. 1. Central part of the media of rabbit's aorta (from the "control group") on the 11th day of the experiment (1st day 8 mg AT 10).
Total destruction of the cellular (My) and extracellular structural elements with massive calcification (Ca). × 5.000 (direct magnification)

Fig. 2. Central part of the media of rabbit's aorta (from the "preventive" Chelaton III application) on the 11th day of the experiment. (1st day 8 mg AT 10, 1st—10th day 120 mg Chelaton III intravenously each day).
Note but less damaged structural elements (myocytes — My, and elastic membranes – EM) without lipid inclusions and without calcium deposits. × 3.000 (direct magnification)

preventive and with therapeutical administration of Chelaton III) were *sacrificed* on the 11th and on the 18th day of the experiment.

Results

Massive calcium deposits in the media of rabbit's aorta can be found already on the 3rd day after AT 10 administration (in the form of mediocalcinosis) in light-

-microscopic observation. At the same time the ultrastructure has been characterized with extracellular lipid accumulation and also with lipid inclusions in the smooth muscle cells, often designated as "foam cells". Progressive lipid accumulation in these modified myocytes causes the decrease of contractile myofilaments and the increase of smooth sarcoplasmic reticulum and mitochondria. In some "foam cells" only residual or none contractile myofilaments can be seen in electronmicrographs. Lipid accumulation in the arterial wall is usually accompanied by massive calcium deposits in the damaged fragmented elastic membrane in the media. Granular sarcoplasmic reticulum and Golgi complex increase in quantity.

On the 11th day after AT 10 application total destruction of both cellular and extracellular structural elements can be seen on electronmicrographs from rabbit's aorta, with massive calcifications. (Fig. 1).

After "preventive" Chelaton III aplication at the same time as AT 10, only slight deposits of lipids and calcium can be found. Elastic membranes are less damaged and the hypertrophy of sarcoplasmic reticulum, mitochondria and Golgi com-

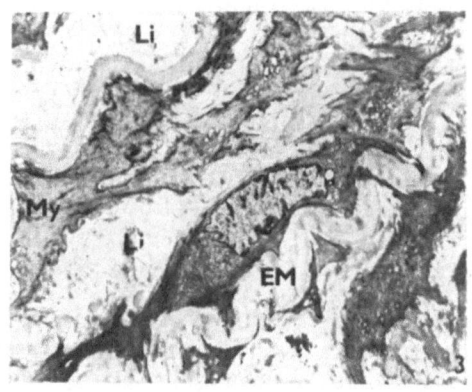

Fig. 3. Central part of the media of rabbit's aorta (from the group with "therapeutical" Chelaton III application) on the 11th day of the experiment. (1st day 8 mg AT 10, 3rd—10th day 120 mg Chelaton III intravenously each day).
Note the extra- and intracellular lipid inclusions (Li), the damaged elastic membranes (EM) and myocytes (My). ×2.000 (direct magnification)

plex is less developed (Fig. 2) on the 11th day of the experiment.

In the group with "therapeutical" application of Chelaton III, there were only residual deposits of calcium but high amounts of lipid inclusions in the media of the aortic wall (Fig. 3) on the 11th day of the experiment.

In the inner part of media adjacent to the intima smooth muscle cells are characterized with hypertrophy of granular sarcoplasmic reticulum and Golgi complex which demonstrate a high proteosynthetic activity.

Conclusions

After "toxic" dosis of dihydrotachysterol (AT 10) the lipids and calcium deposits in the wall of rabbit's aorta increase. Electronmicroscopically calcium deposits are found in the elastic membranes, in collagen fibres, in myocytes in various forms (dispersal deposits, precipitation, crystallized form). The model of aortic changes provoked with dihydrotachysterol (AT 10) seems suitable for the study of the decalcifying or antilipemic effect of drugs.

In a clinical study favourable effect of Chelaton III in occlusive arteriosclerosis has been confirmed according to *Lamar* (1964, 1966). After experimentally provoked changes in rabbit's aorta (with AT 10), cytochemical estimation of the aortic wall in an electronmicroscopic study, using a new method (*Zechmeister*, in press), was performed. The results can be summarized:

1) In experimentally provoked calcification of rabbit's aorta Chelaton III has a significant decalcifying effect on the arterial wall, but a less expressive effect on its lipid content.

2) From the discovery of erythrocytes in the extracellular space of the rabbit's aorta it is evident that Chelaton III increases the permeability of the arterial wall in experimental animals which must be taken in consideration as possible side-effect.

3) The finding of eosinophilic leucocytes in the arterial wall could be correlated with the role of eosinophils perhaps in the process of calcium accumulation and elimination.

REFERENCES

Lamar, C. P. (1964): Chelation therapy of occlusive arteriosclerosis in diabetic patients. Angiology, 15, 9, 379—394.

Lamar, C. P. (1966): Chelation endarterectomy for occlusive atherosclerosis. J. Amer. Geriatr. Soc. 14, 3, 272—294.

Brücknerová, O., Tuláček, J., Krojzl, O.: (1968): Cheláty v léčbě uzávěrových tepenných chorob. Vnitř. lék. 14, 9, 841—845.

Brücknerová, O., Tuláček, J. (1972): Cheláty v léčbě uzávěrové aterosklerosy. Vnitř. lék., 18, 8, 729—736.

Brücknerová, O. (1972): Syndrom intestinální klaudikace. Vnitř. lék., 18, 7, 652—655.

Brücknerová, O. (in press): Contribution to the treatment of occlusive arteriosclerosis with drugs without vasodilating activity. Scripta med. Univ. Brunensis

Zechmeister, A. (in press): A new selective ultrahistochemic method for the demonstration of calcium using N, N-Naphtalylhydroxylamine. Ultrahistochemistry (BRD).

O. G., 3rd Medical Clinic, Department of Anatomy, Department of Pharmacology J. E. Purkynje University, Faculty of Medicine, Brno, Czechoslovakia

AORTIC CHANGES IN SPONTANEOUSLY HYPERTENSIVE RAT (SHR) AS RELATED TO ATHEROGENESIS

P. HADJIISKY, J. RENAIS and L. SCEBAT

Centre for Cardiology Research, Hospital Boucicaut, Paris and Laboratory of Histoenzymology, UER Biomed Sts Peres, Paris, France

The modified structural and/or metabolic behaviour of arterial wall in hypertensive humans and animals may be involved in hypothetic mechanisms by which elevated blood pressure accelerate atherosclerosis.

Recent data suggested that in experimental hypertension, lipid accumulation in aorta depend more upon arterial wall changes than upon direct effect of elevated filtration pressure. Hypertension of spontaneous hypertensive rat (Okamoto Aoki strain) (SHR) mimicks the human one. Hence SHR is a good model for the metabolic and structural study of hypertensive arteriopathy.

The present work deals with morphometric structural and enzymatic changes in SHR aorta during postnatal ontogenesis.

Material and methods

Aortae from 45 SHR and 40 control rats 1, 3, 5—7, 11—13, 16 and 20 month-old were studied according to the technics described in previous works.

Results

The principal data observed are summarized: Figures 1 and 2.

Conclusions

During *prehypertensive stage* (*one-month-old rats*) aortas of Okamoto strain and of Kyoto control rats were identical with regard to morphology, morphometry and metabolism. In two of the four Okamoto rats the only change was the increase of 5' nucleotidase enzyme activity.

In three month-old SHR hypertension was stabilized since one month. The only changes observed were the histoenzymatic ones: 5' nucleotidase and LDH activities generalized increase augmentation of certain oxido-reductases (G6PD) at the edge of the aortic lumen; alkaline phosphatase increase in vasa vasorum.

Arterial behavior in 6 to 9 months-old SHR (*short term hypertension*) was caracterized by the following features:

1) *Metabolic activation of smooth muscle cells* (*SMC*) in the whole media as demonstrated by increase in enzymes activities related to: lipolysis (esterases

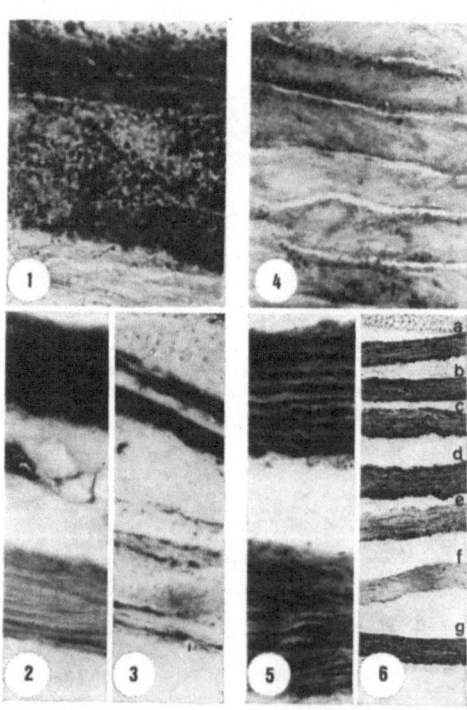

Fig. 1. Area of medial fibrosis in 12 months old SHR, thoracic aorta, × 100000

hydrolyzine indoxyl and naphtyl acetate, acetyl and butyril choline); glycolysis (LDH and GPD); cell respiration; aerobic glucose catabolism and energy production (ICD, SD, MD, G6PD); nucleotides esterolysis (5' Nase, ADPase, ATPases).

2) Ultrastructural changes caracterized by *hyperplasia of cell organelles* in relation to SMC morphogenetic activities: granular endoplasmic reticulum, Golgi apparatus, mitochondria, myofilaments (*Jurukova et al* 1976).

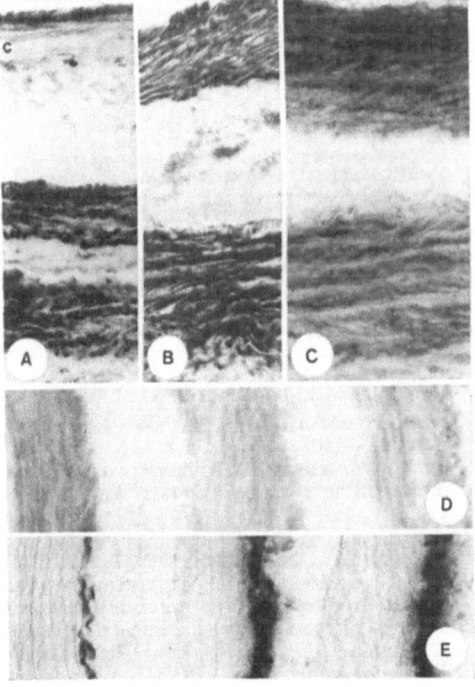

Fig. 2. A. *5'Nucleotidase*, 6 month old rats: increase of activity in SHR abdominal aorta (right); control aorta (left). — B. *5'Nucleotidase*, 12 month-old rats: increase of activity in two SHR thoracic aortas (bottom), control (top). — C. *Glutamate D* — 9 month-old rats: increase of activity in SHR thoracic aorta (bottom) control aorta (top.) — D. *Esterase (naphtyl-acetate)*, 9 month-old rats: decrease of activity in SHR thoracic aorta, medial thickening (bottom); control aorta (top). E. *Butyryl-cholinesterase*, 12 month-old rats; decrease of activity in two SHR thoracic aortas (right), control aorta (left). — F. *Alkaline phosphatase*, 9 month-old rats: increase of activity in vaso vasorum of two SHR thoracic aortas (right); control aorta (left).

3) Activated SMC synthetized the material required for their own growth as well as the matrix scleroproteins: *SMC hypertrophy* and *interstitial connective hyperplasia* became obvious by the 7th month and generalized by the 11th.

4) Presence of a few blood cells and amorphous material within the subendothelial space gave evidence of some *permeability changes.*

5) These structural and metabolic alterations resulted in *media thickening.* Thid was already observed in 18 week-old SHR (21 ± 4% thickness increase compared with control rat of the same age) became more pronounced by the 7th month (35 ± 3%) and worsened by the 12th month (64 ± 2%). Lamellar units were enlarged but their number remained unchanged.

Metabolic and structural arterial changes observed in SHR occur later and are less severe than those observed in experimental hypertension.

In twelve-month-old SHR two new features were found:

1) Generalized decrease of esterases (naphtyl and indoxyl acetate) and cholinesterases (acetyl-butyryl)activities reducing the lipolytic power of arterial wall and compare the metabolic features of SHR aorta with those attributed of aorta in species sensitive to atherosclerosis.

2) Lysosomal acid phosphatase increase. This increase occurs later in SHR aorta than in rat experimental hypertension; it give evidence of the augmentation of SMC lysosomes number, which plays an important role in atherogenesis (*Wolinsky et al* 1973).

In 16—20 month-old SHR severe aortic lesions occured: SMC necrosis and atrophy, cicatricial fibrosis together with foci of decrease or even disappearance of some dehydrogenases and ATPase activities and increase in acid phosphatase activity. Esterases activities decreased still more. Soudanophilic lipids were observed in some intimal esterase-negative foci. Intimal thickening areas were more numerous with regard to the previous stages. Intimal

63

thickness included hypertrophied and metabolically activated cells some of which were catalase-positive and consequently of probable blood origin according to *Adams et al* (1975.).

Conclusions

The aortic changes of SHR developed in three stages:

1) *Latent stage* (1st – 3rd month) during which the only changes were histoenzymatic ones.

2) *Adaptative stage* (3rd – 11th month) with SMC alterations: increased metabolic activities, cell hypertrophy, media thickening.

3) *Degenerative stage* (2d year) with cell necrosis and cicatricial fibrosis.

From these data three factors become apparent which could play a role in atherogenesis, enhancing the risk of lipids accumulation.

Diffuse media thickening which could prolonge the transparietal flow duration.

Interstitial fibrosis acting as a structural barrier.

Decrease in SMC esterases activities, liable to lessen the lipolytic power of arterial wall.

Supported by Grant 77.7.1408 of Delegation générale de la Recherche Scientifique et Technique, France.

REFERENCES

Adams C. W. M., Bayliss O. B., and Turner D. R.: Phagocytes lipid-removal and regression of atheroma. J. Path. 1975, 116, 225—238.

Bretherton K. N., Day A. J., Skinner S. L.: Effect of hypertension on the entry of 125 L-labelled-low density lipoprotein into the aortic intima in normal fed rabbits. Atherosclerosis, 1976, 24, 99—106.

Fuchs U.: Submicroscopy of the arterial vascular wall. Observations in state of hypertension and arteriosclerosis. VEB Gustav Fischer Verlag Jena, 1977.

Gaton E., Benishay D., Wolman M.: Experimentally produced hypertension and aortic acid esterase. Arch. Pathol. Lab. Med. 1976, 100, 527—530.

Hadjiisky P., Renais J., Scebat L.: Etude comparative des enzymes aortiques de rat (athérorésistant) et de lapin (athérosensible). Bull. Assoc. Anat. 1974, 58, 571—584.

Hadjiisky P., Renais J., Scebat L.· Développement etsénescence de l'aorte de rat. Histochimie et histoenzymologie comparative. Atherosclerosis, 1975, 22, 19—38.

Hadjiisky P., Jurukova Z., Renais J., Scebat L.: Artériopathie hypertensive: modifications histométaboliques de l'aorte lors de l'ontogénese postnatale de rat spontanément hypertendu (lignée d'Okamoto-Aoki). Path. Biol. 1976, 24, 401—412.

Hatt P. Y.: Electron microscopic study of arterial lesions in experimental hypertension. p. 196—212, in Hypertension 1972 (Genest J. and Koin E. Eds), Springer 1972.

Jurukova Z., Hadjiisky P., Renais J., Scebat L.: Aortic smooth muscle cells reaction in spontaneous hypertension. Path. Europ. 1976, 11, 105—115.

Lojda Z.: Histochemistry of the vascular wall. p. 364—398. in "Morphologie und Histochemie der Gafäbwand" (Comel M. u. Laszt L. eds), Intern. Symp. Fribourg, 21—22 juin 1965, Karger, ed., Basel, New-york, 1966, vol. I.

Mrhova O., Albrecht I. and Urbanova D.: Vessel wall metabolism in SHR rats in relation to atherosclerosis. Ann. N. Y. Acad. Sci. 1976, 275, 302—310.

Oka M., Angrist A.: Histoenzymatic studies of vessels in hypertensive rats. Lab. Invest. 1967, 16, 25—35.

Okamoto K.: Spontaneous hypertension in rats. Int. Rev. Exp. Pathol. 1969, 1, 227—270.

Postnov J. V.: Histochimie des ferments et taux des électrolytes dans la paroi artérielle au cours de l'hypertension expérimentale et après des agressions (applications) hormonales. Thèse, Acad. Sci. Med., URSS, Moscou, 1969.

Wolinsky H., Goldfischer S., Schiller B., Kasak L. E.: Lysosomes in aortic smooth muscle cells. Effects of hypertension. Am. J. Path. 1973, 73, 727—741.

Woosmann H., Kreher A. C., Nitschkoff S.: Changes of activity of alkaline phosphatase at circulatory system in experimental hypertension of rat. Acta Histochem. 1977, 58/1, 11—16.

Zemplenyi T.: Metabolic intermediates, enzymes and lysosomal activity in aortas of spontaneously hypertensive rats. Atherosclerosis, 1977, 28, 233—246.

P. H., Centre Recherches Cardiologiques — Hôpital Boucicaut, 75730 Paris CEDEX 15, France

ROUND-TABLE DISCUSSION:

"EXPERIMENTAL ATHEROSCLEROSIS. ADAPTATION TO VARIOUS DIETARY REGIMENS"

Chairman: H. C. STARY, L.S.U. School of Medicine, New Orleans, La. U.S.A.

Co-chairman: Z. LOJDA, Research Laboratory of Angiology, Faculty of General Medicine, Charles Univ., Prague, Czechoslovakia.

Participants: C. W. M. ADAMS, Dept. of Pathology, Guy's Hospital Medical School, London U.K.
P. HADJIISKY, Centre of Heart Research, Hospital Boucicout, Paris, France.
W. H. HAUSS, Institute for Medical Information and Biometry, University of Münster, F.R.D.
J. KUNZ, Institute of Pathology, Humboldt University, Berlin, G.D.R.
J. LINDNER, Institute of Pathology, University of Hamburg, F.R.G.
L. VACEK, Laboratory of Pathophysiology of Circulation, IInd Medical Clinic, Brno, Czechoslovakia.
G. WEBER, Institute of Anatomy, Histology and Pathology, Siena, Italy.

The first three speakers centered their attention on the problem of the regression of experimentally induced atheroma in various animals.

ADAMS pointed out conflicting opinions on the regression of human atherosclerosis in connection with dietary restrictions. His experiments on rabbits fed 1% cholesterol diet for 12 weeks from which one group was killed immediately and two other groups received stock diet (one group was fed ad libitum, the other received half of the amount) did not reveal any histological or chemical evidence of a reduction in the atheroma in the restricted group. Surprizingly the blood cholesterol fell more slowly and atheroma appeared worse in animals fed a low caloric diet. These experiments cast some doubts on the postulated anti-atherogenic influence of a severely restricted diet.

WEBER presented results of his investigation using a transmission as well as a scanning electron microscope in vessels of various animal species. His findings favour the regression of atherosclerosis after the withdrawal of the atherogenic diet. The number of smooth muscle cells of plaques was reduced. The cells lost accumulated lipids and endothelial cells regenerated over the residual lesions. He suggested that anti-atherosclerotic dietary and/or drug interventions might aid in the regression of lesions.

STARY described cellular and subcellular events occurring in the regression of lesions in experimental atherosclerosis in Rhesus monkeys. The size of lesions decreased when high serum cholesterol levels dropped. The lesions became progressively less cellular and less rich in lipids. The decrease in the number of

65

macrophage-derived foam cells caused by their death was an early finding. Residual foam cells showed signs of greater activity in the digestion of intracellular lipid droplets. In some animals lesions disappeared completely; however, in animals which had the highest serum cholesterol levels, residual bodies in some intimal smooth muscle cells pointed to incomplete intracellular lipid digestion.

The next three speakers demonstrated the utility of some less commonly used techniques in the study of arterial lesions.

KUNZ presented evidence that endogenous influences could stimulate the atherogenesis in addition to the well known risk factors. Using ^{3}H-thymidine-autoradiography in studies of endothelial plane preparations, a decrease in labelling index with increasing age of animals was found. The endothelium of the aorta near branches of arteries displayed increased labelling indices in comparison to the neighbouring vascular segments. The preferential incidence of atherosclerosis in these areas could be explained by the greater permeability of young endothelium.

HAUSS reported on the usefulness of studies carried out in cultures and sub-cultures of arterial smooth muscle cells and endothelial cells in hypertensive and Streptocotozine diabetic animals and of normal animals. Cell counting and ^{3}H-thymidine-autoradiography was used. LDL and Staphylolysine added to cultures accelerated cell proliferation. On the other hand, acetylosalicylic acid, prednisolone, D-penicillamine, and chloroquine inhibited the proliferation. This treatment can stop the proliferation evoked by LDL and Staphylolysine.

VACEK demonstrated that, in rats with hyperlipidemia and various types of experimental hypertension, no correlation was found either with the adhesivity and aggregabilty of thrombocytes or with the level of serum lipids or lipoproteins in vitro. The same results were obtained on a group of healthy persons and on a group of patients sufferring ischemic heart disease. He arrived at the conclusion that the assessment of thrombocytic functions in vitro does not reflect the real relationship between serum lipids and blood coagulation to atherosclerosis.

The last section was devoted mainly to enzymes.

LINDNER presented results of his extensive biochemical and radiochemical investigations on the regression of the connective tissue components in atherosclerosis. The regression of lesions in experimental atherosclerosis is possible. The turnover rates and content of vascular smooth muscle cells, which areresponsible for the turnover of the ground substance components, decrease with the progress of experimental atherosclerosis. The synthesis of elastin, collagen and glycosaminoglycans which is increased in early stages decreases with the progression of the lesions as well. This concerns also the activities of marker enzymes of the synthesis and breakdown of glycosaminoglycans and collagen (particularly sulphotransferases and protocollagen-proline hydroxylase, β-glucuronidase, specific collagen protease and peptidase, and aminopeptidase). Finally a decrease of proteoglycans, glycosaminoglycans and elastin accompanied by an increase of collagen is found.

Concerning the human atherosclerosis lipid plaques can regress. A decrease of the lipid content of atherosclerotic plaques is also possible. Although exact data particularly on collagen degrading enzymes and enzymes catalyzing the breakdown of proteoglycans and glycosaminoglycans are missing the regression of atherosclerotic lesions seems to be possible. However, further detailed investigation is necessary to clear up this very important problem.

LOJDA pointed out the necessity of studying enzymes biochemically as well as histochemically. He demonstrated in many examples from the field of experimental atherosclerosis the usefulness of enzyme studies from several viewpoints: 1) Enzymes as metabolism markers (necessity of studying as many enzymes as possible). 2) Enzymes as indicators of the susceptibilty or resistence of the arterial wall to atherosclerosis (mainly Krebs cycle enzymes, lysosomal enzymes, alkaline phosphatase). 3) Enzymes as injury markers (chiefly SDH and acid phosphatase). 4) Enzymes as markers of the capillary endothelium for the depiction of vasa vasorum (combined alkaline and DAP IV reaction in the same section). 5) Enzymes as tracers of the permeabilty of the vascular wall (e.g. horse-raddish peroxidase, shawing clearly the necessity of the consideration of both ways: transintimal and transadvential via vasa vasorum). The study of enzymes is very useful in atherogenesis and should also be exploited in relation to the regression of atherosclerotic lesions. Evidence was presented for the possibility of the degradation of lipids and glycosaminoglycans in plaques. However, little is known about the protein catabolism in the vascular wall.

HADJIISKY reported on the usefulness of enzyme histochemical methods (about 20 enzymes were studied) for assessment of the behaviour of smooth muscle cells in the aortae of cholesterol-choline-thiouracil-fed rats oven 7 months (progressive stages) and after removal of the atherogenic diet (regressive stages). Aortic lipoidosis developed in all animals. The muscle cell reaction to the prefence of lipids was very poor: only a progressive decrease of 5.-nucleotidase, acid esterase and cholinesterase was observed. The restitution of activities was observed within 5 months after the removal of the atherogenic diet. However, sudanophilic lipids were present between muscle cells even after 2 years, although the lipolytic activity of the muscle cells was completely restituted.

Conclusions

Due to a lack of time the discussion could not cover all aspects of the very complex problem of experimental atherosclerosis. Most attention from the members of the round-table was devoted to questions concerning permeability, cell proliferation and particularly regression of atherosclerotic lesions. In connection with the regression of lesions, it is necessary to consider possible species differences. The evidence presented concerning the regression of plaques composed of foam cells which are enzymatically very active. However, no evidence was presented that could document the regression of complicated lesions such as occur in human atherosclerosis.

From the participation of the audience in the discussion, the contribution of U. Fuchs (Department of Pathology, Leipzig, DDR) is worth mentioning. He pointed out the increased permeability of the arterial wall after immunologic injury (repeated injections of heterologous proteins) which, in his experiments with rabbits, was particularly high in coronary arteries and could be enhanced even more when some mediators from leucocytes and thrombocytes were injected. It is known that immunologic injury leads to a fibromuscular thickenning of the intima. Such sites may continue to have an increased avidity for lipids for many weeks. The increased permeability of coronary arteries in this situation may explain the frequent occurrence of atherosclerotic changes in these vessels.

THROMBOGENESIS

THE EFFECT OF A NEW INHIBITOR OF PLATELET AGGREGATION (K 3920) ON SOME PLATELET FUNCTIONS IN PATIENTS WITH VASCULAR DISEASES

G. LEONE, G. CORVI, A. DE CRESCENZO, R. LANDOLFI
and L. PARRINELLO

*Department of Internal Medicine, Catholic University of Rome
and Carlo Erba Research Institute, Milan, Italy*

Platelets are considered important in the thrombotic and microembolic complications of atherosclerosis and perhaps also play a role in atherogenesis.

Antiggregating agents have been proposed to prevent thrombus formation; a beneficial therepeutic effect has been reported in a controlled clinical trial with sulfinpyrazone in the prevention of cardiac death after myocardial infarction and administration of dipyridamole and acetylsalicylate improves the reduced mean platelet survival time in coronary atherosclerosis (*Ritchie et al.* 1977).

Increased platelet reactivity has been reported in vasculopathic patients and may be important in the development of thrombotic complications (*Leone et al.* 1974).

The purpose of our investigation was to assess the action of a new antiaggregating agent, 2- [p- (1-oxo-isoindolinyl) phenyl] butyric acid (K 3920 Carlo Erba) (Fig. 1) on the platelet function of vasculopathic subjects.

In vitro K 3920 strongly inhibits platelet aggregation induced by ADP and collagen; the activity is similar to that of indomethacin and may be correlated to thromboxane synthesis inhibition.

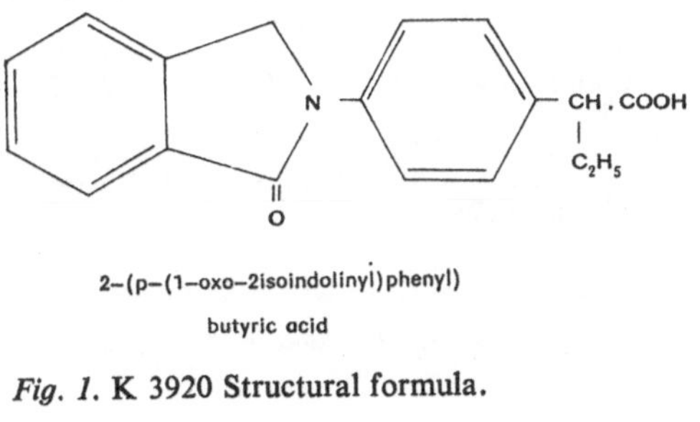

Results and conclusions

K 3920 exhibited antiaggregating activity in subjects with normal and increased platelet aggregability (Fig. 2). The effect was more marked on collagen induced aggregation, particularly on the slope and % maximum aggregation which in every

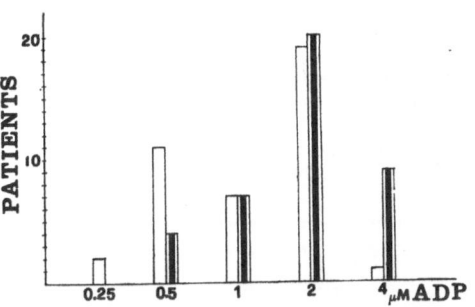

Fig. 2. Sensitivity to ADP (threshold dose) before and after (■■) administration of K 3920.

case differed significantly or higly significantly from basal values.

The compound had maximal effect between 2 and 4 h, normally wearing off 12 h after administration (Fig. 3).

A pharmacological effect was achieved with a/100 mg B.I.D. dose and was not greater with the larger dose.

No significant change was found in other platelet functions, such as platelet adhesiveness, PF 3 and PF 4 release, or in other parameters studied: platelet count, prothrombin time, fibrinogen and thromboelastogram.

2−(p−(1−oxo−2isoindolinyl)phenyl)

butyric acid

Fig. 1. K 3920 Structural formula.

No allergy or other drug related complication was observed. In conclusion, K 3920 has been shown to be suitable for clinical use for its effectiveness on platelet aggregation and its tolerance.

Further studies must be performed in order to determine whether it has a clinical effect in the prevention of arterial thromboembolism.

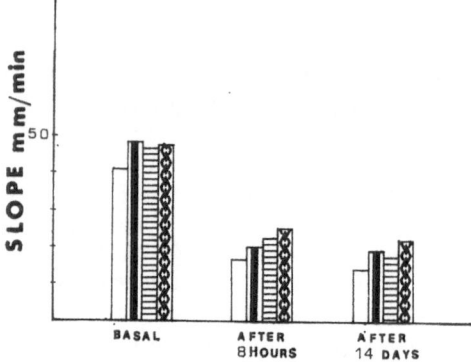

Fig. 3. Effect of administration of K 3920 on collagen induced aggregation (slope) at various times; first and third column: normo and hyperaggregating patients treated with the 100 mg B. I. D. dose; second and fourth column: normo and hyperaggregating patients treated with the 200 mg B.I.D. dose.

Patients and methods

The study was conducted on 40 patients with vascular diseases of various types (myocardiosclerosis, diabetes mellitus, coronary artery disease, peripheral arterial disease).

Platelet aggregation was studied using Born's method (*Born* 1962). ADP at final concentrations of 4, 2, 1, 0.5, 0.25 μM, and collagen (Horm) 4 μg/ml were used for platelet aggregation.

ADP induced platelet aggregation was quantified by the minimal dose of ADP required for irreversible aggregation (threshold dose); collagen induced platelet aggregation was quantified by lag phase, velocity (slope) and maximal change of optical density.

Platelet factor 3 was measured according to the method of Spaet and Cintron (*Spaet et al.* 1975). Platelet factor 4 was assayed as described by *Harada and Zucker* (1966). Platelet adhesiveness was measured according to *Salzmann*.

Before the study, the threshold dose of ADP was established in all subjects and those for whom it was greater than 1 μM were considered normoaggregating (Group A); patients with values of 1 μM or less were considered hyperaggregating (Group B). Half the patients in each group received K 3920 100 mg B.I.D. (1 tablet in the morning and 1 in the evening) and the other half 200 mg B.I.D. (2 tablets in the morning and 2 in the evening) for 14 days, following a completely randomized design in open conditions.

At various times the effect on ADP and collagen induced platelet aggregation was determined *in vitro*. Before and at the end of treatment the following examinations were made: platelet adhesiveness, prothrombin time, platelet count, blood fibrinogen, thromboelastogram, bioavailability of PF 3 and release of PF 4.

REFERENCES

Anturane Reinfarction Trial (1978): Sulfinpyrazone in the prevention of cardiac death after myocardial infarction. N. Engl. J. Med. 298: 289—295.

Born, G. V. R. (1962): Aggregation of blood platelets by adenosine diphosphate and its reversal. Nature, 194: 927—929.

Harada, K. Zucker, M. B. (1966): Simultaneous development of platelet factor 4 activity and release of C^{14} Serotonin. Thromb. Diath. Haemorrh., 15: 413—41.

Leone, G., Bizzi, B., Accorrà, F., Boni, P. (1974): Functional aspects of platelets in diabetes mellitus. In "Platelet aggregation and drugs"

ed. by Caprino and Rossi. Academic Press New York 49—61.

Ritchie, J. L., Harker, L. A. (1977): Platelet and fibrinogen survival in coronary atherosclerosis. Response to medical and surgical therapy. Am. J. Card. 39: 595—597.

Salzman, E. V. (1963): Measurement of platelet adhesiveness: a simple in vitro technique demonstrating an abnormality in Von Willebrand's disease. J. Lab. Clin. Med., 62: 724 to 735.

Spaet, T. H., Cintron, J. (1975): Studies on platelet factor 3 availability. Br. J. Haematol. 11: 269—275.

G. L., Dept. of Internal Medicine, Catholic University of Rome, Italy

PATHOGENETIC ROLE OF HUMORAL AGENTS RELEASED BY PLATELET AGGREGATION IN THE GENESIS OF TRANSIENT ISCHEMIC ATTACKS

T. ASANO, A. TAMURA, CH. OCHIAI and K. SANO

Department of Neurosurgery, Hospital of Tokyo University and Takeo Takahashi and Masahiko Kobayashi, Japan Atherosclerosis Research Institute, Tokyo, Japan

It has recently been shown that there is a close relationship between the occurrence of strokes and the increased aggregation ability of platelets. It has been demonstrated in animal experiments that those agents which induce platelet agrregation, such as sodium arachidonate (*Furlow et al.,* 1974) and ADP (*Heuser et al.,* 1976), cause irreversible cerebral lesions by obliteration of capillary networks when they were injected into the internal carotid artery. These clinical and experimental data indicate that platelet aggregation plays a major role in the stroke pathogenesis. (*Barnett.,* 1976).

Platelets release several vasoactive substances such as serotonin, norepinephrine and histamine when they aggregate (*Weiss,* 1975). Recent discovery of tromboxane A_2 (TXA_2) and prostaglandin I_2 (PGI_2), together with the hypothesis of their antagonistic actions on the vessel wall and platelets, (*Moncada et al.,* 1976) indicates that these prostaglandin derivatives generated by platelet aggregation are also involved in the genesis of strokes. Therefore, it seemed relevant to study the effect of these humoral agents released by platelet aggregation on the cerebral circulation and function in animal experiments and to distinguish their role from the mechanical, occlusive effect due to formation of platelet plugs in the vessel lumina.

The platelets prepared from the platelet-rich plasma obtained from fresh rabbit arterial blood were suspended in a calcium-free Krebs solution. The platelets were aggregated by addition of thrombin and the released substances were immediately injected into the internal carotid artery of rabbits while filtering off the elements formed.

In preliminary in vitro experiments, it was confirmed that TXA was liberated in this platelet preparation. (Fig. 1) The cortical CBF (coCBF), EEG and systemic arterial pressure were continuously monitored under artifical ventilation. (Fig. 2) In a total of 29 rabbits, the coCBF decreased markedly for 10−20 minutes following

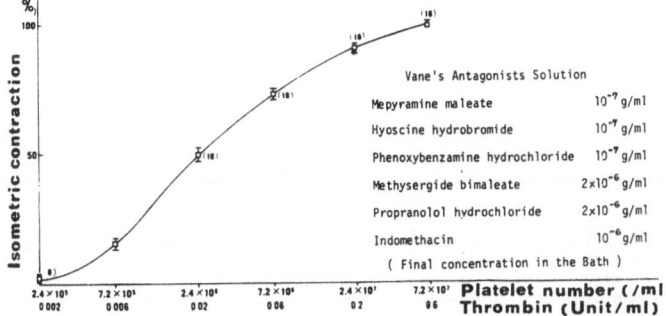

Fig. 1. This dose-response curve was obtained in the presence of Vane's antagonists solution as shown in the right column.

73

injections, accompanied by simultaneous supression of EEG in seven. (Fig. 3-A) In 9 rabbits, the response of coCBF was biphasic, i.e., the initial brief ischemia was followed by the intense hyperemia lasting about 15 minutes. (Fig. 3-B) In the remaining 13 rabbits, only hyperemic responses were oberved without any significanto changes in EEG (Fig. 3-C). All the rabbits were sacrificed 30 minutes after the injections.

In the histological examinations, the intracapillary clot or platelet thrombi were only rarely found in all the specimens. The observed ischemic response of the cerebral hemisphere to the intracarotid injection of the suspension medium of aggregated platelets in the present study is consistent with the current concept that platelet agrregation plays a major role in the genesis of TIAs.

The frequent occurrence of hyperemic responses in the present study, however, indicates that cerebral vasodilation is brought about by some unknown substance. As it is known that the precursors of TXA_2, i.e., the prostaglandin endoperoxides, are liberated in the suspension medium of aggregated platelets, the conversion of these endoperoxides to

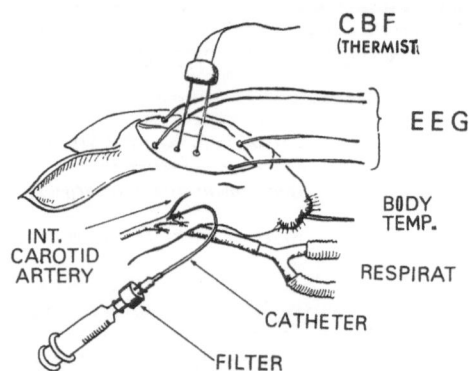

Fig. 2. The experimental set-up is shown. To measure the cortical blood flow in the side of injection, a double-needle type thermocouple (Shincorder) was used.

prostacyclin (PGI_2) in the cerebral vessel wall seems to be a mechanism which may be responsible for the observed hyperemic response.

The results of the present study revealed the complexity of CBF responses to intracarotid injection of humoral agents released by platelet aggregation. The presence of hyperemic responses seems to indicate that there is a protective mechanism in the cerebral vessels preventing thrombo-embolic disorders.

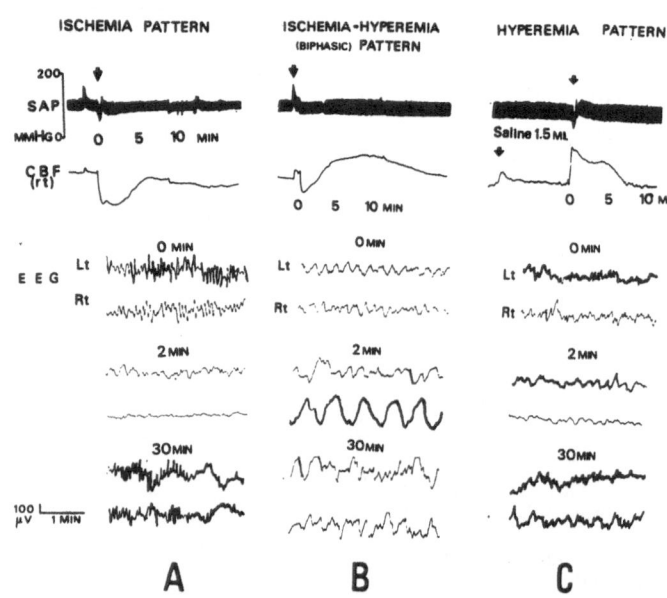

Fig. 3. The three patterns of CBF response to the intracarotid injection of the suspension medium of aggregated platelets (arrows) are shown with their representative EEG changes.

Antiplatelet drugs such as aspirin, which are frequently used at present for prevention of TIAs, are known to inhibit all the synthetic pathways of prostaglandins starting from the platelet membrane and hence will also inhibit the naturally occurring protective mechanism in the prostaglandin system. The clinical importance of further investigation of the mechanism of TIAs and development more specific drugs than aspirin therefore follow from the present study.

REFERENCES

Barnett, J. J. M. (1976): Pathogenesis of transient ischemic attacks. in Cerebrovascular Diseases. Scheinberg P. (ed) Raven Press, New York, 1—22.

Furlow T. W., Bass N. H. (1974): Stroke in rats produced by carotid injection of sodium arachidonate. Science 187, 658—660.

Heuser D., Fieshi C., Volante F. (1976): Platelet emboli and focal cerebral ischemia. An experimental study on the circulatory and metabolic effects on intracarotid infusion of ADP and arachidonic acid in rabbits. in The Cerebral Vessel Wall. Cervos-Navarro (ed). Raven Press. New York: 149—156.

Moncada S., Gryglewski R., Bunting S. (1976): An enzyme isolated from arteries transforms prostaglandin endoperoxides to an unstable substance that inhibits platelet aggregation. Nature 263, 663—665.

Weiss H. J. (1975): Platelet physiology and abnormalities of platelet function. Acta physiol. Scand. 98, 285—294.

T. A., Dept. of Neurosurgery, Tokyo University, Hongo, Bunkyo-ku, Tokyo, Japan

PLATELET HYPOAGGREGABILITY IN SPONTANEOUSLY HYPERTENSIVE RATS RELATED TO THROMBOGENESIS

N. MASHIMO, F. NUMANO, H. MAEZAWA, O. MATSUBARA,
T. MOTOMIYA and H. YAMAZAKI

Third Department of Internal Medicine and Department of Pathology,
Tokyo Medical and Dental University School of Medicine,
Division of Cardiovascular Research, Tokyo Metropolitan Institute
of Medical Science, Tokyo, Japan

Introduction

It is well known that the function of platelets and especially their aggregability are two of the most important factors in thrombogenesis. We have reported an increase in platelet aggregability in thromboembolic diseases (*Yamazaki*, 1975). ADP is known to produce platelet aggregations. Consequently we experimentally produced pulmonary thromboembolism by administering intravenous injections of ADP or collagen, which induce platelet aggregation *in vivo*. (*Kobayashi*, 1973, 1974, 1075). We also reported that pretreatment with antiplatelet drugs such as aspirin and pyridinolcarbamate inhibited the appearence of pulmonary thromboembolism using this animal model (*Kobayashi*, 1973, 1974). In this situation, platelet aggregability may play a key role in thrombogenesis.

A strain of spontaneously hypertensive rats (SHR) was developed by Okamoto and Aoki in 1963 nad has proven to be an excellent experimental animal model for studies on hypertension. Hypertension is one of the greatest factors in thrombotic diseases, yet thrombogenic tendencies in SHR have not been extensively investigated. We used SHR in our experimental model on thrombogenesis and normal Wistar rats as a control.

Materials and methods

30 male SHRs (300 g) and 30 normal male Wistar rats (500 g) were used. Their ages were 20—30 weeks old. SHRs were given a 1% NaCl solution as drinking water over a period of 10 weeks and their blood pressure was higher than that in the control during the experimental period.

1) *In vitro* experiment: A titrated blood sample was taken from carotid cannula of rats in both groups anesthetized by pentbarbital intraperitoneally. Platelet rich plasma (PRP) and platelet poor plasma (PPP) were produced in the normal manner. PRP was diluted nito 30, 000/μl of platelet count with its PPP. Platelet count was measured by a Coulter Counter ZBI. Platelet volume distribution was observed by a Coulter Particle Channelizer. Platelet aggregability induced by ADP (Sigma) 100 μM, 10 μM and 3 μM in final concentration was observed and recorded with a Sienco aggregometer. Platelet ADP and ATP contents were measured by the firefly luciferase method using an ATP photometer (SAI) (*Holmsen*, 1972).

2) *In vivo* experiment: This model was initially described by Kobayashi and Didisheim. Control Wistar rats and SHRs were anesthetized as stated above. They were tracheotomised and cannulated to allow breathing of room air. Two catheters were inserted into the carotid artery and the jugular vein to measure arterial pressure and central venous pressure. Electrocardiogram and respiration were recorded simultaneously. ADP 1 mg/kg was injected rapidly into the jugular vein. Blood samples were taken from the carotid catheter before and after the injection. Platelet count, platelet volume distribution and platelet ADP and ATP contents were measured as stated above. The rat lungs were dissected 1 min after the injection and were studied histologically.

Results

1) Platelet function in SHR and in the control Wistar rat. There wore no significant differences between the two groups in platelet count, platelet volume and platelet ADP and ATP contents. Platelet aggregability, however, was less extensive in SHR (Fig. 1).

2) Changes in platelet count and car-

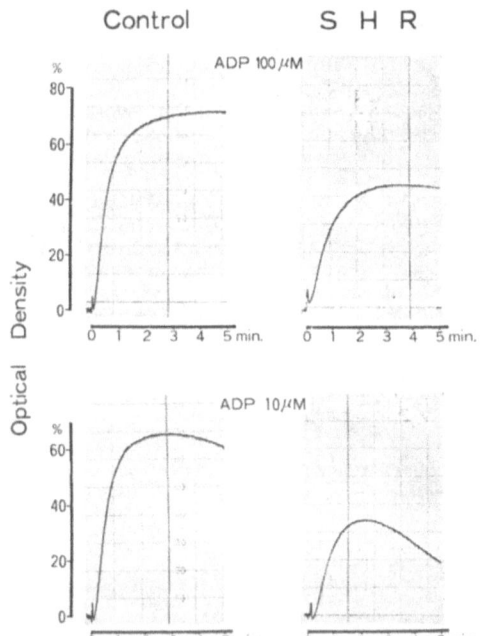

Control   S H R

Fig. 1. Platelet aggregation curves induced by 100 μM and 10 μM of ADP.

diopulmonary function after ADP injection.

In the control, a fall in heart rate and respiratory rate, arterial blood pressure and a rise in central venous pressure were observed 30 sec after the injection and subsided after 3 min. These changes were noted as platelet count decreased. In SHR, however, the changes observed in the control were significantly less marked. Apnea and arrhythmia were observed in all control rats. They were not always seen in SHRs. The duration time of arrhythmia was 34.5 ± 14.9 sec. in the control: 12.4 ± 5.3 sec. in SHR (p < < 0.01). That of apnea was 9.8 ± 14.0 sec. in the control and 1.1 ± 1.4 sec. in SHR (p < 0.01).

3) The changes in platelet ADP and ATP contents.

Platelet ADP and ATP contents were gradually decreased in both groups after the injection. ADP contents in the control significantly decreased to 1.1 ± 0.3 μmoles significantly decreased to 1.1 ± 0.3 μmoles/ $/10^{11}$ pl. at 30 min. in comparison with 1.8 ± 0.6 μmoles/10^{11} pl. in SHR.

4) Rat Lung Histology.

Histological examination revealed thrombi in most of the control pulmonary microvasculature. They were seen less in SHRs.

Conclusions

In this study, intravenous ADP-induced pulmonary thromboembolism, associated with thrombocytopenia and cardiopulmonary disorders, seen in the control, was significantly less severe in SHR. There were no differences in platelet count, platelet volume and platelet ADP and ATP contents between the two groups. However, platelet aggregability induced by ADP was significantly less extensive in SHR. Nagaoka et al. (1971) have already reported platelet hypoaggregability in aged SHR. Our observation was almost indentical with theirs. It is likely that the appearance of pulmonary platelet thrombi induced by intravenous ADP injection is related to platelet reactivities to ADP. Decrease in platelet ADP content after ADP injection was not considerable in the SHR. This change may be related to *in vitro* platelet hypoaggregability in the SHR. It suggests that platelet release response to ADP is far weaker in the SHR. We also compared platelet release phenomenon using ^{14}C-labeled serotonin in the control and in SHR, and a decrease in serotonin release was observed in SHR. This lower platelet reactivity might be a result of platelet exhaustion under hypertensive stress and/or genetic factors. Further investigation is required.

REFERENCES

Okamoto, K., Aoki, K. (1963): Development of a strain of spontaneously hypertensive rats. Jap. Circul. J. 27, 282—293.

Holmsen, H., Storm, E., Day, J. (1972): Determination of ATP and ADP in blood platelets. Anal. Biochem. 46, 489—501.

Kobayashi, I., Didisheim, P. (1973): Systemic effects of ADP-induced platelet aggregation and their modification by aspirin and by pyridinolcarbamate. Thromb. Diathes. haemorrh. 30, 178—190.

Kobayashi, I., Mashimo, N., Herther, K. K., Didisheim, P. (1974): Systemic effects of collagen-induced platelet aggregation and their modification by aspirin and by pyridinolcar-bamate. Thromb. Diathes. haemorrh. suppl. 60, 389—398.

Kobayashi, I., Yamazaki, H., Didisheim p. (1975) Cardiopulmonary dysfunctions caused by ADP-induced platelet aggregation. Jap. Circul. J. 675—682.

Nagaoka, A., Sudo, K., Orita, S., Kikuchi, K., Yoshitomo, A. (1971): Hematological studies on the spontaneously hypertensive rats with special refference to the development of thrombosis. Jap. Circul. J. 35, 1379—1390.

Yamazaki, H., Takahashi, T., Sano, T. (1975): Hyperaggregability of platelets in thromboembolic disorders. Thromb. Diathes. haemorrh. 34, 94—105.

N. M., 3rd Dept of Int. Med., Tokyo Medical and Dental University School of Med. Yushima, Bunkyo-ku, Tokyo, 113, Japan.

PLATELET ADHESION, ON THE INVOLVEMENT OF GLYCOCALICIN, AN EASILY SOLUBLE PLATELET MEMBRANE GLYCOPROTEIN IN THE INTERACTION BETWEEN PLATELETS AND THE FACTOR VIII-RELATED PROTEIN

I. HAGEN and N. O. SOLUM

Institute for Thrombosis Research, University of Oslo, Oslo, Norway

Introduction

The rapid adhesion of platelets to the damaged vessel wall is believed to be the first event in wound healing. New insight into the mechanism of adhesion has been gained during the last few years through the studies of von Willebrand's disease, the Bernard-Soulier syndrome and certain *in vitro* experiments on normal platelets. In the two aforementioned bleeding disorders, the platelet adhesion is impaired, in the former case because of a reduced concentration of the necessary plasma factor (*Weiss et al.* 1973) and in the latter because of a platelet membrane defect (*Nurden and Caen*, 1975). The plasma factor necessary is probably identical to factor VIII-related protein, and adhesion and interaction between the factor VIII-related protein and a receptor on the platelet surface may take place.

Platelet agglutination induced by factor VIII-related protein and the adhesion of platelets to subendothelial tissue are thought to share a common step, namely the binding of factor VIII-related protein to the platelet surface. In the present study, we examined whether the presence of glycocalicin on the platelet surface is a prerequisite for the ability of platelets to agglutinate with factor VIII-related protein.

Materials and methods

The preparation of platelets, platelet ghosts and the agglutination procedure have already been described (*Solum et al.* 1977). Surface labeling of exposed platelet membrane proteins was perfomed by lactoperoxidase-catalyzed (^{125}I) iodination. The proteins were separated by SDS polyacrylamide gel electrophoresis and stained with Coomassie brilliant blue.

Results and discussion

In order to induce agglutination, the factor VIII-related protein must in some way interact with the platelet membrane. In Table I are summarized the results of some experiments performed on modified, normal platelets or platelet ghosts which indicate a correlation between the presence of glycocalicin on the platelet surface and the ability of the platelets to agglutinate with factor VIII-related protein. Removal

Table I. Experiments performed on normal platelets which indicate the role of glycocalicin in the factor VIII-induced agglutination.

1. Storage in Tris-buffered saline 2. Freezing and thawing in Tris-buffered saline 3. Extraction with 3 M KCl	} Elution of glycocalicin; and loss of teh ability to agglutinate with factor VIII.
4. Freezing and thawing in EDTA buffer	No elution of glycocalicin; platelets agglutinate.
5. Partial proteolysis	Destruction of glycocalicin; agglutinate poorly (Jenkins et al. 1976).
6. Incubation with purified glycocalicin	Inhibition of agglutination (Okumura and Jamieson, 1976).

of glycocalicin from the surface membrane of normal platelets is attained by storage in Tris-buffered saline solution, by freezing and thawing in Tris-buffered saline solution or by extraction with 3M KCl. These suspensions of platelets do not agglutinate with factor VIII-related protein. The elution of glycocalicin is prevented by the presence of EDTA and then the platelets retain their ability to agglutinate. Further, partial proteolysis of platelets leads to destruction of glycocalicin (GP I) (*Jenkins et al.* (1976) and incubation of platelets with purified glycocalicin inhibits agglutination (*Okumura and Jamieson,* 1076). However, in the aforementioned situations, the elution or destruction of glycocalicin may not be the only modification of the platelet surface. In order to obtain further information about the protein(s) involved in the interaction between platelets and factor VIII-related protein, platelets from

patients with the Bernard-Soulier syndrome were studied. As demonstrated in Fig. 1, these platelets showed a normal distribution of proteins in SDS polyacrylamide gel electrophoresis, as compared to normal platelets. The surface structure as examined

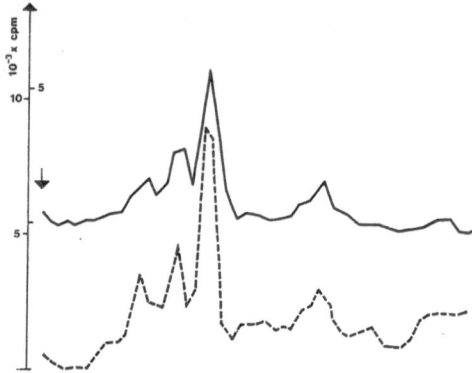

Fig. 2. Distribution of radioactive 125I after SDS polyacrylamide gel electrophoresis of reduced samples of normal platelets (———) and platelets from patients with Bernard-Soulier syndrome (- - - - -).

by the distribution of radioactive iodine after gel electrophoresis was also the same as in normal platelets (Fig. 2). In a previous work it was shown that glycocalicin is absent in platelets from Bernard-Soulier patients. It therefore seems that the absence of glycocalicin from these platelets represent a more specific abnormality than previously recognized (*Jenkins et al.* 1976) and this further emphasizes a possible role for this glycoprotein in platelet adhesion.

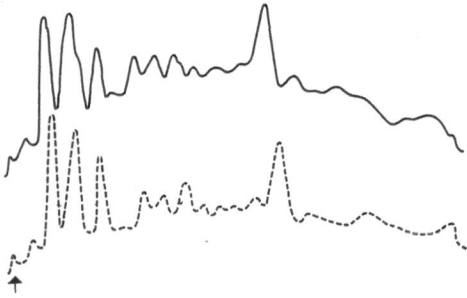

Fig. 1. Distribution of protein after SDS polyacrylamide gel electrophoresis of reduced samples of normal platelets (———) and platelets from patients with Bernard-Soulier syndrome (- - - - -).

REFERENCES

Jenkins, C. S. P., Phillips, D. R., Clemetson, K. J., Meyer, D., Larrieu, M.-J. and Luscher, E. F. (1976): Platelet membrane glycoproteins implicated in ristocetin-induced aggregation. J. Clin. Invest. 57, 112—124.

Nurden, A. T. and Caen, J. P. (1975): Specific roles for platelet surface glycoproteins in platelet function. Nature 255, 720—722.

Okumura, T. and Jamieson, G. A. (1976): Platelet glycocalicin: A single receptor for

platelet aggregation induced by thrombin or ristocetin. Thromb. Res. 8, 701—706.

Solum, N. O., Hagen, I. and Peterka, M. (1977): Human platelet glycoproteins. Thromb Res. 10, 71—82.

Weiss, H. J., Rogers, J., and Brand, H. (1973): Defective ristocetin-induced aggregation in von Willebrand's disease, and its correction by factor VIII. J. Clin. Invest. 52, 2697—2707.

I. H., Inst. for Thrombosis Research, University of Oslo, Rikshospitalet, Oslo 1, Norway.

PLATELET REGENERATION TIME IN CARDIOVASCULAR PATIENTS

R. RONCUCCI, R. DEPERON, J. DESTAILLEUR, J. DOUMONT,
G. LAMBELIN, J. LANSEN, F. VAN STALLE, R. VERHAEGHE

*Continental Pharma, Research Laboratories, Brussels, Institut Médico-Chirurgical
d'Anderlecht, Brussels, Laboratory of Blood coagulation, Medical Research
Dept., University of Leuven, Leuven, Belgium*

Introduction

The determination of platelet survival time (PST) has been widely used for the assessment of drugs affecting platelet function; more recently, this test has also gained interest for its potential use as an early detection method for increased tendency to thromboembolism (*Genton et al.*, 1977). In most of the techniques proposed for the assessment of PST, platelets are labelled with radioisotopes and their disappearance rate from the circulation is assessed by radioactive measurements; the well-known ^{51}Cr-technique is certainly the most popular method (*Aster*, 1971). However a simple, less invasive and non-radioactive technique for the determination of platelet turnover was introduced in 1975 by Stuart et al. This new method is based upon the fact that acetylsalicylic acid (ASA) irreversibly inhibits *in vivo* platelet cyclooxygenase and thus impairs the production of malondialdehyde (MDA) — a biodegradation product of the endoperoxides — when thrombocytes are challenged *ex vivo* with the appropriate aggregation inducers. A single ingestion of 500 mg of ASA has definite inhibitory effect on platelet MDA production which lasts for the life-span of the platelets that have been in contact with the drug. In contrast, MDA production in new platelets injected into the circulation after elimination of ASA from the body is not impaired and therefore daily determinations of MDA before and after one single intake of ASA, make possible the measurement of platelet turnover or, rather platelet regeneration time (PBT).

In order to speed up MDA determinations by the thiobarbituric acid method (*Stuart et al.*, 1975), an appropriate manifold was devised for the adaptation of this assay procedure to an autoanalyzer system (*Roncucci et al.*, 1977).

Using this semi-automated technique, the usefulness of PRT determination was assessed in normal subjects and in patients with an increased thromboembolic tendency; in some cases direct comparison with the ^{51}Cr-technique was carried out.

Methods

Platelet-rich-plasma (PRP) was prepared in the usual manner from citrated whole blood. Platelets were centrifuged and then resuspended in phosphate buffer pH 7.4. Platelet suspensions obtained by this way were incubated with either 1 mN N-ethylmaleimide (NEM) or 0.64 mM arachidonic acid (AA). Platelets were sonicated and debris eliminated by filtration through Seraclear filters. Assessment of MDA by the thiobarbituric acid method using the automated autoanalyzer technique was carried out either immediately or on samples kept at 4 °C. For the calculation of platelet regeneration half-time (PRT - t/2), MDA production in post-ASA samples was expressed as percent inhibition of the pre-ASA value and these data were analyzed with both linear and exponential regression obtained using an appropriate computer program. The best value of PRT t/2 was choosen according to the lowest values of the residual sum of the squares calculated for each type of regression. 5/Cr-PST determinations were achieved according to the technique described by *Aster* (1971). PST t/2 values were obtained using the same calculation methods.

Results

Figure 1 shows the data obtained so far investigating PRT in 9 healthy volunteers (age 22 – 30; 5 males and 4 females); in 15

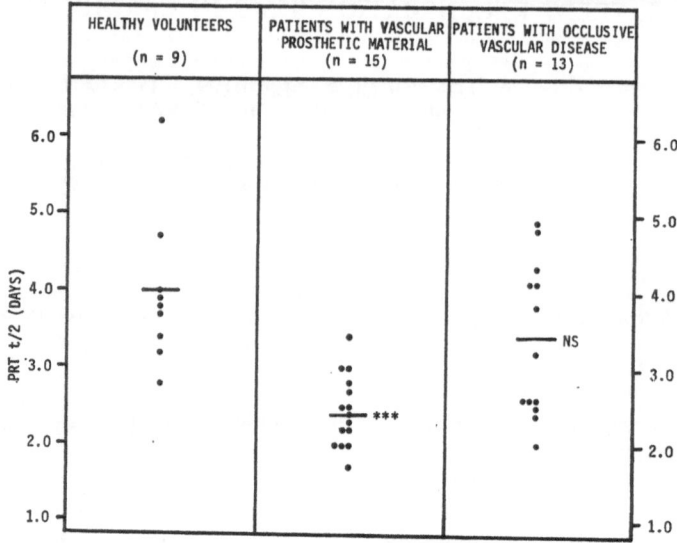

Fig. 1. Platelet regeneration half-time (PRT t/2) in healthy volunteers, patients with vascular prosthetic material and patients-with occlusive vascular disease.

*** Significantly different from the healthy volunteer group (p < .001).
NS Not significantly different from the healthy volunteer group (p > .05).

patients with vascular prosthetic material (age 40–72; 8 males and 7 females) and in 13 patients with occlusive vascular disease (age 58–82; all males). In the group of healthy volunteers (considered here as the control group) the return to the pre-ASA MDA levels was completed within 7 to 8 days and the mean PRT t/2 was found to be 4.0 ± 0.3 days. In the group of patients with vascular prosthetic material (mainly heart valves) the mean PRT t/2 was significantly reduced (2.4 ± 0.1 days) compared to the control group ($p < 001$). In patients with occlusive vascular disease, the mean PRT t/2 was also shorter but the difference was not statistically significant (3.4 ± 0.3 days; $p < .05$). However, six out of these 13 patients exhibited a shortened PRT t/2 value compared to that observed in patients with vascular prosthetic material.

In order to assess the reproducibility of PRT determinations, duplicate measurements were performed on 5 patients within a three week to five month interval. No significant differences between the two sets of data were observed (Table Ia). On the other hand, it should be noted that the induction of platelet aggregation by NEM as well as by AA leads to comparable PRT t/2 values (Table 1b).

Finally, in eight subjects PST was determined concomitantly to PRT. Nearly identical results were obtained in seven of them (Table II). In one subject, however, PRT t/2 was clearly abnormal while PST t/2 was normal.

Conclusions

Platelet malondialdehyde (MDA) production assessed *ex vivo* before and

Table Ia. Duplicate determinations of PRT t/2 (days).

Subject	1	2	3	4	5
Initial PRT t/2	3.7	3.4	2.7	2.3	2.0
Repeat PRT t/2	3.9	3.5	2.8	2.1	2.8

Table Ib. Comparison of PRT determined using either N-ethylmaleimide (NEM) or arachidonic acid (AA) as platelet aggregation inducers.

Subject PRT t/2 (days)	1	2	3	4	5	6
NEM (1 mM)	3.0	2.2	4.1	4.9	2.4	4.3
AA (0.64 mM)	3.2	2.4	3.6	3.6	2.8	4.0

Table II. Simultaneous determinations of PRT t/2 and PST t/2 (days).

Subject	1	2	3	4	5	6	7	8
PRT t/2	3.8	3.9	3.4	1.7	2.2	2.0	2.0	3.8
PST t/2	3.5	4.1	4.2	0.8	1.7	2.0	4.4	3.1

repeatly after one single oral intake of acetylsalicylic acid is a reliable method for the determination of what can be called platelet regeneration time (PRT). The reproducibility of the method seems to be quite acceptable. Compared to the widely used ^{51}Cr-method, PRT determinations do not involve radioactive hazards and are less invasive. Because of these factors, the platelet regeneration time technique seems to be a promising method for the pharmacological assessment of drugs affecting platelet turnover. The data reported in this paper seem to indicate that PRT t/2 is dramatically reduced in cardiovascular patients and especially in those with vascular prosthetic material.

REFERENCES

Aster, R. H. (1971): Factors affecting the kinetics of isotopically labeled platelets. in: Platelets kinetics (Ee. J. M. Paulus) North Holland Publ. Co., 3—23.

Genton, E. and Steele, P. (1977): Platelet survival: value for the diagnosis of thromboembolism and evaluation of antithrombotic drugs. In: Platelets and Thrombosis (Ed. D. C. B. Mills and F. I. Pareti) Academic Press, 157 to 166.

Roncucci, R., Deperon, R., Lansen, J., Destailleur, J., Verhaeghe, R., Doumont, J., Lambelin, G. and Van Stalle, F. (1977): Nonradioactive semi-automated determination of platelet survival time in man. Thromb. Haemostas., 38 (1), 92.

Stuart, M. J., Murphy, S., Oski, F. A. (1975): A simple nonradioisotope technic for the determination of platelet life-span. N. Engl. J. Med., 293, 1310—1313.

R. R., Research Laboratories Continental Pharma, 30 chaussée de Haecht, B-1830 Machelen, Belgium

ATHEROSCLEROSIS AND FACTOR XIII. A NEW TECHNIQUE FOR THE DETERMINATION OF FACTOR XIII USING A LASER NEPHELOMETER

P. POLA, S. SAVI, A. DAL LAGO and J. SHAMI

Catholic University of the Sacred Heart, Dept. of Internal Medicine and Centre for the Study, Prophylaxis and Cure of Angiopathies, Roma, Italy

Parietal damage, fatty infiltration of the walls and disruption of the balance in the coagulation-fibrinolysis system followed by platelet activation are all important changes that often lead to atheroma formation.

They reciprocally influence each other, so that the presence of one inevitably leads to the appearance of the others.

Whatever the initial change, the chain of events leading to the atheroma is always the same, ending with the intra-parietal deposition of fibrin.

This step is very important in as much as it brings about the action of Factor XIII of the coagulation system. This factor stabilizes the fibrin, thus rendering its removal through the fibrinolytic system difficult. Therefore, Factor XIII conditions the sequence of events that leads from the thrombus to the atheroma (Fig. 1).

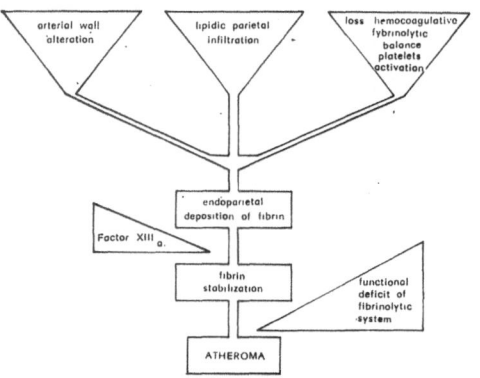

Materials and methods

The determination of Factor XIII was carried out with a new technique prepared in our laboratory (Fig. 2).

— Rabbit serum anti-factor XIII Subunit A Behring Werke
— Citrated plasma 1/10. This was obtained centrifuging blood at 4000 rpm for 15 minutes.

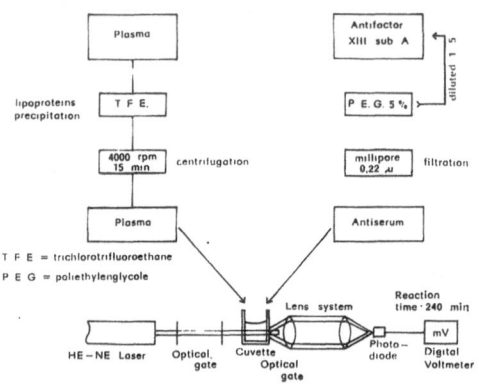

Principle and technique for the determination of factor XIII

The light source is a laser (Helium-Neon) with a wave-length of 633 nm (nanometers). The laser beam passes through two diaphragms, the cuvette and is finally absorbed in a special "trap".

The light is distributed on the immuno-complexes present in the cuvette and is diffused very intensly in the direction of propagation of the ray of light.

In contrast to common nephelometers, in which the light diffused at an angle of 90° with respect to the incident ray is measured, the laser nephelometer measures only the light in the original direction, concentrated by a lens system on a photo-detector.

The electric signal coming from the photo-detector is directly proportional to the intensity of the diffused light striking it and can be measured by means of a digital voltmeter.

To each plasma, trichlorotrifluoro-ethane is added in a ratio of 1/1 to precipitate lipoproteins that can render the plasma turbid. These treated plasmas are energically agitated for 3 minutes and then centrifuged for 15 minutes at 4000 rpm.

From the supernatant a plasma pool is prepared and the following dilutions are made with filtrated physiologic solution 1/1, 1/1.5, 1/2, 1/4.

The anti-serum anti-Factor XIII subunit A is diluted 1/5 with 5% polyethylene-glycol and left to rest for about 1 hour before filtering with Millipore filters of 0.22 micron size.

As a control, the anti-serum is replaced with physiologic solution diluted 1/5 with 5% PEG.

200 μl of sample and 100 μl of diluted anti-serum or control solution are placed in cuvettes for laser nephelometry. Each cuvette is immediately placed in the laser nephelometer and the magnitude of the luminous signal on the voltmeter before the start of the reaction is noted. After 240 minutes the operation is repeated and the luminous signal, produced by the interaction between the light and the antigen-antibody complexes formed, is read.

Reading of the results is done on a curve constructed on graph-paper, with the intensity of diffused light expressed in millivolts, corresponding to the four dilutions of the reference plasma (Fig. 3).

Important characteristics of this technique are the simplicity, the extreme sensitivity and the repeatability of the data. Its validity has been confirmed by numerous comparative determinations using other methods.

Clinically, the technique was used to evaluate Factor XIII in 31 subjects 33 – 75 years old. The subjects were patients of

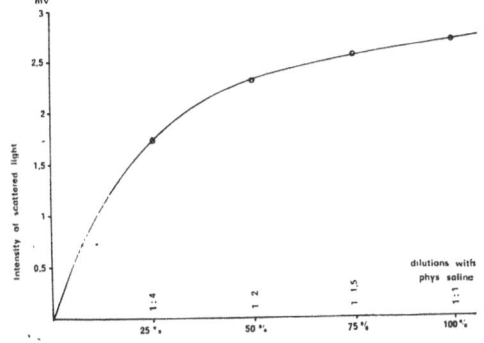

the Department of Clinical Medicine at the Catholic University of the Sacred Heart of Rome.

10 of these subjects were normal and 21 subjects had atherosclerotic vasculo-pathy. 1/3 of these subjects had diabetes mellitus.

Results and conclusions

The results are shown schematically:

subjects	average	increase	t	p
n: 10	81.6 ± 2.61			
a: 21	96.09 ± 7.87	17.74	4.86	<0.01

n = normal subjects
a = atherosclerotic subjects

These results do not permit conclusive deductions because of the limited number of cases studied, but they show the higher values of Factor XIII in arteriopathic subjects compared to normal subjects. This leads us to consider the role of Factor XIII in atherosclerotic vasculo-pathy. Knowledge on this subject is still limited and imprecise. Increased interest in the subjet on the part of researchers is necessary.

The possibility of using a new, sensitive and accurate technique can certainly render research easier.

P. P., Centre of Angiopathies, Department of Internal Medicine, Cath. University, Via Aurelia 239, 00165 Roma, Italy

FIBRINOLYTIC ACTIVITY OF THE ARTERIAL WALL OF PATENT AND OCCLUDED ARTERIES

L. DONNER and L. VODÁKOVÁ

2nd Department of Medicine, Charles University, Prague, Czechoslovakia

Numerous human tissues, including the arterial wall, contain an activator of plasminogen which is postulated to function in the removal of blood clots or other fibrin deposits from tissue parenchyma. In our study we tried to investigate the plasminogen activator of fibrinolysis both in patent and occluded arteries.

Materials and methods

The histochemical method of *Tood* was used in our modification.

734 specimen of various patent, normal and atherosclerotic arteries, thoracic and abdominal aorta and carotic, pulmonary, renal, basilar and coronary arteries were examined. 105 cadavers 1—18 hours post mortem aged 272 days to 85 years were used.

In 20 main coronary and 20 main pulmonary arteries occluded with complete thrombi or emboli, displaying fresh clinical signs of death, the plasminogen activator within the vessel wall was examined. The arteries were obtained 1 to 18 hours after death.

The mean fibrinolytic activity, the confidence limits, analyses of variance and the Duncan test were estimated.

Results

Our results are shown in Table I. The highest fibrinolytic activity of the patent normal arterial wall was within the adventitia. The mean fibrinolytic score was 4.5 to 6.5 points. No significant difference in fibrinolysis was established between the various arteries examined. However a statistically significant increase of fibrinolysis was found within the adventitia of atherosclerotic arteries. The fibrinolytic score was 5.5 to 7.5 points. No correlation was found between the degree of atherosclerosis and the increase

Table I. The fibrinolysis in patent normal (I), atherosclerotic (II) and occluded (III) main coronary and pulmonary arteries.

Coronary A.	Adventitia		
	n	mean score	
I	25	5.66 ± 0.79	I—II (p < 0.01)
II	20	7.77 ± 1.06	I—III (p < 0.01)
III	20	3.92 ± 1.14	II—III (p < 0.01)
	Intima		
I	25	1.40 ± 0.94	I—III (p < 0.01)
II	20	0.95 ± 1.09	II—III (p < 0.05)
III	20	0.32 ± 0.34	
Pulmonary A.	Adventitia		
	n	mean score	
I	34	4.99 ± 1.12	I—II (p < 0.01)
II	11	7.73 ± 0.61	I—III (p < 0.01)
III	19	1.74 ± 0.82	II—III (p < 0.01)
	Intima		
I	34	0.84 ± 1.02	I—III (p < 0.01)
II	5	1.20 ± 1.10	II—III (p < 0.05)
III	19	0.11 ± 0.27	

of fibrinolysis within the adventitia. Intima only occasionally displayed very little fibrinolytic activity or none at all. In normal arteries the fibrinolytic score was 0 to 3.5; in atherosclerotic arteries the fibrinolytic score was o to 3.5 points.

In occluded arteries the results were different. In most occluded arteries there was a generalised atherosclerosis where a higher plasminogen activator within the arterial wall could be postulated. Nevertheless the plasminogen activator within the the adventitia of occluded main coronary and pulmonary arteries was diminished in comparison with normal and atherosclerotic arteries. In coronary arteries with stenosis an increase of fibrinolysis due to atherosclerosis was not present.

In occluded coronary arteries the fibrinolysis within the adventitia was one and half to 6 points; in occluded pulmonary arteries the score was 0 to 4 points.

The plasminogen activator within the intima in occluded arteries is difficult to evaluate. The intima both of patent and occluded arteries generally displayed low fibrinolytic activity or none at all. However, our observations suggest that even in the intima of occluded arteries there is a tendency of fibrinolysis depression in comparison with the intima of patent arteries.

Conclusions

1) The highest fibrinolysis of normal, patent arteries is within the adventitia. Intima display very low or no fibrinolytic activity.

2) There is no statistical difference in the fibrinolytic activity of the different types of arteries examined.

2) There is no statistical difference in the fibrinolytic activity of the different types of arteries examined.

3) A statistically significant increase of fibrinolysis within the adventitia of atherosclerotic arteries in comparison with normal arteries was established.

4) Occluded main coronary and pulmonary arteries by complete thrombi or emboli showed a statistically significant decrease of fibrinolysis within the adventitia.

REFERENCES

1. *Donner L., Klener P., Roth Z. (1977):* The plasminogen activator of the arterial wall. Thrombos. Haemostas. (Stuttg.) 37, 436.
2. *Pandol M., Robertson B., Isacson S., Nilsson I. M.:* Fibrinolytic activity of human veins in arms and legs. Thrombosis et Diathesis Haemorrh. (Stuttg.) 20, 247.
3. *Todd A. S. (1958):* Fibrinolysis autographs. Nature 181, 495,
4. *Todd A. S. (1964):* Blood vessel wall and fibrinolytic activity. In: Johnson S. A., Guest M. M. (Eds) Dynamics of thrombus formation and solution. Lippincot, Philadelphia pp. 321.

L. D., U nemocnice 2, 12808 Prague 2, Czechoslovakia

FIBRINOLYTIC ACTIVITY IN HYPERLIPOPROTEINAEMIAS

HANNA BERENT and Z. RYMASZEWSKI

*Department of Angiology, Institute of Internal Medicine,
Academy of Medicine, Warsaw, Poland*

Introduction

According to some studies, defective fibrinolytic activity can promote vascular complications (*Andersen*, 1976; *Peabody et al.*, 1974). Lipids and lipaemia were found to inhibit fibrinolysis, although there were no apparent correlations be-

to 63 years. Type II was found in 13 patients, IV in 21 and V in 12 patients (WHO classification). 46 subjects matched in age, sex and weight were used as a control group. The effect of physical exercise on fibrinolysis was studied in 30 males with hyperlipoproteinaemias, aged 29 to 52 years. Type II was present in 10 cases, type IV in 20 cases. Twenty healthy men, age and weight matched were used as controls. 70% maximal exercise for 15 minutes was performed on

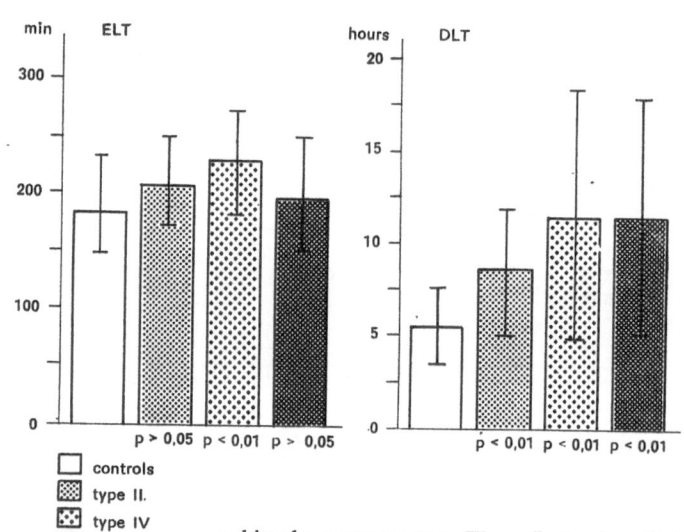

Fig. 1. Fibrinolytic activity at rest in patients with primary hyperlipoproteinaemias and in controls. ELT-euglobulin clot lysis time. DLT-diluted blood clot lysis time.

□ controls
▒ type II.
▨ type IV
▓ type V

tween measures of fibrinolytic activity and plasma lipids observed (*Holzknecht et al.*, 1970). The present study was undertaken to assess fibrinolytic activity in patients with primary hyperlipoproteinaemias at rest and after physical exercise and to evaluate the effect of a high carbohydrate diet on fibrinolysis.

Material and methods

Fibrinolytic activity at rest was studied in 46 patients with hyperlipoproteinaemias, aged 26

a bicycle ergonometer. The effect of a high carbohydrate diet on fibrinolysis was studied on 16 volunteers aged 26 to 60 years. A diet consisting of 2500 calories containing 70% simple carbohydrates was used for one week during the hospital stay.

Fibrinolytic activity was measured by means of euglobulin clot lysis time-ELT, diluted blood clot lysis time-DLT (*Fearnley et al.*, 1957) and on unheated fibrin plates (*Brakman*, 1967). The last test was performed only in the group subjected to exercise.

Results

Statistically significant prolongation of fibrinolysis at rest in ELT was observed

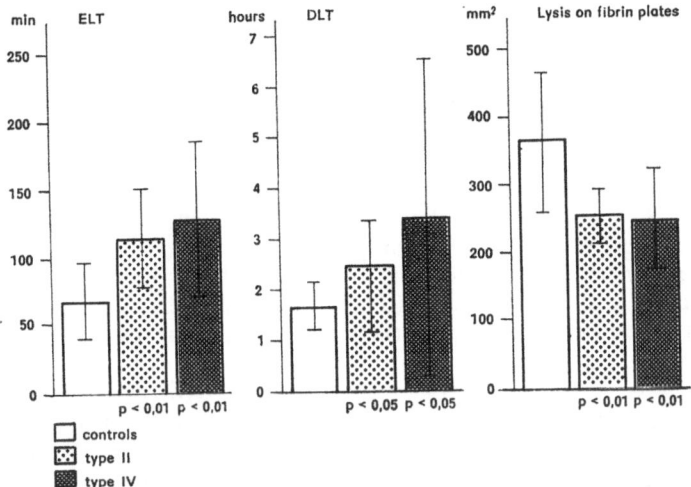

Fig. 2. Effect of physical exercise on fibrinolytic activity in patients with primary hyperlipoprotein-aemias.

in patients with type IV, whereas in DLT in all types, but more pronounced in type IV and V than in type II (Fig. 1). Linear regression analysis did not reveal a signifi-

cant correlation between fibrinolysis time-lipid levels and fibrinolysis time-overweight.

Inhibition of exercise-induced enhan-

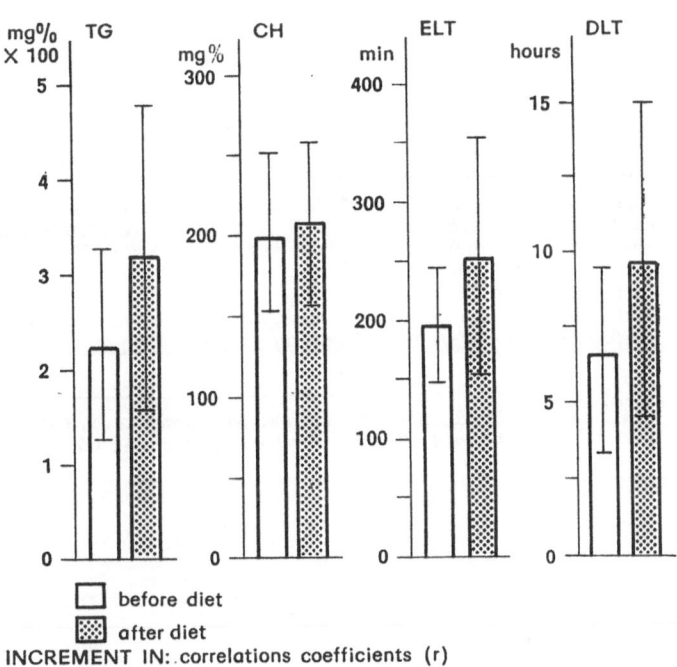

Fig. 3. Effect of high carbohydrate diet on fibrinolytic activity. TG-serum triglycerides level. CH-serum level.

INCREMENT IN:	correlations coefficients (r)	
TG – DLT	+ 0,842	p < 0,01
TG – ELT	+ 0,622	p < 0,01
CH – DLT	– 0,105	NS
CH – ELT	– 0,117	NS

cement of fibrinolytic activity was marked in patients with hyperlipoproteinaemias compared to controls (Fig. 2). Fibrinolytic activity after exercise was lower in hypertriglyceridaemic (type IV) than hyper-cholesterolaemic (type II) patients, but this difference was not significant.

High carbohydrate diet induced hyper-triglyceridaemia was accompanied by a prolongation of fibrinolysis in ELT and DLT, with significant positive correlation to the increase in triglycerides level (Fig. 3).

Discussion

This study confirms that, in primary hyperlipoproteinaemias, fibrinolytic activity is slightly but significantly depressed at rest and physiological enhancement of fibrinolysis after exercise is diminished. This latter finding has been previously reported in patients with type IV (*Epstein et al.*, 1970). According to our results, impaired fibrinolytic response to exercise occur also in patients of type II. Despite the lack of significant correlations of resting values between indices of fibrinolytic activity and plasma lipids level, an association between the increment of serum triglycerides induced by a high carbohydrate diet and fibrinolysis time was observed, in agreement to one study (*Stevenson et al.*, 1970) and in contrast to a other (*Korsan-Bengtsen et al.*, 1972). The importance of these changes in pathology is still disputed and more prospective clinical studies relating fibrinolytic activity to vascular complications are needed.

REFERENCES

Andersen, P. (1976): Hyperlipidaemia and reduced fibrinolytic activity associated with thromboembolic complications in a family. Acta Med. Scand. 200, 289—291.

Brakman, P. (1967): Fibrinolysis: A Standarized Fibrin Plate Method and a Fibrinolytic Assay of Plasminogen. Amsterdam, Scheltema and Halkema NV.

Epstein, S., Rosing, D., Brakman, P., Redwood, D., Astrup, T. (1970): Impaired fibrinolytic response to exercise in patients with type-IV hyperlipoproteinaemia. Lancet, 2, 631—634.

Fearnley, G., Balmforth, G., Fearnley, E. (1957): Evidence of a diurnal fibrinolytic rhythm, with a simple method of measuring natural fibrinolysis. Clin. Sci., 16, 645—650.

Holzknecht, F., Spottl, F., Steinmetz, U., Braunsteiner, H. (1970): A basic study on global coagulation and fibrinolysis of haperlipemic and atherosclerotic patients. Atherosclerosis, 12, 415—426.

Korsan-Bengtsen, K., Gustavsson, A., Sjostrom, L. Bjorntorp, P. (1972): Effects of carbohydrate feeding on blood coagulation, fibrinolysis and platelet adhesiveness — relations to serum lipids and lipoproteins. Thromb. Res. 1, 407—426.

Peabody, R., Tsapogas, M., Kwang-Tzen Wu, Devera), K., Karmody, A., Eckert, C. (1974): Altered endogenous fibrinolysis and biochemical factors in atherosclerosis. Arch. Surg. 109, 309—313.

Stevenson, M., Harper, L., Davidson, P., Albrink, M. (1970): Effect of low and high carbohydrate diets on fibrinolysis. Circulation, 42, suppl. 3, 91.

H. B., 02—006 Warsaw, Nowogrodzka 59, Department of Angiology, Institute of Internal Medicine, Academy of Medicine, Warsaw, Poland

INTERACTION OF ANGIOGRAPHY WITH THE BLOOD COAGULATION AND THE FIBRINOLYTIC SYSTEM

W. H. KRAUSE and A. LANG

Justus-Liebig-Universität, Giessen, F.R.G.

Bernstein and Gans (1966) found that commercial contrast media are strongly anticoagulant *in vitro*. In animals transient anticoagulation was produced by doses many times greater than those used clinically. The basic pathophysiology observed in their experiments was a defect in the clotting of fibrin. They concluded that the media had an antithrombin action. Contact between blood and catheter compound *in vitro* activates coagulation and it has been shown in dogs that the presence of a polyethylene catheter in the circulation stimulates intravascular coagulation. The purpose of the present study was to find out whether an anticoagulant effect can be demonstrated in patients undergoing an angiographic procedure.

Material and methods

The clinical series consisted of 50 randomly selected patients referred for abdominal aortography. The most common indication was occlusive disease, hypertension and suspected malignant disease. 40 men and 10 women were studied; their ages ranged from 20 to 80 years (Fig. 1). The mean age was 66.4 years. The catheter (Desilet, Vygon, size of catheter 2.0 mm) was introduced percutaneously according to Seldinger's method into the femoral artery. The contrast media used were Conray 60 (meglumin-iotalamat) and Conray 70 (sodium-iotalamat, meglumin-iotalamat). The mean volume of contrast medium for angiography was 122.5 ml, the iodine concentration was 38.6 g. All patients were in the fasting state before angiography. The renal function was tested by measuring the serum creatinin concentration. This was normal in 47 patients, there was one patient with 2.1 mg/100 ml and two patients with 1.4 mg/100 ml.

Blood samples were obtained before the introduction of the catheter and 30, 60 minutes and 6 hours after angiography. The following coagulation tests were made: haematocrit, platelet count, activated PTT, normotest, thrombin-, thrombin coagulase, reptilase time, fibrinogen Plasminogen and antithrombin III concentrations are found by the immunological method (partigen plate) and staphylococcal clumping test and latex agglutination test was used for determining FDP. Platelet-poor plasma was obtained with 3.8% trisodium citrate solution containing aprotinin, serum was obtained with thrombin (20 U/ml and aprotinin 50 U/ml). The results were corrected to the measured haematocrit. Statistical method: the two factor variance analysis for dependent variables was used.

Results

The results are represented as mean values of the 50 patients undergoing abdominal aortography. The haematocrit fell from sample I to sample II by 4% of the original value.

The platelet count showed no significant decrease but a significant increase 6 hours after angiography.

The fibrinogen concentration showed a borderline significant decrease 30 min after angiography.

A significant decrease was found for antithrombin III and plasminogen only in the samples taken 30 min after angiography.

No significant changes were found in the activated PTT and normotest.

The thrombin coagulase times (TC) showed a significant increase, the reptilase times were also significantly prolonged and, similarly, the thrombin time was also significantly prolonged. The plasma conray concentration had maxima after 30 and 60 min.

The plasma conray concentration revealed a significant correlation between TC times (40, 60 min p 0.05), reptilase times (30, 60 min p 0.01, r = 0.5) and thrombin times (30, 60 min p 0.01, r = 0.38).

The serum FDP concentration measured with the latex test and the stap. clumping test showed a significant increase up to 6 hours after angiography.

There was no correlation between reptilase time, thrombin-coagulase time and the FDP concentration.

In summary, a significant increase of the thrombin-, reptilase and thrombin-coagulase times was found with a significant correlation to the plasma conray concentrations at the given times. It is concluded that the prolongation of the coagulation times is caused in the first place by the contrast-medium in terms of an inhibition of fibrin polymerization.

There was no correlation for the coagulation times (reptilase, thrombin coagulase) with the serum FDP. The increase of the degradation products up to 6 hours after angiography suggest activation of the fibrinolytic system, set up by the process of catheterisation and the injection procedure with a shortlasting local hypoxaemia. Indications of activation of intravascular coagulation may be a discerete reduction of fibrinogen, plasminogen and antithrombin III levels 30 min after angiography. Thrombo-embolic complications were not seen in the patients investigated and similarly no signs of increased bleeding tendency were observed. The anticoagulant effect was demonstrated by the increased thrombin and reptilase times which show a significant correlation to the contrast media concentration in plasma.

W. H. K., Zentrum Innere Medizin, Justus-Liebig-Universität, Giesen, F.R.G.

SOLUBLE FIBRIN IN PLASMA AND ENDOPEROXIDE-FORMATION IN PLATELETS AS AN INDICATION OF PRETHROMBOTIC STATES FOLLOWING MYOCARDIAL INFARCTION

F. R. MATTHIAS, D. L. HEENE and TH. SCHÖNDORF

Department of Medicine, Justus Liebig University, Giessen, F.R.G.

Following myocardial infarction the blood of the patient generally shows a tendency to hypercoagulability. As a consequence, deep vein thrombosis is observed in up to 30% in such cases. Thrombosis is significantly reduced by heparin administration (*Gallus et al.*, 1973; *Warlow et al.*, 1973). The plasmic coagulation system as well as the platelets are involved in the mechanism of venous thrombus formation (*Walsh*, 1975). Many attempts have been made to gather analytical criteria to detect thrombotic states. As intravascular thrombin action is the decisive event, the detection and quantification of soluble fibrin and fibrinopeptides seem to be convincing parameters for an activated coagulation system. In order to predict the thrombogenic activity of platelets, the extent of platelet aggregation, the liberation of β-thromboglobulin and the production or liberation of other platelet constituents were determined. In the experiments described the soluble plasma fibrin was measured by affinity chromatography and correlated to the prostaglandin-endoperoxide production of platelets under standardized conditions.

Methods

The procedure of blood sampling, preparation of platelet-rich plasma and platelet suspensions in plasma and buffer as well as the isolation of soluble fibrin from plasma and its quantification have already been described (*Heene, Matthias*, 1973; *Matthias et al.*, 1977; *Matthias* 1978). After incubation with N-ethylmaleimide (NEM) over a defined period of time, prostaglandin-endoperoxides of platelets were measured as n moles of malondialdehyde (MDA) per 10^9 platelets (*Stuart et al.*, 1975; *Smith et al.*, 1976).

Results and discussion

In all patients investigated no signs of venous thrombosis could be detected by clinical and doppler sonic examination. In Figure 1 the plasma fibrin content in two patients following myocardial infarction is demonstrated over a period of time. After 4 to 5 days soluble fibrin has declined to normal values. As shown on the left part of the figure, in many of our cases the plasma fibrin increases for some time despite continuous heparin infusion of 20 − 30 000 NIH units per day and despite a thrombin time prolongation to over 2 1/2 times the control value. This phenomenon is more pronounced in shock

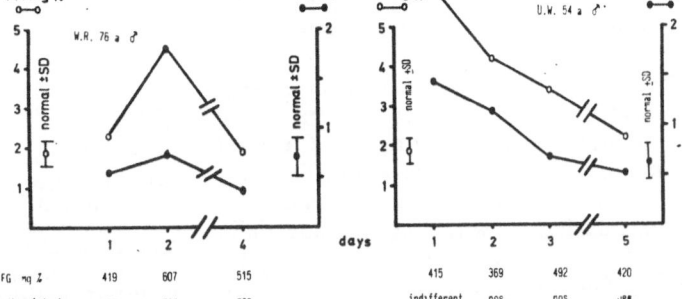

Fig. 1. Myocardial infarction: soluble plasma fibrin (FM) in mg% and % of plasma fibrinogen (FG). Normal donors: n = 27

93

	A	B	C
SOLUBLE FIBRIN MG / 100 ML PLASMA	1.5 ± 0.5	5.0 ± 1.6	8.2 ± 2.4
n MOLES MDA PER 10^9 PLATELETS	8.9 ± 1.5	11.9 ± 2.5	9.9 ± 3.2

Fig. 2. Soluble fibrin in plasma and prostaglandin endoperoxides (measured as n moles MDA) per 10^9 platelets after 10 min. incubation in buffer together with NEM. Basal level before incubation: $0.4-1.2$ n mol MDA/10^9 platelets. Mean values $\pm$ SD.
A = healthy donors (n = 11); B = patients after myocardial infarction (n = 7) C = patients after myocardial infarction suffering from circulatory insufficiency under norepinephrine and/or dopamine administration (n = 7).

patients with DIC (*Reinicke et al.*, 1977).

Figure 2 demonstrates the soluble plasma fibrin of control persons, of patients with myocardial infarction without any complications, from which blood was take complications, from which blood was taken 1 hour after hospitalization before any treatment, and, thirdly, of patients following infarction and suffering from circulatory insufficiency under norepinephrine and/or dopamine infusion. In the last group other drugs were also administered; blood was taken during the first 3 days of hospitalization. All patients received heparin. The plasma fibrin content is elevated in the patient groups and highest in those patients suffering from circulatory insufficiency. All differences are significant. In comparison, formation of prostaglandin-endoperoxides of platelets is shown. Endoperoxide production is augmented in the patient groups; compared to the control group, however, the increase is significant only in the patients of group B, where no drugs were given before taking the blood samples. Despite the more activated coagulation system indicated by the higher plasma fibrin concentration, platelets of group C exhibit a minor endoperoxide elevation. This may be due to the different drugs administered and interfering with the prostaglandin system — such as analgetics and furosemide. On the whole, the results demon-

strate that, together with increased fibrin formation, the arachidonic acid-prostaglandin system is stimulated after myocardial infarction and probably producing thrombus promoting activities. Similar results were obtained by other workers (*Abbate et al.*, 1977).

Figure 3 shows the soluble fibrin in plasma and the plasma's prostaglandin-endoperoxide promoting activity in a patient over a period of 3 days. This patient received no drugs besides heparin and norepinephrine. Platelets of a normal donor and the patient's platelets were suspended in the patient's plasma. The value of endoperoxides obtained by control platelets and patient's platelets supended in normal plasma, respectively, was taken

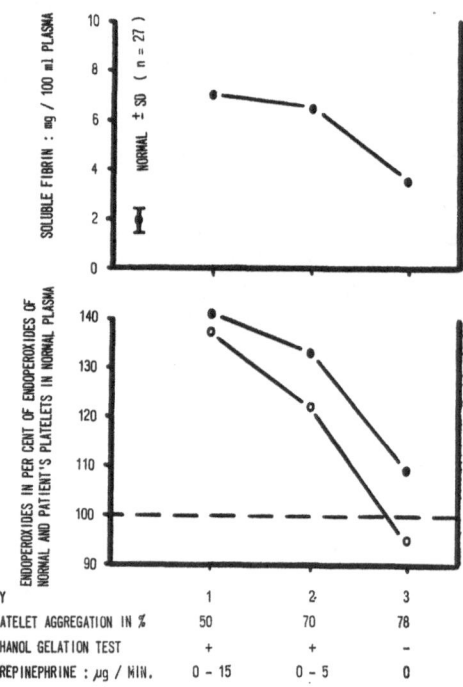

DAY	1	2	3
PLATELET AGGREGATION IN %	50	70	78
ETHANOL GELATION TEST	+	+	-
NOREPINEPHRINE : µg / MIN.	0 - 15	0 - 5	0

Fig. 3. Upper diagram: Soluble fibrin in plasma of a patient after myocardial infarction.
Lower diagram: Prostaglandin endoperoxide formation in patient's plasma after 60 min. of incubation at 37° together with NEM.
o = normal platelets in patient's plasma; o = patient's platelets in patient's own plasma. 100% = normal or patient's platelets in normal plasma, respectively.

as 100%. As can be seen, the endoperoxide stimulating potency of the patient's plasma declines together with the decrease in the soluble plasma fibrin. This may be due mainly to the diminihsing plasma thrombin and catecholamine action with time.

Conclusions

Following myocardial infarction, soluble plasma fibrin is elevated, mainly in patients suffering from circulatory insufficiency. Heparin does not stop thrombin activity and fibrin formation immediately in every case. Concomitantly, a stimulated prostaglandin system of platelets indicated by the increase in endoperoxide formation can be assumed. The plasma's endoperoxide-producing activity declines together with the soluble plasma fibrin content. Various drugs administered to the patient may depress the prostaglandin system, but probably do not always influence the thrombus forming ac.ivities of the platelets. It remains to be found to what an extent antiplatelet drugs of the aspirin-like type may prevent deep vein thrombosis. It was shown that acetylsalicylic-lysine could not diminish postoperative thrombo.ic events (*Schöndorf, Hey*, 1977). To inhibit the release of procoagulant platelet factors 3 and 4, relatively high amounts of acetyl-salicylic acid have to be administered (*Vinazzer*, 1975). High aspirin doses, however, may induce an opposite, thrombosis stimulating effect by blocking the prc stacyclin formation of the vessel walls (*Burch et al.*, 1978).

REFERENCES

Abbate, R., Gensini, G. F., Prisco, D., Valeri, A., Serneri, G. G. (1977): Increased formation of malondialdehyde by N-ethyl-maleimide and thrombin in patients with cerebrovascular disorders and with history of myocardial infarction. I. Florence Conf. Thrombos. Haemostas. abs. p. 131.

Burch, J. W., Stanford, N., Majerus, P. W. (1978): Inhibition of platelet prostaglandin synthetase by oral aspirin. J. clin. Inve(t. 61, 314—319.

Gallus, A. S., Hirsh, J., Tuttle, R. J., Treblicock, R., O'Brien, S. E., Carroll, J. J., Minden, J. H., Hudecki, S. M. (1973): Small subcutaneous doses of heparin in prevention of venous thrombosis. N. Engl. J. Med. 288, 545—551.

Heene, D. L., Matthias, F. R. (1973): Adsorption of fibrinogen derivatives on insolubilized fibrinogen and fibrinmonomer. Thrombos. Res. 2, 137—154.

Matthias, F. R., Reinicke, R., Heene, D. L. (1977): Affinity chromatography and quantitation of soluble fibrin from plasma. Thrombos. Res. 10, 365—384.

Matthias, F. R. (1978): Soluble plasma fibrin and platelet prostaglandin endoperoxides following myocardial infarction. Haemostasis 7, in press.

Reinicke, R., Matthias, F. R., Lasch, H. G. (1977): Content of soluble fibrin in plasma of patients after myocardial infarction, with carcinomas and consuption coagulopathy. Thrombos. Res. 11, 365—375.

Schöndorf, T., Hey, D. (1977): Modified 'low-dose' heparin prophylaxis to reduce thrombosis after hip joint operations. Thrombos. Res. 12, 153—163.

Smith, J. B., Ingerman, C. M., Silver, M. J. (1976): Malondialdehyde formation as an indicator of prostaglandin production by human platelets. J. Lab. clin. Med. 88, 167—172.

Stuart, M. J., Murphy, S., Oski, F. A. (1975): A simple non-radioisotope technic for the determination of platelet life-span. N. Engl. J. Med. 292, 1310—1313.

Vinazzer, H. (1975): Beeinflussung der Thrombozytenfunktion und Gerinnung nach intravenöser Verabreichung von Acetylsalicylsäure. Colfarit — Symposion III, Köln, FRG, pp. 28—45.

Walsh, P. N. (1975): The possible role of platelet coagulant activities in the pathogenesis of venous thrombosis. Thrombos. Diathes. haemorrh. 33, 435—445.

Warlow, C., Terry, G., Kenmure, A. C. F., Beattie, A. G., Ogston, D., Douglas, A. S. (1973): A double blind trial of low doses of subcutaneous heparin in the prevention of deep-vein thrombosis after myocardial infarction. Lancet II, 934—936.

F. R. M., Dept. of Medicine Justus Liebig-University, Klinikstr. 36, D 6300 Giessen, F.R.G.

ERYTHROCYTE MEMBRANES AS A TARGET FOR ANTITHROMBOTIC AGENTS

J. ROBA, M. CLAEYS, R. ROET, W. VAN OPSTAL
and G. LAMBELIN

Continental Pharma, Research Laboratories, Brussels, Belgium

The role of erythrocytes in arterial thrombogenesis is so far poorly understood, although there is experimental basis for their active participation (*Wiedeman*, 1973). It has been recently suggested that erychrocytes can release significant amounts of an aggregating agent, possibly ADP, and subsequently activate platelet aggregation and thrombus formation (*Born et al.*, 1976). Such a release may be triggered by mechanical deformations of red cells in turbulent flow areas, as in atherosclerotic arteries. Drugs stabilizing the erythrocyte membrane can prevent this release under certain circumstances. In order to assess the potential role of such a mechanism, we have compared 4 antithrombotic drugs, namely acetylsalicylic acid (ASA), dipyridamole, sulfinpyrazone and suloctidil for their activity

Figure 1

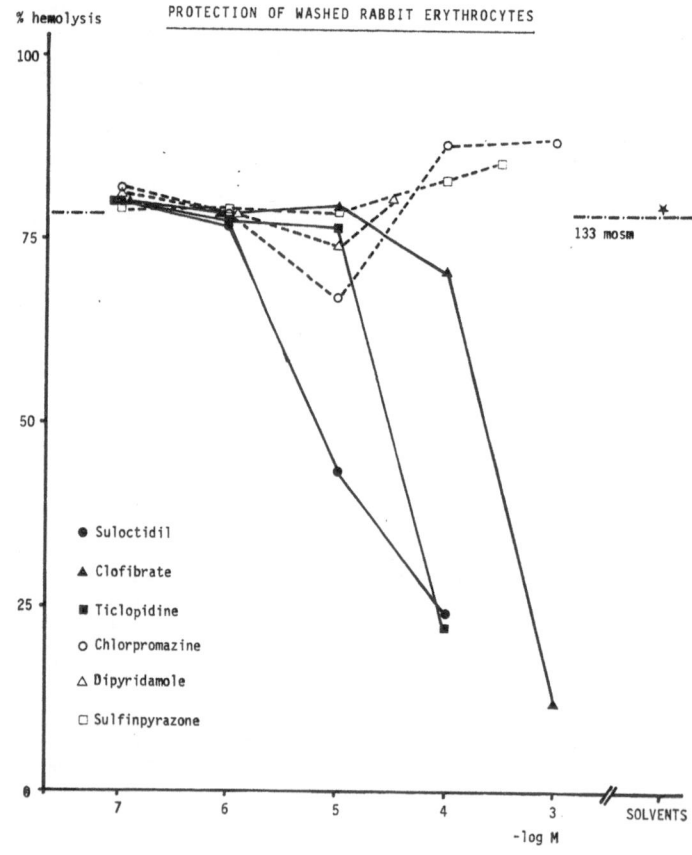

Fig. 1. Erythrocytes were obtained from heparinized (10 U/ml) rabbit venous blood, washed thrice in phosphate buffer and adjusted to 40% hematocrit. Aliquots of 0.3 ml were suspended in 10 ml of 133 mOsm NaCl solution which sometimes contained solvents or tested compounds at the indicated concentrations (−log. M) Results shown are from a typical experiment.

96

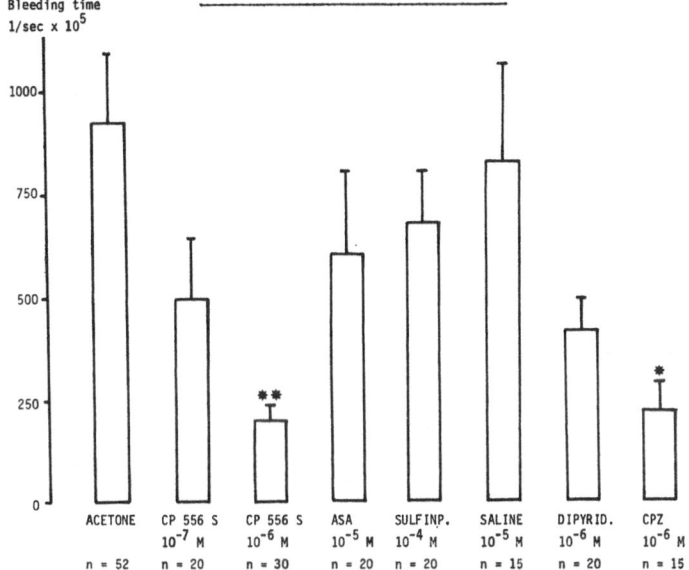

Fig. 2. The in vitro bleeding time of canine citrated blood, incubated with drugs or solvents, is expressed as 1/t. * or ** indicate values significantly different from the corresponding controls (t test and Wilcoxon non-parametric test) at the thresholds p = 0.05 and 0.01.

a) on erychrocyte membrane, b) on *in vitro* bleeding time erythrocytes mediated thrombus formation), and c) on *in vivo* ADP-induced platelet aggregation (filter loop technique).

Methods

Erythrocyte membrane protection

Venous blood was obtained from anesthetized rabbits. Erythrocytes were washed thrice in neutral isotonic phosphate buffer. Concentration of cells was adjusted to 40% hematocrit. 70% hemolysis was obtained by dilution in hypoosmotic NaCl solutions (130 to 140 mOsm), which may contain tested drugs or vehicle.

In vitro bleeding time

The method was that described by Born (*Born et al.* 1976). Canine or human citrated (0.38 g/10 ml) blood, incubated for 20 min with ASA, dipyridamole, sulfinpyrazone, chlorpromazine, suloctidil or vehicles was perfused at 150 µl/min through a polyethylene tubing system. Bleeding time through a standardized incision was measured under microscopic observation.

ADP — induced platelet aggregation in rats (filter loop technique).

The method and the results have been published (*Roba et al*, 1976).

Results

As show in Fig. 1, dipyridamole has lower activity and sulfinpyrazone is devoid of protecting effect on erythrocyte membrane. ASA has very weak activity at $10^{-5}M$ (results not shown). In contrast, suloctidil exhibits a marked protective

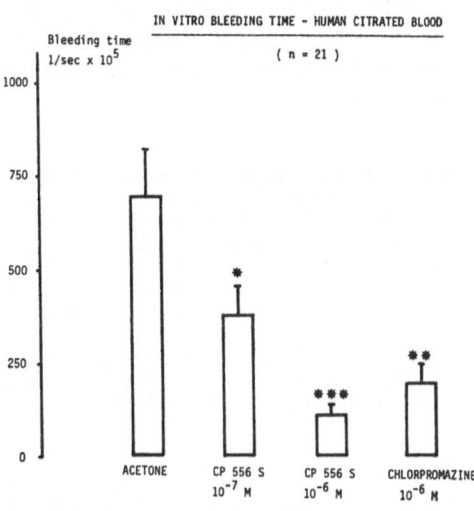

Fig. 3. Similar experiments as in fig. 2. using human citrated blood.

activity from 10^{-6}M. In other experiments, using a range of hypoosmotic solutions, it appears that this drug is about 10 times as potent as chlorpromazine.

The *in vitro* bleeding time of dog blood is not significantly altered by ASA (10^{-5}M), sulfinpyrazone (10^{-4}M) and dipyridamole (10^{-6}M), although a trend to increased values was noted, particularly with dipyridamole (Fig. 2). The proportion increased in that group, compared with the controls ($p < 0.05$). Suloctidil is signi-with dipyridamole (Fig. 2). The proportion of values higher than 8 min is significantly increased in that group, compared with the controls ($p < 0.05$). Suloctidil is significantly active at 10^{-6}M ($p < 0.01$), as is chlorpromazine ($p < 0.05$). In human blood, a significant effect of suloctidil is observed at 10^{-7} and 10^{-6}M (Fig. 3). The results of the filter loop experiment show that ASA is not active in doses up to 3 mg/kg i.v. The minimal active dose of dipyridamole is 3 mg/kg and that of suloctidil is 0.1 mg/kg.

Discussion

These experiments confirm the observations by *Born et al* (1976) that drugs stabilizing the erythrocyte membrane prevent *in vitro* platelet aggregation and adhesion triggered by red cells. Chlor-promazine effectiveness in preventing this mechanism is tentatively explained by inhibition of ADP leakage from erythrocytes. It appears that suloctidil has a potent protecting effect on erythrocytes which can explain its potent activity in preventing in vitro thrombus formation at 10^{-7} and 10^{-6}M. The weak inhibition by suloctidil of *in vitro* ADP induced platelet aggregation (*Mills and Macfarlane*, 1977) cannot be supposed to play a significant role. The marked inhibition by suloctidil of ADP-induced obstruction of a filter loop and the weak activity of dipyridamole and ASA would suggest the participation of erythrocytes in this model. This would explain why the pressure changes across the filter during about 30 sec after local ADP injection, which is certainly longer than needed for washout by blood.

The results obtained are consistant with the hypothesis of a significant but secondary participation of erythrocytes in the mechanisms of thrombus formation in arteries. Whether or not ADP release is involved, rather than another factor or mechanical alteration of the red cells, remains to be determined. It must be kept in mind that the amount of ADP present in 1 mm^3 of blood is about 75 pM in erythrocytes and 7 pM in platelets (calculated from *Pfeiffer and Mücke*, 1977 and *Holmsen et al*, 1972).

REFERENCES

Born, G. V. R., Bergquist, D. and Arfors, K. E. (1976): Evidence for inhibition of platelet activation in blood by a drug effect on erythrocytes. Nature, 259, 233—235.

Holmsen, H., Horm, E. and Day, J. H. (1972): Determination of ATP and ADP in blood platelets. Analyt. Biochem., 46, 489—501.

Mills, D. C. B. and Macfarlane, D. E. (1977): Depletion of platelet amine storage granules by the antithrombotic agent, suloctidil. Thromb. Haemostas., 38, 1010—1017.

Pfeiffer, H. J. and Mücke, D. (1977): Die Adeninnukleotidkonzentration des menschlichen Erythrozyten unter besonderer Berücksichtigung physiologischer Altersunterschiede. Kinderarztliche Praxis, 45, 249—256.

Roba, J., Bourgain, R., Andries, R., Claeys, M., Van Opstal, W. and Lambelin, G. (1976): Antagonism by suloctidil of arterial thrombus formation in rats. Thrombos. Res., 9, 585 to 594.

J. R. Department of Pharmacology, Research Laboratories Continental Pharma, 30 chaussée de Haecht, B-1830 Machelen, Belgium

DIFFERENT FORMS OF SOLUBLE FIBRIN MONOMER COMPLEX INDICATING THEIR DIFFERENT DEVELOPMENTAL PROCESSES IN HYPERCOAGULABLE STATES

T. ABE, M. KAZAMA, K. NAKAMURA, I. NAITO and J. MATSUDA

Department of Medicine, Teikyo University, Tokyo, Japan.

Introduction

The soluble fibrin monomer complex (SFMC) is the one of the coagulation parameters which reflect hypercoagulability by an increase in plasma. SFMC was quantified by the chromatography of test plasma on Bio-Gel A-15 m column (*Alkajaersig*, 1973), and the arbitralily defind "hypercoagulability (HC) score" was used to express the amount of SFMC eluted at the void volume of the column (*Kazama*, 1976).

Results

A) *Characterization of SFMC produced in vitro and in vivo.*

The formation of SFMC was attempted *in vitro*, (1) by adding a small amount of thrombin to normal plasma or mixing soluble fibrin with normal plasma, and (2) in the process of fibrin clot degradation with plasmin. These SFMC's were separated from the parent plasmas by gel exclusion chromatography. SFMC produced by the procedure (1) was thrombin clottable, paracoagulable and sometimes cold precipitable, containing intact fibrinogen/fibrin (FBG/fb), which was revealed by SDS-PAA disc electrophoresis.

In contrast, another SFMC produced by the procedure (2) did not show any of these properties but consisted of FDP of different degradation (Table I).

The experimental DIC were induced in dogs by injecting canine thromboplastin extract and the process was modified by the combination of either one of heparin, urokinase or t-AMCHA. SFMC was formed in all these experiments regardless of the modification and each SFMC was isolated from the plasma by paracoagulation with protamine sulfate and analysed by SDS-PAA electrophoresis.

The SFMC formed in the acute DIC by a single injection of thromboplastin extract was composed of FBG/fb, intact and slight-was composed of FBG/fb, intact and slightly degraded, and partial crosslinking was revealed by the presence of a small amount of the γ-γ dimer. The main component of SFMC's formed in the other modifications were also FBG/fb, although a slight variation were noted; the absence of crosslinked complexes in DIC treated with heparin, a slight increase of degraded FBG/fg in DIC treated with UK/and the absence of this degradation in DIC treated with t-AMCHA (Table) were obeswed.

B) *Characterization of SFMC appeared in the clinical specimens*

SFMC's were isolated by cold precipitation or paracoagulation with protamine sulfate from the plasma of 9 cases showing high HC scores, i.e. cerebral thrombosis, DIC complicated by malignancies and rheumatoid arthritis. They were analysed by SDS-PAA electrophoresis. In the first two cases of old cerebral thrombosis, SFMC was com-

CHARACTERIZATION OF "SFMC" PREPARED IN VITRO EXPERIMENTS

	Fibrinogen	Fbg/fb complex		FDP	fdp complex	
		stabilized	non-stabil.		stabilized	non-stabil.
HMW complex	-	+	+	-	+	+
clottability	+	+	+	-	-	-
PS	-	+	+	-	-	+
EG	-	+	+	-	-	-
cold Ppt.	-	+	+	-	-	-
components	Fbg	Fbg/fb crosslink. complex	Fbg/fb	fdp X Y D E	fdp X,Y,D,E crosslink. complex	fdp X,Y,D,E

99

posed of slightly degraded FBG/fb complex. In the following five cases of DIC, SFMC's were composed of intact FBG/fb with partial crosslinking, except the seventh case of acute promyelocytic leukemia, in which degradation of the α-chain was apparent in the reduced specimen.

Discussion and conclusions

1) Two types of SFMC were reproducible *in vitro*. One was by the addition of a small amount of thrombin to plasma and the another was produced in the process of clot dissolution. They were different each other in thrombin-clottability, paracoagulation and the grade of degradation by plasma. (*Graff*, 1975).

2) It was found from the experimental DIC that the thrombin activation in blood was prerequisite for the formation of SFMC and its component was basically intact FBG/fb with partial crosslinking, which was slimilar to the SFMC produced with thrombin *in vitro*.

3) SDS-PAA electrophoresis of SFMC's isolated from the clinical specimens revealed that the main component in cases of cerebral thrombosis was partly degraded FBG/fb, whereas it was intact FBG/fb in cases of DIC, and they were partly crosslinked.

It is expected that further information on the process of hypercoagulability states would be available from the quantitative analysis by comparison of HC score with PS or EG test and subunit analysis of SFMC on SDS-PAA electrophoresis.

REFERENCES

Alkajaersig, N., Roy, L., Fletcher, A. P. and Murphy, E. (1973)[2] Analysis of gel exclusion chromatographic data by chromatographic plate theory analysis: Application of plasma fibrinogen chromatography. Thromb. Res. 3: 525—544.

Graeff. R., von Hugo, R. and Mafter, R. (1975) The elevation of hypercoagulability and DIC by quantitative gel filtration and by chain analysis of isolated soluble fibrin monomer complexes. Thromb Diath. Haemorrh. 34: 355.

Kazama, M. and Abe, T. (1976) Change of the molecular mass of fibrinogen in circulation blood, as an index of the hypercoagulable states. Thromb. Res. suppl II, 133—142.

T. A., Dept. of Medicine Teikyo University, 11—1, Kaga 2 chome, Tokyo, Japan.

VASCULAR OPERATIONS WITH THE AID OF AN AUTOTRANSFUSION-SYSTEM: CHANGES IN BLOOD COAGULATION

H. DENCK, M. FISCHER, P. HOPMEIER, M. LURF,
E. CHOWANETZ and G. PRENNER

*1st Surgical Department, Central Laboratory, Institute of Anaesthesiology.
Municipal Hospital, Lainz, Vienna, Austria*

With the intraoperative autotransfusion (IOAT) of patient's blood, a promising approach for optimal acute blood substitution has been established in vascular surgery.

From 1975—1977 31 patients of the 1st Surgical Department underwent vascular surgery with Bentley's autotransfusion pump being used. Pre-, per- and post-operative blood coagulation was checked by the Institute of Anaesthesiology and the Central Laboratory. As with certain cases coagulation disorders have been described when using the IOAT-system, we were interested in further investigation.

Patients, IOAT-System, Methods

Using Bentley's autotransfusion pump, 31 patients with the following indications were operated.

For the majority of the patients the intraoperative use of the IOAT pump was pre-planned, whereas for 10 of the 31 patients it was an acute necessity.

For autotransfusion Bentley's full occlusive roller pump system combined with the one way autotransfusion unit ATS-200 was used. The extra-corporal system contained 5.000 I.U. heparin in 500 ml of Ringer's lactate solution and all patients were given 75 I.U. heparin/kg body weight intravenously. Due to the long duration of the operation and due to polytransfusions, intraoperative heparin injections were necessary in some cases.

Different changes in hemostasis have already been described when using extra-corporal circulation systems (cardiopulmonary bypass, artificial kidney system etc.). We were specially interested in the consumption coagulopathy which represents one cause for hemostatic disorder. Criteria for the diagnosis of a consumption coagulopathy were: thrombocytopenia, hypofibrinogenemia, occurence of fibrin monomers (positive ethanol test), decrease in antithrombin III and, especially a progressive increase in the coagulation disorder.

Results

Out of the 31 patients, who were operated with the IOAT-system, it was possible to check the blood coagulation of 22 before and after operation and on the following days. Table I. shows that there were 2 different treatment groups, one where the use of the IOAT-system was pre-planned and another where it was an emergency. There was a significant difference in the pumping volume, the

Table I.		pre-planned	acute	total
venous thrombectomies		15	2	17
arterial reconstructions		5	7	12
aneurysma of the aorta (5 cases)				
traumatic injury (5 cases)				
vascular reconstructions				
in the pelvic region (2 cases)				
porto-caval shunts		1	1	2

pumping time and the substitution of volume and blood.

Blood coagulation tests

The fall in the platelet count was considerably greater in the group where the IOAT-system was used in an emergency than in patients with the IOAT-treatment being pre-planned. The average decrease in the platelet count (approx. 58% and 30% respectively) was clearly stronger than the fall between the pre-and postoperative hematocrit values (35% and 20% respectively). There is no direct connection between the thrombocytopenia and the hematocrit changes which were caused by intraoperative volume and blood substitution.

In the treatment group where the IOAT-system was used in an emergency the mean fibrinogen values decreased by 70%, in the group where the use was pre-planned they only decreased by 31%. Even here both groups showed a more pronounced decrease than one would expect from the effect of possible blood dilution with reference to the changes in hematocrit values.

There were no signs of hyperfibrinolysis.

In spite of the fact that by means of intraoperative thrombin time tests the ATS-system as wel as the patient seemed to be sufficiently anti-coagulated with heparin, an activation of blood coagulation (tissue thromboplastin, non-physiological surfaces, foam etc.) and consequently a consumption reaction took place.

Additional facts were the finding of fibrin monomers through positive ethanol tests (in the emergency group in all patients and in the group with pre-planned treatment in 5 out of 13) as well as a decrease in antithrombin III during the time of IOAT. The longer the operation lasted the more pronounced were the changes. From the different intraoperative changes in blood coagulation and platelet count in each patient one can see that the blood dilution effect only plays a minor part. For all the patients a low dosis heparin infusion therapy (250 – 500 I.U./h) made it possible to bring all values back to normal in due course. There was no postoperative bleeding complication.

Conclusions

Intraoperative autotransfusion has proved especially useful in vascular surgery. 31 patients were treated with this system. In spite of a heparin therapy the risk of a consumption coagulopathy in IOAT-treatment still exists. The extent of changes in blood coagulation in emergency or pre-planned use depends on the pumping time and the duration of the operation. A low dosis heparin infusion was very successful; within 24 to 48 hours after operation the hemostasis went back to normal.

The IOAT-system represents an important new way for acute blood substitution. Nevertheless, continual coagulation tests are necessary.

REFERENCES

1. *Feist H. W., E. Götz, G. Warth, G. Baumann, H. M. Becker.* Autotransfusion bei Beckenvenen Thromboseoperationen. Prakt. Anästh. 11. 214, 1976.
2. *Fekete L. F., Bick Rl.* Laboratory Modalities for Assessing Hemostasis During Cardiopulmonary Bypass. Sem. Thrombos. Hemostasis. III, 83, 1976.
3. *Fischer M.* Diagnose der Verbrauchskoagulopathie Wien. Klin. Wschr. 85, 319, 1973.
4. *Homann B., Klaue P.* Erfahrungen mit der intraoperativen Autotransfusion in der Erstversorgung Unfallverletzter. Anästhesiol. Inform. 18, 117, 1977.
5. *Homann B., P. Klaue, S. Hauptvogel* Erste Erfahrungen mit der maschinellen intraoperativen Autotransfusion. Anaesthesist 26, 606, 1977.
6. *Kienninger G., M. Junger, W. Neugebauer, K. Schmidt* Die intraoperative Autotransfusion. Prakt. Anästh. 11, 203, 1976.
7. *Rakower Sr., Worth M. H., Bermans J., Lackner H.* Hämostatic and homeostatic changes following massive autotransfusion in the dog. J. Trauma. 14, 594, 1974.

M. F., Municipal Hospital Vienna-Lainz, Centrallaboratory, Wolkersbergenstr. A-1130, Vienna, 1, Austria

THROMBOGENIC AND ATHEROGENIC INFLUENCE OF CASTRATION IN WOMEN

A. NOVOTNÝ and V. DVOŘÁK

Clinic of Obstetrics and Gynaecology of Faculty of Medical Hygiene, Charles University, Prague, Czechoslovakia

The relationship between the incidence of atherosclerosis, ischaemic heart disease and venous thromboembolism and sex, i.e. the higher incidence of atherosclerotic diseases in men and higher rate of thromboembolic disease in women has been known for a long time.

We tried to establish whether the incidence of atherosclerotic disease and ischaemic heart disease is higher in women after artificial surgical elimination of ovarian function by castration than in other women with intact activity of the ovaries. To this end a group of 372 patients (159 men and 213 women) were subjected to a detailed medical examination. This group comprised 18 women who had undergone surgical castration, i.e. 8.4% of the total mumber of women. This percentage is relatively high and may be explained by the fact that some time ago for fear of possible malignant reversal of ovarian tissue during gynaecological laparotomies in a large percentage so-called preventive castration was performed.

Atherosclerosis was revealed in a relatively high percentage: in 76 men (48.1%) and 109 women (50.3%). The percentage was very high in castrated women where it was diagnosed in 13 of 18 women, i.e. in 72.2%. This higher incidence as compared with the frequency of atherosclerosis in the whole group, was statiscally significant. When attempting to divide the investigated group according to age, we observed that after castration women developed signs of atherosclerosis at a younger age than the remaining patients and the frequency rose steeply. According to our findings in castrated women where the ovarian function was suddenly interrupted atherosclerosis begins at an earlier age and is more frequent than in noncastrated women.

Ischaemic heart disease was recorded in 75 patients of our group: in 18.9% of the men and 21.3% of the women. In the group of castrated patients the rate of ischaemic heart disease was highest, i.e. 55.5% (10 of 18 women). The differences in the incidence of this disease in castrated and non-castrated women was statistically significant. When analyzing these data with regard to age we recorded a rise of the disease in men and women up to the age of 65 years; then in men a decline was recorded while in women the rate continued to increase up to the oldest age groups. The curve of incidence of IHD in castrated women was high above the corresponding curve for men and noncastrated women. Based on these findings we may that obviously the ovary plays an important part in the pathogenesis of atherosclerosis and ischaemic heart disease.

Next we were concerned with the influence of avarian function on venous thrombogenesis, i.e. on the rate of thromboembolic disease of venous origin. In our previous work we revealed some important facts indicating for instance an increased incidence of this disease at the time of decline or cessation of ovarian activity. Our findings of the incidence of thromboembolic complications after gynaecological operations associated with castration are of great interest.

There are clearly marked differences in the incidence of venous thromboses (9.18% in operations incl. castration and 4.39% in operations without castration).

It is very difficult to explain the above great and significant differences otherwise than by the preservation or removal of the ovaries. Castration performed along with hysterectomy practically does not protract the operation, it does not involve greater traumatization or devastation of tissues. Patients where the ovaries are preserved are somewhat younger than castrated women, but the difference is not big enough to explain the revealed differences in the incidence of thromboembolic complications. These facts are in our opinion evidence that ovarian hormones influence not only the arterial and cardiac but also the venous part of the circulation. We found that removal of the ovaries has late sequelae such as higher incidence of atherosclerosis and ischaemic heart disease. It has also early sequelae which are manifested by a greater risk of the development of postoperative thromboembolism.

We examined under strictly standard conditions total serum lipoproteins and the lipoprotein spectrum by electrophoresis on paper, where three fractions were assessed (alpha, beta and the start fraction ypsilon). The estimations were made closely before the operation and than on the 1st and 3rd and 6th day after operation. We examined thus a total of 50 women who were divided into three groups. The group included 20 women after abdominal hysterectomy with castration on account of uterine myomas, 15 women after minor laparotomies where the ovaries were preserved and 15 patients after vaginal plastic operations.

In the first group of patients (hysterectomy with castration) we observed an initial decline of lipoproteinaemia, resembling the decline in the concentration of other substances (e.g. total proteins). This decline was, however, followed starting on the first day by a rise up to the sixth day. Assessment of the lipoprotein spectrum revealed that the observed rise of lipoproteinaemia was due above all to a change of the electrophoretic lipoprotein fraction L-beta. The variations in group II (laparotomy without castration) were as expected and in group III we observed only irregular variations.

We investigated this important finding of early post-castration dyslipoproteinaemia further by examining a larger group of operated women (70 operated patients, incl. 40 castrated women). We used a simpler method, described by Burnstein, where only coarsely disperesed lipoproteins, in particular fraction beta, is assessed. After operations associated with castration we observed immediately after operation a brisk decline of the lipoprotein concentration, followed from the first day onwards by a rapid rise. In the remaining laparotomies (group II) there was a slight rise starting only on the 3rd day. After plastic operations (group III) we observed a considerable variation of values.

The immediate consequence of this dyslipoproteinaemia is a certain deviation in the coagulation balance which leads to an increased risk of the development of thromboembolic complications.

The assessed changes of serum lipoproteins are of an adverse character and they may be regarded as changes which later lead to the development of metabolic disorders causing atherosclerosis and ischaemic heart disease. Both these diseases are encountered according to our findings more frequently in castrated women than in the other patients.

The ovaries thus appear to be important organs the function of which – in particular oestrogenic steroidogenesis – influence the lipid metabolism, on the condition of the venous and arterial wall and blood clotting. After their removal several phenomena develop which we include under the term of postcastration syndrome.

A. N., Clinic of Gynaecology, Šrobárova 50, 10034 Prague 10, Czechoslovakia

METABOLISM OF VASCULAR WALL

METABOLIC DISTURBANCES
HEMODYNAMIC FACTORS
PSYCHOLOGICAL STRESS

SERUM LIPOPROTEIN ABNORMALITIES IN EARLY STAGES OF PERIPHERAL ATHEROSCLEROSIS

P. KIRSTEIN and A.G. OLSSON

King Gustaf V Research Institute and Department of Medicine, Karolinska Hospital, Stockholm, Sweden

Introduction

Many studies have been published in the last ten years concerning serum lipids and atherosclerosis of the lower limbs. Almost all these studies have dealt with total cholesterol and triglycerides. To our knowledge no study has as yet been published on analyses of quantitatively determined serum lipoproteins, particularly high density lipoproteins (HDL). We have analysed serum lipoproteins in patients referred for the first time with the disease. No patient had already been treated for the disease. This is a report of the results from the first 51 patients.

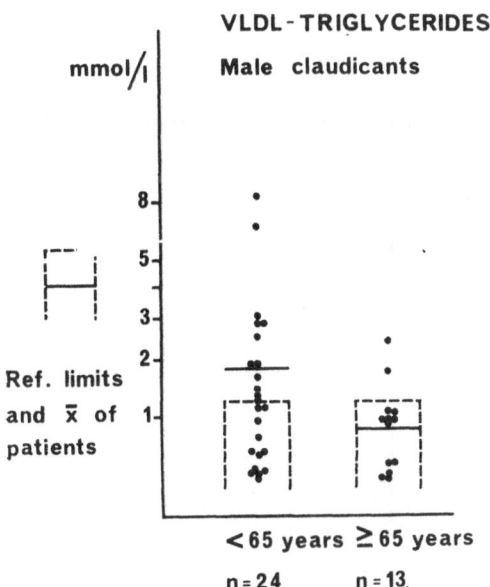

VLDL - TRIGLYCERIDES

Male claudicants

mmol/l

Ref. limits and x̄ of patients

<65 years   ≥65 years

n = 24   n = 13

Fig. 1.

Material

All the patients (37 males, 14 females, mean age 62 for both sexes) had recently suffered from the symptoms of atherosclerosis in the legs. Diabetics were excluded.

Methods

The diagnosis was made by non-invasive methods: digital pulse plethysmography, quantitative segmental pulse volume recording, ancle and toe blood pressures at rest and after treadmill exercise.

After an overnight fast venous blood was withdrawn for measurement of serum lipids and lipoproteins. Cholesterol and triglycerides were measured in the lipoprotein classes of very low (VLDL), low (LDL) and high (HDL) density. After ultracentrifugation at d = 1.006 and precipitation of LDL (bottom fraction) with heparin and $MnCl_2$ agarose gel electrophoresis was carried out on whole serum and top and bottom ultracentrifugal fractions.

Results and discussion

About 1/4 of the men had type IV. Type II A + II B and type III were found in less than 10%. 50% of the women had type II A or II B. Thus about half of the men and women were normal. Taking a VLDL cholesterol/triglyceride ratio of ≥0.78 as a sign of altered VLDL metabolism we found another 16% of male patients with lipoprotein abnormalities. Late pre-β (PLβ) bands seen in agarose gel electrophoresis of VLDL (*Olsson et al.* 1977) were found in just over 50% against 40% in a population of healthy 40 year old men (n.s. difference). LPβ bands are thought to represent intermediary lipoprotein particles.

The mean serum VLDL triglyceride concentration of the men, 1.47 ± 0.27

107

(SEM) mmol/l, was higher than that of the women, 0.89 ± 0.08 mmol/l (p < < 0.05). Men <65 years had higher serum VLDL triglyceride level compared to older men, 1.82 ± 0.40 mmol/l versus 0.83 ± 0.16 mmol/l (p < 0.05). (Fig. 1.)

The mean serum LDL cholesterol concentration for the men, 4.37 ± 0.16 mmol/l, was within our reference limits but lower than that for the women, 5.43 ± 0.34 mmol/l (p < 0.01) which was elevated in all age groups. (Fig. 2.)

The serum HDL cholesterol concentration in men increased with age (Fig. 3). HDL cholesterol in males <65 years was 1.15 ± 0.05 mmol/l versus 1.72 ± 0.17 mmol/l in older males (p < 0.005). Normal materials giving reference levels for HDL cholesterol in older men is lacking but Carlson and Ericsson, 1975, gave a mean concentration of 1.33 mmol/l for the age group 50−59. In the present material the mean HDL cholesterol of that age group was significantly lower, 1.14 ± ± 0.06 mmol/l (p < 0.01). The mean HDL cholesterol in women which generally tends to be higher than that in men was 1.55 ± 0.08 mmol/l in our patients.

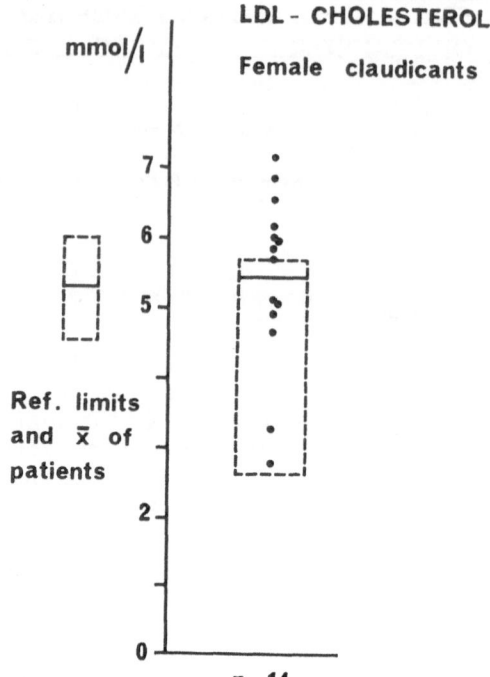

Fig. 2.

Conclusions

These preliminaty data on serum lipoprotein analyses in patients with new symptoms of atherosclerosis of the legs have shown: 1) Men <65 years had significantly elevated VLDL triglycerides compared to older men. 2) Women had significantly elevated mean LDL cholesterol compared to men for all age groups. 3) Men 50−59 years had significantly lower mean HDL cholesterol compared to normal men of the same age. Men had increasing HDL cholesterol with age. 4) There was a tendency to increased frequency of late pre-β (LPβ) bands.

In younger men low HDL cholesterol might be a risk factor for peripheral atherosclerosis of the legs as has been shown for coronary and cerebral atherosclerosis.

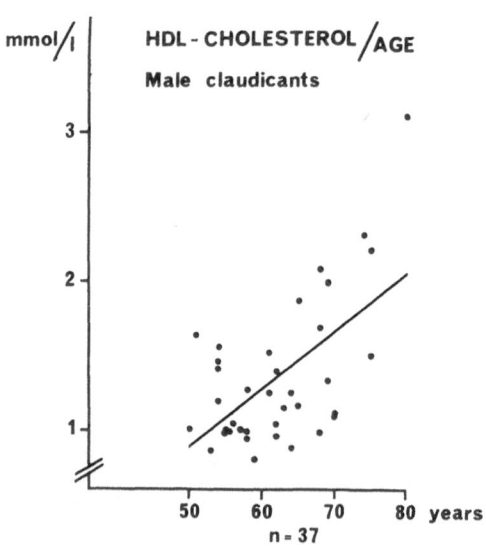

Fig. 3.

REFERENCES

Carlson, L. A., Ericsson, M. (1975) Quantitative and qualitative serum lipoprotein analysis. Atherosclerosis 21, 417.

Greenhalgh, R. M., Rosengarten, D. S., Mervart, I., Lewis, B., Calnan, J. S., Martin, P. (1971) Serum lipids and lipoproteins in peripheral vascular disease. Lancet II, 947.

Olsson, A. G., Carlson, K., Carlson, L. A. Late pre-β lipoproteins (LPβ) of serum very low density lipoproteins. Proceedings of Conference on Atherosclerosis, Milan 1977. Raven Press. In press.

P. K., King Gustaf V Research Institute, Karolinska Hospital, S-104 01 Stockholm, Sweden

HYPERLIPOPROTEINEMIA AND PERIPHERAL ARTERIAL DISEASE

D. SIEVERS, H. M. SAHLENDER and W. SCHOOP

Aggertalklinik, Engelskirchen, G.F.R.

Numerous studies on the risk profile of peripheral arterial occlusion disease (PAD) have shown an increased incidence of disorders of lipid metabolism. However, the data on the frequency and types of the disorders of lipid metabolism exhibit great differences. The present study performed on a large collective using lipoprotein electrophoresis and the preparative ultracentrifuge is conceived as a further contribution to evaluation of the role of hyperlipoproteinemia (HLP) and its types as risk factors in PAD.

Over a period of 6 months HLP was sought in almost all of the 1198 inpatients of a clinic for vascular diseases. A cholesterol value of 300 mg/dl and/or a triglyceride value of 200 mg/dl was fixed as the upper normative limit of lipid concentration in serum. From the group of patients with demonstrated lipid metabolism disorders, 160 patients were selected on a random basis and their lipoproteins analysed and typed according to the Fredrickson scheme. In this collective, further risk factors, such as cigarette smoking, hypertension and diabetes mellitus were also determined.

The control group consisted largely of patients with venous conditions or degenerative diseases of the spine.

The first lipid determination was made one week after inpatient admission at the end of a 12–16 hour period of fasting. For typing of a lipid metabolic disorder after Fredrickson, fasting blood was taken again on the following day and a lipoprotein electrophoresis performed on agaragarose gel as well as a preparative ultracentrifugation. A value of 190 mg/dl was fixed as the upper normative limit for the β-cholesterol concentration.

The angiological findings were based on anamnesis, measurement of the pulse, vascular auscultation and mechanical oscillogram of the legs at rest and in exercise. In about 2/3 of the patients of the group with determination of the lipoprotein type and PAD, the vascular finding was checked angiographically.

	n	HLP	%
PAD	683	316	46,3
CONTROLS	443	122	27,5
TOTAL	1126	438	38,9

Table: Frequency of hyperlipoproteinemia (HLP) in patients with peripheral arterial occlusive disease of the lower limbs (PAD) and in controls (cholesterol $\geq$300 mg/dl and/or triglycerides $\geq$200 mg/dl.

Table I. This table depicts the frequency of HLP in patients with PAD and in control subjects. In the PAD group the percentage rate was 46,3 and in the controls 27.5. The frequency of HLP in the PAD group is nearly twice as high as in the controls. The total collective consisted of 1126 persons, 438 of them suffered from HLP.

Hypercholesterolemia, hypertriglyceridemia and a combination of both of 438 patients with HLP subdivided into a PAD group (n = 316) and control group (n = 122). The combination of hypercholesterolemia and hypertriglyceridemia was predominant in the PAD group, $p < 0.01$. In the control group, on the other hand, patients with hypercholesterolemia predominated ($p < 0.05$). The serum lipid concentrations did not differ appreciably in the two collectives.

Figure 1: This figure depicts the distribution of HLP types after Fredrickson of 160 patients taken from a total HLP collective of 438 persons. The PAD

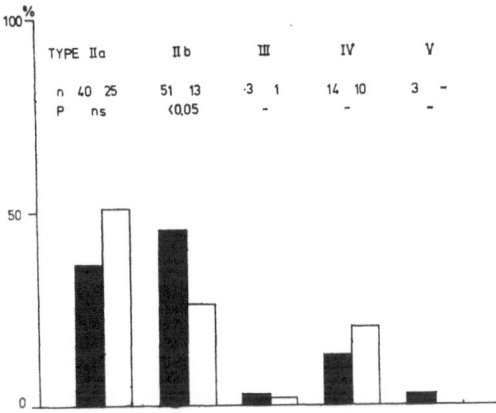

Fig. 1. Distribution of the hyperlipoproteinemia types according to Fredrickson in 111 patients with peripheral arterial occlusive disease of the lower limbs ■ and 49 controls □.

group (black columns) consisted of 111 patients, the control (white columns) of 49 patients. A prevalence of type II b was found in the PAD group (p < 0.05). The incidence of type II a did not show any

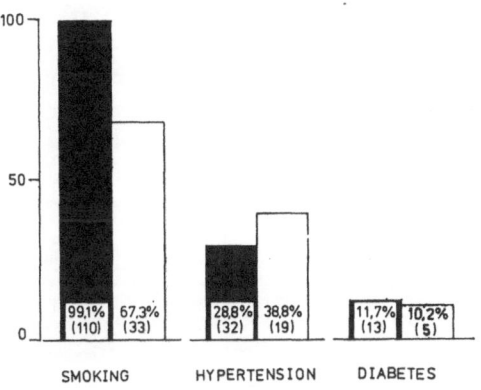

Fig. 2. Distribution of further risk factors in 111 patients with peripheral arterial occlusive disease of the lower limbs ■ and 49 controls □.

significant difference between the two groups.

Figure 2: This figure demonstrates the frequency of further risk factors for 160 patients with HLP typing after Fredrickson: Black columns PAD group, white columns control group. Except a different rate of cigarette smoking in the two collectives, no differences were found as regards hypertension and diabetes mellitus. In the PAD group, the age was 53.2 ± 7.3 years, and in the control group 49.7 ± 9.1 years; the body weight was 78.3 ± 10.9 kg and 84.4 ± 15.7 kg and the proportion of male patients 95.5% and 67.3% respectively.

Three aspects must be considered when evaluating the results of studies of disorders in lipid metabolism.

1. The structure of the investigated collective with regard to age, sex and body weight.

2. Living habits, food, alcohol consumption and medication.

3. The criteria for fixing the normative range of serum lipid concentrations.

Any alteration in one of these points leads to a shift in the frequency of occurrence and distribution of the HLP types. This may explain the appreciable variations in the findings of various authors.

In a review, Kremer (1973) states that the mean frequency of disorders of lipid metabolism in arterial occlusive disease is 45% (range $25-74\%$). The frequency of 46.3% which we found is in agreement with this value. There is further agreement with other authors in the finding that disorders in lipid metabolism are demonstrable twice or several times as frequently in patients with arterial occlusions as in corresponding control groups.

In patients with arterial occlusions and HLP, some authors have observed a higher frequency of Fredrickson type II whereas others more frequently found type IV HLP. These differences are probably attributable to the different examination procedures, especially with regard to different settings of upper normal values of lipids in serum. Our high triglyceride value of 200 mg/dl may well explain the low frequency of type IV which we found. Our results show a significant increase in the combination of hypercholesterolemia and hypertriglyceridemia and corresponding a higher frequency of type II b in PAD patients as compared to a control collective. A similar finding is indicated in the study by Kremer (1973), which was performed using a similar methodology. The study of Skrede (1975) also shows a similar tendency with a higher frequency of the combination of hypercholesterol-emia and hypertriglyceridemia in PAD patients as compared to controls. On the other hand, a series of studies shows an increase in type IV in PAD patients. In the interpretation of these differences, the background of further atherogenic risks must be taken into account; their importance may be greater than that of HLP. A cumulation of one of these risk factors in a certain HLP type may be responsible for the higher frequency of arterial occlusions in this type.

D.S., Aggertalklinik, Engelskirchen, G.F.R.

SERUM LIPOPROTEIN DISTRIBUTION IN 103 NONAGENARIANS

H. HECKERS, W. BURKHARD, D. PLATT and W. FUHRMANN

Center of Internal Medicine and Institute of Human Genetics,
Justus-Liebig University, Giessen, F.R.G.

Introduction

Data on blood lipid and lipoprotein concentrations in relation to different age groups covering the range up to 70 eyars of life are available from many epidemiological studies (*Svanborn et al.*, 1977; *Gordon et al.*, 1977; *Kritchevsky*, 1978). Comparable studies on representative groups of very old people are almots completely missing (*Franke*, 1978) although they may contribute some important information on the mechanism of an uncommonly high life expectancy. Repeatedly it has been demonstrated (*Franke*, 1978) that a very high life expectancy is, among other things, a consequence of a weak tendency to atherosclerotic complications. These observations suggest the hypothesis that the risk factor profile of this age group is exceedingly low. Moreover it can be speculated that an unusually high life expectancy may, in part, be due to some syndromes of lipoprotein metabolism which have lately been investigated in detail, i.e. familial hyper-alpha- and/or hypobeta-lipoproteinemia.

Both are said to represent "antirisk" factors with regard to atherosclerosis and to facilitate distinctive longevity (*Glueck et al.*, 1977).

As part of a retrospective study on cardiovascular risk factors in a statistically representative group of 103 nonagenarians, the results of the fasting lipid and lipoprotein values are described here.

Methods

Blood was taken from the subjects receiving their usual diets after an overnight fast. Lipid and lipoprotein determinations were performed after one ultracentrifugal separation of serum at d 1.006 for 18 hours at 40 000 rpm (105 000 × g) in a rotor 40.3 (Spinco model L5.50 preparative ultracentrifuge, Beckman Instruments GmbH, München, Germany), followed by precipitation (*Burstein and Samaille*, 1960) of LDL (low density (beta) lipoproteins), lipid electrophoresis (*Gret.n et al.*, 1970) of whole serum, top and bottom fractions after ultracentrifugation and HDL (high density (alpha) lipoproteins) fraction after precipitation and chemical analysis of cholesterol (*Röschlau*, 1974) and triglycerides (*Eggstein and Kreutz*, 1966). All values are given as mean values of a duplicate analysis. Data on the lipid moieties of VLDL (very low (pre-β) lipoproteins) and LDL were obtained by the subtraction method.

Tab. 1 Mean fasting lipoprotein composition in unselected more than ninety years old people. Triglyceride (mmol/1) and cholesterol (mg/100 ml) concentration in the 3 LP classes, ratio of LDL-cholesterol/HDL-cholesterol and presence of sinking pre ß LP. Mean value ± S.E.M.

	TOTAL		VLDL		LDL		HDL		LDL/HDL	SINKING PRE ß
	TG	Chol	TG	Chol	TG	Chol	TG	Chol	Chol	
Males	1.06±	203.5±	0.62±	18.3±	0.23±	133.8±	0.21±	51.8±	2.76±	18 (n)
(n=33)	0.38	42.1	0.34	8.2	0.09	38.5	0.07	14.3	1.15	
Females	1.64±	219.0±	1.04±	26.6±	0.35+	137.8±	0.27±	54.4±	2.76±	40 (n)
(n=70)	1.15	46.4	1.03	26.6	0.27	37.5	0.09	15.5	1.14	
All	1.46±	214.6±	0.90±	24.0±	0.31±	136±	0.25±	53.6±	2.76±	48 (n)
(n=103)	1.01	45.4	0.89	22.7	0.23	37.7	0.09	15.1	1.14	

TG = triglycerides; Chol = cholesterol

113

Results and discussion

The female/male ratio of all people over 90 years of age living in the Federal Republic of Germany in 1975 was 2.16, whereas the sex ratio in our study was 2.25 in favour of the females. In Tab. I. the mean concentration of cholesterol and triglycerides in total serum and in the 3 LP (lipoprotein) classes is given for each group (of males and females) and for the whole group of nonagenarians, completed by the data on sinking pre-β lipoprotein (Lp (a) lipoprotein). The high incidence of sinking pre-β LP in very old subjects does not confirm the assumption that Lp (a) might represent a genetic risk factor with respect to coronary heart disease (CHD) (*Dahlen*, 1974).

Our results indicate that mean lipid and lipoprotein values in nonagenarians are rather low. Though the average difference is small, the mean values of HDL cholesterol and LDL cholesterol are higher in female than in male nonagenarians. Based on the atherogenic index LDL cholesterol/ /HDL cholesterol, which takes into account that LDL cholesterol is positively and HDL cholesterol is negatively correlated to the risk of CHD, no difference exists between the two sexes. Compared to the results of the cooperative lipoprotein phenotyping study (*Castelli et al.*, 1977) nonagenarians do not have higher mean HDL cholesterol levels than septuagenarians. In addition, our study does not confirm the finding that hyperalpha-and/or

hypobeta-lipoproteinemia is of special importance in distinctive longevity (*Glueck et al.*, 1977 (see Figrs 1 and 2). None of the very old people investigated had a LDL cholesterol value greater than 225 mg%.

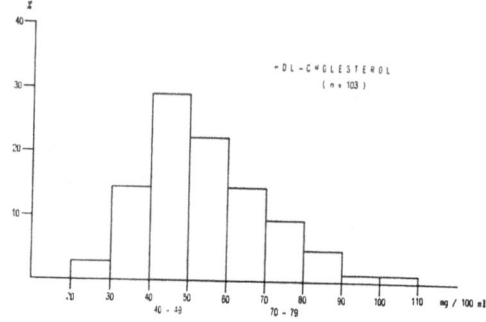

Fig. 1. Distribution of HDL cholesterol in an unselected group of 103 nonagenerians.

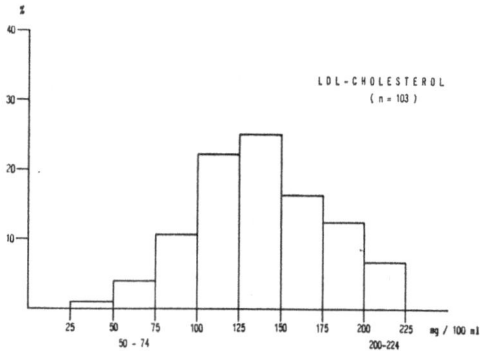

Fig. 2. Distribution of LDL cholesterol in an unselected group of 103 nonagenerians.

REFERENCES

Castelli, W. P., Doyle, J. T., Gordon, T., Hames, C. G., Hjortland, M. C., Hulley, S. B., Kagan, A., Zukel, W. J. (1977) HDL cholesterol and other lipids in coronary heart disease. The cooperative lipoprotein phenotyping study. Circulation 55, 767—772.

Franke, H. (1978) Kriterien der Langlebigkeit mit entsprechenden klinischen Beobachtungen bei 356 Überhundertjährigen der Bundesrepublik Deutschland. Internist 19, in press.

Glueck, C. J., Gartside, P. S., Steiner, P. M., Miller, M., Todhunter, T., Haaf, J., Pucke, M.,

Terrana, M., Fallat, R. W., Kashyap, M. L. (1977) Hyperalpha- and hypobeta-lipoproteinemia in octogenarian kindreds. Atherosclerosis 27, 387—406.

Gordon, T., Castelli, W. P., Hjortland, M. C., Kannel, W. B., Dawber, T. R. (1977) High density lipoprotein as a protective factor against coronary heart disease. Am. J. Med. 62, 707—713.

Kritchevsky, D. (1978) How aging affects cholesterol metabolism. Postgr. Med. 63, 133—135.

H. H., Center of Internal Medicine, Justus-Liebig-University, D-6300 Giessen, F.R.G.

ARTERIO-VENOUS DIFFERENCES OF VARIOUS PLASMA PROTEINS IN PERIPHERAL VASCULAR DISEASE

F. S. FERUGLIO, A. PEZZOLI and E. PASCALI

Institute of Medical Clinic and Therapy, University of Trieste, Italy

In a study of the behaviour of the plasma protein pattern in vascular disease, the results of 15 plasma protein quantitative determinations simultaneously carried out in the arterious and venous blood of a group of patients with chronic obstructive arterial disease of the lower limbs — are presented.

The plasma proteins were selected because of their biological role as acute phase reactants (ceruloplasmin, haptoglobin, orosomucoid, C-reactive protein, fibrinogen), protease-inhibitors (α_1 antitrypsin, α_1 antichymotrypsin, $\varkappa_2$ macroglobulin, antithrombin III) Ig's (IgG, IgA, IgM), albumin, prealbumin and transferrin. 21 subjects (17 males, 4 females) with a mean age of 60 (47—78) years with chronic untreated obstructive arterial disease of the lower limbs were examined. According Lériche, 10 patients (48%) were classified in the 2nd stage, 2(9%) in the 3rd stage and 9(43%) in the 4th stage. Clinical and laboratory investigations excluded any association with other disease; none of the patients was diabetic. As controls 10 normal subjects (5 males, 5 females) of the same age group (mean 57 years) without any vascular and coagulative alteration were examined.

In patients blood samples were simultaneously obtained from the femoral vein draining the limb mainly affected by lesion and from the femoral artery. In the control group blood was drawn under the same conditions from femoral vein and artery.

For all the samples the determination of individual proteins was preceded by agarose zone electrophoresis in order to point out abnormalities which could interfere with the immunochemical determination. The presence of M-components, hemolysis, α_1 antitrypsin deficiency (and heterozygosity for the gene for deficiency) and differences of haptoglobin genotypes were particularly excluded. The immunochemical determination was carried out on plasma samples for fibrinogen and antithrombin III and on serum samples for the other proteins by the single radial immunodiffusion method. Immunodiffusion plates prepared in our laboratory with monospecific antisera were used. The system adapted allows simultaneous duplicate determination of 12 samples with double calibration curves for 5 standard dilutions and double internal control. For each plasma protein tested the difference between the arterial and venous concentration obtained in patients was compared with controls. The significance of the differences between the mean values was calculated by the Student t-test. „p" values lower than 0.05 were considered as significant.

Tables I and II summarize the results. The lack of correlations between reduction of protein levels in venous blood and molecular weights (Table III) is in disagreement with the presence of passive and aspecific "trapping" phenomena at the peripheral level. It is therefore unlikely that a "molecular sieving" effect is associated with the vascular lesion that controls the venous concentration of plasma proteins in relation to their size. The reduced concentrations in venous blood appear justified when the biological role of the plasma proteins, which present the most significant arterio-venous differences, is considered. For many of the studied proteins, such differences could be considered as an expression of "consumtion". Such a mechanism could explain the results obtained from the quantization of the main protease inhibitors (α_1 antitrypsin, α_2 macroglobulin, antichymotrypsin, antithrombin III). Particularly the interference of α_2 macroglobulin with coagulative and fibrinolytic systems is well known. This polyvalent protease inhibitor, moreover, seems to be specifically bound to human vascular endothelium. The relationship between hemostasis and atherosclerosis could explain the arterio-venous differences observed for antithrombin III and fibrinogen which both could have an important role in initiating and/or per-

115

Table I.

PROTEINS g/l	sample	PATIENTS n = 21			CONTROLS n = 10			
		R	x̄	SD	R	x	SD	
PREALBUMIN	A	0.09— 0.37	0.24	0.07	0.10— 0.30	0.19	0.07	$p < 0.01$
	V	0.08— 0.36	0.23	0.07	0.10— 0.30	0.19	0.07	
ALBUMIN	A	33.1 —43.7	38.9	3.0	33.2 —49.0	39.4	5.1	NS
	V	33.1 —43.1	37.9	3.0	33.2 —49.0	39.1	4.9	
TRANSFERRIN	A	1.66— 4.10	2.68	0.58	1.71— 3.44	2.42	0.53	NS
	V	1.66— 4.10	2.66	0.57	1.60— 3.43	2.37	0.53	
CERULOPLASMIN	A	0.30— 0.61	0.41	0.08	0.30— 0.61	0.42	0.10	$p < 0.01$
	V	0.26— 0.57	0.39	0.09	0.30— 0.61	0.42	0.10	
HAPTOGLOBIN	A	1.02— 5.71	2.74	1.27	1.46— 5.44	3.00	1.54	NS
	V	0.83— 5.33	2.65	1.23	1.46— 5.11	3.00	1.52	
OROSOMUCOID (α_1 ac. glycoprot.)	A	0.69— 1.49	1.02	0.22	0.59— 1.86	0.95	7.40	$p < 0.001$
	V	0.65— 1.49	0.93	0.22	0.59— 1.86	0.95	0.40	
C-REACTIVE PROT. mg/l	A	3.0 —87.5	15.4	19.5	2.2 —61.7	12.0	19.5	$p < 0.05$
	V	2.0 —86.3	14.1	18.6	2.2 —61.7	12.0	19.5	
FIBRINOGEN	A	2.6 — 5.6	3.9	0.9	2.2 — 4.5	3.1	0.8	$p < 0.001$
	V	2.1 — 5.1	3.5	0.9	2.2 — 4.5	3.1	0.8	

Table II.

PROTEINS g/l	sample	PATIENTS n = 21			CONTROLS n = 10			
		R	x̄	SD	R	x̄	SD	
α_1 ANTITRYPSIN	A	2.06— 5.04	3.34	0.84	1.80— 5.16	3.37	1.09	$p < 0.01$
	V	1.88— 4.82	3.14	0.80	1.80— 5.16	3.36	1.09	
α_1 ANTICHYMO-TRYPSIN	A	0.40— 1.17	0.64	0.20	0.21— 1.44	0.63	0.40	$p < 0.001$
	V	0.40— 1.14	0.62	0.19	0.21— 1.44	0.63	0.40	
α_2 MACRO-GLOBULIN	A	1.26— 4.90	2.43	0.97	1.33— 2.77	2.14	0.50	$p < 0.01$
	V	1.14— 4.64	2.27	0.98	1.33— 2.77	2.14	0.50	
ANTI-THROMBIN III	A	0.17— 0.39	0.30	0.05	0.21— 0.28	0.25	0.03	$p < 0.001$
	V	0.17— 0.39	0.27	0.05	0.21— 0.28	0.25	0.03	
IgG	A	7.9 —25.0	14.1	4.6	6.2 —18.0	10.4	4.3	NS
	V	7.6 —25.0	13.9	4.5	6.2 —18.0	10.2	4.3	
IgA	A	0.8 — 6.4	3.5	1.3	0.7 — 4.3	2.3	1.1	$p < 0.01$
	V	0.8 — 6.4	3.3	1.3	0.7 — 4.3	2.3	1.1	
IgM	A	0.7 — 3.7	1.7	0.9	0.7 — 3.9	1.5	1.0	NS
	V	0.7 — 3.7	1.6	0.9	0.7 — 3.9	1.5	1.0	

petuating arterial lesions. Orosomucoid (or α_1 acid glycoprotein, reviewed by *Schmid* 1975) seems to have functions which do not limit its biological role to that of a simple APR. Interferences have been proposed with cell proliferation, with the formation of collagen fibers, with platelets (which seem to have significant amounts of the protein bound tightly to their membrane) and with the blood clotting mechanism (primarily at the level of the prothrombin activation). CRP is a trace constituent of normal plasma which acts as a very sensitive and early APR. Its function as a fagocytosis-promoting factor and the interactions with the complement system are known.

The interpretation of the results obtained

Table III.

PROTEINS	MW (after Putnam 1975)	A—V differences
OROSOMUCOID	40.000	$p < 0.001$
α_1 ANTITRYPSIN	54.000	$p < 0.01$
PREALBUMIN	54.980	$p < 0.01$
ANTITHROMBIN III	65.000	$p < 0.001$
ALBUMIN	66.000	NS
α_1 ANTICHYMOTRYPSIN	68.000	$p < 0.001$
TRANSFERRIN	76.500	NS
C-REACTIVE PROTEIN	118.000	$p < 0.05$
CERULOPLASMIN	151.000	$p < 0.01$
IgG	160.000	NS
IgA	160.000	$p < 0.01$
FIBRINOGEN	340.000	$p < 0.001$
HAPTOGLOBIN 2-2	400.000	NS
α_2 MACROGLOBULIN	725.000	$p < 0.01$
IgM	950 000	NS

for prealbumin, ceruloplasmin and IgA could be more difficult. In particular, the decreased venous concentration of IgA does not seem sufficient for immunological interpretations. At the present time, moreover, there does not seem to be coherete direct evidence that immune mechanisms actually promote human atherogenesis (with the exception, perhaps, of the graft rejection reactions).

An approach to vascular dissease from a protidological point of view seems very useful, in the explanation of etiopathogenesis of atherosclerosis, because of possible physiopathological, clinical and therapeutical implications. We therefore feel justified in pursuing this kind of investigation.

Further information could be obtained
— from study of a greater number of patients and from comparison of arteriovenous differences among more homogeneous groups (single clinical stages, cases with atherosclerotic and non atherosclerotic arteriopathy, cases of acute arterial obstruction, cases with peripheral tissue lesion of non arteriopathic origin);
— from extension of the investigation to other plasma proteins (blood coagulation proteins, fibrinolytic and complement systems);
— from evaluation of the modified biological activity of proteins.

Apart from the etiopathogenesis of the lesion, we consider important, from a clinical point of view, to obtain further information (in terms of protidology) about the progress of the lesion with time and its metabolic consequences. It is not unlikely that the spontaneous and progressive worsening of the vascular disease has physiopathological causes different and independent from the etiological agents.

If this kind of investigation were extended, plasma protein studies could become essential for more correct clinical staging, for monitoring the course of the disease and in the choice of a more suitable (pharmacological or surgical) treatment.

The progress of knowledge about the behaviour of the plasma protein pattern in vascular disease could contribute to conditioning therapeutical alternatives which consider the protein physiopathology.

A STUDY OF LOW AND VERY LOW DENSITY LIPOPROTEINS PENETRATION, A RADIOACTIVE LABEL IN THE CORE OF THE LIPOPROTEIN PARTICLE, INTO THE ARTERIAL WALL

A. N. KLIMOV

The Anitchkov Department of Biochemistry of Lipids and Atherosclerosis, Institute of Experimental Medicine, Leningrad, USSR

Introduction

In our experiments carried out earlier it was shown that, after administration of VLDL and LDL, containing a radioactive label in the lipid and protein moieties of the lipoproteins, into rabbits with experimental hypercholesterolemia the lipid/ /protein radioactivity ratio in the lipoproteins of the plasma and aorta in rabbit-recipients was rather simular.

Thus it was concluded that the lipoproteins penetrate into the arterial wall rather without preliminary splitting, i. e. as intact particles.

When studying penetration into the aorta by labelled lipoproteins, containing a label on the surface of the lipoprotein particle (in unesterified cholesterol, phospholipids, and apoproteins), one cannot exclude the physico-chemical exchange of these components between the lipoproteins of the plasma and vascular wall, which complicates interpretation of the data obtained. In connection with the latter we prepared rabbit VLDL and LDL, containing a radioactive label (^{14}C-palmitic acid) predominantly in the core of the lipoprotein particle — in trriglycerides (TG) and ethers of cholesterol (ECh). Part of the label was contained in the lipoprotein phospholipids (PL).

Methods and materials

In order to prepare such lipoproteins ^{14}C-palmitic acid in a complex with albumin in a dose of about 5mCi was administered intravenously into rabbits with experimental hypercholesterolemia. In 48 hours the animals were decapitated and as much blood as possible was collected. VLDL, LDL or the total fraction of these lipoproteins were isolated from the blood plasma by the method of preparative ultra-

Table I. Percentage distribution of radioactivity among PL, ECh, and TG in rabbit plasma and aorta lipoproteins 24—48 hours following intravenous administration of homologous lipoproteins labelled by ^{14}C-palmitic acid

Class of lipoproteins	Number of experiments	Distribution of radioactivity in U (mean)		
		PL	ECh	TG
VLDL + LDL used for administration	3	16	13	71
VLDL + LDL of the plasma		37	44	19
VLDL + LDL of the aorta		57	27	16
VLDL used for administration	2	21	19	60
VLDL of the plasma		57	29	14
LDL of the plasma		65	26	9
VLDL + LDL of the aorta		63	26	11
LDL used for administration	2	36	18	46
VLDL of the plasma		37	28	35
LDL of the plasma		64	25	11
VLDL + LDL of the aorta		65	15	20

centrifugation. After dialysis against a physiological solution an aliquota of isolated lipoproteins was delipidated with a mixture of chloroform-methanol, and the lipid extract was treated by thin layer chromatography. Sections of the chromatogram corresponding to PL, TG, and ECh were scraped off to determine the radioactivity in a scintillation counter. The basal volume of the dialysate, containing labelled lipoproteins, was used for intravenous administration into rabbit-recipients, which also had experimental hypercholesterolemia. Lipoproteins of the aortic wall were isolated by adding heparin and calcium ions to the buffer extract of the tissue with subseqent precipitation of the total fraction of VLDL and LDL. The procedure has been described in detail in earlier publications.

Results and discussion

In all cases the isolated labelled lipoproteins from the blood plasma of rabbit-donors contained the highest percentage of label in the TG component (from 46 to 71%), then followed the by PL component (from 16 to 36%); ECh contained the least label (from 13 to 19%).

After intravenous administration of these lipoproteins into rabbits with experimental hypercholesterolemia the following regularities were found.

In 24—48 hours of circulation of labelled lipoproteins in the blood ot the rabbit-recipients a redistribution of the label was observed both in VLDL and in LDL. In the first place we noted a sharp decrease (on an average, by approximately 4 times) of the TG radioactivity percentage. PL and ECh radioactivity percentage increased correspondingly. The radioactivity drop in the TG component of the lipoproteins can more readily be explained by its splitting under the action of blood plasma lipoprotein-lipase.

The label redistribution taking place in the plasma lipoproteins was also reflected in the character of label distribution in aorta lipoproteins. Thus, if the radioactivity revealed in aorta lipoproteins is compared with the radioactivity of lipoproteins administered to rabbits (Table II), it can be a concluded that there is greater VLDL and LDL penetration into the aorta per phospholipid label than per label localized in the core of the lipoprotein particle (ECh, TG).

It cannot, of course, be excluded that a certain part of the radioactive PL in the

Table II. Penetration of labelled VLDL and LDL into the aortic wall of recipient rabbits 24—48 hours after their intravenous injection

No.	The class of lipo-proteins injected	The site of radioactivity in VLDL and LDL	Dose of radioactivity administered, cpm	Time of circulation of the radioactive lipoproteins, hours	Radioactivity found in the same site of VLDL+ isolated from the aorta, cpm	% of dose administered
1	VLDL + LDL	ECh, TG	$93.8 \cdot 10^5$	24	885	0.009
		PL	$19.8 \cdot 10^5$	24	475	0.026
2	VLDL + LDL	ECh, TG	$122.4 \cdot 10^5$	24	2001	0.016
		PL	$43.2 \cdot 10^5$	24	7081	0.164
3	VLDL + LDL	ECh, TG	$136 \cdot 10^5$	48	1558	0.011
		PL	$6.96 \cdot 10^5$	48	1956	0.281
4	VLDL	ECh, TG	$49.2 \cdot 10^5$	48	296	0.006
		PL	$9.6 \cdot 10^5$	48	396	0.041
5	VLDL	ECh, TG	$111.4 \cdot 10^5$	48	188	0.002
		PL	$36.2 \cdot 10^5$	48	1912	0.053
6	LDL	ECh, TG	$11.3 \cdot 10^5$	48	232	0.021
		PL	$5.98 \cdot 10^5$	48	536	0.090
7	LDL	ECh, TG	$37.2 \cdot 10^5$	48	514	0.014
		PL	$24 \cdot 10^5$	48	2241	0.093

plasma lipoproteins could have passed over into the aorta lipoproteins as a result of physico-chemical exchange.

From Table II it can also be seen that LDL penetrates into the rabbit aorta more rapidly than VLDL, both according to the determination of the phospholipid label and to the label, localized inside the lipoprotein particle (Ech, TG).

Comparison of radioactivity distribution (at the end of the experiment) showed that in the majority of experiments distribution of radioactivity among PL, ECh, and TG in plasma and aorta lipoproteins was relatively similar. Particularly clear results were observed when pure fractions of VLDL or LDL were administered to the rabbits. Single-valued radioactivity figures shared by TG in lipoproteins of the plasma and aorta attract particular attention.

As a whole the obtained data confirm the earlier expressed point of view that the arterial wall takes up plasma lipoproteins in the form of intact particles.

A. N. K., The Anitchkov Dept. of Biochemistry of Lipids and Atherosclerosis. Inst. of Experim. Med., 12 Pavlov St., Leningrad 197022, USSR.

PROTEIN COMPONENTS OF EDEMA FLUID AND SERUM

A. HIROTA, K. CHANG, H. SAWAI, T. SAKAI, T. SAKAI,
K. ISHIDA, SO YABUKI, K. SEKI

3rd Dep. of Internal Medicine, Toho University, Tokyo, Japan

Previously, protein components of edema fluid and serum were examined by disc-electrophoresis and the relationship between them has already been reported by us. All the protein components of serum appeared in edema fluid, but their concentration in edema fluid was much smaller than in serum, and generally the larger their molecular weight, the smaller their concentration in edema fluid. However, this was not always so. As our previous method is semi-quantitative, in the present study, single radial immuno diffusion was used. In order to get a relationship between edema fluid and serum, the concept of selectivity index was applied.

Method and materials

Subjects were 53 patients with various edema, 23 males and 30 females, 62.1 years old on an average, ranged from 19 to 92 years old; they were cardiac, hepatic, nephrotic, cachectic and lymphedema.

Edema fluid was obtained with Sourthey's needle from the subcutaneous tissue of the distal portion of the leg,

The concentration of α_1-acid glycoprotein (α_1-AGP), albumin (Alb), transferrin (Tr), Ig-G and α_2-macroglobulin (α_2-M) was measured by single radial immuno diffusion. These 5 protein components were chosen by comparing the phorogram in edema fluid and serum by disc-electrophoresis.

The E/S ratio of each protein component was obtained, that is, the ratio of protein component in edema fluid to that in serum. Then the E/S ratio of each protein component was divided by the E/S ratio of transferrin. The relationship of the quotient (Q) against the molecular weight was plotted on a bi-logarithmic scale. This height may, therefore, mean the degree of passage of each protein component through the capillary walls, compared with that of transferrin.

In this study, the degree of the passage of transferrin was used as a standard, and was expressed as a 100%, according to the concept of selectivity index by Cameron et al.

Table 1
The protein component concentrations and the edema fluid / serum of them

		α₁-acid glycoprotein	albumin	transferrin	Ig-G	α₂-macroglobulin
CACHECTIC EDEMA	serum	180.05	2241.18	154.08	1790.45	76.52
	edema fluid	37.78	625.77	30.59	209.41	13.67
	E/S ratio	24.02	25.06	22.77	14.23	10.84
CARDIAC EDEMA	serum	155.85	3065.00	196.58	2428.00	324.80
	edema fluid	32.33	425.30	110.20	208.60	11.31
	E/S ratio	20.38	14.80	17.29	8.48	4.21
HEPATIC EDEMA	serum	70.35	2492.00	218.52	2510.00	272.60
	edema fluid	5.26	228.18	15.35	75.61	8.23
	E/S ratio	8.12	9.38	7.50	3.49	3.25
LYMPH-EDEMA	serum	105.57	3114.29	256.46	1865.71	251.43
	edema fluid	42.25	1672.00	80.13	649.43	31.56
	E/S ratio	40.39	53.94	31.34	36.36	14.63
NEPHROTIC EDEMA	serum	133.80	1288.80	104.92	1380.00	276.80
	edema fluid	13.50	110.04	13.70	115.80	5.20
	E/S ratio	9.01	6.70	13.41	5.43	1.75
MEAN	serum	146.16	2490.52	232.49	2010.00	235.51
	edema fluid	28.94	617.60	33.50	237.13	14.08
	E/S ratio	22.25	22.98	19.38	13.56	7.98

Results

Table I shows the E/S ratio of each protein component. The ratios of most protein components were low in hepatic

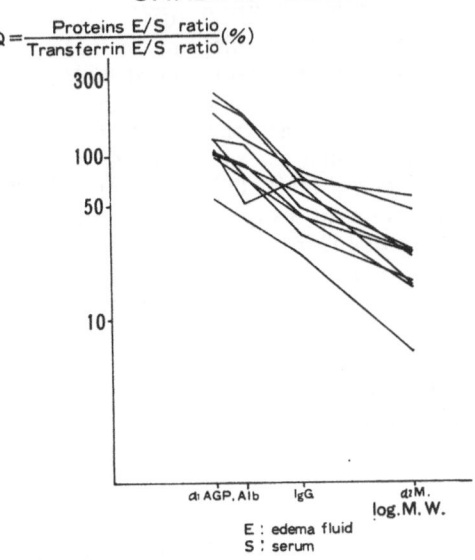

CARDIAC EDEMA

$$Q = \frac{\text{Proteins E/S ratio}}{\text{Transferrin E/S ratio}} (\%)$$

E : edema fluid
S : serum

Fig. 1.

121

edema. Those of Alb and Ig−G were high, and that of Tr was low in lymphedema.

Figure 1 shows the relationship between the Q and the molecular weight in cardiac edema. The ordinate represents the Q. The abscissa shows molecular weight. The curve is almost linear slanting to the

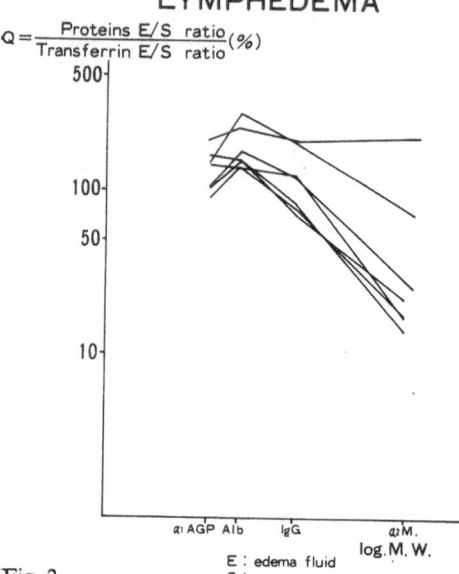

LYMPHEDEMA

$$Q = \frac{\text{Proteins E/S ratio}}{\text{Transferrin E/S ratio}} (\%)$$

E : edema fluid
S : serum

Fig. 2.

right. This may indicate that the passage of protein molecules depends mainly upon molecular weight and almost not upon other factors, such as electric charge etc.

In liver cirrhosis, the height of α_2-M is almost as high as that of Ig−G, that is, α_2-M with a molecular weight of 820,000 leaked as easily as Ig−G with a molecular weight of 168,000.

In nephrotic edema, the curve is almost linear similar to cardiac edema. The height of each protein component is lower

than 100%, that is, the height of Tr. This may indicate that the passage of Tr through the capillary walls is the easiest among these 5 protein components. However, the number of cases examined here is only 4, therefore, it is impossible to make a general statement.

In cachectic edema, α_1-AGP with a molecular weight of 44,000 is lower than that of Alb. Factors other than molecular weight may play some role here. The height of α_2-M varies greately. This may be due to the kind of diseases, complications and/or degree of cachexia.

Figure 2 shows lymphedema. The height of α_1-AGP is lower than that of Alb, and the height of Ig−G is higher than that of Tr. Therefore, factors other than molecular weight may affect the passage of proteins through the capillary walls. These 6 cases have very similar curves. But, in this disease, the effect of metabolism must be taken into consideration.

Conclusions

Protein components of edema fluid and serum were measured by single radial immuno diffusion in various edematous diseases and were compared with each other.

1) The passage of protein components through the capillary walls seemed to depend mainly upon molecular weight, that is, generally speaking, the larger the molecular weight, the smaller its degree of passage through the capillary walls. This, may, however, also be influenced by other factors such as electric charge etc.

2) The pattern of the passage of protein components through the capillary walls seems to differ according to the cause of the edema.

REFERENCES

Wolstenholme, G. E. W. & Cameron M. P., (1961): Renal biopsy, J. & A. Churchill, London p. 32.

Cameron J. S. & Blandford, G., (1966): The simple assessment of selectivity in heavy proteinuria, Lancet II: 242.

A. H.,: 3rd Department of Internal Medicine, Toho University Hospital, 2-17-6 Ohashi, Meguroku, Tokyo, Japan.

DNA TEMPLATE ACTIVITY OF AORTIC WALL CELLS IN EXPERIMENTAL DIABETES

R. LEHMANN and R. DÉNES

*Institute of Arteriosclerosis Research, University of Münster, F.R.G.
and 3rd Medical Clinic, Semmelweis University, Budapest, Hungary*

Introduction

Diabetes mellitus is one of the most important risk factors in vascular diseases. Because it is generally believed that the nuclei of eucaryotic cells are capable of responding to a variety of extrinsic factors, this study was carried out to evaluate the alteration of DNA template activity within artery wall cells of rats exposed to short time experimental diabetes.

Methods and material

For this purpose an ultracytochemical method was employed which has been tested previously in other systems (*Frenster*, 1971; *Lehmann and Slavkin*, 1976; *Lehmann et al.*, 1977; *Lehmann et al.* 1978). This method is based on the property of acridine orange (AO) to interact with DNA resulting in electron-dense AO chromatin interaction products which can be visualized in the electron microscope. Further details of the method have been published elsewhere (*Lehmann and Slavkin*, 1976). Experimental diabetes (Dénes et al., 1978) was produced with streptozotocin (75 mg/kg) in male rats weighing 200 to 250 g. The rate of elimination of glucose was 0.232% glucose/min (SD 0.057, SE 0.009) in experimental and 1.817% glucose/min (SD 0.301, SE 0.052) in control animals. The rate of secretion of insulin was 5.30 μE/ml/min (SD 2.20 SE 0.33) in experimental and 40.13 μE/ml/min (SD 5.45, SE 0.93) in control animals.

Results

As early as 2 weeks after injection of streptozotocin the distribution patterns of AO positive cells were determined in 5 differential regions of the aorta of experimental and control animals: Regio intercostalis superior and posterior, regio renalis superior and posterior

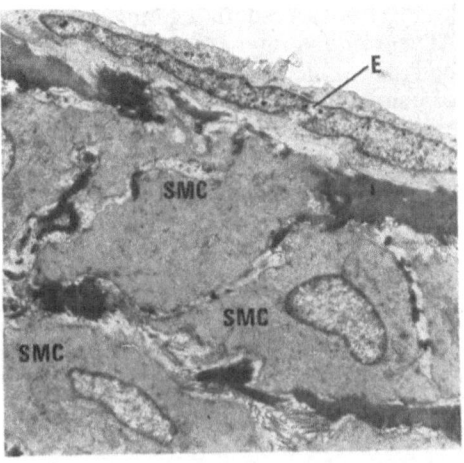

Fig. 1. Electron-dense AO chromatin interaction products are found in the endothelial nucleus (E). Adjacents smooth muscle cells (SMC) are AO negative. Aorta, regio renalis inferior. 9.300×.

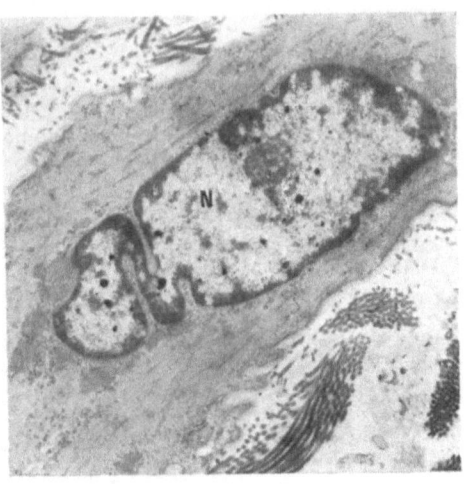

Fig. 2. AO positive nucleus (N) of a smooth muscle cell of the media of a control animal. Aorta, regio renalis superior. 14.000×.

123

and a region of the abdominal aorta below the AO renalis. The highest number of AO positive cells were found in regions 5 and 11. 41% of the intimal cells and 64% of the adventitial cells in region 5, and 56% of the intimal cells (Fig. 1) and 38% of the adventitial cells (Fig. 2) in region 11 exhibited AO chromatin interaction products. In the media only in region 5 could a few AO positive cells (<1%) be observed. In region 10 and 12 no AO chromatin interaction products could be seen. Similarly in comparable regions of control animals no or only a few AO

positive cells could be detected. An exception was region 10 of a control animal where several AO positive smooth muscle cells were found (Fig. 3). The AO positive cells appeared either as small cell groups or as individual cells adjacent to AO negative cells.

Discussion

In the present study as well as in previous papers (*Lehmann et al.* 1977, 1978) it has been shown that artery wall cells are capable of responding to extracellular factors such as experimental diabetes, experimental hypertension, and atherogenic diet with an altered DNA template activity. Although there are differences in species and regions of the aorta, the results obtained indicate that cell nuclei of the intima and adventitia are more responsive to extracellular factors than medial cell nuclei. Further analysis of these findings should increase our understanding of the clinical experience that vascular disease is a frequent complication in human diabetes. The results suggest the preferential role of hemodynamic predilection in the development of arteriosclerosis.

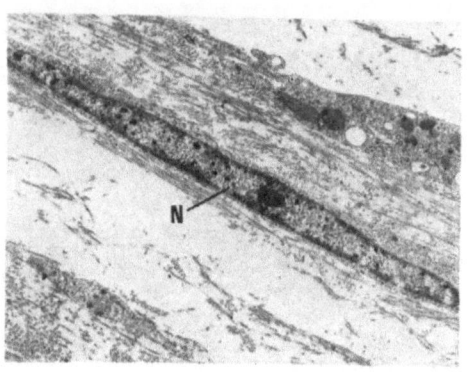

Fig. 3. AO positive (N) of a fibroblast of the adventitia. Aorta, regio renalis inferior. 14.000×.

REFERENCES

Dénes, R., Mey, J., Lehmann, R., Hauss, W. H. (1978): Vascular smooth muscle cells in culture after experimental diabetes. In: "State of prevention and therapy in human arteriosclerosis and in animal models" (eds. W. H. Hauss, R. W. Wissler, R. Lehmann). Abh. Rhein.-Westf. Akad. Wiss. 63, 249–266.

Frenster, J. H. (1971): Electron microscopic localization of acridine orange binding to DNA within human leukemic bone marrow cells. Cancer Res. 31, 1128–1133.

Lehmann, R., Slavkin, H. C. (1976): Localization of "transcriptively active" cells during odontogenesis using acridine orange ultra-

structural cytochemistry. Developm. Biol. 49, 438–456.

Lehmann, R. Dénes, R., Kerényi, T. (1977): Distribution of DNA template activity in artery wall cells. Prog. biochem. Pharmacol. 13, 271–275.

Lehmann, R., Dénes ,R., Kerényi, T., Hauss, W. H. (1978): Alteration of DNA template activity in artery wall cells induced by risk factors. In: "State of prevention and therapy in human arteriosclerosis and in animal models" (eds. W. H. Hauss, R. W. Wissler, R. Lehmann). Abh. Rhein.-Westf. Akad. Wiss. 63, 267–283.

R. L., Institute of Arteriosclerosis Research at the University of Münster, Westring 3, 4400 Münster, F.R.G.

STIFFNESS OF THE ARTERIAL WALL IN RESPONSE TO POTASSIUM AND PHARMACOLOGICAL ACTIVATION

G. PFITZER and J. W. PETERSON

2nd Institute of Physiology, University of Heidelberg, F.R.G.

Introduction

Recent work in muscle physiology has shown that the muscle's ability to resist sudden changes in length reflects basic actomyosin cross-bridge properties rather than those of an inert series elastic element unrelated to the molecular mechanism of force generation (*Huxley and Simmons*, 1972). Characteristic plots of instantaneous forces resulting from rapid length changes (Tl curves) extrapolate to a single value of quick shortening needed to discharge all active force. That this value is independent of the absolute force developed indicates that Tl curves are representative of a "quantized" unit of force development (the Ca^{++}-activated actomyosin cross-bridge) and that total stiffness therefore measures the relative numbers of available cross-bridges which have been activated in skeletal (*Ford, et al.*, 1977) and in heart (*Yamamoto and Herzig*, 1978) muscle. Our determinations of Tl curves in arterial smooth muscles have yielded quantitatively similar results (*Paul and Petersen*, 1977).

Methods

Swine carotid arteries were prepared in Krebs-Henseleit physiological saline solution (PSS) pH 7.4 bubbled with 40% O_2/5% CO_2. Arteries were slit open longitudinally and small segments of media dissected out parallel to the muscle orientation (*Paul, Glück and Rüegg*, 1976). Tissue segments, typically 5—7 mm long and 3×10^{-3} cm^2 cross-section area, were then attached by means of a tissue cement to two small glass rods connected to a force transducer and the moveable core of a vibrator and incubated in 2 ml glass cups which were maintained at 37 °C, continually exposed to the gases and could be changed in about 10 seconds. Small rectangular stretches and releases of up to 2% of the tissue rest length (the zero passive tension length Lô) were applied by the vibrator, ob-taining smooth length steps with a rise time of about 1.5 millisecond.

A few experiments were performed on other arterial preparations. Spiral strips of rat tail artery were prepared and were mounted as described above; 1 mm rings of rabbit renal artery were cut and looped over platinum wires glued to the glass rods. All other procedures were identical to those used with the carotid artery.

Results

Near maximal but unstable contractures in the swine carotid artery were obtained in K$^+$-PSS (50% substitution of Na$^+$-salts

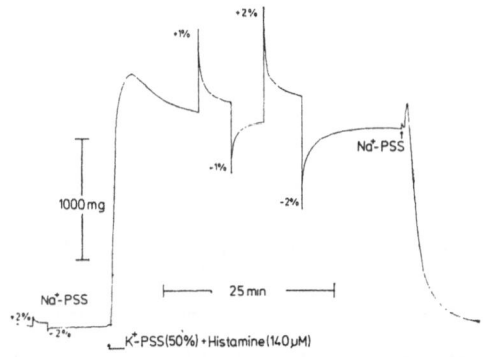

Fig. 1. A maintained maximal contracture with K$^+$-histamine and subsequent relaxation in swine carotid artery, with periods of stretch and release of the sizes indicated (as % of the resting length). The biphasic contracture seen here is more pronounced than usually observed. Before activation, the passive force changes in response to stretch/release are quite small.

by K$^+$-salts). Maximal and stable contractures about 3—4× greater were produced by adding 10^{-4}M histamine (e. g., *Hudgins and Weiss*, 1968). The rat tail artery and rabbit renal artery were maximally activated by 3×10^{-6} and 1.5×10^{-5}M

125

norepinephrine respectively in Na$^+$-PSS.

Figure 1 illustrates a stable maximal contracture with K^+-histamine at various times during tension maintenance, sustained stretches and releases of the indicated magnitudes were imposed. Because of slow recorder pen response time (300 ms), initial force changes were also measured with a storage oscilloscope, thus giving the extreme instantaneous force change at the instant the stretch/release was complete. After attaining the peak force change, the tension at first very rapidly then increasingly slowly equilibrates towards a final value in agreement with the force-length relation of the arterial muscle.

when normalized to relative isometric force and resting length. The Tl curves are linear for stretches and give an extrapolated value for the total force discharge of about 1%, not substantially greater than that for skeletal muscle. The Tl curves are, however, rather more nonlinear for releases, perhaps indicating the presence of a small series elasticity not contained in the actomyosin cross-bridges alone.

A comparison of Tl curves measured in swine carotid artery with K^+, histamine, and K^+-histamine activation are shown in Figure 3. Because the 3 modes of activation give various stable isometric

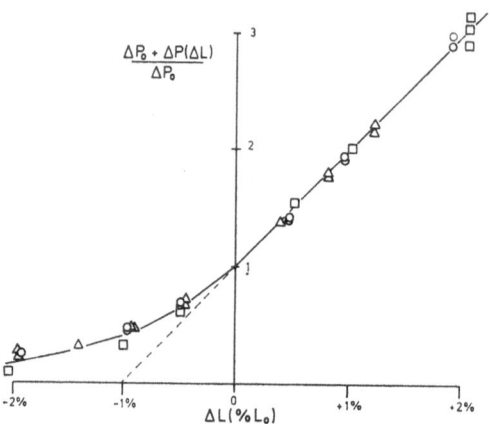

Fig. 2. A plot of the extreme force changed ($\Delta P(\Delta L)$) attained with various size stretches and releases, expressed relative to the active isometric force (ΔPo) developed with maximal activation (i. e., Tl curve) for swine carotid artery (squares), rat tail artery (triangles), and rabbit renal artery (circles).

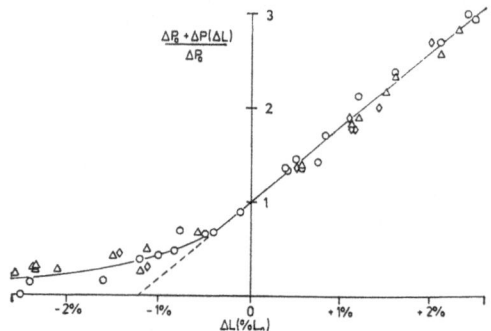

Fig. 3. A Tl curve as in Figure 2 for swine carotid artery activated to varying levels of isometric force development with K^+ (triangles), histamine (diamonds), and K^+-histamine (circles). Data for this 3-fold comparison was accumulated from samples from 5 arteries.

To ascertain that the observed stiffness measurements (Tl curves) are a general arterial property, similar measurements were made with different preparations representing a range of artery types from larger conductance vessels to smaller resistance vessels. The results of such a comparison are seen in Figure 2. Even though the absolute dimensions, methods of activation, and isometric force development of the 3 preparations differed largely, plots of the data superimpose

tensions, force changes upon stretch/release are again expressed relative to absolute force. A linear Tl curve, extrapolated to essentially the same value as in Figure 2, is again seen. No consistent difference with the various stimulants was detected.

Conclusions

Measurements of stiffness in various arterial preparations yield Tl curves very similar to those found in skeletal muscle. The fact that the extrapolated value for complete tension discharge does not depend on the relative tension developed argues that a similar interpretation of the data prevails; i.e., arterial stiffness results primarily from the differing numbers of activated actomyosin cross-bridges obtained with the various stimulants used, rather than from changes in a series elastic component. These findings differ from other reports in the literature (e.g. *Mulvaney and Halpern*, 1976).

The source of activator Ca^{++}, whether external as with K^+-stimulation or primarily internal as with histamine or norepinephrine stimulation, makes no difference. Thus, the ability of the arterial wall to resist rapid deformative stresses most strongly depends upon the level of activation of the smooth muscle within.

REFERENCES

Ford, L. E., Huxley, A. F., Simmons, R. M. (1977): Tension respones to sudden length change in stimulated frog muscle fibres near slack length. J. Physiol. 269, 441—515.

Hudgins, P. M., Weiss, G. B. (1968): Differential effects of calcium removal upon vascular smooth muscle contraction induced by norepinephrine, histamine and potassium. J. Pharmacol. Exp. Therap. 159, 91—97.

Huxley, A. F., Simmons, R. M. (1972): Mechanical transients and the origin of muscular force. Cold Spring Harb. Symp. quant. Biol. 37, 669.

Mulvany, M. J., Halpern, W. (1976): Mechanical properties of vascular smooth muscle cells in situ. Nature 260, 617—619.

Paul, R. J., Glück, E., Rüegg, J. C. (1976): Cross bridge ATP utilization in arterial smooth muscle. Pflügers Arch. 361, 297.

Paul, R. J., Peterson, J. W. (1977): Smooth muscle energetics. in: Excitation-Contraction coupling in smooth muscle (ed. Casteels, R. et al.) Elsevier, Amsterdam.

Yamamoto, T., Herzig, J. W. (1976): Series elastic properties of skinned muscle fibres in contraction and rigor. Pflügers Arch. 373, 21—24.

G. P., II Physiologisches Institut Universität Heidelberg Im Neuenheimer Feld 326 D-6900 Heidelberg 1., G.F.R.

PROSTAGLANDIN-LIKE ACTIVITY IN PATIENTS SUFFERING FROM OCCLUSIVE ARTERIAL DISEASES

M. BIELAWIEC. A. BODZENTA and H. LUKJAN

Department of Haematology, Institute of Internal Medicine,
Medical School, Białystok, Poland

Introduction

The naturally occurring, biologically active substances, prostaglandins, are now known to be formed in a variety of tissues, including blood vessels and platelets.

The concept of the potential role of prostaglandins in atherogenesis is new and there are only a few reports concerning this problem (*Subbiah*, 1978).

The vasodilator and anti-aggregatory properties of prostaglandins in patients with occlusive arterial disease seems to be of particular interest. The present study was carried out to investigate the effect of nicotinic acid derivatives on the fibryolytic, kininogenic and prostaglandin-like activity in the blood of patients with occlusive arterial disease.

Material and methods

The investigations were carried out on 30 patients (4 females and 26 males) aged 42—72 years with obliterative arteriosclerosis of the lower limbs and 10 healthy persons aged 20—30 years.

The following determinations were made in the plasma:

1. Extraction of prostaglandin-like material (*Unger et al.*, 1971)

2. Kinins and kallikrein activity (*Buluk et al.*, 1970)

3. Kininogen level (*Briseid et al.*, 1967)

4. Euglobulin fibrinolysis time (*Chakrabarti et al.*, 1968)

Biologically active substances were assayed on rat stomach strips (*Vane*, 1957; *Gilmore et al.* 1968) and the small intestine of a guinea pig. The results were analysed statistically with the aid of the Student test.

Results

Fig. 1 shows the mean values and standard deviations of the level of pros-

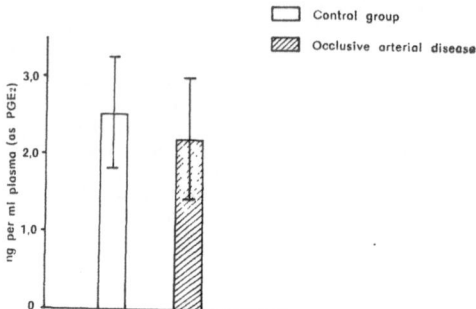

Fig. 1. The level of prostaglandin activity in the peripheral venous blood of patients suffering from occlusive arterial disease and in healthy subjects.

taglandin activity in patients with occlusive arterial disease. The level of prostaglandin activity in peripheral venous blood from 30 patients was found to be 2.0 ± 0.8 µg//ml plasma as PGE_2. Similar values were

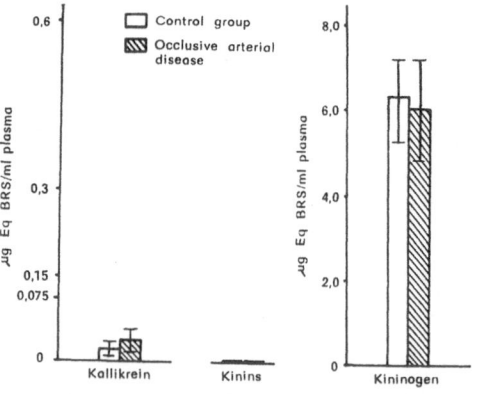

Fig. 2. Mean levels of kallikrein, kinins and kininogen in the peripheral venous blood of patients suffering from occlusive arterial disease and in healthy subjects.

found in healthy subjects, $2.5 \pm 0.79\ \mu g/ml$ plasma ($p < 0.25$).

Fig. 2 illustrates the mean values and standard deviations of the level of kallikrein, kinins and kininogen in the patients investigated. The level of plasma kallikrein was barely recordable in the patients and healthy subjects ($0.04 \pm 0.07\ \mu g$ Eq. BRS/ /ml plasma). No plasma kinins were found in either of the groups investigated. The level of kininogen in the patients was 6.2 ± 1.3 and in the healthy persons it was only slightly higher $6.4 \pm 1.5\ \mu g$ Eq. BRS/ml plasma ($p < 0.5$).

Fig. 3 depicts the behavior of fibrinolytic kininogenic and prostaglandin-like activity after intravenous infusion of 300 mg Sadamin ('Polfa''). 10 minutes after the infusion of Sadamin a transient shortening of the euglobulin fibrinolysis time to 68 ± 8 min. ($0.01 < p < 0.001$) was observed together with a fall in the kininogen level to about $5.0 \pm 1.2\ \mu g$ Eq. BRS/ml plasma, an increase in the kallikrein titer to about $0.3 \pm 0.2\ \mu g$ Eq. BRS/ml plasma, a higher level of prostaglandin activity $4.4 \pm 0.6\ \mu g/ml$ plasma as PGE_2 and the appearance of a measurable amount of free kinins. During the next 30 minutes observation a gradual fall in the activity of the systems studied occurred.

Discussion

The results presented above show that there were no statistically significant differences in the levels of prostaglandin activity, kallikrein and kininogen in the venous blood obtained from patients with occlusive arterial disease and from healthy subjects. However administration of Sadamin caused an increase in the fibrinolytic, kininogenic and prostaglandin-like activity in both the groups studied.

Previous investigations showed that nicotinic acid derivatives have a favourable, therapeutic effect on patients with occlussive arterial disease. It was thought that these good results are brought about by the effect kinins exert on the microcirculation and formation of collateral circulation (*Bielawiec et al.*, 1971). As the present studies show, it appears that this mechanism is connected with another group of strongly acting substances, prostaglandins. Some authors have drawn attention to the close relation ship between kinins and the release of prostaglandins (*McGiff et al.*, 1975). The prostaglandins thus released, especially PGE_1 and prostacyclin, cause vasodilation and, as potent inhibitors of platelet aggregation and adhesion, prevent arterial trombus formation. From our results it seems that the higher level of prostaglandin-like activity occurring in patients with occlusive arterial disease after administration of nicotinic acid derivatives indicates a relationship between the prostaglandins and the fat balance, which may play a role in atherogenesis. This problem however requires further study.

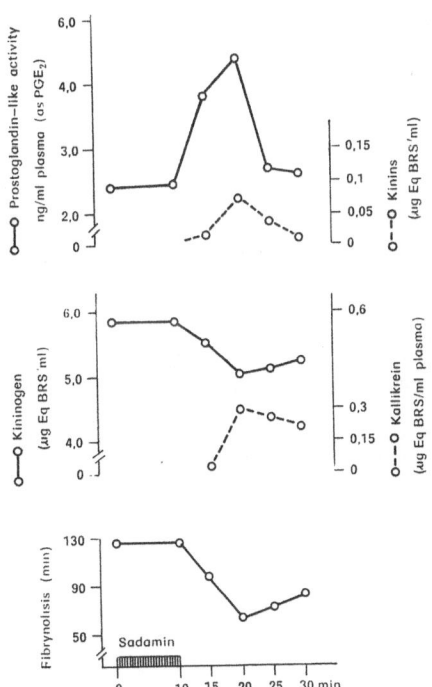

Fig. 3. Behaviour of fibrino- lytic, kininogenic and prostaglandin-like activity after intravenous infusion of 300 mg Sadamin.

REFERENCES

Bielawiec, M., Łukjan,' H. (1971): Der Einfluss der Fibrinolyse-Activierung auf den peripheren Kreislauf bei obliterieren den Gefässkrankheiten. Med. Wschr. 7, 312—314.

Briseid, K., Dyrud,O. K., Rinvik, S. F. (1967): In vitro estimation of the rate of release of kinin in human plasma. Acta pharmac. et toxic. 25, 201—213.

Buluk, K., Czokało, M., Małofiejew, M. (1970): Contact and plasminforming systems in the blood. Thromb. Diathes. Haemorrhag. 24, 548—558.

Chakrabarti, R., Bielawiec, M., Ewans, J. F., Fearnley, G. R. (1968): Methodological study and a recommended technique for determing the euglobulin lysis time. J. Cl. Path. 21, 698—701.

Gilmore, N., Vane, J. R., Wyllie, J. H. (1968): Prostaglandins released by the spleen. Nature, Lond. 218, 1135—1140.

McGiff, J. C., Itskovitz, H. D., Terragno, A., Wong, P. Y-K. (1975): Modulation and medation of the action of renal kallikrein-kinin system by prostaglandins. Fed. Proceed. 35, 175—180.

Subbiah, M. T. R. (1978): Prostaglandins and the arterial wall: an avenue for research in the pathogenesis of atherosclerosis. Mayo Cl. Proceed. 53, 60—62.

Unger, W. G., Stamford, I. F., Bennett, A. (1971): Extraction of prostaglandins from human blood. Nature, Lond. 233, 336—337.

Vane, J. R. (1957): A sensitive method for assay of 5-hydroxytryptamine Br. J. Pharmac. Chemother. 12, 344—349.

M. B., Haematology, Institute of Internal Medicine, Medical School, Białystok, Poland

PROSTAGLANDINS AND MOTILITY OF HUMAN VEINS

H. P. BRUCH, E. SCHMIDT and R. LAVEN

Department of Surgery, University of Würzburg, Würzburg, F.R.G.

In the areas of the venous and arterial vascular regions, confusing PG-effects have been described, depending on the place dealt with and the mode of application. In experiments on animals vascular dilating effects were mostly observed. For this reason it is said that prostaglandins have an essentially anti-hypertensive power, but it was the vessels where the differences in individual considerable species were observed.

Therefore we examined the direct effect of prostaglandins on the smooth muscle system of human vessels. As the sympathetic autonomous system plays an essential role in the regulation of the vascular motility, the interplay of adrenergically stimulating and inhibiting substances with prostaglandins were taken into consideration.

Immediately after resection during operation, fresh human saphenous veins were cut into spiral strips and incubated in a Tyrode bath. The isometric tension changes were continually registered. All tension changes were related to the muscle cross-section of the specimen. The relative references were the maximum contraction of the vessel strips in a potassium solution (135 mval/l). The examination of the specimen took place at a 30% tension which corresponds to the state of tension *in vivo*.

As representative for prostaglandins F_2 alpha and E_1, which are quantitatively and qualitatively greatly similar, Figure 1 shows the dose-response graph of prostaglandin E_2 on human venae saphenae and, in comparison, on human spleen arteries. There is always an increase in tension according to the dosage. Especially remarkable, however, is that the prostaglandin-induced contractions, in com-

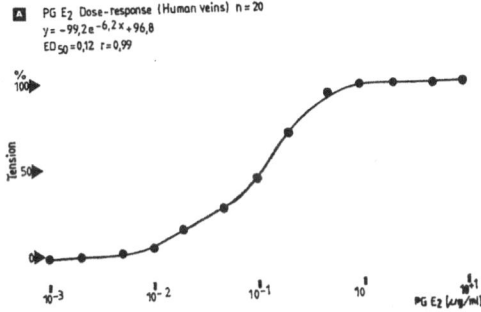

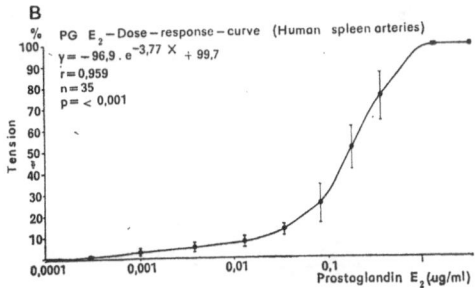

Fig. 1.

parison with the noradrenaline-induced contractions, are not tonic but peristalsis-like and practically indefatigable as you can see from the original registration (Fig. 2.)

Human saphenous veins and human mesenteric arteries react insignificantly to concentrations under 10^{-3} µg/ml PG E_2. The first noticeable contractions take place at a concentration of 5×10^{-3} µg/ml. The relaxative effects of the lower concentrations (below 10^{-3} µg/ml), often described, were never observed. The maximum effective concentration of 1µg/ml, however, remains the same.

In Figure 3 one can see the prostaglandin-induced contractions of arteries

131

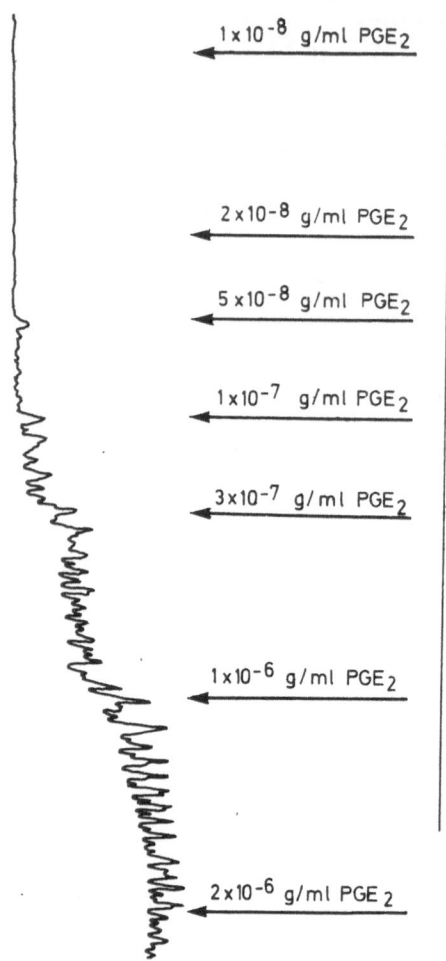

Fig. 2.

against those of the veins. Compared with the contraction in potassium solution, a contraction of 57, 9%, plus or minus 8%, under a maximum effective prostaglandin E_2 dose takes place, under prostaglandin F_2 alpha a contraction of 78%, plus or minus 6.4%. Thus, veins react visibly stronger to prostaglandins than do the arteries. Prostaglandin F_2 alpha can cause a contraction of 115% plus or minus 20% in the human vena saphena magna. Prostaglandin A_1, on the other hand, leads to a dose-dependent relaxation of minus 11%, plus or minus 7.6%.

As many researchers can prove, prosta-

glandins are synthesized in the arterial and venal vascular walls and influence there the tone of the smooth vascular muscles. On the other hand, a humoral effect of prostaglandins on the vascular system is also possible. Prostaglandins are set free especially during the reduced supply of blood to the kidneys as well as after sympathetic stimulation and an adrenaline dose from the spleen into the venal blood. The largest prostaglandin producer of the body is, however, the human intestine. Prostaglandins are transported from here into the mesenteric venal blood. They are then removed from the venal blood, partly in the liver and, especially the vascular constricting prostaglandins, in the lungs. Thus it is

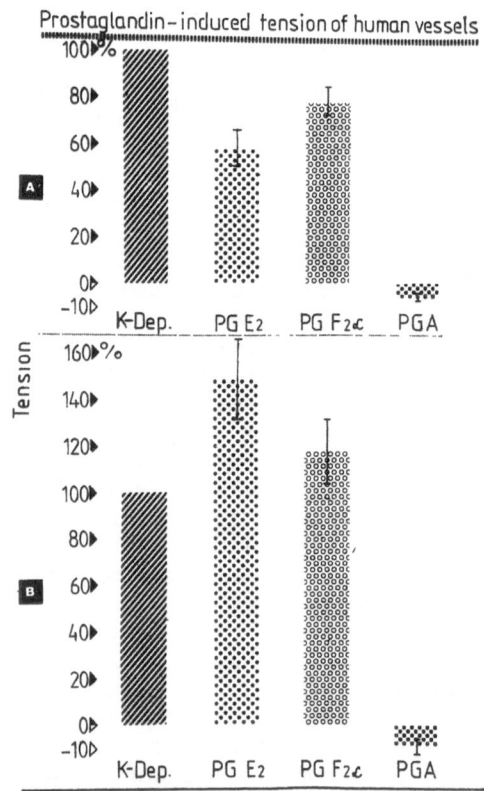

A = Art. lienalis
B = Vena saphena magna

Fig. 3.

avoided that large quantities are carried into the arterial system.

Summarizing one can speculate

1. A high dosage of prostaglandins of the groups E and F, which are transported into the lungs, must lead to a contraction of the pulmonary vascular system and consequently to a drop in blood pressure. The mechanism could play an important role in various forms of shock, especially in septic shock caused by gram-negative bacteria, because the endotoxin of gram-negative bacteria functions as a potent inhibitor of the prostaglandin-dehydrogenase.

2. Under pathophysiological conditions large quantities of prostaglandins could pass the lungs, enter humorally into the arterial system and cause the blood pressure there to increase considerably.

3. Prostaglandins of the group A, which are to a small extent vascular-dilating and can be metabolized in the liver, could be released into the arterial system in cases of serious disorders of the liver metabolism. Unsolved hypotonic conditions in serious liver ailments which have not yet been pathogenetically explained, could support this assumption.

B. H. P., University of Würzburg Department of Surgery, Jos. Schbeiderstr. 2 D-87 Würzburg, F.R.G.

A RATIONAL BASIS FOR THE USE OF DRUGS WITH ENDOTHELOPROTECTIVE ACTIVITY IN PERIPHERAL ISCHAEMIA

J. HLADOVEC

Cardiovascular Research Centre of the Institute for Clinical and Experimental Medicine, Prague 4, Czechoslovakia

The ultrastructural damage of endothelium is a common finding in ischaemic tissue lesions produced in various ways, for instance by occlusions of arteries, carbon monoxide inhalations, etc. Endothelial lesions have the usual consequences, such as increased permeability, platelet activation and adhesion to the vessel wall and activation of the blood clotting system by thromboplastic material, subendothelium and collagen. What is the mechanism of this endothelial damage? Endothelial cells have, of course, their oxidation metabolism. In acute situations several intermediary mechanisms are important for the development of lesions. One of them is the accumulation of lactate. Lactate has an enhancing effect on endothelial desquamation as demonstrated by the increased level of circulating endothelial cells after intravenous administration in rats (1). Endothelial cells were counted in Bürker's chamber by an original method based on isolation of a nuclear cell bodies together with platelets by differential centrifugation and the subsequent removal of platelets aggregated by addition of adenosine-diphosphate (2). The cell numbers were also increased after the release of femoral artery ligations in rats (Fig. 1). Lactate probably acts by changing the consistency of the endothelial cementing material. In addition to the lactate effect, there may be a contribution of the released catecholamines which may also produce an endothelial contraction with all the consequences of endothelial desquamation.

Endothelial cells are very sensitive structures which may be damaged by many agents of physical, physico-chemical, chemical and biological character (1) (Tab. I). On the other hand, a list of endotheloprotective agents may be defined on the basis of our experimental studies (3) (Tab. II). Many drugs, of course, appear at the same time in several subgroups, for instance acetylsalicylic acid belonging to analgetics-antipyretics and simultaneously to "antiplatelet" drugs, hydroxychloroquin being an antirheumatic, "antiplatelet" drug as well as an antimalaric. Most endotheloprotective drugs show a marked dose optimum, i.e. they have a two phase effect with the dose. In fact, many drugs produce an adverse effects on the endothelium after doses above this optimum and this may help to expalin some of their side-effects.

According to our hypothesis, all endotheloprotective drugs act by influencing the dynamic equilibrium of calcium ions available at the endothelial membranes and some of them also at the membranes of other tissue cells and their organelles.

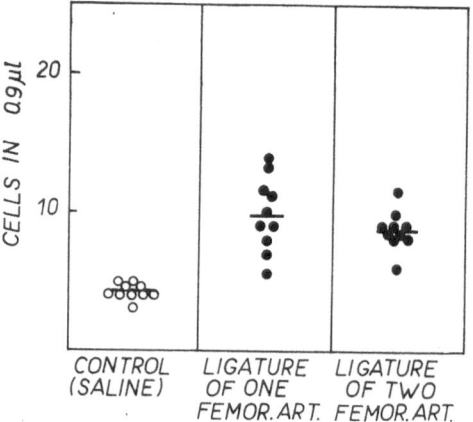

Fig. 1.

Table I.

NOXIOUS INFLUENCES

PHYSICAL	MECHANICAL
	THERMIC
	RADIANT
PHYS.-CHEMICAL	OSMOTIC
CHEMICAL	TOXIC (ENDOTOXIN, NICOTIN, HOMOCYSTEIN, METHIONIN, BILE ACIDS, OXID. LIPIDS, FATTY ACIDS)
	ACIDS
	MEDIATORS (CATECHOLAMINES, HISTAMINE, 5-HT, PROSTAGLANDINS, PEPTIDES.)
	ANOXIA (LACTATE?)
	IMMUNOLOGIC
	HORMONAL (CONTRACEPTIVES)
BIOLOGIC	INFECTIOUS (VIRUSES)

Table II.

ENDOTHELOPROTECTIVE DRUGS

VITAMINS	(FLAVONOIDS, COUMARIN)
„VENOTONICS"	(TRIBENOSIDE, CALC. DOBESILATE)
CALCIUM ANTAGONISTS	
CARDIOTONICS	(DIGITALIS)
ANTIARRHYTMICS	(NITRITES, QUINIDINE)
ANTIATHERO-SCLEROTICS	(CLOFIBRATE, PYRIDINOLCARBAMATE)
„ANTIPLATELET" DRUGS	(SULPHINPYRAZONE, HYDROXYCHLORO-QUINE, DIPYRIDAMOLE)
ANALGETICS-ANTIPYRETICS	ANTIPHLOGISTICS, ANTIRHEUMATICS
HORMONES	(GLUCOCORTICOIDS)
ETHANOL	

Depending on the ability of the drug to enter such deeper structures, its activity may be demonstrated predominantly at the endothelial level or at the level of tissue cells and their organelles where it affects their specific functions. This is probably the common link in the mechanism of all cardiovascular drugs. Calcium is the most important agent forming molecular bridges in the cementing substance between endothelial cells and thus regulating the consistency of this material. Thus, it regulates also the intercellular adhesion. Moreover, calcium ions are the mediator of endothelial contraction which contributes to the loss of endothelial integrity. There is a marked concentration optimum for calcium ions in this respect. It may be easily demonstrated with our method for the estimation of circulating endothelial cells that calcium itself has a two-phase effect dependent on the dose and that the protective effects of endothelotropic drugs may be inhibited by high doses of calcium repeatedly by alternately increasing the doses of the drug and calcium. This supports the assumption of the competitive character of both drug and calcium activities. Many drugs with an endotheloprotective activity have either a weak chelating activity for calcium ions or interfere with the transmembrane transport of these ions.

It may be concluded that, according to our hypothesis, endotheloprotective drugs have a stabilizing effect on the endothelium against various noxious agents including anoxia and may be used for the prevention of ischaemic injury with satisfactory rational justification.

REFERENCES

1. *Hladovec J. (1978):* Circulating endothelial cells as a sign of vessel wall lesions. Physiol. bohemoslov., 27, 140—144.
2. *Hladovec J., Rossmann P. (1973):* Circulating endothelial cells isolated together with platelets and the experimental modification of their count in rats. Thrombosis Res., 3, 665—674.
3. *Hladovec J. (1977):* Vasotropic drugs — a sruvey based on a unifying concept of their mechanism of action. Arzneim.-Forsch./Drug Res., 27, 1073—1076.

J. H., IKEM, Vídeňská 800, I46 22 Prague 4, Czechoslovakia.

BIOMECHANICAL PROPERTIES OF HOG CAROTID ARTERIES

A. G. HUDETZ, G. MÁRK, E. MONOS, JUDIT SZUTRÉLY
and A. G. B. KOVÁCH

*Experimental Research Institute, Semmelweis Medical University,
Budapest, Hungary*

Introduction

Recently, increasing attention has been
paid to passive and active nonlinear
mechanical properties of large arteries.
This growing interest has been motivated
by the fact that understanding the role
of the arteries in normal circulatory
control and the hemodynamic consequences of vascular lesions demands
detailed knowledge of the relationship
between the structure and function of the
vessel wall. Previously, we studied the
passive mechanical properties of human
anterior cerebral and internal carotid
arteries (*Márk et al.*, 1977, 1978). For
interpretation of our results the influence
of the smooth muscle tone on the mechanical properties of arteries should also
be considered. As arteries isolated from
cadavers could be actived only in a few
cases, a systematic study of their active
mechanical properties was not possible.
Our previous studies revealed that active
strain response of hog carotid arteries was
similar to that of the human carotids.
Therefore hog carotid arteries were
choosen to study the effect of smooth
muscle activation on the mechanical
properties of carotid arteries *in vitro*.

Methods

Carotid arteries were isolated 15 minutes
after slaughtering the pigs, immersed into an
oxygenated Krebs-Ringer solution and transported to the laboratory within half an hour.
15—20 cm long segments of the arteries were
dissected. stretched to their *in vivo* length and
mounted in the experimental apparatus (*Cox*,
1974) in oxygenated Krebs-Ringer solution
thermostated at 37 °C. Measurements were performed after an incubation time of at least 2
hours. Arterial segments were subjected to

a quasi-static mechanical test consisted of slow
(100 Hgmm/min) and cyclic inflation and deflation of the segments by air in the range of
0—250 mmHg intraluminal pressure, while pressure and external diameter were recorded. This
procedure was repeated in the passive state and
after activation of the smooth muscle by
0.5 μg/ml norepinephrine. Mechanical parameters were computed at 10 mmHg pressure

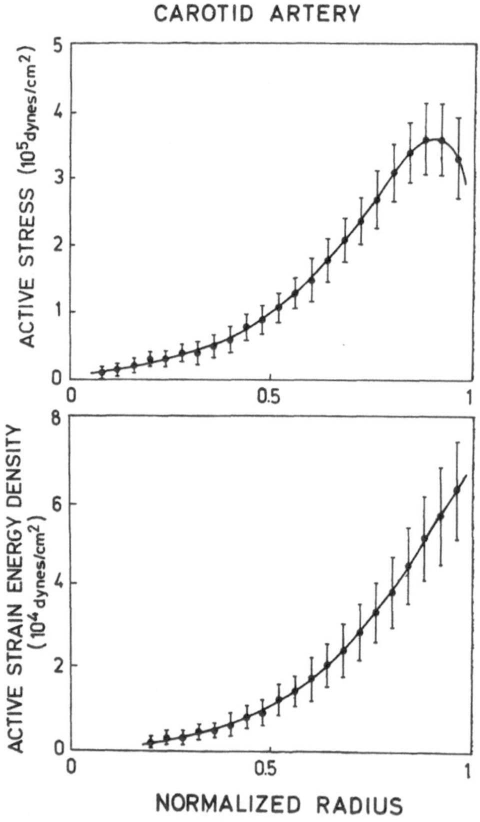

Fig. 1. Dependence of active stress and active
strain energy density developed in smooth muscles on the normalized radius of the arteries.

136

steps from the diameter/pressure *inflation* curves according to the following definitions:

average wall stress:

$$S = \frac{P}{2} \frac{R_e + R_i}{R_e - R_i},$$

strain energy density:

$$W = \frac{1}{R_o h_o} \int_{R_{io}}^{R_i} PR_i' dR_i',$$

incremental elastic modulus (Hudetz, 1978):

$$H = \frac{\Delta P}{\Delta R_e} \frac{2R_i^2 R_e}{R_e^2 - R_i^2} + \frac{2PR_e^2}{R_e^2 - R_i^2},$$

incremental distensibility:

$$D = \frac{2}{R_i} \frac{\Delta R_i}{\Delta P},$$

characteristic impedance:

$$Z_o = \frac{1}{R_i^2 \pi \sqrt{(\varrho D)}},$$

where R_i and R_e are the internal and external radii of the vessel at the intraluminal pressure P.

Results and conclusions

Fig. 1 shows the average values ($\pm$ SE) of the mechanical quantities characterising contractile properties of the smooth muscle computed from 24 measurements on 15 carotids. The average maximal active isometric stress was $(4.36 \pm 0.60) \times$ $\times$ 10 dynes/cm^2, developed at a tangential stretch of 1.64 ± 0.04. The strain energy density in the smooth muscle reached an average maximal value of $(6.8 \pm 1.2) \times$ $\times$ 10^4 dynes/cm^2.

Changes in the geometry and elastic properties of the arteries are compared in *Fig. 2*. A relative decrease in the internal radius (active isobaric strain) had a maximum of 8.8 ± 1.2 percent at very low internal pressure levels (24 ± 3 mm Hg). The incremental modulus decreased markedly with a maximum of 39.5 ± 3.3 percent in the normal physiological pressure range (117 ± 9 mm Hg). Similar characteristics were found for incremental distensibility and characteristic impedance (*Fig. 3*). Maximum changes in these quantities were 79 ± 10 percent (at $122 \pm$

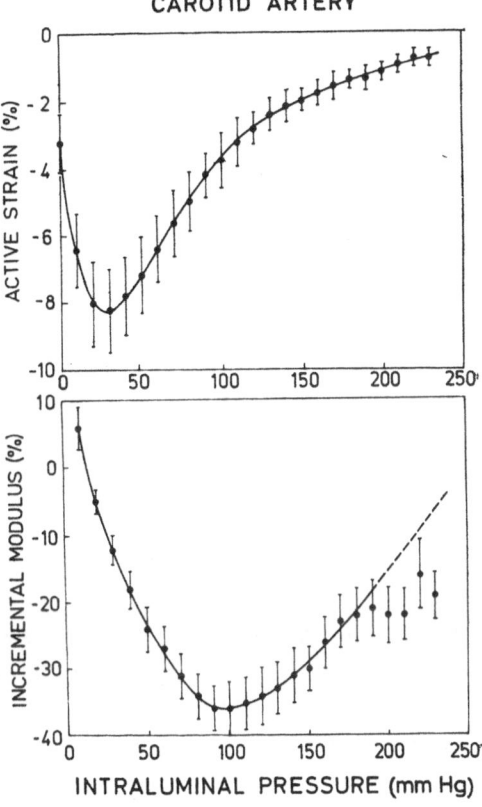

CAROTID ARTERY

Fig. 2. Comparison of average relative changes in internal radius and incremental elastic modulus of arteries due to smooth muscle activation. Deviations from the broken line are artefacts originating from slight buckling of the vessel when inflated over 180 mmHg internal pressure.

$\pm$ 9 mm Hg) and 18.7 ± 1.8 percent (at 136 ± 9 mm Hg) respectively.

It has been shown that smooth muscle contraction decreases the incremental elastic modulus and increases the incremental distensibility of hog carotid arteries at each level of intraluminal pressure. Other studies revealed that the passive incremental modulus of fibrosclerotic human internal carotid arteries was $40-56$ percent smaller than that of the normal vessels (*Márk et al.*, 1978). If our present results could be extrapolated to human carotid arteries, then the difference in the incremental modulus of fibrosclerotic and

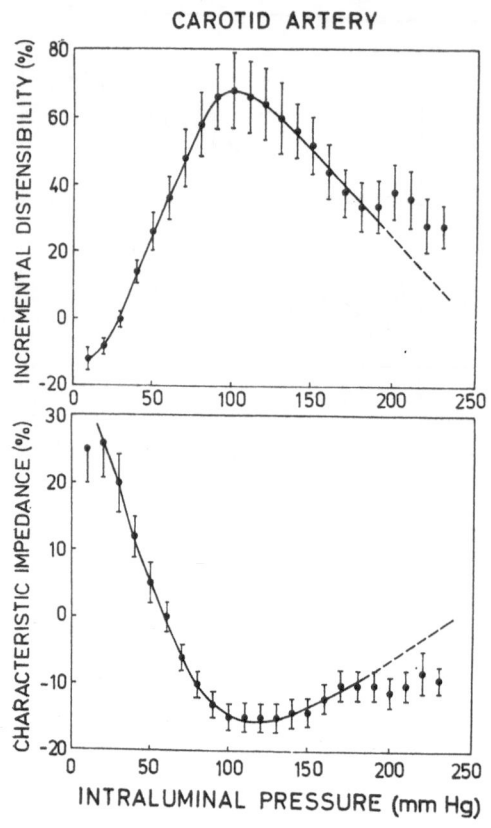

CAROTID ARTERY

INTRALUMINAL PRESSURE (mm Hg)

normal arteries may be smaller *in vivo* than was observed *in vitro* due to decreased smooth muscle tone of the fibrosclerotic vessels.

Existence of a local compensatory process tending to maintain certain hemodynamically important properties of fibrosclerotic arteries has been suggested recently (*Márk et al.*, 1977, 1978). However, these controlled properties have not yet been specified unanimously. It was found in the present work that the maximum active isobaric strain developed at pressure levels well below the physiological range. Active control of the elastic modulus, distensibility and impedance, however, may be most effective at normal physiological blood pressure levels. This suggests that in optimization of circulatory functions not the diameter but incremental distensibility and characteristic impedance of large arteries are the main controlled variables.

Fig. 3. Influence of smooth muscle activation on incremental distensibility and characteristic impedance at different internal pressure levels. Note that maximum changes develop in the normal physiological pressure range.

REFERENCES

Cox, R. H. (1974): Three-dimensional mechanics of arterial segments *in vitro:* methods. J. Appl. Physiol. 36, 381—384.

Hudetz, A. G. (1978): Incremental elastic modulus for orthotropic incompressible arteries. J. Biomechanics (to be published).

Márk, G., Hudetz, A. G., Kerényi, T., Monos, E., Kovách, A. G. B. (1977): Is the sclerotic vessel wall really more rigid than the normal one? Prog. biochem. Pharmacol. 13, 292—297, Karger, Basel.

Márk, G., Hudetz, A. G., Monos, E., Fódy, L., Kovách, A. G. B. (1978): Biomechanical properties of normal and fibrosclerotic human internal carotid arteries. (published in this book).

A. G. H. Experimental Research Dept., Semmelweis Medical Univ. 1082 Budapest, Üllöi ut 78/a, Hungary

BIOMECHANICAL PROPERTIES OF NORMAL AND FIBROSCLEROTIC HUMAN INTERNAL CAROTID ARTERIES

G. MÁRK, A. G. HUDETZ, E. MONOS, L. FÓDY
and A. G. B. KOVÁCH

*Experimental Research Institute, Semmelweis Medical University,
Budapest, Hungary*

Introduction

It is obvious that the mechanical properties of blood vessels play a decisive role in both physiological and pathological cardiovascular events. Several researchers have experimentally studied the possible connection between pathomechanism of arteriosclerosis and local hydrodynamic effects at certain predilection sites such as bends, orifices and bifurcations of the arterial tree (*Patel et al.*, 1974). Much less effort has been devoted to quantitative evaluation of the changes in elastic properties of arteries due to arteriosclerotic processes, though the mechanical state and elasticity of an injured artery are of ultimate importance in controlling local hemodynamics.

It is generally accepted that fibrosclerotic processes are accompanied by an increase in the wall thickness and rigidity of the arterial wall. The results of experimental studies are, however, contradictory (*Newman et al.*, 1971). Furthermore, only few data (*Márk et al.*, 1977) have been published concerning the elastic properties of fibrosclerotic human cranial arteries, a problem having special importance with respect to human pathology. Our earlier studies (*Márk et al.*, 1977) revealed that elasticity of fibrosclerotic human anterior cerebral arteries was 34—45 percent *greater* than that of the normal vessels. To validate this surprising result for other cranial arteries, the passive mechanical properties of human internal carotid arteries were studied in this work.

Methods

The arteries were excised not later than 2 days after death from 18 cadavers. A straight 15 to 20 cm long cylindrical segment was dissected, stretched to its *in vivo* length and mounted in the experimental apparatus (*Cox*, 1974). Vessels were immersed into an oxygenated Krebs-Ringer buffer solution thermostated at 37 °C. The intraluminal pressure was changed slowly (100 mmHg /min) from 0 to 250 mmHg by cyclic inflation and deflation with air, while the pressure and external diameter of the vessels were recorded continuously. To find the wall thickness of the artery the net weight of the segment was determined. After measurement, the arteries were examined histologically under a light microscope and classified into fibrosclerotic (N = 10) and normal (N = 8) groups according to the relative increase in collagen content of the media, intimal proliferation and smooth muscle damage. The fibrosclerotic specimens contained no plaques.

After digitalizing the diameter/pressure curves, several quantities characterising the mechanical properties of the vessels were computed, e. g. the incremental elastic modulus (Cox, 1977):

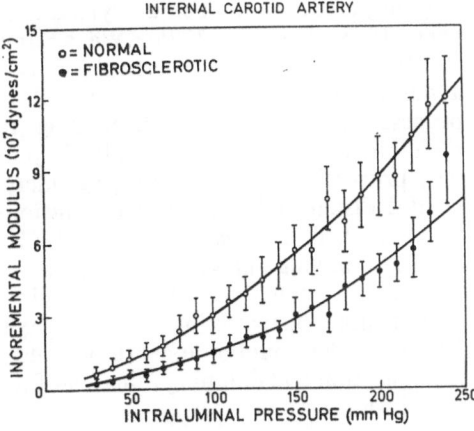

Fig. 1. Comparison of the average incremental elastic moduli of 10 fibrosclerotic and 8 normal human arteries at identical internal pressure levels.

$$E = \frac{\Delta P}{\Delta R_e} \frac{2R_i^2 R_e}{R_e^2 - R_i^2},$$

and incremental distensibility:

$$D = \frac{2}{R_i} \frac{\Delta R_i}{\Delta P},$$

where R_i and R_e are the internal and external radii of the segment and Δp is the pressure increment (10 mmHg) respectively.

Results and conclusions

Fibrosclerotic arteries were found to be more elastic than the normal ones, that is their incremental elastic modulus was $40-56$ percent smaller ($p < 0.05$) than that of the normal ones at identical internal pressure levels in the range of $90-250$ mm Hg (Fig. 1). The internal radius to wall thickness ratio was $37-38$ percent smaller in the fibrosclerotic group ($p < 0.05$, $40-250$ mm Hg) than in the normal one (Fig. 2). The internal radius and strain energy density were equal in the two groups. There was no significant difference in the incremental distensibilities

of the two groups (Fig. 3), due to the opposite changes in elastic modulus and wall thickness.

Taking into consideration our similar results for the anterior cerebral artery (*Márk et al.*, 1977) we suppose that neither

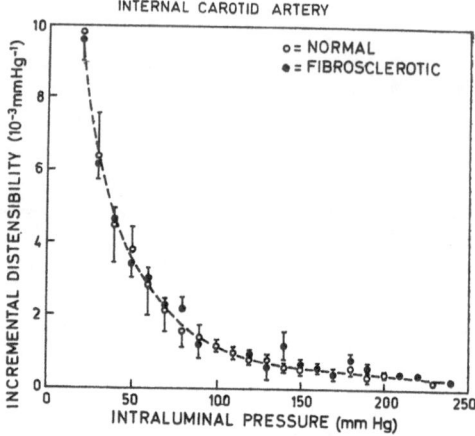

Fig. 3. Dependence of average incremental distensibilities of fibrosclerotic and normal human arteries on the internal pressure.

the elasticity nor distensibility of human cerebral arteries decrease, at least in a certain period of fibrosclerosis. Changes in the structure of the vessels are usually considered as pathological processes but they may also have compensatory character (*Fry*, 1973; *Rodbard*, 1975). We assume that the observed increase in the elasticity is a consequence of a local compensatory process in the vessel wall, tending to maintain some hemodynamically important properties of the arteries, eg. incremental distensibility. Similar conclusions were reached by *Thind* (1974) and *Cox* (1977) studying elasticity changes of arteries in experimental hypertension. Incremental distensibility is the main factor in determining local blood flow configuration and damping function of the vessel wall.

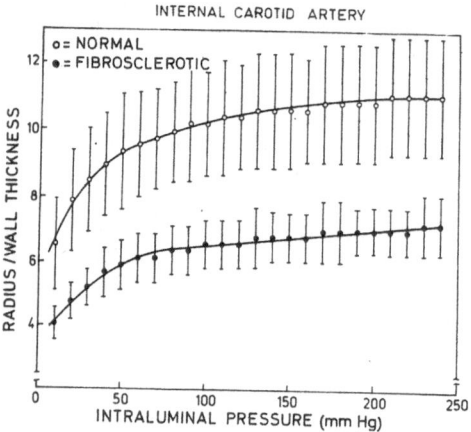

Fig. 2. Comparison of the average radius to wall thickness ratio of fibrosclerotid and normal human arteries at identical internal pressure levels.

REFERENCES

Cox, R. H. (1974): Three-dimensional mechanics of arterial segments *in vitro:* methods. J. Appl. Physiol. 36, 381—384.

Cox, R. H. (1977): Carotid artery mechanics and composition in renal and DOCA hypertension in the rat. Cardiovasc. Medicine 2, 761—766.

Fry, D. L. (1973): Responses of the arterial wall to certain physical factors. In: "Atherogenesis: Initiating Factors". CIBA Found. Symp. 12, 127—164. Assioc. Sci. Publ., Amsterdam.

Márk, G., Hudetz, A. G., Kerényi, T., Monos E., Kovách, A. G. B. (1977): Is the sclerotic vessel wall really more rigid than the normal one?

Prog. biochem. Pharmacol. 13, 292—297, Karger, Basel.

Newman, D. L. Gosling, R. G. Bowden, N. L. R. (1971): Changes in aortic distensibility and area ratio with the development of atherosclerosis. Atherosclerosis 14, 231—240.

Patel, D. J., Vaishnav, R. N., Gow, B. S., Kot, P. A. (1974): Haemodynamics. Ann. Rev. Physiol. 36, 125—154.

Rodbard, S. (1975): Vascular Caliber. Cardiology 60, 4—49.

Thind, G. S. (1974): Blood vessel wall characteristics in experimental hypertension. Angiology 25, 752—763.

G. M. Experimental Research Dept., Semmelweis Medical Univ., 1082 Budapest, Üllöi út 78/a, Hungary

BIO-MECHANICAL AND HISTOLOGICAL RESEARCH ON HEALTHY AND VARICOSE HUMAN VEINS

E. SCHMIDT, H. P. BRUCH, R. LAVEN, G. WINTER and P. KUJATH

Department of Surgery, University of Würzburg, Würzburg, F.R.G.

The pharmaceutical industry offers today a wide range of drugs to which venal tonic qualities are ascribed. It seemed therefore to be of use to examine the physiological parameters of healthy and varicose veins and to compare them with histological findings, in order to be able to draw conclusions about the muscular activity of the vessels. Indeed, drugs which influence the muscle tone can only produce an effect when based on an intact muscle system.

Thirty spiral strips of varicose human saphenous veins were examined, ten parallel studies were carried out on healthy saphenous veins. The muscle spiral strips were suspended between two hooks in a circulating Tyrode bath and the isometric tension development was continuously registered. (The tension development related to the muscle cross-section). The quantitative reactions of different specimen were thus comparable. With the aid of a digital computer, length/tension diagrams were approximated. Using the least squares method, the following equation was formed.

$$T = a \cdot e^{bx.L-L}o + c$$

T = tension related to the muscle cross-section (dyn/mm^2)

Lo = length of the muscle strip in mm (tension 10 dyn/mm^2)

L = actual muscle length in mm.

The maximum tension development per muscle cross-section (dyn/mm^2) (100%) resulted from the depolarization in a potassium Tyrode solution (135 mval/l). Working graphs were drown up for all the strips. The quotient LN 2 : B was applicable to all specimen. LN 2 : B refers

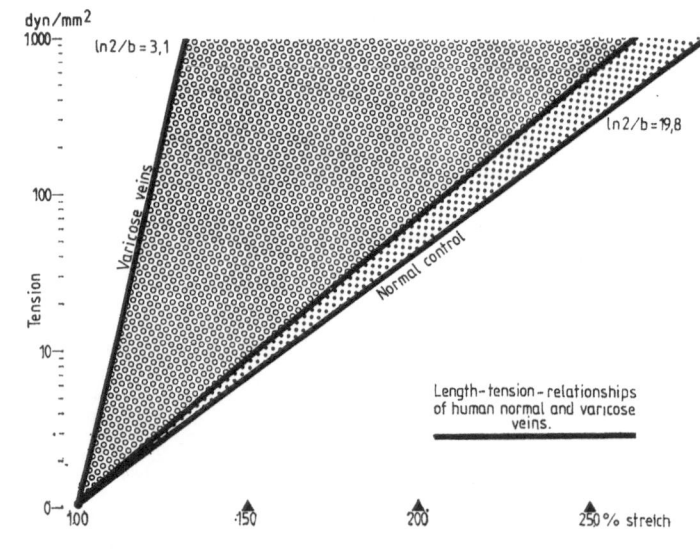

Fig. 1.

142

to that change in length in per cent which is necessary in order to doubly increase the tension of a muscle strip.

In histological examinations we tried to compare this physiological parameter

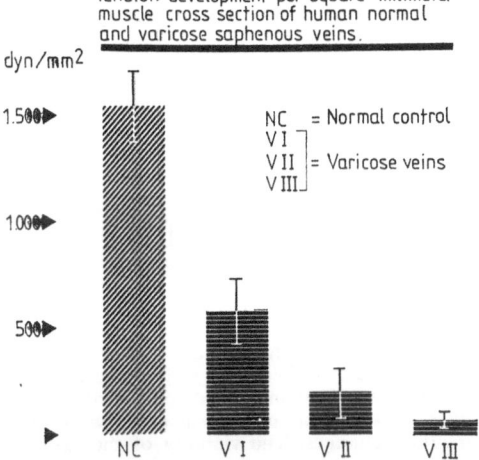

Fig. 2.

with morphological changes. Using Elastica-van Gieson colouring of the strips, the specimens were ordered according to their morphological changes without referring to the previous physiological parameter. The result showed that the elastic-muscular wall-sections of the varicose veins were replaced fibrously according to the degree of varicosity. In extreme cases almost complete fibrosis of the venous walls took place resulting in

a binding of the muscular elements still present. In closer correlation to the histological findings the physiological parameters changed. The healthy vena saphena was easily expandable. LN 2 : B = = 18 to 19.8%, while the extremely varicose veins showed a high rate of rigidity, LN 2 : B = 3 to 5%. (Fig. 1) The length tension diagrams, which, in semi-logarithmical presentation impress as a straight line, show that very high tension is necessary in order to expand varicose vessels even only a little. With increasing sclerosis of the venous walls the active tension also decreased. While the healthy vena saphena magna reached a tension of ~1500 (dyn/mm^2), the active tension development of varicose vessels only reached 50−400 dyn/mm^2 (Fig. 2.)

From this research we can see that, parallel to the histological changes in the varicose veins, deviations of the physiological parameters also take place. The active tension functions imparted through the muscular elements of the venous wall decreased greatly. On the other hand, the fibrous structures increased. In the course of development from the healthy to the extremely varicose veins the rigidity also increases while the active muscular function is finally completely lost.

Presuming the effectiveness of the drugs, a therapy which influences the venous tone is only then of value if it treats vessels which are, for a great part, still healthy. A strongly varicose vein no longers offers a physiological basis for pharmacological therapy.

S. E. University Department of Surgery, Jos. Schneiderstr. 2 D-78 Würzburg, F.R.G.

THE INFLUENCE OF CIGARETTE SMOKING ON HUMAN ARTERIAL EXPLANTS IN VITRO

K. FEESER, R. EBERT and A. K. HORSCH

Med. Univ.-Klinik Heidelberg, F.R.G.

Introduction

Cigarette smoking is a well established risk factor for atherosclerosis and its sequelae, namely peripheral vascular disease, coronary heart disease and stroke. Epidemiological, experimental and clinical studies have clearly demonstrated the atherogenic effect of cigarette smoking, but very little is known of the underlying pathogenic mechanisms. Nicotine, carbon monoxide with the resulting hypoxia and other substances in cigarette smoke have all been suggested as the primary causative agent. Indirect effects of cigarette smoke inhalation such as the release of catecholamines and free fatty acids have also been considered, but the decisive link for this association has so far not been found.

The lipid metabolism of human arteries incubated in human serum drawn before and after cigarette smoke inhalation was studied *in vitro*. In atherogenesis the lipid metabolism is altered in a typical way and we hoped to see if substances present in the serum after cigarette smoke inhalation would also influence this metabolism *in vitro*.

Material and methods

Serum: After fasting overnight, blood was drawn from young healthy men at rest 30 and 15 min before smoking. Smoking conditions were standardized. 1 min and 20 min after smoking blood was drawn again and nicotine and carbon monoxide levels were determined. Blood samples were pooled and the serum was sterilized by filtration and inactivated. The blood drawn before smoking was treated similarly. To each type of incubation medium — fasting serum or smoking serum — an equal amount of tissue culture medium and ^{3}H-oleic acid (2Ci/mmol spec. activity, 10 μCi/ml incubation medium), ^{14}C-linoleic acid (60 mCi/ml

spec. act., 4 μCi/ml incub. medium) and ^{32}Phosphate (30-100Ci/mg, 50 μCi/ml incub. medium) were added.

Tissue culture

Four human femoral arteries in different stages of atherosclerosis (WHO I—II,II, II—III and III) were removed immediately post mortem and divided into explants of approximate 20 mm. These explants were randomised and distributed to either the fasting or the after smoking incubation medium. After 24 h all explants were washed, part of them taken down and the other part incubated for a further three days in a nonradioactive medium with daily medium changes. The viability of the explants was checked by glucose uptake and lactate

UPTAKE OF ^{3}H-OLEIC ACID INTO EXPLANTS OF VARIOUS HUMAN
FEMORAL ARTERIES IN TISSUE CULTURE
(dpm/mg protein · 10^6 dpm in incubation medium)

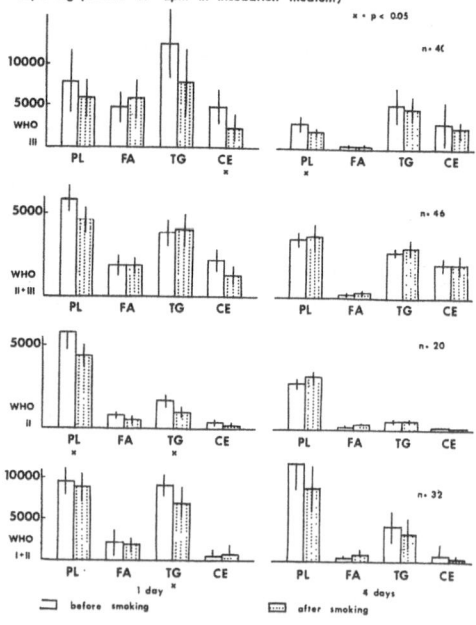

Figure 1 and Figure 2. PL = phospholipids; FA = free fatty acids; TG = triglycerides; CE = cholesterol esters.

production. Controls of sterility were also done. All media were stored for further examination. At the end of tissue culture all explants were washed, intima and parts of the media stripped off, homogenized and lipids and proteins extracted for subsequent analysis.

Details of the methods have been described elsewhere (*Horsch et al.*, 1977a.)

Results

In all the experiments the uptake of all labels seems to be higher after one day in the fasting incubation system. As would be expected, after four days the activity has decreased, but the difference between the two incubation systems persists. The decrease of activity in the explants is due to the release of labelled lipids into the incubation medium. The released lipids were recovered quantitatively, primarily as fatty acids and to a lesser extend as phospholipids. Only marginal amounts of cholesterol esters and triglycerides were mobilized.

The incorporation of ^{3}H-oleic acid into different lipids of the explants after one

INCORPORATION OF ^{14}C·LINOLEIC ACID INTO LIPIDS OF HUMAN ARTERIAL EXPLANTS IN TISSUE CULTURE
(dpm / mg protein · 10^6 dpm in incubation medium)

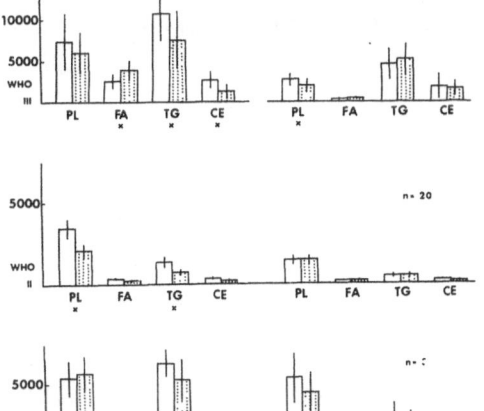

Fig. 2.

UPTAKE OF ^{32}P·PHOSPHATE INTO PHOSPHOLIPIDS BY HUMAN FEMORAL ARTERIES IN TISSUE CULTURE

(dpm / mg Protein · 10^6 dpm in incubation medium)

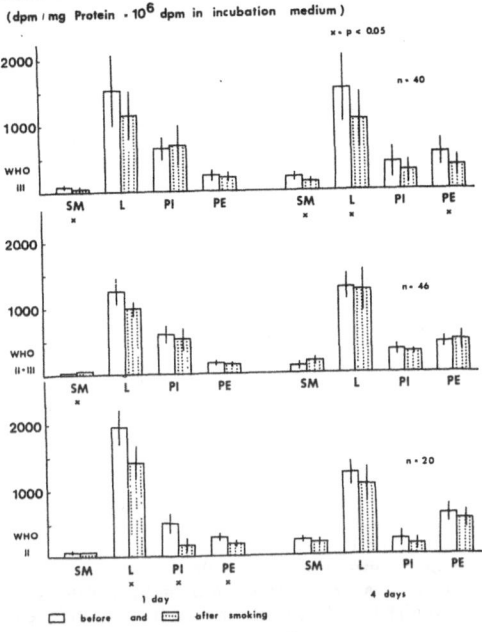

Figure 3. SM = sphingomyelin; L = lecithin; PI = phosphatidyl inositol; PE = phosphatidyl ethanolamine.

and four days is shown in Table I. The individual data for all four arteries are given. In some lipid fractions the synthesis is significantly higher in the fasting incubation system. Additionally, it should be noted that the incorporation of the labelled fatty acids into phospholipids and triglycerides seems to be dependent on the atherosclerotic involvement of the arteries. In advanced lesions phospholipid synthesis seems to be lower, whereas triglyceride and cholesterol ester synthesis seems to be increased. Similar data were obtained for the incorporation of ^{14}C-linoleic acid (Table II). Again significantly more activity is present in some lipid fractions after incubation in the fasting serum. Cholesterol esterification again is considerably higher in the artery with advanced lesions compared to the early lesions.

The highest incorporation of ^{32}Phosphate occurs into lecithin followed by phosphatidyl inositol (Table III).

Surprisingly, there is only a slight

decrease in the activity in lecithin after four days; while phosphatidyl inositol decreases, the activity in the phosphatidyl ethanolamine fraction increases approximately in the same proportion as the former decreases. In the 4 day period in both incubation systems there is a constant increase in the sphingomyelin synthesis.

Conclusions

There seems to be a decrease of lipid synthesis in the smoking system, but the significance of these findings is difficult to evaluate (*Horsch et al.*, 1977 b). In atherogenesis, phospholipid synthesis and cholesterol esterification are increased and while the phospholipid synthesis and especially lecithin synthesis are considered to be a protective mechanism, the esterification of cholesterol is the important and sclerogenic cellular event in the development of the lesion. However, we could not conclude from our findings that the decreased phospholipid synthesis after incubation in the smoking serum is an explanation of the well documented atherogenic effect of cigarette smoking. Further experiments in our incubation system are necessary to establish more decisively the *in vitro* effect of cigarette smoke inhalation.

REFERENCES

Hill, P., Wynder, E. L. (1974): Smoking and Cardiovascular Disease. Effect of Nicotine on the Serum Epinephrine and Steroids. American Heart Journal 87, 491—496.

Horsch, A. K., Eber, H. G., Römmele, U. (1977a): Langfristige Gewebekultur von menschlichen normalen und atherosclerotischen Arterien-explantaten. Virchows Arch. A. Path. Anat. and Histol. 375, 287—301.

Horsch, A. K., Koch, A. Heuck, C. C., and Mörl, H. (1977b): Effect of Cigarette Smoking on Uptake of ^{3}H-Oleic and ^{14}C-linoleic Acid by Human Arteries in Vitro. Atherosclerosis IV, 172.

Kershbaum, A., Bellet, S., Hirabayaski, M., Feinber, J. J. (1966): Regular, filtertip, and modified cigarettes. Nicotine excretion, free fatty acid mobilization, and catecholamine excretion. Journal of the American Medical Association 195 (13), 1095—1098.

Strong, J. P., and Richards, M. L. (1976): Cigarette Smoking and Atherosclerosis in Autopsied Men. Atherosclerosis 23, 451—476.

US Department of Health, Education and Welfare. The Health Consequences of Smoking. A Report to the Surgeon General 1971.

A. K. H., Med. Univ.-Klinik Bergheimerstr. 58, D-6900 Heidelberg, F.R.G.

POSTISCHEMIC HYPERRESPONSIVENESS OF CANINE CAROTID ARTERIES

E. MONOS and A. G. B. KOVÁCH

Experimental Research Institute, Semmelweis Medical University, Budapest, Hungary

Introduction

Physiological responses to smooth muscle activation in large arteries are mediated by changes in diameter and in elastic wall properties. As a result, changes in strain energy density, distensibility, characteristic impedance and, to a certain degree, also in the peripheral resistance of the arterial tree will influence the performance of the whole cardiovascular system (*Cox*, 1975a; *Monos and Szücs*, 1978; *Monos et al.*, 1978a). These variables should be under close physiological control to minimize short-term arterial pressure fluctuations, the pulsatile energy of the heart, etc. The above geometric and elastic responses of the arteries are functions of the intraluminal pressure. The pressure dependent response characteristics of large arteries are influenced by several factors, such as structural-geometrical properties reflected by regional differences in vascular control, hormonal interactions and pathological alterations (*Cox*, 1975b; *Hudetz et al.*, 1977; *Márk et al.*, 1977). The present work was carried out to explore the effect of transient local ischemia on the active response characteristics of canin common carotid arteries.

Methods

Experiments were carried out on 10 dogs anesthetized with pentobarbital sodium (33 mg/kg bw.). Both carotids were exposed on the neck. One of them was subjected to one hour local ischemia by squeezing the blood out of the lumen and clamping both ends of an 8—10 cm section. The vessel was covered with body warm paraffin oil. After this ischemic period the blood was allowed to recirculate through the carotid for an additional one hour period. Then large-deformation active and passive mechanics of the arteries were tested using an *in vitro* technique (*Cox*, 1973). The excised cylindrical segment of the artery was mounted in a temperature controlled tissue bath at its *in vivo* length. The intraluminal pressure was changed slowly (100 mmHg/min) in the 0—250 mmHg range while the outer diameter and axial extending force were recorded at both relaxed and activated (0.5 μg/ml norepinephrine) states of smooth muscle. The diameter versus pressure and axial force versus pressure curves were digitalized in 10 mmHg pressure steps; the average passive and active mechanical properties (e. g. strains, normal stresses, incremental elastic modulus, incremental distensibility, strain-energy density) of the arterial wall were computed. The contralateral artery served as normal control.

Results and conclusions

It was found that the reactivity of the smooth vascular muscle was markedly enhanced after one hour transient ischemia. *Fig 1.* demonstrates that, though the shape of the response curves was essentially the same, active strain (i.e. a relative

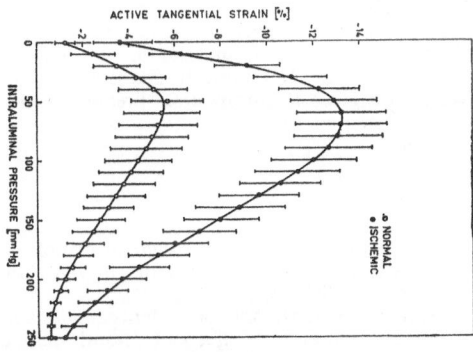

Fig. 1. Effect of one-hour transient ischemia on active tangential strain elicited by 0.5 μg/ml norepinephrine in canine carotids. The active strain is defined as the relative change in the outer diameter through smooth muscle contraction at identical intraluminal pressure values.

change in the outer diameter) elicited by norepinephrine was at least twice as large in the ischemic group than in the normal one at each pressure level studied. The maximum of this geometric response (normal: $-5.7 \pm 1.5\%$; ischemic: $-13.2 \pm \pm 2.0\%$; $p < 0.01$) developed at relatively low (50 mm Hg) intraluminal pressure, while the maximum elastic reponse, that is the decrease in elastic modulus (normal: $15-20\%$; ischemic: $40-45\%$; $p < 0.05$) was observed at higher pressure (100 to 200 mm Hg in both groups), or stretch levels (*Fig. 2.*). The same dose or norepinephrine elicited larger elasticity increase in the ischemic than in the normal artery, but no differences between the two groups

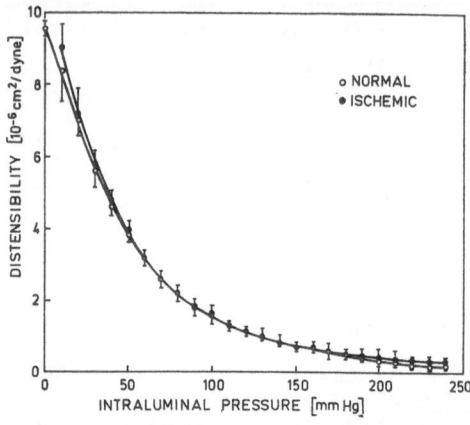

Fig. 3. Distensibility of normal and postischemic carotid arteries as a function of intraluminal pressure. The distensibility is inversely proportional to the elastic modulus and to the wall thickness/radius ratio.

could be found in the elastic moduli of passive wall elements. Similarly, the mean incremental distensibility (*Fig. 3.*) and strain-energy density of the passive wall elements did not differ as radius to wall thickness ratios were the same in the two groups.

Thus, after transient local ischemia, an increased vascular smooth muscle response to norepinephrine was found for which alterations in the average mechanical properties of passive wall elements seemed not to be responsible. It is supposed that the increase in the reactivity of arteries after ischemia may enhance vascular effects of both sympathetic hyperactivity and elevated levels of constrictor substances in blood found during or after hypotensive states.

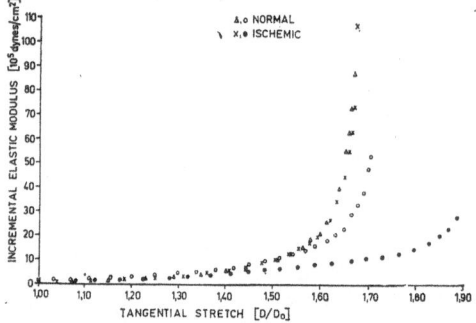

Fig. 2. Incremental elastic moduli of normal and postischemic carotid arteries as function of tangential stretch (dog: No. 3.). The elastic moduli characterize the specific stiffness of the arterial wall for 10 mmHg pressure increments. Δ, x: relaxed smooth muscle; o, o: activated smooth muscle; D: midwall diameter of the vessel at a given P_i intraluminal pressure value; D_o: diameter of the vessel at zero intraluminal pressure.

REFERENCES

Cox, R. H. (1975a): Pressure dependence of the mechanical properties of arteries in vivo. Am. J. Physiol. 229, 1371—1375.
Cox, R. H. (1975b): Arterial wall mechanics and composition and the effects of smooth muscle activation. Am. J. Physiol. 229, 807—812.
Hudetz, A. G., Márk, Gy., Monos, E., Szutrély, J., Kovách, A. G. B. (1977): Biomechanical properties of human cerebral arteries. Proc. Internat. U. Physiol. Sci. 13, 337.
Monos, E., Cox, R. H. Peterson, L. H. (1978a) Direct effect of physiological doses of arginine vasopressin on the arterial wall in vivo. Am J. Physiol. 234, H167—H172, or Am. J. Physiol.: Heart Circ. Physiol. 3, H167—H172.

E. M. Experimental Research Institute Semmelweis Medical University, 1082 Budapest Üllöi ut 78/a., Hungary

VOLUME AND SURFACE AREAS OF SOME VASCULAR SMOOTH MUSCLE CELL ORGNELLES IN RAT

V. LEVICKÝ and A. V. LOUD

Institute of Normal and Pathological Physiology, Slovak Academy of Sciences, Bratislava and New York Medical College, Valhalla, New York, U.S.A.

Considerable attention has been devoted in pertinent literature to ultrastructures of the blood vessel smooth muscle cell presumed to be the beare of the functional phenomenon of excitation-contraction coupling (*Bohr*, 1964, *Devine et al.*, 1972). Nonetheless, hardly any quantitative data are available as yet on the size of the cell volume occupied by these structures, or about the areas of the various membrane surfaces involved in ion movement during contraction. The present work has for aim to fill up some of the gaps in our knowledge on the quantity of some ultrastructural components in the vascular smooth muscle cell and to put the data into relation with the function of the ultrastructure under study.

Methods

The quantitative evaluation has been made on portal vein of 5 white rats. The tissue were

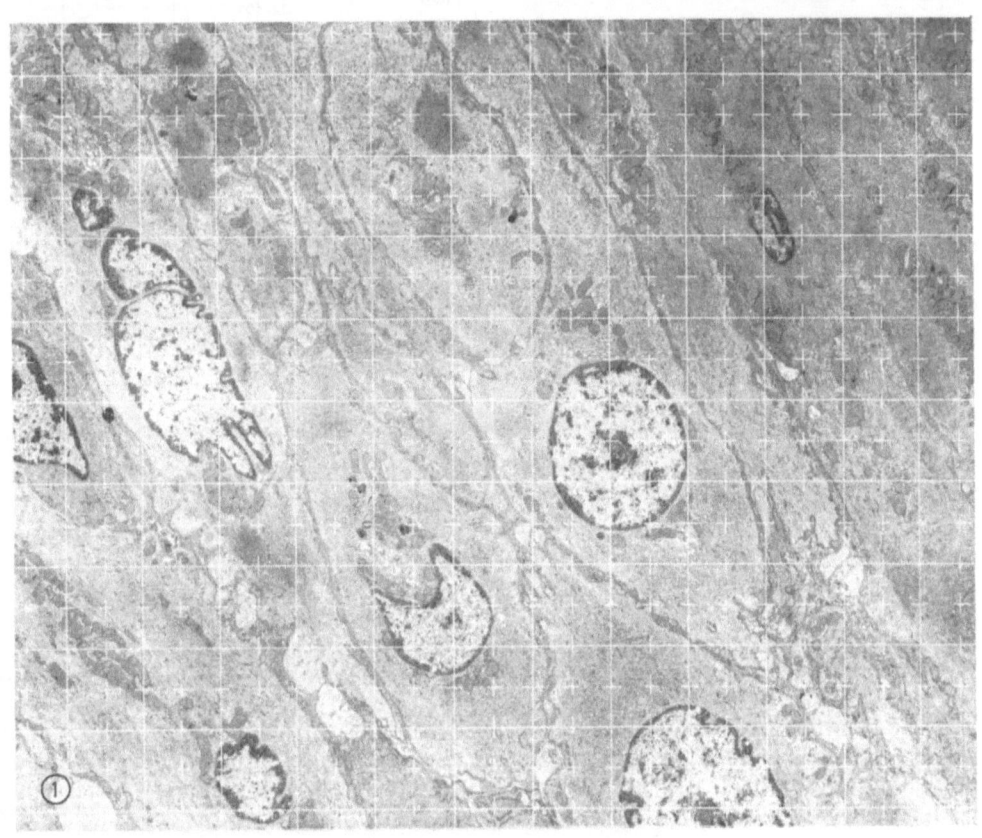

fixed according to Karnovsky and Millonig, dehydrated in acetone and embedded in Durcupan ACM.

The quantitative stereological analysis was made on photographic prints of electron micrographs. In connection with the ultrastructure, two sizes of the resulting print magnification were used: a) 10.000× for calculating the volume fraction of nuclei in the cytoplasm, the surface area of the cell membrane and the surface area of the cell nucleus; b) 70.000× for calculating volume fraction of mitochondria, sarcoplasmic reticulum, surface vesicles and surface areas of the membranes of these structures. The theoretical aspects and the use of stereological techniques have already been described earlier (*Loud et al.*, 1965, *Underwood*, 1970). For the ultrastructure evaluation proper, prints were prepared on which the square grid was simultaneously imprinted (Figure). The latter consists of lines whose mutual intersections constitute test points for point counting (the total count being 500 points). To evaluate the size of the areas with the aid of the linear integration method, use was made of horizontal lines.

Results

As shown in Table I, the volume of sacroplasm is made up of 8.051 percent of mitochondria, 3.785 percent of sarcoplasmic reticulum, 1.799 percent of surface vesicles; the remaining part of sarcoplasm, including myofilaments, represents 86.401 volume percent. As evident from Table II, nuclei make up 5.362 percent of the entire smooth muscle cell volume. Therefore, the true volume values of the evaluated ultrastructures in the whole cell are lower by about 1/20. Table I also gives the surface areas per unit of cell volume in three types of membranes. The data reveal that the values of the surface areas of mitochondrial, sarcoplasmic reticulum and surface vesicles membranes are relatively close.

Discussion

These results make it clear that of all the components of cytoplasm, mitochondria occupy the greatest volume in the smooth muscle cell. This also applies to cells of other tissues — a fact related to their function, as the principal energy source of cell activity.

From a morphological (and probably also a functional) aspects, cell membrane is made up of two regions: a) the membrane proper; b) surface vesicles which represent inpocketings of sarcolemma into the interior of the cell. Their function still remains fairly obscure. It was assumed that they serve to a substantial expanding of the surface of the cell membrane (*Gabella*, 1971). However, from the values

Table I.

Organelle	Percent of Sarcoplasm. Volume ± S.E.	Membrane Area (μm²) Sarcoplasm. Volum (μm³) ± S.E.
Mitochondria	8.015 0.332	0.085 0.013
Sarcoplasm. reticulum	3.785 0.571	0.125 0.022
Surface vesicles	1.799 0.350	0.070 0.017
Rest sarcoplasm	86.401 2.210	—

Table II.

Percent of Cell Volume ± S.E.		Membrane Area (μm²/μm³) ± S.E.	
Nuclei	Sarcoplasm	Nucl. membr. Nucl. volume	Cell. membr. Sarcoplasm. volume
5.362 0.523	94.638 0.523	2.716 0.282	1.670 0.285

of the ratio of their surface to 1 μm³ of cytoplasm (0.070 μm²/μm³) in view of this ratio in the case of the whole membrane (1.670 μm²/μm³), this surface enlargement appears to be negligible — a mere 4.2 percent.

Sarcoplasmic reticulum is the only structure of the vascular smooth muscle cell whose volume was determined with the aid of the "integration-by-weight" method (*Somlyo et al.*, 1975). This volume in the tonic smooth muscle of the great elastic arteries (pulmonary artery and aorta of the rabbit) was found to be 5%, while in the more phasic smooth muscles (portal vein and taenia coli of the rabbit) it was only 2%. This difference is attributed to an increased protein synthesis in the elastic type arteries. Our data — 3. 785% — determined by means of the stereological technique is much more precise and is a better basis for judging the function of sarcoplasmic reticulum under altered conditions.

It may be presumed that analogously to other tissues, the various ultrastructures of the vascular smooth muscle cell also have their own quantitative characteristics, which change when the function becomes altered through both physiological and pathological factors. The change in these quantitative relationships is so sensitive an indicator that it enables to detect an altered cell function at the ultrastructural level already in the early stages of the process.

REFERENCES

Bohr, D. F. (1964): Electrolytes and smooth muscle contraction. Pharmacol. Rev. 16, 85.

Devine, C. E., Somlyo, A. V., Somlyo, A. P. (1972): Sarcoplasmic reticulum and excitation-contraction coupling in mammalian smooth muscles. J. Cell. Biol. 52, 690.

Gabella, G. (1971): Caveolae intracellulares and sarcoplasmic reticulum in smooth muscle. J. Cell. Sci. 8, 601.

Loud, A. V., Barany, W. C., Pack, B. A. (1965): Quantitative evaluation of cytoplasmic structures in electron micrographs. Lab. Investig 14, 996.

Somlyo, A. P., Somlyo, A. V. (1975): Ultrastructure of smooth muscle. In: Methods in Pharmacology, pp. 3—45. Ed. by Daniels, E. E., Paton, D. M., Plenum, New York.

Underwood, E. (1970): Quantitative Stereology. Addison Wesley Publ. Co., Reading, Massachusetts.

V. L. Institute of Normal and Pathological Physiology, Slovak Academy of Sciences Sienkiewiczova 1, 884 23 Bratislava, Czechoslovakia

FLOW — RESISTANCE RELATIONSHIP FOR THE CEREBROVASCULAR SYSTEM OF RABBITS UNDER NORMAL AND PATHOPHYSIOLOGICAL CONDITIONS

H. HUTTEN and P. VAUPEL

Institute for Physiology, University of Mainz, F.R.G.

Introduction

Cerebrovascular autoregulation, i.e. the ability of the brain to maintain a constant blood flow despite changes in perfusion pressure, has been investigated in man and in various animals by many groups using different methods such as inert gas clearance, thermoclearance, electromagnetic flow meters and bypass systems. Most of the results support the widely accepted hypothesis that cerebrovascular autoregulation exists over a large range of blood pressures if it is not disturbed by such factors as anesthesia, hypoxia, hypercapnia, and total ischemia (*Hirsch,* 1971; *Bés and Géraud,* 1974). However, there is also strong experimental evidence agasinst cerebrovascular autoregulation (*Sagawa and Guyton,* 1961; *Gercken and Roth,* 1961; *de Valois and Peperkamp,* 1971).

Methods

Cerebrovascular resistance (CVR) in rabbits (slight anesthesia induced with ketamine and maintained with urethane) is measured by means of an extracorporeal by-pass system consisting mainly of a pressure-equalizer, a heat-exchanger and a roller pump with pressure-independent output. Decoupling systemic and infusion pressure is achieved by the pressure-equalizer. Blood is withdrawn from the aorta through a femoral catheter and reinfused into both internal carotid arteries (*Hutten and Vaupel,* 1977). All accessible arteries to extracerebral regions including both external carotid arteries are carefully ligated. The vertebral arteries and the spinal arteries are not ligated. Different flow values (CBF), i. e. flow input into both internal carotid arteries, can be set by means of the pump. The established infusion pressure (IP) is measured at the site of reinfusion by a Statham transducer. CVR is calculated from IP divided by CBF according to OHM's law.

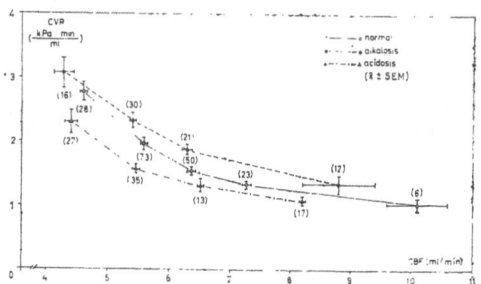

Fig. 1. CBF-CVR relationships in rabbits with normal hematocrit values during normal acid-base-balance (curve in the middle), during acidosis (lower curve) and during alkalosis (upper curve).

Results

Measurements are performed on a total of 92 normal rabbits in 5 groups:

group I: normal acid-base-status and normal hematocrit;

group II: normal acid-base-status, but during acute hemodilution;

group III: acidosis, combined with normal hematocrit values;

group IV: alkalosis, combined with normal hematocrit values;

group V: hypoxia, combined with normal hematocrit values.

Additionally, measurements were performed on 17 rabbits with provoked systemic atherosclerosis (group VI).

In all groups I — VI, CVR decreases with increasing CBF. Fig. 1 shows that CVR is shifted to lower values by acidosis and to higher values by alkalosis. The shape of the CBF − CVR relationship, however, remains unchanged. In Fig. 2, CVR is compared for normoxia nad hypoxia. Hypoxia yields a lowering of the CBF to

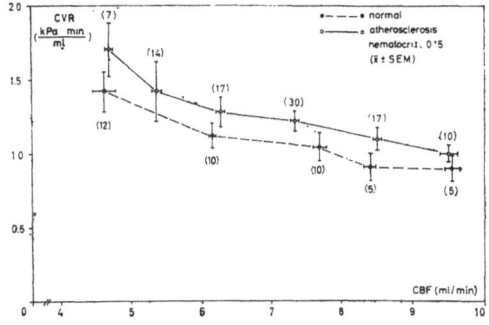

Fig. 2. CBF-CVR relationships in rabbits with normal hematocrit during normoxia (upper curve) and hypoxia (lower curve).

CVR relationship without changing its shape. Fig. 3 shows that, in comparison with normal rabbits with undisturbed acid-base-status and corresponding hematocrit values, CVR is shifted to higher values in rabbits with systemic atherosclerosis.

Discussion

Within the autoregulatory range, the vascular system should respond to an increase of the perfusion pressure with a corresponding increase of the vascular resistance in order to maintain constant flow. Therefore, raising the flow against autoregulation by means of the pump output should cause a drastic rise of both infusion pressure and vascular resistance. However, the experiments show that IP is only slightly increased with increasing CBF, whereas CVR, on the contrary,

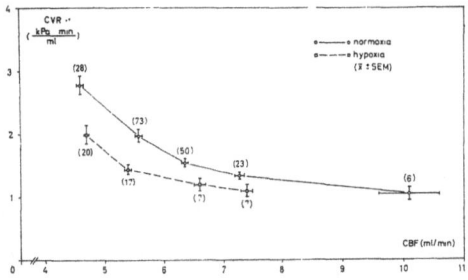

Fig. 3. CBF-CVR relationships in normal rabbits with undisturbed acid-base-status and in rabbits with provoked systemic atherosclerosis.

is reduced with increasing CBF. Auto-regulation proponents feel that the lack of autoregulation is caused by:

1. Anesthesia: Anesthesia, however, is very slight as could be demonstrated by provocation tests.

2. Hypoxia: No significant deviation in the shape of the CBF-CVR relationship occurs if normoxia is changed to hypoxia and during different degrees of acute hemodilution.

3. Ischemia: Total ischemia, i.e. stopped flow during connection of both internal carotid arteries with the extracorporeal by-pass system, was kept less than 1 minute in most cases. Partial ischemia for one single hemisphere was less than 2 minutes, i.e. less than the critical value.

4. Hypercapnia: The shape of the CBF-CVR relationship is not significantly affected by changes in the pH-value. Subgroups assigned to respiratory and nonrespiratory acidosis did not show significant differences.

Additionally, the following arguments must be discussed:

5. Supply of extracerebral tissue cannot be excluded totally. However, the total mass of extracerebral tissue supplied from the internal carotid arteries through anastomosis must be very small compared with intracerebral tissue mass, as could be demonstrated by dye injection.

6. Supply of intracerebral tissue, normally supplied from the verterbal arteries, can also not be excluded because in nearly all experiments IP was slightly higher than the systemic pressure which was lowered due to the withdrawal of blood from the aorta. However, it can be expected that the vessels in the brain stem manifest similar behaviour to those in the hemispheres.

7. Retrograde flow into the aorta through the vertebrobasilar system can occur if IP is considerably elevated above the systemic pressure. However, addition of bicarbonate to the reinfused blood always caused a significant reduction of CVR due to vasodilation. Furthermore, hemodilution lowered CVR considerably. There-

153

fore, it must be concluded that the retrograde shunt is negligible.

8. CBF-CVR relationships in rabbits with provoked systemic atherosclerosis are not different from those in normal rabbits with corresponding low hematocrit values. This can be expected as atherosclerosis is restricted to those large vessels which do not significantly determine the total vascular resistance. The shift to higher CVR values in the atherosclerotic rabbits may be caused mainly by excessive hyperlipidemia (*Leonhardt and Arntz*, 1977).

Conclusions

The results presented here do not support the hypothesis of cerebrovascular autoregulation in rabbits.

REFERENCES

Bés, A., Géraud, G.: Circulation Cérébrale (Vol. 1), Edition Sandoz 1974.
Gercken, G., Roth, E.: Pflügers Arch. 273, 589—603 (1961).
Hirsch, H.: In: Physiologie des Kreislaufs. Ed.: E. Bauereisen, p. 145—184, Springer-Verlag Berlin—Heidelberg—New York 1971.
Hutten, H., Vaupel, P.: Med. Welt 28, 1567 to 1572 (1977).

Leonhardt, H., Arntz, H.-R.: Rheologica Acta 16 (4), 369—377 (1977).
Sagawa, K., Guyton, A. C.: Amer. J. Physiol. 200, 711—714 (1961).
Valois, J. C, de, Peperkamp, J. P. C.: In: Brain and Blood Flow. Ed.: R. W. Ross Russell, p. 254—257, Pitman Publishing Company, London 1971.

H. H., Institute for Physiology, University of Mainz, Saarstr. 21, D-6500 Mainz, F.R.G.

CELL-KINETICAL INVESTIGATIONS IN THE PERIPHERAL ARTERIAL VESSELS OF RATS WITH DEPOT-ANGIOTENSIN-HYPERTENSION BETWEEN 3 HOURS AND 14 DAYS

E. ENGLER, D. MATTHIAS and C.-H. BECKER

Academy of Sciences, Central Institute for Heart and Circulatory Regulation Research, Berlin, G.D.R.

The increase in peripheral resistance in the region of arterioles and small arteries is an essential basis for arterial pressure increases in hypertension (*Folkow*, 1971). However, knowledge of structural alterations of the vessels, especially of hypertrophic and hyperplastic processes in hypertension is still incomplete. Thus,

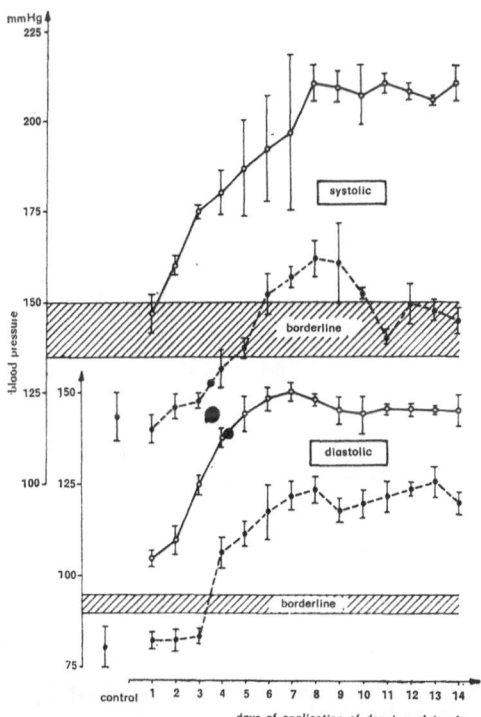

Fig. 1. Time course of systolic and diastolic blood pressure. Daily basal value before injection (— — — —) and daily mean value after injection (————). The blood pressure was measured eight times in 6 hrs after each injection. n = 6—30 experimental animals and 16 controls

induced hypertension, the development of morphological and proliferative behaviour of peripheral arterial vessels was investigated and correlated with the change in blood pressure.

For this purpose 30 rats received daily 1.25—2.5 mg A II s.c. for 1—14 days (*Engler et al.*, 1976). Between the 1st and 14th day the animals were killed and pancreas, gastro-intestinal tract and mesenterium were examined histologically and autoradiographically. To determine the proliferation rate, the labeled cells of capillaries and arterial walls as well as mitoses, were counted on an organ sectional area of 50 mm² each, following pulse labeling with 3H-thymidine.

In all animals the A II injections led to an immediate increase in blood pressure (Fig. 1). With every new injection the blood pressure rose further and persisted longer, and was finally established at a highly raised level. The daily basal value also increased and the diastolic basal pressure remained constant in the hypertensive region from the 4th day on (Fig. 1). Thus, the prevailing diastolic reaction shows that the increase in the peripheral resistance is in the foreground, suggesting a longlasting effect of A II on the resistance vessels.

The latter revealed — depending on the size and function — distinct differences in the time course of the pathological and proliferative alterations and the involvement of different wall layers. The pathological alterations are described here only in correlation with changes in blood pressure and with the distribution and time course in rats with depot — angiotensin (A II) of proliferative behaviour

155

of the arterial wall. With the pathological and proliferative alterations 3 distinct reaction phases were observable, generally connected with proliferation in the media.

In the first 3 hrs, before light microscopical alterations were observable, the first changes in the proliferation rate occured. Thus, the number of labelled capillaries rose, though they otherwise behaved normally over the whole period. The pericytes were labelled predominantly. The precapillaries and arterioles also displayed more frequent labeling (Fig. 2). Increased adventitial proliferation was observable. In the precapillaries the media cell proliferation was most important. Thus, all the small vessels were involved in this first reaction. The capillaries and precapillaries seem to have been stimulated to an immediate adaptative response by the high angiotensin doses. In the whole further course of the experiment these arterial terminal vessels appeared unaltered.

On the second day there was no difference in the proliferation rate, compared to the controls, though single arterioles showed pathological alterations. With a further rise in the blood pressure and the formation of pathological alterations increased proliferation is seen first in the arterioles and prearterioles and later also in diffrently large arteries (Fig. 2). There the media and adventitia were also labeled more frequently. The media frequently proliferated in its outer third at the media-adventitia-junction. From this reactive zone a granuloma like adventitia proliferation occured with advancing damage. Then the endothelial cell proliferation increased intensively.

This second phase in repair processes of vascular wall damage is then followed after 14 days by marked proliferation of the media, while only minor reactions occured in the endothelium and adventitia. Striking were numerous larger cross-sections of vessels in which the media was thickened, and numerous media cells were labeled with 3H-thymidine. In this

3rd stage, in which the increased blood pressure reached a constant level, the peripheral vessels react predominantly with media hyperplasia and both arterioles and arteries are involved in the process.

Parallel to the 3H-thymidine incorporation rate, we could also observe an increase in the number of labelled mitoses.

In summary, we can conclude that, with establishment of stable resistance hypertension, the proliferation pattern of the arterial vascular wall cells is dependent on the size of the vessels, the time course of the hypertension and the presence of pathological alterations.

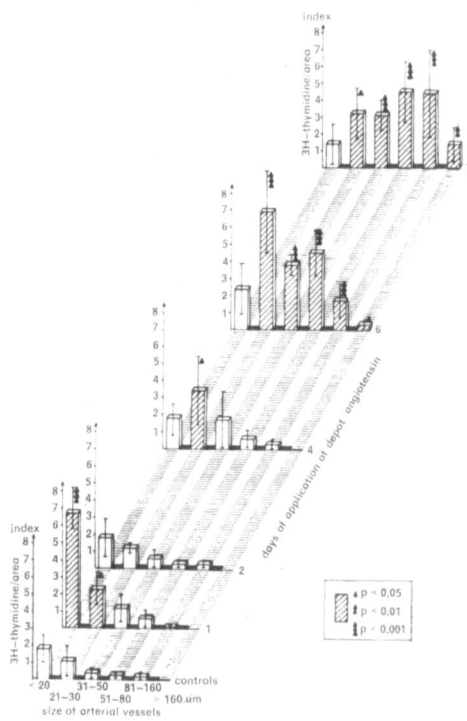

Fig. 2. Time course of the number of 3H-thymidine labeled arterial vessels with different size following depot angiotensin. Area unit: 2.5 mm^2 organ sectional field. n = 6 hypertensive and 2 vehicle controls in each time period and 6 normal rats.

E. E., ZI Herz-Kreislaufforschung, 1115 Berlin, Wiltbergstr. 50, G.D.R.

THE REACTIVITY OF ISOLATED VENOUS PREPARATION FROM RABBITS PRETREATED WITH RESERPINE

J. TÖRÖK and R. TÖRÖKOVÁ

*Institute of Normal and Pathological Physiology, Slovak Academy of Sciences
Bratislava, Czechoslovakia*

Introduction

Hughes and Vane (1967) demonstrated that transmural nerve stimulation produced a contraction in isolated rabbit portal veins with high spontaneous tone. In the presence of alfa-adrenergic blocking agents, this response has been converted to relaxation. The present study was undertaken to investigate the existence and evaluate the functional role of inhibitory response to transmural nerve stimulation in the portal vein with low initial tone from rabbits pretreated with reserpine.

Methods

A rabbit isolated portal vein was longitudinally divided in half and mounted vertically in an organ bath containing 20 ml Krebs bicarbonate solution bubbled with 95% O_2 + 5% CO_2 and maintained at 37 °C. The strips were connected to a force displacement transducer for continuous isometric recording. The initial tension was set at 1 or 2 g. For studies of responsiveness to transmural nerve stimulation (TS), the strip was placed between a pair of platinum electrodes and stimulated with rectangular pulses of 0.5 msec duration, delivered at 35 V, with varying frequencies (2—16 Hz). To deplete catecholamine stores in the portal vein, reserpine (1 mg/kg) was injected intraperitoneally into the rabbit 48 and 24 hours prior to sacrifice.

Results

As shown in Fig. 1, TS at 8 Hz caused the contraction of a portal vein strip from untreated animals. The preparation partially contracted by noradrenaline (NA, 10^{-7}M) was further contracted with TS.

There was a higher amplitude of spontaneous mechanical activity in the portal vein from a reserpinized animal. In this preparation TS at 8 Hz caused an inhibition of spontaneous rhythmic activity. After the vein was partially contracted by NA (10^{-7}M), TS produced relaxation. This response was also observed when active tone was produced by histamine (Fig. 2) and other vasoactive drugs (adrenaline, acetylcholine, $SrCl_2$ and $BaCl_2$). Inhibitory response to TS was observed in all 57 preparations examined and could be obtained in both completely and partially NA-depleted vessels.

The relaxation induced by TS was not affected by guanethidine ($10^{-6} - 10^{-5}$M)

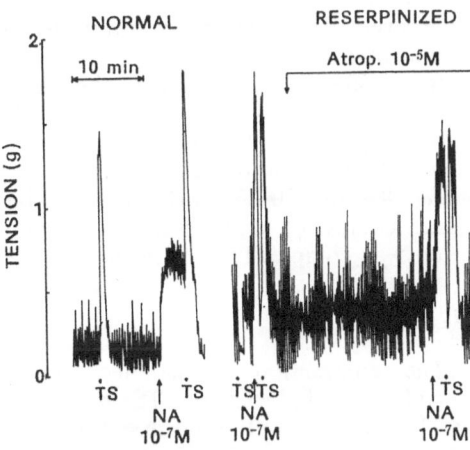

Fig. 1. Isometric tension recording from a portal vein strip removed from untreated (left) and reserpine pretreated rabbits (right). Transmural nerve stimulation (TS) at 8 Hz for 30 sec with 0.5 msec duration pulses at 36 V. Active muscle tone was produced by noradrenaline (NA).

157

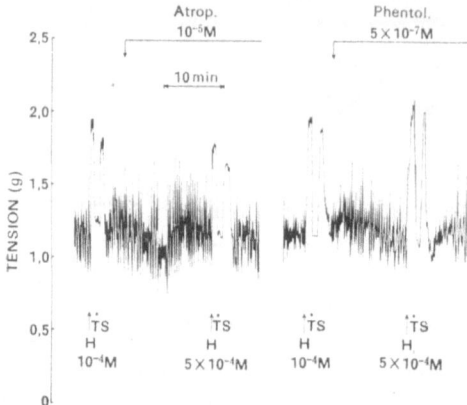

Fig. 2. Effect of atropine (Atrop.) and phentolamine (Phentol.) on relaxation of portal veins partially contracted by histamine (H) induced by transmural nerve stimulation (TS) at 8 Hz for 60 sec.

and atropine $(10^{-6} - 10^{-5}M)$. Moreover phentolamine $(10^{-7} - 10^{-6}M)$ did not prevent relaxation of vessel partially contracted by histamine, $SrCl_2$ and $BaCl_2$.

Relaxations induced by TS in the presence of antagonists of alfa-adrenergic receptors were also observed in both reserpine pretreated and untreated preparations. Ergotamine $(5 \times 10^{-6} \text{ g/ml})$ produced a sustained contraction (Fig. 3); the relaxation induced by TS at 8 Hz was not prevented by guanethidine, propranolol and atropine.

By adding KCl $(1-5 \text{ mM})$ to the organ bath the tone was decreased and rhythmic activity increased. TS-induced relaxation, however, was not prevented. On increasing K^+ to $30-35$ mM the vascular tissue contracted and TS-induced relaxation was completely abolished.

Discussion

The contraction of isolated rabbit portal veins induced by TS has been attributed to excitation of the sympathetic adrenergic nerve terminals (*Hughes and Vane*, 1967). These results support this view.

The relaxation of partially contracted vessels induced by TS was probably produced by excitation of the noradrenergic, noncholinergic nervous mechanism; it was obtained in preparations from reserpinized rabbits in the presence of adrenergic neuronal blocking agent guanethidine and of both alfa- and beta-receptor blocking agents, phentolamine and propranolol. The relaxation to TS was resistent to atropine in concentrations much higher than necessary to abolish the response to exogenous acetylcholine. The fact that relaxation was obtained in veins contracted by acetylcholine indicates that the cholinergic mechanism is not involved.

Neurogenic relaxation is not limited to the portal vein alone; it has also been observed in isolated perfused central arteries of rabbit ears (*Kalsner*, 1974) and in isolated intracranial vessels (*Lee et al.*, 1975) partially contracted by NA and other agents.

Demonstration of nonadrenergic, noncholinergic relaxation in blood vessels, which becomes manifest when sympathetic adrenergic control is eliminated, signifies that an additional vascular tone modulating mechanism enables vascular adaptation to a change in the local environment.

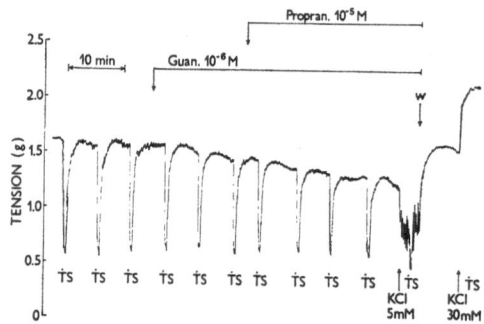

Fig. 3. Effect of guanethidine (Guan.), propranolol (Propran.) and potassium chloride (KCl) on relaxation of portal veins induced by transmural nerve stimulation (TS) at 8 Hz for 30 sec. Active muscle tone was produced by ergotamine $(5 \times 10^{-6} \text{ g/ml})$.

J. T. Inst. Norm. Pathol. Physiol. Slovak Academy of Sciences, 884 23 Bratislava Sienkiewiczova 1, Czechoslovakia

EFFECTS OF OXYGEN, HYPOXIA, METABOLIC INHIBITORS, NITRITE, INDOMETHACIN, AND ADENOSINE ON THE SPONTANEOUS TONE OF A NERVE-FREE VESSEL, THE HUMAN UMBILICAL ARTERY

G. L. NADÁSY, E. MONOS, E. MOHÁCSI, J. CSÉPLI and A. G. B. KOVÁCH

Experimental Research Institute and 2nd Department of Gynecology, Semmelweis Medical University, Budapest, Hungary

Introduction

Human umbilical arterial segments and strips are in a contracted state in an O_2-bubbled Krebs-Ringer solution, and this contraction is not affected by thorough washing of the specimens. A direct contracting effect of raising pO_2 on the umbilical artery has not been prove unambiguously (*Eltherington et al.* 1968, *Panigel* 1962, *Tuvemo* 1975). On the other hand, PGE_2, $PGF_{2\alpha}$ as well as endoperoxides PGG_2 and PGH_2 were found to be synthesized in human umbilical cord and artery, and the same agents had contracting effects on umbilical arterial strips (*Tuvemo* 1975). The remaining contraction of the umbilical arterial strips previously treated with 5-HT and then washed out was inhibited by PG synthesis blocker indomethacin in concentration of 8 µg/ml (*Strandberg and Tuvemo* 1975). The studies presented here were performed in an attempt to obtain more information on spontaneous contraction and on its mechanism using a technique that allows measurement of fine mechanical changes on cylindrical segments without damaging the wall structure (*Cox* 1974). No contracting agent except oxygen was used during the experiments.

Methods

67 cylindrical arterial segments were prepared from the middle (nerve-free) part of the umbilical cords within 20 minutes after delivery. The 1.5—2.5 cm long segments were thoroughly washed with cold Krebs-Ringer solution, cannulated at both ends, axially estended by 10% of their excised length and mounted in Krebs-Ringer bicarbonate solution at 37 °C. The solution was bubbled with a gas mixture of 95% O_2 and 5% CO_2. Duration of the preincubation period was 1 hr. All of the segments were in a maximally contracted (closed) state at the end of the preincubation. Then either of the following substances was added to the incubation solution: KCN (3.5 mM), oligomycin (2.8 µg/ml), 2-deoxy-glucose (10 mM, no glucose added), indomethacin 1 µg/ml), to inhibit cytochrom oxydase, oxydative phosphorylation, phosphohexose isomerase and prostaglandin synthethase, respectively. Furthermore, dilatatory action of $NaNO_2$ (mM), adenosine (10 µM) and Ca^{2+} free Krebs-Ringer solution (0.5 M EGTA added) was investigated. Normal Krebs-Ringer solution bubbled with 95% O_2 and 5% CO_2 was used for control segments. In hypoxic experiments, a gas mixture containing 95% N_2 and 5% CO_2 was used. At the end of the incubation period (2 hrs) the intraluminal pressure was raised to 100 mm Hg in 20 seconds and then maintained at that level. The outer diameter of the segments was continuously measured with a cantilever trans-

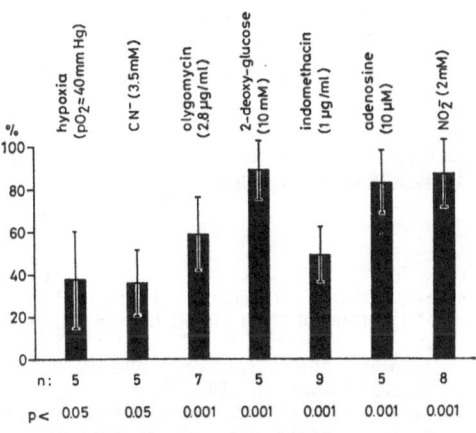

Fig. 1. Inhibition of spontaneous smooth muscle tone in the human umbilical artery *in vitro* (as a percentage of relaxation effect induced by a Ca^{2+}-free Krebs-Ringer solution with 0.5 mM EGTA). $\bar{x} \pm$ SEM. The statistical significance of the dilatatory effect expressed in p values is denoted.

159

ducer (resolution: 40 μm). In response to the intraluminal pressure rise there was a sudden increase in external diameter followed by a slow exponentially decreasing dilatation. External diameters reached in 24 minutes were taken to characterize contraction-relaxation states of the segments. The dilating effect of the different agents was expressed in percentage of the dilation effect of a Ca^{2+} free solution.

Results and conclusions

All substances were applied and hypoxia also dilated the segments compared to the controlgroup. (Fig. 1.) Segments dilated in hypoxic solution were equilibrate date 50 mmHg intraluminal pressure. A slow but distinct contraction was found when the bubbling was changed for 95% O_2 and 5% CO_2. (Fig. 2.)

The hypothetic mechanism of oxygen-dependent spontaneous tone and sites of action of some inhibitors used are shown in Fig. 3.

According to these results the spontaneous tone of the umbilical artery depends at least partly on a) the molecular oxygen, b) the extracellular Ca^{2+}, c) the intactness of mitochondrial electron transport chain and oxidative phosphorylation, d) the intactness of the prostaglandin synthetase system. The spontaneous tone of the segments can be inhibited by vasodilator agents e)nitrite and f) adenosine. Both mitochondrial cyt aa$_3$ and non-mitochondrial oxygenisation of arachidonic acid into PG endoperoxides may account for sites of contractile action of oxygen on the human umbilical artery.

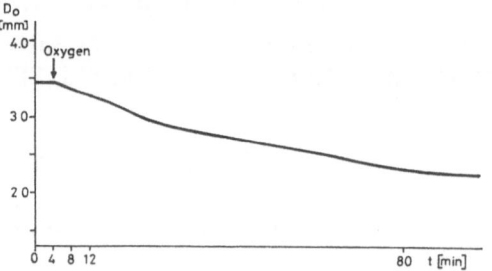

Fig. 2. Oxygen-induced contraction of a human umbilical arterial segment. At the point denoted by the arrow 95% N_2, 5% CO_2 bubbling (p$O_2 \approx$ 40 mmHg) was changed for 95% O_2, 5% CO_2 (p$O_2 \approx$ 360 mmHg). D_o: outer diameter. Intraluminal pressure = 50 mmHg.

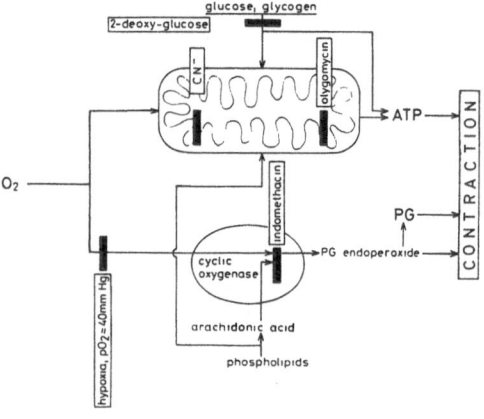

Fig. 3. Hypothetical mechanism of the O_2 dependent spontaneous tone of the human umbilical artery. Assumed sites of action of some inhibitors used are denoted.

REFERENCES

1. *Cox, R. H. (1974):* Three-dimensional mechanics of arterial segments in vitro: methods. J. Appl. Physiol. 36, 381—384.
2. *Eltherington, L. G., Stoff, J., Hughes, T., Melmon, K. L. (1968):* Constriction of human umbilical arteries Circ. Res. 22: 747—752.
3. *Panigel, M. (1962):* Placental perfusion experiments Am. J. Obstet. Gynecol. 84, 1664 to 1683.
4. *Strandberg, K., Tuvemo, T.* (1975): Reduction of the tone of the isolated human umbilical artery by indomethacin, eicosa-5,8,11,14-tetraynoic acid and polyphloretin phosphate Acta Physiol. Scand. 94, 319—326.
5. *Tuvemo, T. (1975):* Prostaglandins and the regulation of the tone of the human umbilical artery. An experimental study Acta Univ. Ups. 225.

G. L. N., Experimental Research Institute, Semmelweis Medical University, Budapest 1082 Budapest, Ulloi ut 78/a, Hungary

NEURO-VASCULAR TRANSMISSION RELATED TO THE RATE
AND NUMBER OF STIMULATION IMPULSES

J. GERO and M. GEROVÁ

*Institute of Normal and Pathological Physiology, Slovak Academy
of Sciences, Bratislava, Czechoslovakia.*

Hitherto knowledge on sympathetic control of peripheral circulation has refered almost exclusively to values of maximal response: the time course of vascular contraction or BF reduction is generally negleted. Thus pertinent data, characterizing the range of total vascular response (as reflected e.g. by blood flow debt) related to individual stimulation parameters are lacking.

In order to obtain analytical data on 27 anesthetized dogs, the blood flow (Statham electromagnetic flowmeter), diameter of the femoral artery (displacement transducer) and blood pressure (Statham electromanometer) were monitored; the peripheral stump of the decentralized homolateral sympathetic trunc ($LG_3 - LG_4$ level) was stimulated by supramaximal rectangular impulses of 5 msec duration. In individual series the number of impulses varied in exponential order (from 2^3 to 2^{11}); within each stimulation series consisting of an equal number of impulses, the frequency varied from 0.1 to 300 Hz.

The vascular response to each individual stimulation has been evaluated as A) Maximum BF change (ΔBF_M), i.e. the difference between resting (BF^0) and minimal (BF_{Min}) blood flow, as well as B) Total BF reduction, which will be referred to as blood flow debt (BF_D), i.e. the difference between resing BF and the BF reduced by sympathetic stimulation.

A) Relating maximum BF changes to stimulation frequency (Fig. 1.), it was revealed that the validity of the generally accepted hyperboloid frequency-response curve is limited except for stimulations in which a minimum number (300 and 2100 for resistant and conduit vessels, respec-tively) of impulses is exceeded; in trains of substantially lower number (less than 60 and 200, respectively) of impulses the frequency-response ratio is inverted.

B) Whatever the range of impulses applied within each range (the number of impulses being equal) the total BF reduction (blood flow debt) is inversely proportional to the stimulation frequency. (Fig. 2.) At any rate of stimulation, on augmenting the number of impulses the

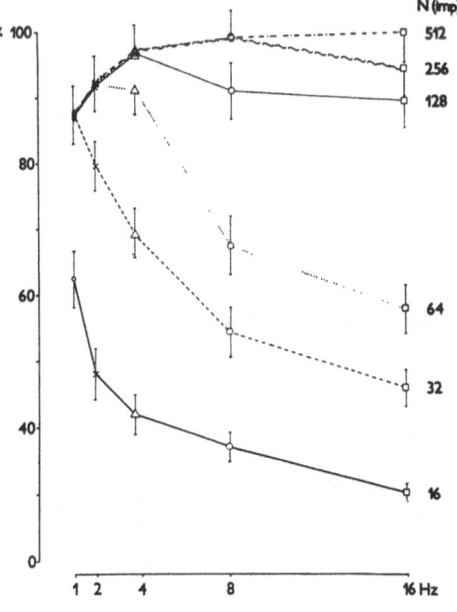

Fig. 1. Frequency — response curve to sympathetic stimulation consisting of on increasing number (N) of impulses (imp) — numerals on the right margin Abscissa: frequency of stimulation (Hz). Ordinate: maximal BF change (ΔBF_M) in percent; ΔBF_M at N = 512 imp, Fr = 16 Hz is taken as 100%. Each symbol represents the mean value ($\pm$SE, vertical bars) of at least 6 individual values (range 6—12).

value of the blood flow debt increases. Relating the total BF change to one impulse, however, revealed (Fig. 3.) that this value declines at low (0.1 – 0.4 Hz), exponentially increases at high (1 – 8 Hz) and linearily rises at very high (16 – 300 Hz) frequencies.

Similar sets of stimulation were applied after administration of cocaine hydrochloride (1 – 2 mg/kg i.v.). The results indicate that there are variations in the rate of the re-uptake of the transmitter which underlie changes of the frequency-response ratio. The rate of re-uptake is to be considered as a damped-wave series function, its amplitude being determined by the gradient of the increase and its damping ratio by the total amount of the transmitter within the neuro-vascular synapse.

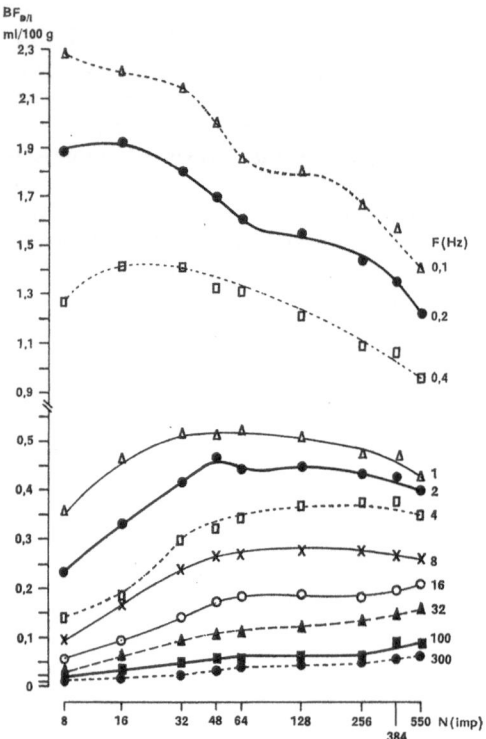

Fig. 2. Blood flow debt (BF in ml/100 g — ordinate) induced by sympathetic stimulation consisting of an increasing number of impulses (N imp — abscissa), applied at increasing frequency — see numbers at the righthand margin. Each symbol represents the mean value of at least 6 (range 5–13) individual values; SE in all values is less than 11.2% (range 5.9–11.2) of the mean.

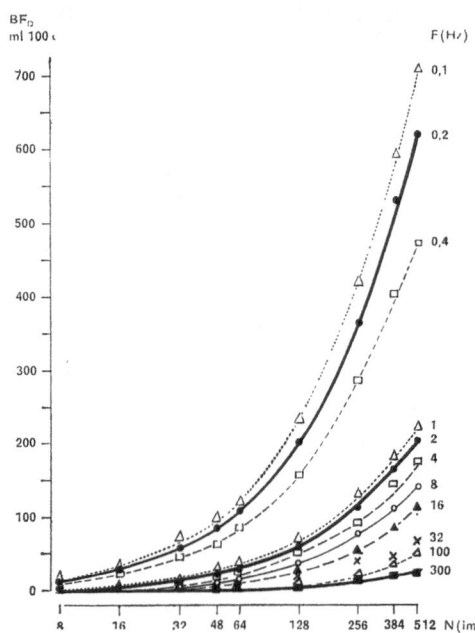

Fig. 3. Blood flow debt related to one impulse (BF$_{DI}$, in ml/100 g — ordinate) induced by sympathetic stimulation consisting of an increasing number of impulses (N imp — abscissa), applied at increasing frequency — see numerals at the righthand margin. For explanation of symbols see legend for fig. 2.

J. G., Sienkiewiczova 1, 884 23 Bratislava, Czechoslovakia

IMMUNOLOGICAL ASPECTS OF VASCULAR DISEASES

IMMUNOLOGICAL STUDIES IN CHRONIC OCCLUSIVE ARTERIAL DISEASES

K. INADA, A. OKADA and R. MIYAMOTO

Dept. of Surgery, Gifu University, School of Medicine, Gifu, Japan

It is well known that the frequency of vascular diseases is definitely low in Japan compared to Europe and America. This is ascribed to the fact that arteriosclerosis is generally mild in Japanese. On the contrary, pulseless disease or Takayasu's arteritis and Buerger's disease or thrombo-angiitis obliterans are frequently seen in Japan. These two diseases contrast in many aspects and the etiology is not clarified in either of them.

Materials and methods

Immunological studies were performed on 19 patients with aortitis syndrome (Takayasu's arteritis, AOS), 41 cases of Buerger's disease (TAO) and 44 cases of arteriosclerosis obliterans. The following investigations were carried out:
1) Skin tests using PPD and DNCB were performed. 2) The content of T-cells in peripheral blood was determined by the microplate method (Tachibana). 3) Blast formation of lymphocytes by PHA was measured by a scintilation counter using ^{3}H-thymidine. 4) Protein fractions were analysed by single radial immunodiffusion and crossed immunoelectrophoresis. 5) Serum complement was measured by Mayer's method.

Results

1) The tuberculin reaction was negative in five of 19 cases with AOS, in six of 41 with TAO and in eleven of 44 with ASO. There was no difference between the three groups, although in four of six cases the reaction was negative in patients with AOS in active stage. There was no difference between patients with ischemic ulcer and without ulcer either in TAO or ASO.
2) The skin test by DNCB was negative in five of 12 cases in AOS, in three of 29 in TAO and in five of 32 in ASO. All patients with AOS in active stage showed a negative reaction, while in three of ten it was negative in chronic stage. There

was no difference between patients with ischemic ulcer and without ulcer either in TAO or ASO.
3) The perecentage of T-cells in peripheral blood was significantly decreased in all three diseases, especially prominent in AOS compared to TAO and ASO. No difference was found between the latter two. There was no difference between patients with AOS in active stage and in chronic stage. The decrease of T-cells was more prominent in patients with ulcer compared to those without ulcer in TAO.
4) The stimulation index was significantly reduced in AOS compared to TAO and ASO, although there was no difference between patients in active stage and in chronic stage. No difference was found between patients with ulcer and without ulcer either in TAO or ASO.
5) The increase of α-antitrypsin, haptoglobin, hemopexin and $\beta_{/A}/\beta_{/C}$ globulin (C3) was significant in AOS. The increase of all fractions of serum protein was prominent and persisted during the active stage of AOS. The increase of haptoglobin, hemopexin and C3 was significant in TAO, although the increase of haptoglobin, hemopexin, transferin and C3 was significant in ASO. IgG, IgA and IgM

Table I.

		Skin test		
		No.of cases	(+)	(−)
PPD	Aortitis	19	14	5*
	Buerger	41	35	6
	Arterios.obl	44	33	11
DNCB	Aortitis	12	7	5**
	Buerger	29	26	3
	Arterios.obl.	32	27	5

    * 4 in active stage
    ** 2 in active stage

165

increased significantly in AOS compared to other diseases. aortitis, although participation of the same mechanism is not denied in cases of both TAO and ASO.

Representative cases will be briefly described. The figure shows the serum protein pattern by immunoelectrophoresis of a 26-year-old female with aortitis syndrome in active stage. A significant increase of all fractions is noted compared to normal.

The next figure shows the serum protein pattern of a 34-year-old man with Buerger's disease who has a skin ulcer in the right foot. The increase of α_1-antitrypsin and haptoglobin is significant.

6) The level of serum complement is significantly raised in AOS compared to TAO and ASO.

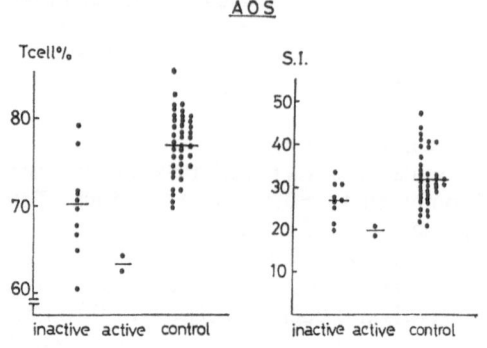

Fig. 1.

Discussion

The aortitis syndrome is a clinical entity known as Takayasu's arteritis or young female arteritis named by Ross and McKusick. The etiology is still unknown. It is well known that clinical signs suggesting inflammation, such as fever, positive C-reactive protein and increase of blood sedimentation rate, are frequently found and also changes in immunoglobulin are characteristic in patients with aortitis especially in active stage. Autoimmune mechanism is considered to be related to the development of the disease.

The etiology of Buerger's disease or thromboangiitis obliterans is unknown, too. We believe in the existence of a group of patients, distinctly different from those with ASO, who fit into the condition that Buerger originally described. Contrary to aortitis, clinical signs suggesting inflammation are usually absent in patients with both TAO and ASO.

In the present study a decrease of cell-mediated immunity was noted in all three diseases, especially significant in patients with AOS. It is apparent that the immunological mechanism plays an important role in the development of

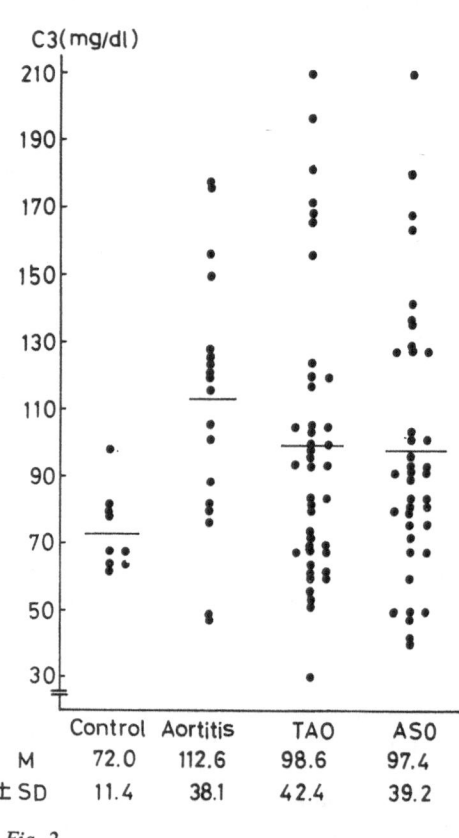

	Control	Aortitis	TAO	ASO
M	72.0	112.6	98.6	97.4
±SD	11.4	38.1	42.4	39.2

Fig. 2.

I. K., Dept. of Surgery Gifu Univ. School of Med, 40 Tsukasa-cho, Gifu-shi, Gifu Ken 500, Japan

SIGNIFICANCE OF IMMUNOLOGICAL STUDIES OF PERIPHERAL ARTERIAL DISEASES

J. POKORNÝ and Z. JEŽKOVÁ

Laboratory of Angiology, Charles University and Institute of Haematology and Blood Transfusion, Prague, Czechoslovakia

This study was carried out to obtain information on the possible role of immunologic mechanisms in the pathogenesis of peripheral vascular diseases. A large number of investigators have found evidence that immunologic mechanisms influence the etiopathogenesis of inflammatory arterial diseases; it is, however, far more difficult to determine whether these mechanisms also exert a pronounced effect in atherogenesis. In our studies we have examined antibodies against the blood vessel wall and other materials not only in patients suffering from peripheral vascular diseases but also in clinically healthy subjects. The complement consumption test for determination of antibody positivity was used in our investigations.

Results

Initially, attention was centred principally on the positivity of antibodies against the whole blood vessel wall in the inflammatory spastic stage of thrombangiitis obliterans characterized by typical migratory phlebitis (mostly histologically verified). These antibodies were demonstrated in 97,5 per cent of 120 cases. Further investigation here revealed the highest finding of antibodies against adventitia and the lowest against intima. The positivity of antibodies in the chronic obliterative stage of thrombangiitis obliterans against the individual blood vessel coats (adventitia, muscularis and intima) was practically identical. However, compared to the spastic inflammatory stage of thrombangiitis obliterans, the percentage of antibody positivity against the whole vessel decreased significantly in this stage of the disease (to 50%) and corresponded to the findings in atherosclerosis obliterans with the signs of heavier ischemia of the lower limbs (53.6%). In contrast, the positivity findings of antibodies against the blood vessel wall in healthy subjects was confirmed in 1 per cent of 200 blood donors. The difference in these findings is statistically significant. (Fig. 1).

Our attention in the second group of immunological investigations was turned

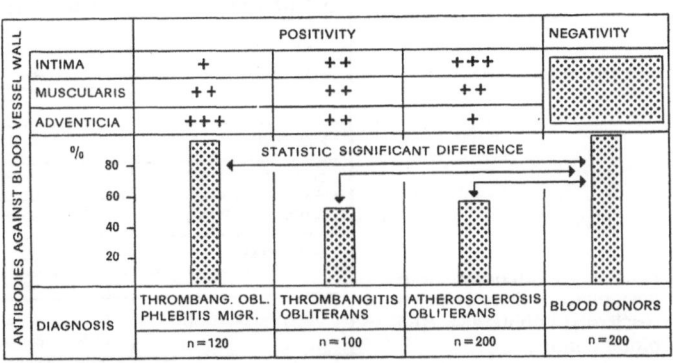

Fig. 1. Antibodies against blood vessel wall in inflammatory spastic stage of thrombangiitis obliterans, obliterative stage of thrombangiitis obliterans, atherosclerosis obliterans and in blood donors.

Fig. 2. Antibodies and fibrinolytic activity in cases with atherosclerosis obliterans and blood donors.

ANTIBODIES AGAINST (IN % OF CASES)	ATHEROSCLER. OBLIT. n = 86	BLOOD DONORS n = 200
HYALURONIC ACID	69	2.5
HYASE	36	1.5
HEPARIN PRECURSOR	37	1.0
HEPARIN	17	0.5
CHOLESTEROL	77	2.0
PHOSPHOLIPIDS	44	1.5
CHOLIC ACID	34	1.0
COLLAGEN	52	1.0
		$p < 0.05$
FIBRINOLYTIC ACTIVITY	83 % > 250'	95 % < 250'

to the role of mucopolysaccharides in atherosclerosis obliterans. In this group of 86 patients suffering from atherosclerosis obliterans, we found antibodies in a very high percentage. These findings were completed by observation of the following antibodies: against the blood vessel wall, cholesterol, phospholipids. (Fig. 2). In these patients the fibrinolytic activity decreased strikingly.

Finally, in the last group attention was focussed on the antibodies in atherosclerosis obliterans against antigens which can be related to hemocoagulation. Here we stated the antibody positivity (from 87 patients of another group with atherosclerosis obliterans) against fibronogen, thrombin, albumin, collagen, blood vessel cholesterol. On the other hand, in 200 healthy subjects a negligible percentage of antibody positivity was found. (Fig. 3). Assessing the occurence of the positive response of antibodies regardless of a single antigen, we can conclude that a total positive antibody finding appeared in 53%. The extent of fibrinolysis is strikingly prolonged here.

Discussion

We assume that the above findings of antibodies against mucopolysaccharides can signify an immunological reaction to antigenic process affecting mucopolysaccharide or glycoprotein components against heparin and its precursors. This can be an indication of the possibility that, due to a metabolic disturbance, a bio-

ANTIBODIES (% CASES)	ATHEROSCLER. OBLIT. n = 87	BLOOD DONORS n = 200
FIBRINOGEN	36	3
ALBUMIN	29	2
THROMBIN	26	0.5
COLLAGEN	43	1
BLOOD WESSEL WALL	50	0.5
CHOLESTEROL	53	1
FIBRINOLYTIC ACTIVITY	66 % > 250' 17 % ≥ 300'	95% < 250'

Fig. 3. Antibodies and fibrinolytic activity in atherosclerosis obliterans and blood donors.

chemical disorder can occur. The organism begins to respond to this change at the stage of heparin precursors. From these antibody findings, due to pathologic changes in the organism, we can suppose that insufficient or altered heparin production is involved. Certainly also metabolic disorders in more systems and not only in the blood vessel alone must be considered in the course of atherosclerosis. Such processes can be manifested immunologically as nonphysiological action which can respond through the production of antibodies.

From the antibody findings against antigens in relation to the hemocoagulation it can be concluded that these antibodies, as mentioned above, can be an expression of nonphysiological actions. It is assumed that an antibody finding can be considered a very sensitive indicator of temporary changes in the hemocoagulation system.

A defective fibrinolytic mechanism could play a role in the atherogenesis, enabling fibrin deposition in the arterial wall. According to the current hypotheses, all components which influence atherogenesis or development of atherosclerotic processes must be in equilibrium in order to maintain an appropriate or normal arterial state and adequate blood vessel permeability. If one factor changes, the others will adjust accordingly as this constitutes a determinant for the production of antibodies. Every increase in arterial immunologically mediated permeability could then facilitate lipid deposition in the blood vessel wall. Finally the finding of various antibodies could probably yield information about the activity of an inflammatory or atherosclerotic process. This can, to a certain degree also contribute to differential diagnosis of peripheral vascular processes.

REFERENCES

Chudomel, V., Ježková Z., Libánský J. (1959): Detection of leucocyte antibodies by the complement consumption test. Blood 14: 920.

Ježková Z., Pokorný J. (1967): The appearence of a wide variety of antibodies in atherosclerosis. Angiologica 4: 359.

Pokorný J., Ježková Z. (1962): Significance of immunological studies in peripheral obliterating vascular diseases. Circular. Res. 11: 961.

J. P., IVth Int. Clinic FVL KU, U nemocnice 2, 128 08 Prague 2, Czechoslovakia

VASCULAR CHANGES OF LOW CALCIUM DIET FED ANIMALS AGAINST SOLUBLE IMMUNE COMPLEX

H. YAMAGUCHI, H. TAKEUCHI and CH. TORIKATA

Department of Pathology, School of Med. Keio Univ., Tokyo, Japan

Introduction

Basement membrane (BM) is composed of mucopolysaccharide (MP) and so far the morpho-functional behaviour of BM has been studied using special staining techniques and chemical analysis. The common chemical characteristics of MP are its polymeric structure and strong negative electron charges. When these negative charges are saturated with cations, MP yields a flocculent precipitate. The molecular structures repel each other resulting in a loosened and elongated molecular structure. These chemical characteristics are usually utilized in fixation and staining in histo-chemical studies. (*Meyer* 1959, *Pearce* 1960) Biological alteration of these characters seriously affects the morpho-functional reactions of the vascular wall against injurious stimuli.

Among cationic materials, calcium is the most common and widely distributed bivalent salt and is easily ionized. Fragmentary but significant facts suggest a relationship between MP and calcium. Tissues in which circulated a low calcium medium showed hyperexudation and the cellular movement in the matrix of connective tissues was enhanced. In hypocalcemia, calcium ions incorporated in MP pass into the blood more easily than bone calcium.

In this paper, SIC was intravenously administered into guinea pigs, fed a low calcium content diet, 0.2% weight, for five weeks. The serum calcium dropped to 3.5 mEq/l from 4.3 − 5.5 mEq/l in controls. 1.3 − 1.5 gm% of calcium content is thought to be the nutrient requirement for normal development in guinea pigs (*O'Dell* 1957).

Results

With SIC administration in the lungs, interstitial pneumonia is sometimes observed and these changes disappeared spontaneously within several weeks. Angiitis of angiolytic changes of the vascular wall were observed; these are the desquamation of vascular endothelia, the loosening of intermuscular and for perivascular connective tissue and the eroded vascular wall, crowded with leucocytes (Fig. 1). The vascular wall became thinner. With EM examination, loosening and duplication of BM of the blood vessel were observed (Fig. 2) and the cytoplasmic processes and/or the nucleus of the smooth muscle cells protruded into the subendothelial space with activated muscle cells accentuated the dequamation of the endo-

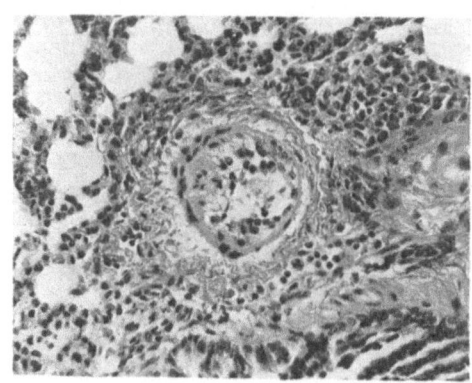

Fig. 1. Four weeks after administration, desquamation of the vascular endothelia associated with loosening of intermuscular connective tissue was demonstrated. In the eroded site, smooth muscle cells of the vascular wall were crowded with leucocytes and the vascular wall became thinner.

170

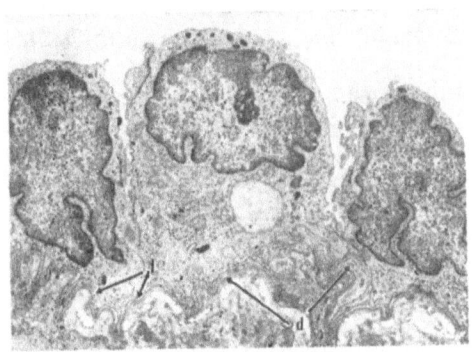

Fig. 2. With E. M. examination, the most characteristic morphological manifestation is the loosening (e) and duplication (d) of the basement membrane of the vessel wall.

thelial cells from the vessel wall and resulted in erosion of the vessel wall.

Discussion

A large number of works have been devoted to the biological role of IC in living animals but the formative pathogenesis of IC diseases is still difficult to clarify experimentally. The reasons why experimental IC diseases, similar to spontaneously induced ones, are difficult to produce, are numerous and include the comsumption rate, entrapment mechanism and biological activities. On the other hand, disposition for the provocation of IC diseases is also an important factor.

In the vascular wall BM is not only important for the structural and functional differentiation of endothelial cells and smooth muscle layers but may also act as an important filter for exudation. In various allergic diseases, it may be the deposition site.

In the previous paper, guinea pigs fed a low calcium diet displayed mesangiolytic changes of the glomeruli, and additional IC administration exaggerated the amount of deposition in the BM and a mesangial matrix was demonstrated. (*Yamaguchi* 1978).

In this paper in which the animals were fed low calcium diet plus S.I.C. administration, angitis or angiolytic changes

of the vascular wall in the lungs was noted.

These changes in the vascular wall are probably related to the morpho-functional alteration of BM which is mainly composed of MP.

The vacuolarisation of the endothelial cells, usually demonstrated in IC, administered to animals fed a normal diet, are rather smaller in number in this experiment. It is felt that in animals fed a normal diet, exudate, produced by IC, administration penetrates into the vascular wall (*Yamaguchi* 1972). On the other hand, in the animals fed a low calcium diet, BM and the connective tissue in the vascular wall became loosened and the exudated fluid would be able to flow out through loosely connected vascular components. The regurgitation of exudate would not occur.

The protrusion of the smooth muscle

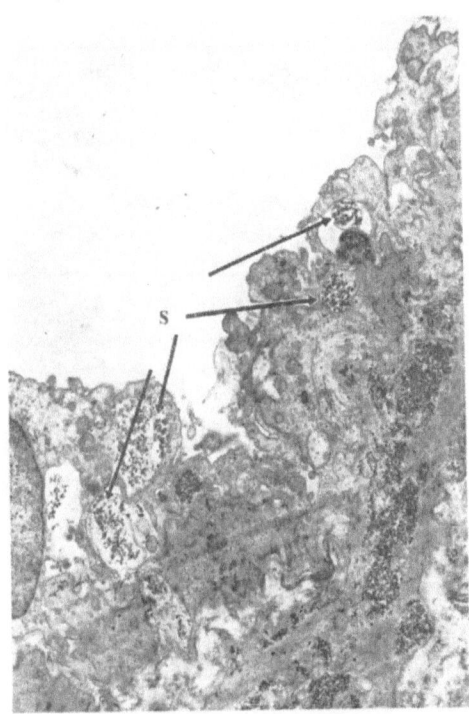

Fig. 3. Activation of smooth muscle cells and their cytoplasmic processes was observed and/or the nucleus of the smooth muscle cells (s) protruded into the subendothelial space across the basement membrans.

171

cells across BM and dedifferentiation into endothelial cells, resulting in the desquamation of pre-existing endothelial cells may also indicate the loosining of MP.

IC deposition along BM, as seen in the kidney and reported in the previous paper (*Yamaguchi* 1978), were not demonstrated in the vascular wall in the lung. It is supposed that, compared with kidney where a lot of blood is filtered, one IC administration is not enough to demonstrate deposition in the vascular wall. So with EM examination, IC deposition along the BM is not demonstrated in the vascular wall.

REFERENCES

Meyer, K., Hoffman, P. and Linker, A. (1959): In connective tissue. Thrombosis and atherosclerosis ed by Page, J. H. 86—96, Academic press.

O'Dell, B. L., Morris, E. R., Rickett, E. E. and Hogan, A. G. (1957): Diet compostion and mineral balance in guinea pigs, J. Nutr. 63. 65.

Pearce, A. G. E. (1960): Histochemistry; Theoretical and applied. Churchill, London.

Yamaguchi, H., Takeuchi, H., Torikata, C., and Sakaguchi, H. (1978): Studies on the formative mechanim of mesangiolytic changes of renal glomerulus induced by a low calcium diet breeding. Exp. Path. (in Print).

Yamaguchi, H., Takeuchi, H., Torikata, C. and Sakaguchi, H. (1978): Mechanisms of immune deposition in relation to a loosened molecular structure of A. M. P. caused by a low calcium diet — especially to their negative charges. Exp. Path. (in Print).

Yamaguchi, H., Nakajima, S., Torikat, C. and Takeuchi, H. (1972): Studies on the morphological changes of artery caused by exudation — initial changes of arteritis. Acta Path. Jap. 441—455 22, 3.

H. Y., Depart. of Path. Sch. of Med. Keio Univ., Tokyo, Japan.

BLOOD SERUM PROTEINS AND FREE SH GROUPS IN THE DIAGNOSIS OF CLASSICAL POLYARTERITIS NODOSA

Z. HRNČÍŘ, M. TICHÝ and LIBUŠE HRNČÍŘOVÁ

2nd Department of Medicine, Faculty of Medicine, Charles Univ., Hradec Králové and 2nd Department of Medicine, Faculty of Medicine, Purkyně Univ., Brno, Czechoslovakia

Classical polyarteritis nodosa (P. N.) is generalized necrotizing arteritis. Hitherto, the diagnosis of P. N. is based on histological criteria. A survey of clinical literature on classical P. N. for the past two decades shows that (1) there are relatively few studies on this subject, (2) they are usually case histories drawing attention to less frequent or misleading manifestations of the disease and (3) no symptom has yet been defined in laboratory diagnostics, the sensitivity, specificity and accessibility of which would help in making the diagnosis. The role of immunological changes, especially in relation to the circulating immune complexes HB_sAG − anti HB_s, is accentuated pathophysiologically in part of the patients. Liver and vascular changes in some patients can be explained in this way.

In this situation we wish to evaluate the laboratory findings in 17 patients with histologically verified classical P. N. from the diagnostic point of view. This is a prospectively studied series gathered over the last ten years. All these patients were subjected to the following tests: total protein, electrophoretic analysis on cellulose-acetate membranes, levels of IgA, IgG and IgM by means of radial immunodiffusion according to Mancini et al. (1965 and the levels of free SH groups according to Ellman (1959). The control group consisted of 30 blood donors of corresponding age and sex.

Evaluation of the results of total proteinaemia and the electrophosphoreograms (Table I.) revealed a significant decrease in albumin and an increase in alpha-2 globulin and especially in alpha-1 globulin levels in the disease tested. Levels of IgA, IgG and IgM in P. N. did not differ significantly from findings in the control series; however, the levels of free SH groups were significantly reduced (Table II.). We consider an evaluation of the observed changes to be topical from

Table I.

NON-PAIRED T-TEST FOR BILATERAL ALTERNATIVE FOR TOTAL PROTEIN (TP) AND ELECTROPHORETIC PATTERN (g/100ml) IN POLYARTERITIS NODOSA (P.N.) AND IN CONTROL GROUP (C.G.)						
INDEX	GROUP	No	x̄	SIGMA	t	p
TP	C.G.	30	7,05	0,87	0,1359	N S
	P.N.	17	6,97	2,13		
ALBUMIN	C.G.	30	3,41	0,44	2,317	0,0316*
	P.N.	17	2,80	1,01		
ALPHA-1GLOB.	C.G.	30	0,29	0,14	3,523	0,0018**
	P.N.	17	0,50	0,22		
ALPHA-2GLOB.	C.G.	30	0,76	0,21	2,552	0,0142*
	P.N.	17	0,95	0,31		
BETA GLOBULIN	C.G.	30	1,02	0,22	1,1249	N S
	P.N.	17	0,93	0,31		
GAMMA GLOBULIN	C.G.	30	1,55	0,29	1,481	N S
	P.N.	17	1,80	0,66		

Table II.

NON-PAIRED T-TEST FOR BILATERAL ALTERNATIVE FOR IgA, IgG, IgM (mg/100ml) AND SH-GROUPS (mmol/l) IN POLYARTERITIS NODOSA (P.N.) AND IN CONTROL GROUP (C.G.)						
INDEX	GROUP	No	x̄	SIGMA	t	p
IgA	C.G.	30	390,0	138,8	1,128	N S
	P.N.	17	457,6	160,1		
IgG	C.G.	30	1317,2	337,8	1,740	N S
	P.N.	17	1507,1	353,7		
IgM	C.G.	30	118,6	12,5	2,001	N S
	P.N.	17	87,8	48,6		
SH-GROUPS	C.G.	30	0,3708	0,157	3,901	0,0003***
	P.N.	17	0,2292	0,091		

the diagnostic point of view. An indispensable starting point for this is the finding of a highly significant increase in alpha-1 globulin (p = 0.0018) and a simultaneous highly significant decrease in the levels of free SH groups (p = 0.0003).

There is still no sensitive and easily accessible guideline in the clinical and laboratory diagnostics of classical P. N. We therefore used the described deviation in alpha-1 globulin and free SH groups for the formulation of an auxiliary diagnostic index which we termed the polyarteritis nodosa index (PN$_i$). It has the following formula:

$$\frac{\text{alpha-1 globulin (g/100 ml)}}{\text{SH groups (mmol/l)}} \times 10$$

The mean value of PN$_i$ in P. N. was 25.8 while in the blood donors it was only 10.4 (Tab. III.). This difference was of high statistical significance (p = 0.0038). The value of PN$_i$ in P. N. patients was significantly higher even in comparison with a group of positive rheumatoid arthritis patients, 72 ankylosing spondylitis patients and 34 patients with gout (Tab. III.). No statistical differences were found when compared with findings in 50 persons suffering from acute myocardial infarction on the 7th and 14th day after occurrence. This, however, is a disease which practically does not come into consideration in differential diagnosis compared to P. N.

We are fully aware of the fact that the PNi thus defined is not a marker specific for the disease being examined or a marker which would solve the biochemical diagnosis of this disease. On the other hand, we believe that, in the given situation, the calculation of the PN$_i$ is of practical help in the difficult diagnosis of this disease.

Table III.

POLYARTERITIS NODOSA INDEX (PN$_i$)					
DIAGNOSIS	No	$\bar{x}$	95% CONFIDENCE LIMIT		
POLYARTERITIS NODOSA	17	25.8*	35.0	–	16.6
BLOOD DONORS	30	10.4	14.5	–	6.2
RHEUMATOID ARTHRITIS RF SEROPOSITIVA	50	15.5	18.1	–	12.9
ANKYLOSING SPONDYLITIS	72	11.7	13.4	–	9.9
GOUT	34	13.6	17.7	–	9.6
MYOCARDIAL INFARCTION (7-th day)	50	19.8	23.0	–	16.5
MYOCARDIAL INFARCTION (14-th day)	50	17.3	20.3	–	14.3

*p : 0.0183 − 0.0038

Z. H., 2nd Dept. of Med., Faculty of Med., 500 36 Hradec Králové, Czechoslovakia

THE EFFECT OF AUTOLOGOUS SERUM AND SOME DRUGS ON CELLULAR IMMUNE REACTIONS IN VASCULAR DISEASES

MÁRIA HORVÁTH, KLÁRA ÓNODY and S. GERÖ

3rd Dept. of Med. Semmelweis University, Nat. Inst. of Haematology and Blood Transfusion, Arteriosclerosis Research Group of the Min. of Health, Budapest, Hungary

Introduction

In our earlier works, a significant cellular and humoral immune response were demonstrated under both experimental and clinical conditions using human vascular antigens. Histological changes reminiscent of those found in atherosclerosis could also be observed in immunized guinea pigs.

Materials and methods

Patients: 30 patients were investigated. The first group consisted of 10 patients with acute myocardial infarction, the second group contained 10 patients with arteriosclerosis obliterans and the third contained 10 patients suffered from superficial thrombophlebitis. The control group consisted of 5 persons without detectable vascular disease.

$CaCl_2$-Tris-Citrat (shortly CTC) buffer-extracts from human aortic wall with lipoid plaques and from intact venous wall prepared by the method of Robert et al. (1968) were used as antigens. The protein concentration of vascular extracts was determined according to Lowry. The aortic-CTC in 250 µg/ml and the venous-CTC in 300 µg/ml doses, respectively, were used.

The autologous serum after inactivation at 56° C for 30 minutes was applied in a 25 µl dose.

Oradexon (fluoromethylprednisolon) in a 125 µg/25 µl and Heparin in a 125 IU/25 µl dose were employed.

Methods: 1. The leukocyte migration test was applied the by method of Bendixen and Søborg (1970). Results were expressed in migration indices and were always compared to the migration observed in the control chambers.

2. The antibody titre was determined from inactivated sera by the passive hemagglutination technique.

Results

The autologous serum could essentially block the migration-ihnibitory effect of vascular antigens in all the groups of patient.

(Fig. 1). The blocking effect proved to be more effective at higher than at lower levels of antibodies in the sera. The correlation coefficients were calculated and shown.

(Fig. 2). Oradexon affected the migration-inhibition induced by vascular extracts in a similar way as autologous serum,

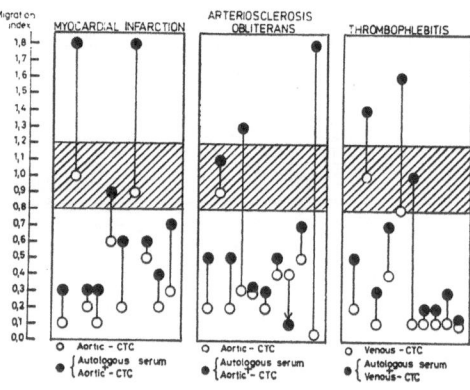

Fig. 1. Effect of autologous serum on leukocyte migration-inhibition induced by vascular antigens.

mainly in patients with myocardial infarction and thrombophlebitis.

(Fig. 3). Heparin also reduced the migration-inhibition induced by aortic CTC extract in the majority of patients with myocardial infarction and arteriosclerosis obliterans, but such an effect could not be seen in patients with thrombophlebitis receiving Heparin therapy.

(Fig. 4). In the control group vascular extracts could not induce migration-

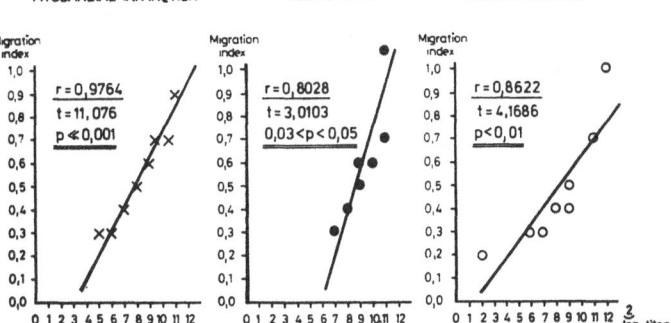

Fig. 2. Correlation between the blocking effect of autologous serum on migration-inhibition and antibody titre.

inhibition and neither autologous serum nor Oradexon or Heparin could influence the cell-migration.

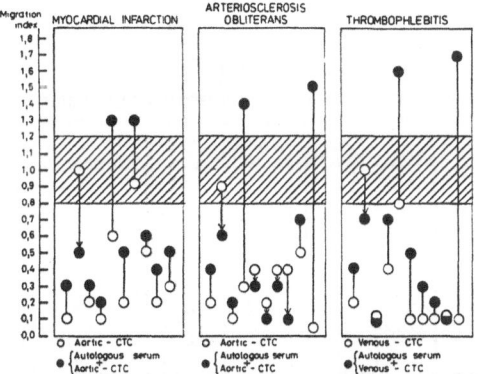

Fig. 3. Effect of Oradexon on leukocyte migration-inhibition induced by vascular antigens.

Discussion

The immune processes have a particular significance in the substitution of diseased arteries and coronaries by veins and after experimental and human heart transplantations.

Several authors have reported the blocking effect of autologous serum on cell-mediated immune reactions, mainly in autoimmune illnesses.

It is known that corticosteroids reduce the blastic transformation induced by mitogens and moderate the migration-inhibition and the cytotoxic reaction.

In our studies the reduction of cellular immune response caused by Oradexon has also been demonstrated.

Data concerning effects of Heparin on the cell-mediated immune response are controversial. It also influences the afferent and the efferent branches of immune response (*Ting*, 1976.). In our examinations, Heparin could decrease the migration-inhibition only in patients with myocardial infarction and arteriosclerosis obliterans. The decrease in thrombocyte count, the influencing of interaction between lipoprotein-lipase and endothel and the development of Heparin-antithrombin III. complexes may be suggested as the manner in which Heparin acts in vascular diseases.

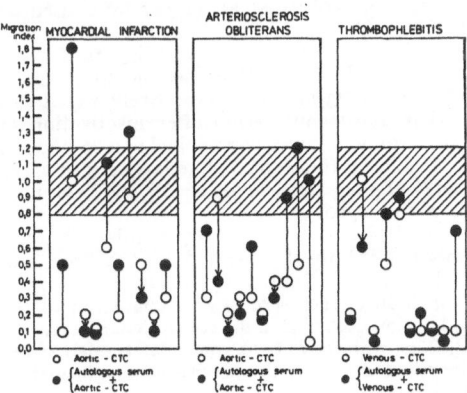

Fig. 4. Effect of Heparin on leukocyte migration-inhibition induced by vascular antigens.

M. H., Lenin krt. 93., 1067, Budapest, Hungary

IMMUNOLOGY OF ENDOTHELIAL CELLS. ACTION OF TICLOPIDINE

B. LACAZE, C. FERRAND, and O. PEPIN

PARCOR Recherche et Développement — Toulouse, France

The injection of rat endothelial cells into rabbits produces an arterial immunologic pathological condition, (*Scebat et al.*, 1967), which, at the moment of apparition of the specific antibodies, induces a decrease in the enzymatic activity of the endothelial cells and an increase in the platelet aggregant properties tested according to the Vane technique, (*Bunting et al.*, 1973).

An increase in the complement levels was also observed in all immunized animals. The administration of Ticlopidine to immunized animals results in an increase in the enzymes involved in the cyclic AMP synthesis, the inhibition of platelet aggregation and a collapse of the complement levels.

Materials and methods

Animals: — common rabbits weighing about 2 kg
     — Sprague Dawley rats weighing about 250 g.
Treatment : Ticlopidine : 150 mg/kg/day orally.

The rats were sacrificed and the aortas removed under sterile conditions after ligature of the efferent blood vessels. The aortas are then inverted in order to place the endothelial cells on the outside, treated with collagenase at 37 °C for 20 minutes and centrifuged. The isolated endothelial cells are washed with tyrode solution.

The immunizing injections of the cells, to which a complete Freund adjuvant was added, are injected by intra or hypodermic route on days O, 8, 15 and 30.

On day 30 a serum immunoelectrophoresis is carried out in order to verify the presence and the concentration of the antibodies.

The semi-quantitative enzymatic evaluations are obtained by the Apizym technique for β-glucosaminidase, β-glucuronidase and adenyl cyclase, (*Gilman*, 1970).

The inhibitory effect on the platelet aggregation is estimated by the Born method, (*Born*, 1962), carried out on part of the aorta according to the technique of Bunting (*Bunting et al.*, 1973).

The complement is evaluated by the haemolysis technique of 50% sheep R.B.C.

Three groups of animals are used:

Group I: 6 rabbits (controls) receiving no medical treatment,

Group II: 6 rabbits mmunized with endo, elial cells,

Group III: 6 rabbits immunized with endothelial cells and treated daily from the 30th day after immunization unti, their sacrifice wi 150 mg/kg/day of Ticlopidine by oral administration.

The sacrifice is carried out on the 45th day.

Results

1) Immunologicity: the antigen used in the rabbit serum immunophoresis is composed of rat endothelial cells. Depending on the animals, one or two precipitation arcs are observed.

2) Semi-quantitative enzymatic estimations show a significant decrease of β-glucosaminidase and adenyl cyclase in the immunized rabbits of Group II compared to the control group. But the Group III animals (immunized, but treated with Ticlopidine) show a significant increase of β-glucosaminidase and adenyl cyclase while the β-glucuronidase decreased.

3) The average values (and S. E. M.) of the complement levels are 88 (± 5), 145 (± 4) and 38 (± 4) for Groups I, II and III respectively. The differences among all the groups are highly significant ($p < 0.001$).

4) The technique of Bunting & Vane, (*Bunting et al.*, 1973), applied to the endothelium of the Group II animals, show an increase of the ADP induced aggregation of the platelet compared with the control group. On the other hand, the immunized rabbits treated with Ticlopidine (Group III) show a response similar to the control group (inhibition

177

of the aggregation induced by the endothelial cells).

Discussion

Rat endothelial cells injected in rabbits induce the formation of antiendothelium antibodies, resulting in a decrease in the amounts of adenyl cyclase involved in the cyclic AMP and thus in the synthesis of the prostaglandin system involved in the inhibition of platelet aggregation. On the other hand, the administration of Ticlopidine increases the adenyl cyclase levels, thus allowing increased cyclic AMP synthesis. The decrease of the complement levels in the rabbits inhibits the reaction of its fixation on the Ag—Ac complex and therefore also its pathogenicity.

Finally the inhibitory activity of the aorta on platelet aggregation is suppressed in immunized animals but not in the animals treated with Ticlopidine.

REFERENCES

Born, G. V. R. (1962): Aggregation of blood platelets by adenosine diphosphate and its reversal. Nature, 194, 297.

Bunting, S., Gryglewski, R., Moncada, S. and Vane, J. R. (1973): Arterial walls generate from prostaglandin endoperoxydes a substance which relaxes strips of mesenteric and coeliac arteries and inhibits platelet aggregation. Prostaglandins, 12, 6, 897.

Gilman, A. G. (1970): A protein binding assay for adenosine 3'—5' cyclic monophosphate. Proc. Nat. Acad. Sci. U.S.A., 67, 305.

Jaffe, E. A., Nachman, R. L., Becker, C. G. and Minick, C. R. (1973): Culture of human endothelial cells derived from umbilical veins. J. Clin. Invest., 52, 2745.

Scebat, L., Renais, J., Groult, M. (1967): Pouvoir immunogène et pathogène de la paroi artérielle. Arch. Mal. Cœur, 9, (1), 50—61.

B. L. — Immunology PARCOR R & D, B., P. 3005 Toulouse, France

IMMUNOLOGICAL AND FUNCTIONAL RESULTS OF ALLOGENEIC VEIN TRANSPLANTATION IN THE LOW PRESSURE SYSTEM

R. ENGEMANN, H. H. KÖRNER and A. THIEDE

Department of Surgery, Christian-Albrecht-University, Kiel, F.R.G.

Introduction

So far, autologous veins have been transplanted in peripheral artery reconstruction or as a coronary bypass, while homologous replacements have seldom been attempted. The extended radical operation of malignant tumors as well as the increasing number of traumatic vascular lesions of peripheral veins require prosthetic and biological material for repair or replacement (*Vollmar et al.* 1978). This work was carried out to investigate veins allografted into the low pressure system. Using inbred rat strains with well known immunogenetical species difference in the RtH-1-system — comparable to the human HLA-system — we were able to coordinate the reactions appearing at the grafts to a definite immunogenetical difference and also to reproduce them at any time.

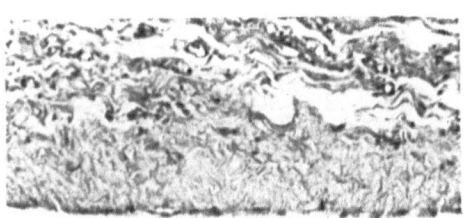
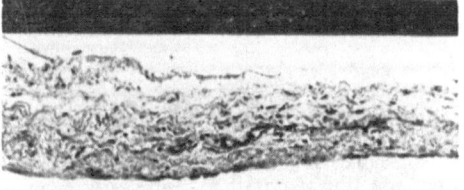
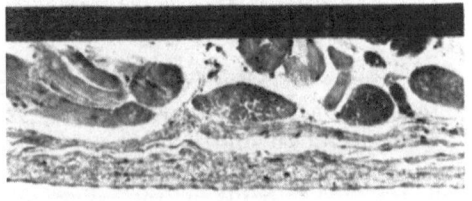

Fig. 2. Vessel wall 100 days after vein transplantation (from left to right syngeneic, weakly and strongly allogeneic combination).

Materials and methods

A syngeneic control group (n = 15), a weakly allogeneic (n = 15) and a strongly allogeneic (n = 15) combination were formed from the inbred strains F 344, LEW and CAP which are bred and maintained at Kiel. With microsurgical techniques and under sterile conditions we replaced the infrarenal vena cava by an 1.2—1.5 cm long piece of intrathoracic vena cava (Fig. 1). After 50 and 100 days the animals were examined macroscopically and microscopically. At intervals of 14 days transplantation antibodies were assayed using a modified hemagglutination test

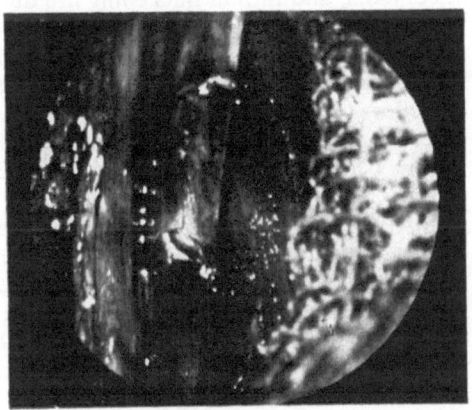

Fig. 1. Vein segment (arrow) grafted into the vena cava inf.

179

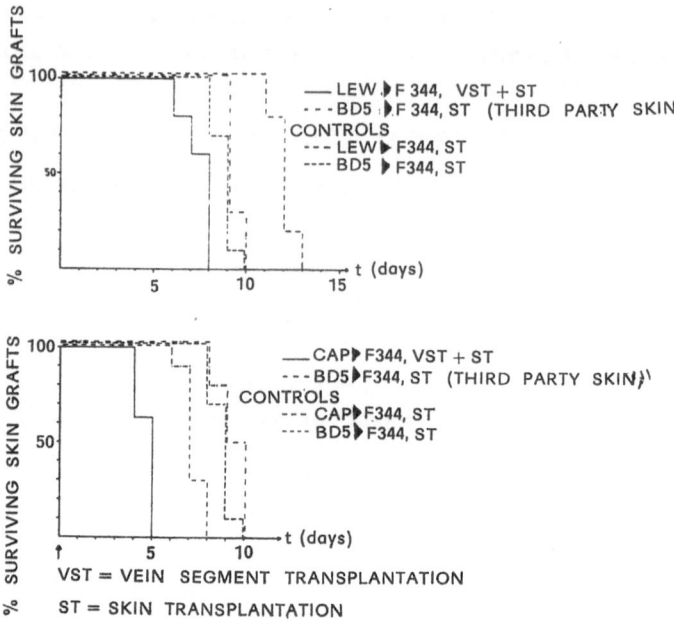

Fig. 3. Rejection of additional skin grafts after vein in vein transplantation representing cell mediated immune reaction.

VST = VEIN SEGMENT TRANSPLANTATION

ST = SKIN TRANSPLANTATION

(*Askenase* 1973). Skin grafts in additional sub groups were transplanted for evaluation of the cell mediated immunological reaction 14 days after vein transplantation. Controls were made by third party skin grafts (strain BD5).

Results

The grafts of all three combinations were functioned for up to 100 days. Macroscopically and microscopically, there was no difference after 50 and 100 days between the syngeneic and the two allogeneic combinations. Notably, we could not find any histological evidence for an immunological reaction consisting of mononuclear cell infiltration of the adventitia (Fig. 2). In our test, transplantation antibodies were found only in the strongly allogeneic combination. The medium survival time of donor specific skin grafts as an indicator of sensitisation of the cell mediated immune reaction after vein transplantation was 7.4 ± 0.3 days for the LEW to F344 group (normal skin graft survival 12.0 ± 0.4 days) and 4.3 ± 0.3 days for the CAP to F344 combination (normal skin graft survival 7.2 ± 0.4 days) (Fig. 3).

Third party skin was rejected at normal intervals.

Discussion

Long term results of allografted fresh rat veins as arterial replacement show a high percentage of graft destruction (*Deltz et al.*, 1977). The alterations found in the transplanted vessels as thromboses, aneurysms, and intima thickening are due to the increased pressure and to immunological reactions which occur to the vessel wall. Our data, based on experiments in inbred rat strains, give evidence of the fact that allogeneic vein grafts transplanted in the central vein system also survive against a strong difference in the Major Histocompatibility Complex (MHC). We emphasize that, in contrast to earlier investigations which supposed veins to be less antigeneic than arteries, we have found evidence of normal sensitization of the afferent part of the immune reaction, as the titres of the humoral antibodies and the shortened medium survival time of donorspecific skin grafts are comparable with the results of transplantation of aorta in aorta (*Thiede* 1977) or vein in aorta (*Deltz et al.*, 1977). We suppose that the missing reactions of the efferent part of the immune reaction after vein in vein transplantation are due to a different equipment of vena cava and aorta in rats with vasa vasorum which provides the vein with some sort of a "priviliged position". Summarising our results, we can say that allogeneic veins used as venous replacement in rats are not rejected.

REFERENCES

Askenase, R. P. (1973): Augmented agglutination of erythrocystes in the presence of macrophages, a new assay for antibody. Immunology 25, 47.

Deltz, E., H.-G. Sonntag and A. Thiede (1977): Funktionelle und morphologische Untersuchungen bei allogenen Venentransplantaten. VASA 6, 211.

Thiede, A. (1977): Gefässtransplantation. Die Bedeutung immunologischer Reaktions-mechanismen. Untersuchungen an standardisierten Ratteninzuchtstammkombinationen. In: Ergebnisse der Angiologie, ED N. Klüken, Schattauer Verlag Stuttgart—New York.

Vollmar, J., H. Loeprecht und S. Hutschenreiter (1978): Rekonstruktive Eingriffe am Venensystem. Chirurg 49, 296.

R. E. Abteilung für Allgemeine Chirurgie, Chirurgische Univ.-Klinik, Hospitalstr. 40, D-2300 Kiel, F.R.G.

IMMUNOLOGICAL AND FUNCTIONAL RESULTS OF ALLOGENEIC VEIN TRANSPLANTATION WITHIN THE ARTERIAL SYSTEM

E. DELTZ and A. THIEDE

Department of Surgery, Christian-Albrecht-University, Kiel, F.R.G.

Allogeneic vein grafts have been used for surgical reconstruction of veins and arteries in cases in which autogenous grafts could not be obtained. These operations had varying long-term results. Many studies have been carried out in different animal species in order to detect the immunological mechanisms which had been assumed to be responsible for the unconvincing results. In most of these investigations, however, the animals were not typed genetically, so that the studies were not based on exact immunological data. In order to demonstrate the significance of immunological factors, transplantations of vital allogeneic veins were carried out within inbred rat strains.

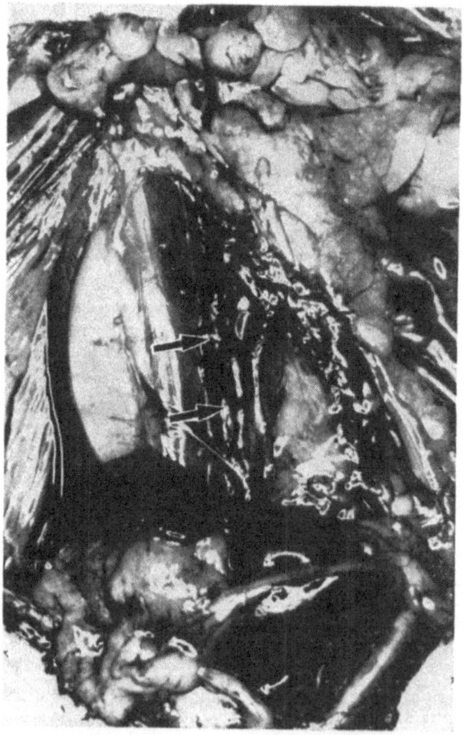

Grafting procedure

A segment of inferior vena cava with a length of $1-1.5$ cm was removed from the donor and then grafted into the abdominal aorta of the recipient below the renal arteries after an adequate segment of the recipients aorta had been removed (Fig. 1).

The following strain combinations have been used.
1. Syngeneic control
CDF → CDF
2. Weakly allogeneic (RtH 1 identical)
LEW → CDF
3. Strongly allogeneic (RtH 1 incompatible)
BD_5→CDF

Histological findings

100 days after transplantation the grafts were removed and examined histologically. All grafts remained patent during this period. The syngeneic graft showed no infiltration by round cells whereas there was slight infiltration in the weakly allogeneic combination. Massive infiltration can be seen in the strongly allogeneic group of vein grafts. Moreover, the vein wall seemed to be almost completely destroyed. Comparison of these pictures shows that increasing infiltration and destruction of the wall of the graft is dependent on immunogenetic differences between donor and recipient.

Fig. 1. Vein segment (arrows) grafted into the abdominal aorta.

Hemagglutination antibody titre

The hemagglutination antibody titre was determined in the two allogeneic strain combinations. Maximum titre were found on about the 56th day. Antibodies against the weakly allogeneic donor were not found (Fig. 2).

Cellular immune reaction

In order to demonstrate the cellular immune reaction, skin grafting of the donor strain was carried out in addition to vascular grafting. In the weakly and in the strongly allogeneic strain combination subsequent skin grafts of the donor strain were rejected in an accelerated manner. Skin grafts of control groups were not rejected earlier (Fig. 3).

Booster effect of subsequent skin grafts

Subsequent skin grafts used as an indicator demonstrate changes in cellular immunological reactivity. Furthermore they cause an additional booster effect which is demonstrated by the increasing titres of transplantation antibodies. In the strongly allogeneic group venous grafts alone lead to slightly increasing titres. The titres were much higher when skin grafts were performed 28 days after vessel transplantation.

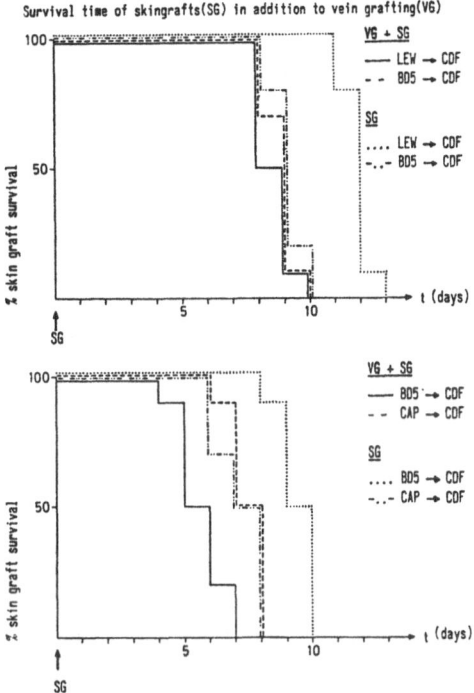

Fig. 3. Rejection of subsequent skin grafts in addition to vein grafting representing cellular immune reaction

Results

The long term results of vein grafting in the arterial system in rats show that in weakly allogeneic strain combinations vein grafts were tolerated well over a long period. The immunological response to weakly allogeneic grafts is slight and does not lead to complete destruction of the graft. In strongly allogeneic strain combinations the immunological response is intense and leads to biological destruction of the graft. These findings however can only be made following transplantation of vital veins into the arterial system. Formalin preserved veins implanted in immunogenetically different rats do not cause an immunological response (*Anders et al.*, 1976; *Deltz et al.*, 1978), nor do allogeneic veins transplanted into the venous system (*Thiede et al.*, 1978).

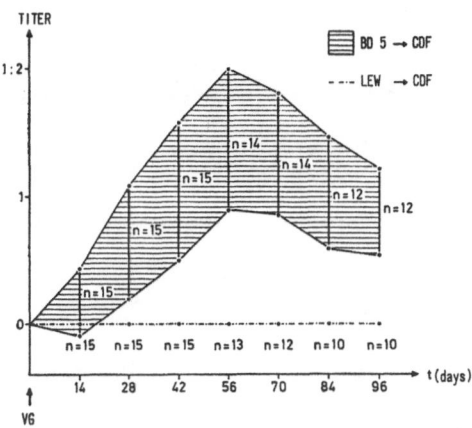

Fig. 2. Hemagglutination antibody titre following vein transplantation

183

REFERENCES

Anders, A., A. Thiede (1976): Der Wert for-
malinfixierter, allogener Venen für den Ge-
fäßerrsatz im Langzeitversuch. Langenb.
Arch. Chir. Suppl., 163.

Deltz, E., A. Anders, H. G. Sonntag, A. Thiede
(1978): Vergleichende immunologische und
morphologische Untersuchungen nach Transplantation frischer und konservierter allogener
Venen im Rattenexperiment. Zschr. Exper.
Chir. 11 (in press).

Thiede, A., R. Engemann, H. Körner, W. Müller-
Ruchholtz (1978): Die Bedeutung der Hämo-
dynamik für die Stärke der Abstoßungsreak-
tion. Vergleich der immunologischen Reak-
tionen bei Arterientransplantation im Hoch-
und Venentransplantation im Niederdruck-
system bei entsprechenden Ratteninzucht-
kombinationen, Langenb. Arch. Chir. Suppl.
313.

E. D., Abteilung Allgemeinchirurgie, Zentrum Operative Medizin I, Christian-Albrechts
-Universität, D 2300 Kiel, F.R.G.

ADAPTABILITY OF VASCULAR TISSUE

RECONSTRUCTIVE SURGERY
ADAPTATION OF VASCULAR WALL TO CHANGES
IN ARTERIAL CIRCULATION

RECONSTRUCTION OR AMPUTATION IN OLD PEOPLE WITH AORTOLIAC OCCLUSIVE ARTERIAL DISEASE?

G. SANOUDOS, P. TSAKONAS and N. TSAGANOS

N.I.M.T.S. Hospital, Athens, Greece

Surgical management of aortoiliac occlusive arterial disease is well established, although there remains a certain variation in operative procedures (*Moore et al.,* 1968, *Szilagyi* 1969, *Perdue et al.,* 1971). With increasing age of the population, the disorder appears with increasing frequency. This communication discusses the treatment of elderly patients with aortoiliac occlusive disease.

Materials and methods

A series of 52 patients were operated at the Nosileftikon Hospital from January 1973 through December 1976 for aortoiliofemoral arterial occlusive disease. There were 46 men and 6 women; ages ranged from 56 to 84, the average was 70. The frequency of patients with very advanced symptoms of ischemic rest pain, pregangrenous lesions, or actual tissue necrosis was noteworthy and many patients with claudication were severly incapacited. Approximately 92% of these patients had one or more associated diseases (Table I).

Table I. Associated disease

	No. of patients	percentage
Arteriosclerotic heart disease	37	76
Bronchopulmonary disease	30	60
Diastolic hypertention	17	36
Azothemia	6	12
Cerebral vascular disease	10	20
Cancer of bladder	2	4

Each patient with complaints of lower extremity ischemic symptoms ranging from moderate claudication to severe rest pain and ulceration was assigned a functional grade on a scale which ranges from A to F, according to *Imparato and Sanoudos* (1970, Table II) Angiographic visualization of the terminal aorta and its ramifications

Table II. Indications for operation

Category	Descriptions	Number of patients	percentage
F	Ischemic ulcers	8	15
E	Rest pain	16	31
D	Severe claudication	20	39
C	Moderate claudication	8	15
	Total	52	100

was accomplished in all patients (*Haimovici et al.* 1969).

The prefered surgical procedure was bypass grafting with a plastic prosthesis, using a woven dacron bifurcation graft. When the major area of involvement was confined to the aorta and common iliac region a local endarterectomy was carried out, here on three patients. The type of procedure performed is listed on Table III.

Table III.

Procedure	No. of patients
Aortofemoral bypass	27
Aortoiliac bypass	17
Endarterectomy	3
Femorofemoral bypass	3
Bilateral axilofemoral bypass	2
Total	52

The risk of a major abdominal procedure was considered too great for five patients and an extra-peritoneal approach was elected for them.

All the patients were transfered to the Intensive Care Unit (I.C.U.) for three to five days. Postoperative care included E.C.G. monitoring, hourly vital signs, urine output and venous blood gases. Routine follow up consisted of monthly examinations for the first three months and twice yearly thereafter.

187

Results

There were no deaths and the only morbidity was the occurence of acute thrombofiebitis of an upper extremity, from an intravenous catheter which subsided following anticoagulation. Ischemic ulcers were healed in all patients. All patients were discharged with restored femoral pulses.

Follow-up of this series of patients ranges from 4 months to 5 years with an average of 23 months. There were 6 late deaths, 3 from myocardial infarction, 2 from cancer and one from stroke, unrelated to the surgical procedure performed, all with functioning arterial reconstruction, for a late mortality rate of 10% at an average of 17 months after operation. Late thrombosis occured in two patients. This was on one side of the bifurcated graft and the unilateral straight prosthesis of another. In the first case, a crossover femorofemoral bypass was combined with a femoropopliteal reconstruction and profundoplasty, while in the second flow was restored by simple embolectomy. Vigorous femoral pulses, healing of all lesions, and absence of incapacitating claudications were taken as indications of late success and these conditions existed in living patients or up to the time of death in 52 of the original 52 patients.

Discussion

The population treated belongs to the geriatric age group which, in addition to an ischemic foot, commonly also have had lessened muscular strength, lowered cardio-respiratory reserve, generally less ability and balance, and usually decreased motivation for rehabilitation (*Thompson et al.*, 1974). In addition, amputation still involves high morbidity and mortality.

Accordingly, every effort aimed at avoiding amputation has strong merit. We believe that modern care can prevent or handle the loads that an operation of the magnitude of aortoiliofemoral reconstruction imposes on pulmonary, cardiac and renal function in this age group. Vigorous replacement of extracellular fluid volume with balanced saline solutions to prevent postoperative renal complications has been advocated by many investigators, who have recommended the supply of up to 1000 ml. of Ringer's lactate per hour during the operation plus replacement of blood loss. However, such rough treatment may have undesired effects on this fragile age group. Careful attention to preoperative pulmonary and cardiac support and strict adherence to postoperative monitoring in the I.C.U. will minimize the occurence of complications.

Bilateral revascularization is usually recommended, even when symptoms predominate on one side, since progress of disease frequently necessitates secondary operations on the other side. A bifurcation prostheses adds little to an operation that includes aorto-femoral anastomosis. Bifurcated prostheses was the preferred surgical procedure in this series of patients, because it has certain advantages over the endarterectomy. There is less dissection and operative time and trauma, less blood loss and the conduit more adequately circumvents a more extensive diseased area (*Moore et al.*, 1968).

It is concluded that, while amputation of a lower extremity still involves high morbidity and mortality in the geriatric patient and has a strongly undesirable psychological impact, aggresive modern care can prevent or handle the loads that aortoliac reconstruction imposes on pulmonary cardiac and renal function in the elder patients.

REFERENCES

Haimovici, H. and Steinman, (1969): Aortoliac angiographic patterns associated with femoropoplital occlusive disease. Significance in reconstructive arterial surgery. Surgery 65, 232.

Imparato, A M., Sanoudos, G. Epstein, H. X., Abrams, R. M., Beranbamy, E. R. (1970): Results in 96 aortoiliac reconstructive procedures: Preoperative angiographic and functional classifications used as prognostic guides. Surgery 68, 610.

Moore, W. S., Cafferata, H. T., Hall, A. O. and Blaisdell, F. W. (1968): In defense of grafts across the inguinal ligament: An evaluation of early and late results of aortofemoral pass grafts. Ann Surg. 168, 207.

Perdue, G. D., Long, W. D., Smith, R. B. III. (1971): Perspective concerning aortofemoral arterial reconstruction, An Surg. 173, 940.

Szilagyi, D. E., (1963): Some controversial topics on vascular surgery. Amer. J. Surg. 118, 406.

Thompson, R. G., Keagy, R. D., Compere, C. L., Meyer, P. R. (1974): Amputation and rehabilitation for severe foot ischemia. Surg. Clin. N. A. 54, 137.

G. S., Nosileftikon Hospital, Monis Petraki 10., Athens, Greece

189

RESULTS OF RECONSTRUCTIVE SURGERY FOR OCCLUSIVE DISEASE OF AORTOILIAC AND FEMOROPOPLITEAL ARTERIES

E. TÜNDER, K. PODER, H. TIKKO, V. MÖLDER and E. SEPP

Tartu State University, Tartu, U.S.S.R.

In the period of 1960—1978, 1002 reconstructive operations were performed at the Tartu University Hospital for occlusive arterial disease of the lower extremities. There were 928 primary operations. 74 secondary operations were performed for late failures after reconstructive surgery, comprising 7.4% of all the operations.

Aortoiliac reconstructions (572 operations). Reconstructions were mainly performed for disabling claudication (less than 100 m), for rest pain, ulcer or gangrene. The operability also depends on the patient's general condition and on the pattern of his arterial disease.

Different methods of reconstruction with an extensive aortoiliofemoral disease. In order to avoid a second operation, we frequently performed a bifurcation bypass in cases of a moderate stenosis of the opposite iliofemoral arteries.

Open or semiclosed endarterectomy (92 procedures) was usually the operation of choice if the disease was limited to the aorta and to the common illiac arteries. Less frequently we used semiclosed endarterectomy for lesions extending to the external iliac artery.

Although we seldom used eversion endarterectomy (Connolly' first modification) for bilateral operations (10 cases) it proved a highly effective procedure for extensive unilateral iliofemoral lesions

Table I. Results of aortoiliac reconstructions (follow-up 1—10yrs)

Type	Cases	Mortality	Patency Early	Late
Prosthetic bypass	348	3.7%	96%	80%
Eversion endarterectomy	116	3.4%	98%	89%
Open or semiclosed endarterectomy	92	2.2%	98%	80%
Axillofemoral bypass	8	12%	88%	29%
Femorofemoral bypass	8	0%	100%	75%
Total	572	3,7%		

were used, depending on the nature and extent of the disease, the patient's general condition and also on the personal choice of the operating surgeon (Table I).

The largest group of operations (348) consisted of bypass grafting. Bifurcation bypass was used in 239 cases and unilateral aorto- or iliofemoral bypass in 109 cases. Bypass grafting, as the simplest and fastest procedure, was considered to be the most suitable operation on patients

(106 cases). In these patients we used an extraperitoneal approach and always restored the patency of the internal illiac artery. Lumbar sympathectomy was added to all types of aortoiliac operations.

Follow-up studies (Table 1) revealed no significant difference between the results of bypass grafting and different types of endarterectomy. Early patency in the whole group was about 96% and late patency made up 80—89%; hospital

Table II. Results of femoropopliteal reconstructions (follow-up 1—10 yrs)

Type	Cases	Mortality	Patency	
			Early	Late
Femoropopliteal autovenous bypass	147	0.7%	90%	79%
Femorotibial autovenous bypass	38	0%	66%	42%
Femoropopliteal prosthetic bypass	43	2,3%	79%	31%
Open or semiclosed endarterectomy	114	1,8%	81%	48%
Homoarterial or homovenous bypass	14	0%	79%	36%
Total	356	1,1%		

mortality was about 3—4%. Long term success in this region depends greatly on the quality of runoff through the deep femoral artery, the wide patency of which can generally be achieved only by local endarterectomy or patch grafting.

Femoropopliteal and femorotibial reconstructions (356 operations). In recent years reconstructions in these patients were performed mainly for limb salvage and less frequently for disabling claudication. Angiographically, many patients with far advanced ischemia had femoropopliteal occlusions with diminished outflow, i.e. simultaneous occlusions of leg arteries.

The best results in this group were obtained using a reversed autogenous saphenous vein graft, placed along the natural course of the artery (147 operations with early patency in 90% and with late patency in 79% of cases). With 38 femorotibial saphenous vein reconstructions early patency comprised 66% and late patency, 42%. In patients who do not have a saphenous

vein with a satisfactory diameter (4 to 6 mm) endarterectomy was usually performed, with early patency in 81% and late patency in 48% of cases. Femoral profundaplasty alone was effective in some cases. Results of a prosthetic or homologous bypass were less favourable with remote patency in 31% and 36% of cases, respectively. Concomitantly with reconstructions, lumbar sympathectomy was performed, especially in patients with a severe ischemia and a poor run-off.

Most patients with far advanced ischemia had combined aortoiliac and femoropopliteal occlusions. In these cases we usually performed only aortoiliac reconstruction, restoring flow to the profunda femoris artery. However, in 43 patients complete revascularisation of the aortoiliac and femoropopliteal arteries was accomplished in a single operation. This was usually carried out in patients with hypoplastic or diffusely damaged profunda femoris artery and also in cases where the distal, i. e. femoropopliteal lesion, was angiographically more significant than the proximal one.

Reoperations after late complications of aortoiliac reconstructions were performed in 74 patients (Table III), with the reestablishment of flow in 69% of cases. Most complications (54

Table III. Results of reoperations after aortoiliac reconstructions (late failures)

Type	Cases	Results	
		Good	Bad
Thrombectomy of prosthesis with profundaplasty	25	18	7
Resection of anasthomotic aneurysm and replacenent	14	12	2
Implantation of new bypass	19	14	5
Partial excision and ligation of prosthesis	6	0	6
Femorofemoral bypass	5	4	1
Axillofemoral bypass	5	3	2
Total	74	51	23

cases) were reocclusions of the aortofemoral bypass or of endarterectomized arteries. Different surgical methods were used for their correction, such as thrombectomy of a prosthesis with profundaplasty, implantation of a bypass after endarterectomy or of a new bypass after an old one, restoration of flow with a femoro-femoral or axillofemoral bypass. False aneurysms in 14 patients were mostly situated on the common femoral artery. Treatment in these cases commonly consisted of resection and replacement of the distal part of the prosthesis with reanastomosis at the original site. Infection of the prosthesis was encountered in 6 cases. Partial excision and ligation of the prosthesis was usually done without reestablishment of flow.

The presented results of 1002 operations from the Tartu University Hospital confirm the current views in reconstructive surgery for occlusive arterial disease: the applicability of different operative methods in aortoiliac reconstructions with relatively good results, a tendency to restriction of operative indications in patients with relative ischemia and femoropopliteal or femorotibial occlusions and applicability of reoperations in most cases of late complications after aortoiliac reconstructions.

E. T., Tartu State Univ., 8. Puuepa Street, 202400 Tartu, U.S.S.R.

THE HEALING OF VASCULAR PROSTHESES IN A MAN

V. RUŽBARSKÝ and M. KRAJÍČEK

Institute for Clinical and Experimental Medicine, Prague, Czechoslovakia

Introduction

The results of healing of vascular prostheses under experimental conditions have been widely described. This study was undertaken to shed light on healing in patients who received vascular prosthesis at different times in the past, which became occluded and afunctional. Of the total number of 14 patients, comprising 13 men and 1 woman, the material was obtained by biopsy from 5 patients and in autopsy in 9 cases. The investigated vascular reconstructions remained patent from 1 to 14 years. We used 11 dacron prostheses, 2 terylene and 1 collagen knitted prosthesis. In 9 patients the prostheses were used for bilateral and in 2 for unilateral aortofemoral by-pass. Two reconstructions involved the femoropopliteal and one the caroticofemoral area.

Macroscopic findings

Major macroscopic findings were occlusion of the bypass and false aneurysm.

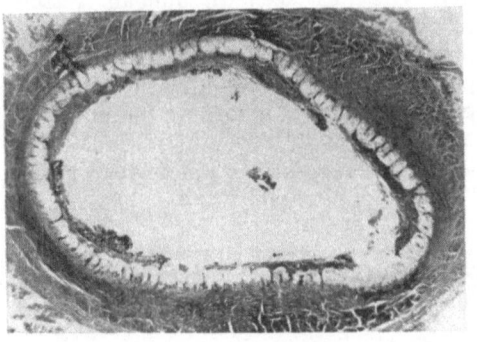

Fig. 1. Histotopogram terylen's prosthesis which was functional twelve years. Fiftysix years old man. Stained according to Mallory, original enlarged 6×.

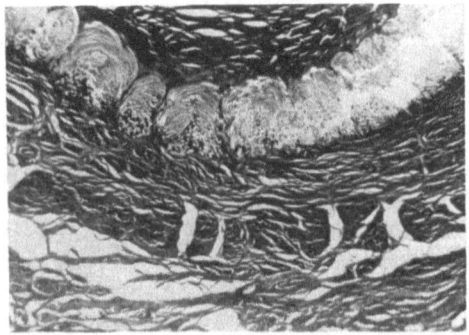

Fig. 2. Fibrous pseudointima (up) and pseudoadventicia (below), dacron's prosthesis that was functional ten years. Sixtysix years old man. Stained according to van Gieson, original enlarged 25×.

Of the 14 reconstructions, only two showed no evidence of thrombosis, five were obliterated by or closed by a new obstructive thrombus. Mural thrombosis at the initial stage of organisation was seen in five cases. False aneurysm occurred in five cases and was unilateral in four and bilateral in one case. A bilateral aortofemoral bypass was involved in all cases.

Histological findings

a) Intima — formation of a low pseudointima was observed in all investigated prostheses irrespective of their life span or type. The pseudointima consisted of lamellar acellular collagen connective tissue completely lacking the upper endothelial surface layer. Smooth muscle cells were also absent. Comparison of the area close to the anastomoses with the central or other segments of the prosthesis did not show any differences. In general, the pseudointima varied in thickness and was somewhat thicker around the anastomosis than in the central part. Regardless of the length of survival or type of prosthesis, some of its areas were completely bald or covered only by fibrin. Usually this was the case at the apex of plications. Generally the pseudointima slightly adherred to the prosthetic tissue, and the intima was connected with the pseudoadventitia by fibrous bridges of varying width only in some cases.

b) Cellular reaction was highly variable and apparently unrelated to the type of substitute used or the length of its patency. It contained mononuclear cells or polynuclear giant cells. These cells were located at the border between the pseudoadventitia and prosthesis or infiltrated the prosthetic fibres. Occasionally we observed a tendency to fibre phagocytosis. On comparing different parts of the prostheses, we found a somewhat higher cellular reaction in the neighbourhood of anastomoses than in central parts. Dacron prostheses displayed a very variable reaction, sites of massive cellular reaction alternating with reaction-free sites. Reaction of terylene prostheses seemed to be more dispersed. The collagen-tissue prosthesis elicited no reaction.

c) Fibrin was observed in all but collagen-tissue prostheses. It formed layers of varying thickness superimposed on the fabric of the prosthesis or infiltrated both the fibre fascicles and their fibres, irrespective of the type or survival time of the prosthesis. There does not seem to be any relationship between fibrin infiltration and cellular reaction, especially in dacron prostheses, in contrast with terylene prosthesis where such a relationship may exist. Since only samples from two patients were available, we cannot draw any definitive conclusion.

d) Pseudoadventitia was well developed in all prostheses regardless of their time of survival and type. Its layer varying in thickness consisted of lamellar acellular collagen connective tissue with poor vascularisation. A higher number of capillaries was seen only close to the anastomoses. The pseudoadventitia generally adherred to the prosthetic fabric. Collagen formed fibrous bridges between fibre fascicles or between its fibres. We found no evidence of smooth muscle cells or elastic fibres in the pseudoadventitia.

e) Infection occurred in two cases and was a causal factor of false aneyurym in one case and separation of the prosthesis from its bed in the other. In one case we also found an abscess in the immediate neighbourhood of the prosthesis deforming it slightly by the pressure exerted on the wall.

f) A major deformation was seen in one case where reconstruction was blocked due to thrombus organisation.

g) Regressive changes were represented by calcification and lipoidosis. There was focal calcification that was confined to the anastomoses area.

Lipoidosis was present in all prostheses regardless of their age and type and involved both the pseudointima and pseudoadventitia similar to bridges inside the prosthesis. Morphological investigation showed that the implanted substitutes failed to develop layers as differentiated and vital as seen in human vessels. In conclusion, despite the fact that some prostheses remained patent for a prolonged period of time, we did not observe perfect biological incorporation and none of the employed types of vascular prosthesis meets the requirements of an "ideal" vascular substitute.

V. R., IKEM, 146 22 Prague 4 - Krč, Vídeňská 800, Czechoslovakia

SECONDARY RECONSTRUCTIVE OPERATIONS IN PATIENTS AFTER AORTOILIAC SURGERY

V. TRIPONIS and DALIA TRIPONIENE

Department of Vascular Surgery, University of Vilnius, U.S.S.R.

Secondary reconstructive operations represent one of the most important subjects in the field of vascular surgery. The vast majority of investigators who have dealt with late complications after aortoiliac surgery continue to advise an aggressive approach to the problem. The most frequent indication for secondary aortiliac repair is graft thrombosis (*Szilagyi et al.*, 1975; *Thompson et al.*, 1977). Anastomotic aneurysms and infection are comparable rare complications which require a secondary procedure. *Neugebauer* (1972) suggests that all the late complications after aortoiliac surgery are derived from two causes; the first lies in the difficulties encountered in choosing the right method of treatment and the second in the further progress of atherosclerosis. Other investigators have pointed out that, among causes due to late complications, errors in surgical technique are not the least important factors (*Cohn et al.*, 1970; *Bernhard et al.*, 1977).

The incidence of anastomotic aneurysms as reported by *Neugebauer* (1972), *Bardos et al.*, (1974) and *Davis* (1975) ranges from 1.8% to 10.5%. Graft infection according to the data presented by *Liekweg and Greenfield* (1977) is encountered in 2.6% of patients operated for aortoiliac occlusions. Similar data were reported earlier by *Jamieson* (1975).

The purpose of this work is to review late complications after aortoiliac reconstructive operations carried out in our clinic, to emphasize some factors expected to be of importance in causing failures and to evaluate methods of secondary operations used in the series.

Over a period of 12 years, 624 patients were operated on for aortoiliac occlusive disease, total number of reconstructive operations being 772. The number of patients who underwent secondary reconstructive operations was 120, or 19.2% of the primarily operated patients. 81 patients (112 operations) were reoperated

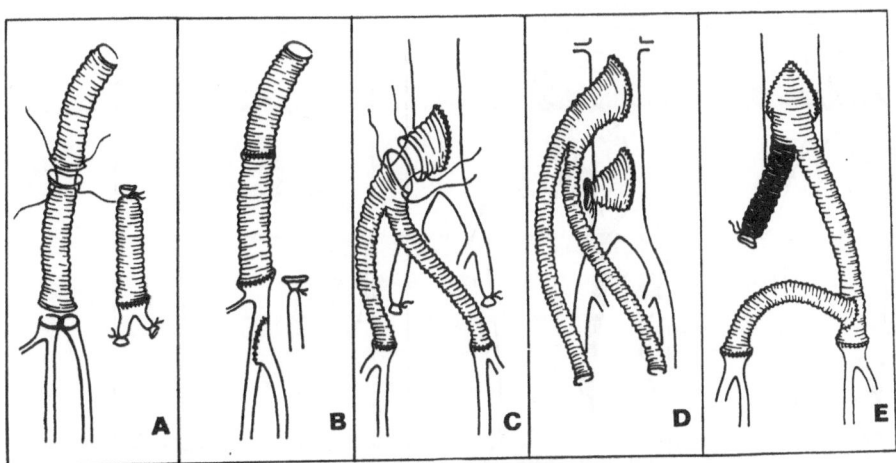

Fig. 1. The most common reconstructive operations used in the clinic.

195

for late postoperative complications: thrombosis, stenosis of anastomosis, anastomotic aneurysm and graft infection. This number of operations does not include 10 cases that required only simple thrombectomy. Of 122 secondary reconstructive operations performed in the late postoperative period, 85 were carried out for thrombosis of vascular grafts and endarterectomized segments. Indications for secondary operations were as follows: graft thrombosis in 56 patients, stenosis of anastomosis in 5, anastomotic aneurysms in 13 and graft infection in 7. Progression of atherosclerosis was discovered in 40 patients with graft thrombosis. In 21 patients, further progress of the disease was traced by examining the deep femoral and the superficial femoral arteries during secondary operations. Stenosis and occlusions in the proximal parts of those arteries were the most evident manifestations of the advancing process. In 9 patients, progression of atherosclerosis in the bifurcation of the aorta and the common iliac arteries was confirmed by angiographic investigations. In 2 patients new signs of the disease were found above the proximal and below the distal anastomosis. 7 patients demonstrated thickened neointima at the site of distal anstomosis. No further devel-

opement of the occlusive process was found by angiography in the main arteries of the legs of these patients. However, increased peripheral resistance after secondary operations could suggest an advanced process in the small arteries. The following secondary reconstructions were employed: reconstruction of distal anastomosis (83), replacement of two side grafts or resuturing of proximal anastomosis (6), replacement of one side iliofemoral bypass graft (8), axillofemoral or femoral-femoral bypass (10), other bypass operations (5). (Fig. 1). The most common reconstructive procedure used for graft thrombosis was the reestablishment of distal anastomosis by a new graft interposition and suturing it to the deep femoral artery or to both femoral arteries below the previous anastomosis (Fig. 1, A–B). Additional femoropopliteal or femorotibial venous bypasses were carried out in 12 patients. In 6 patients major reconstructive operations such as replacement of two side grafts (Fig. 1, D) or insertion of a new one without suturing it directly to the aorta (Fig. 1, C) were carried out. In cases of unsuccessful graft thrombectomy, femoral-femoral or axillofemoral bypasses were the preferred operations (Fig. 1, E). "Other bypass operations" include bypassing of infected

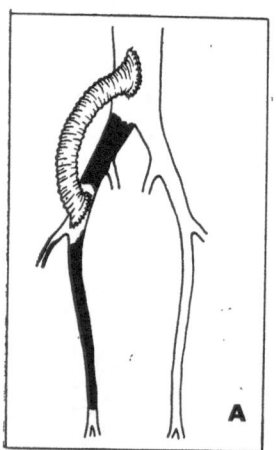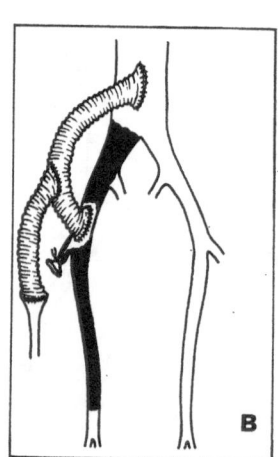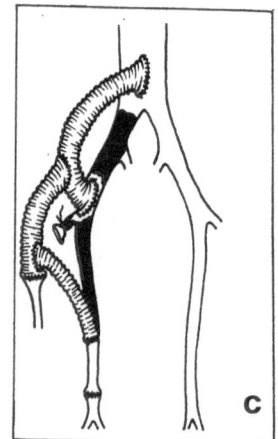

Fig. 2. Stages of on atypical reconstructive operation.

196

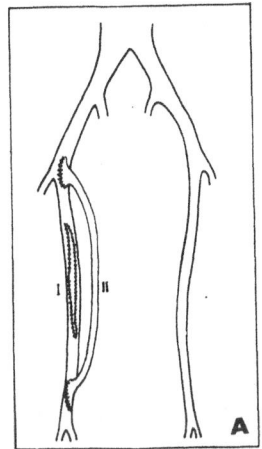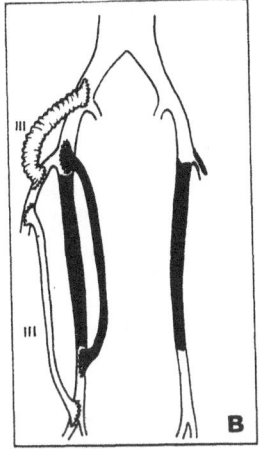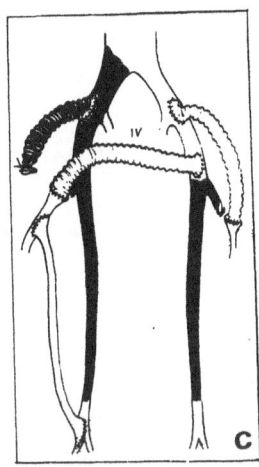

Fig. 3. Stages of an atypical reconstructive operation.

areas with vascular prosthesis as well as with autologous venous bypasses from the external iliac to the superficial femoral artery.

In patients who required more than one secondary operation some atypical methods of reconstruction were applied. The schemes of such operations are depicted in Figures 2 and 3.

In many of our patients who did not required laparotomy, peridural anesthesia was used.

Good results were obtained after 93 reoperations, the revascularization rate being 83%. 8 patients of the 81 reoperated died in the early postoperative period, the overall mortality rate being 9.9%. In the group of patients with graft thrombosis, stenosis of anastomosis and anastomotic aneurysms the mortality rate was 4.9% (3 patients died). In these three patients two side grafts were reinserted. Amputations have been performed in 6 patients. The highest mortality rate was noted in patients with infected grafts. 5 patients of 7 died in this group, an everage of 3 months after reoperation and in one amputation of both extremities was carried out.

REFERENCES

Bardos P., L. Bergdahl, W. E. Meier (1974): Anastomosen-Aneurysmen nach Dacron—Graft im aortoiliakalen Bereich und deren chirurgische Behandlung. Thoraxchirurgie, 22, 461—463.

Bernhard V. M., L. I. Ray, J. B. Towne (1977): The reoperation of choice for aortofemoral graft occlusion. Surgery, 82, 867—874.

Cohn L. H., W. S. Moore, A. D. Hall (1970): Extra abdominal management of late aorto-femoral graft thrombosis. Surg, 67, 775—779

Davis H. J. (1975): Complications of surgery of the abdominal aorta. Amer. J. Surg., 130, 523—527.

Jamieson G. G., J. A. De Weese, Ch. G. Rob (1975): Infected arterial grafts. Ann. Surg., 181, 850—852.

Liekweg W. G., Greenfield L. J. (1977): Vascular prosthetic infections: Collected experience and results of treatment. Surgery 81, 335—342.

Neugebauer J. (1972): Früh und Spätverschlüsse und Nahtaneurysmen nach Rekonstruktionen im aorto-iliakalen Abschnitt. Zbl. Chir., 97, 993—1000.

Szilagyi D. E., J. P. Elliot, R. F. Smith, J. H. Hageman, R. K. Sood. (1975): Secondary arterial repair. Arch. Surg., 110, 485—493.

Thompson W. M., Johnsrude J. S., Jackson D. C., Older R. A. (1977): Late complications of abdominal aortic reconstructive surgery: Roentgen evaluation. Ann. Surg., 185, 326—334.

V. T., Tverečiaus 5—5, 232040 Vilnius, U.S.S.R.

THROMBOSIS OF AORTO-ILIAC RECONSTRUCTION: ORIGIN, PREVENTION AND TREATMENT

J. BARTOŠ, K. TERŠÍP and B. DRUGOVÁ

First Surgical Clinic and Radiological Clinic, Faculty of Medicine, Charles University, Prague Czechoslovakia

At the first Surgical Clinic in Prague, a total of 1187 vascular reconstructions were performed in cases of chronic arterial disease of the lower extremities. Here we will analyse the cases and discuss prevention and treatment of postoperative thromboses following reconstructive operations in the aorto-illiac region. These operations are not only the most frequently performed of all reconstructive operations, but they are also the most successful.

In the majority of cases operated, obliterations of the superficial femoral artery and of tibial arteries were present in addition to obliterations or stenoses of the aorto-iliac region. The revascularisation of the extremity is ensured in these patients only through deep femoral artery collaterals. Therefore, after thrombosis of such a reconstruction, a severe lower extremity ischemia develops, leading to amputation if reoperation is not undertaken.

From the point of view of thrombosis onset, three types of thrombosis can be differentiated: peroperative, early, occuring between the second day to third month after operation and late thrombosis, developing during the later postoperative period.

From 1959 to the end of 1977, 472 aorto-iliac reconstructions were performed. Complications were encountered in 160 patients (33%). The most frequent complications were anastomotic aneurysms and thrombosis, which were observed in 90 of 472 primary operations over the 18 year period (19%). The most frequent thrombosis is late, occuring in 72 patients (15%). (Fig. 1).

The causes of thromboses are depicted in Fig. 2. While peroperative thrombosis is mainly a consequence of faulty operative technique, late thrombosis was in a great majority of cases found to be a result of deep femoral artery obliteration due to the progression of arteriosclerotic changes. After endarterectomies, especially in late

Fig. 1. Complications and reoperations after aorto-iliac reconstructions

Complication	4 7 2 operations			
	Number	Reoperated	Success	Unsuccess
Hemorrhage	1	1	0	1
Infection	13	13	1	12
Perforation (striptor)	4	4	4	0
Anastomoses aneurysms	50	50	44	6
Aneurysms after common femoral artery T.E.	1	1	1	0
Aneurysm common iliac artery T.E.	1	1	1	0
Thromboses peroperative	15	15	9	6
early 90 19%	3	1	1	0
late	72 15%	72	61	11
	160 33%	158	122	36

Fig. 2. Causes of thromboses after aorto-iliac reconstruction

	Number	Operation	Number	Cause	Number
Peroperative	15	by-pass	11	Intimal dissection or deep femoral artery stenosis	8
				prosthesis compression	1
				embolism	2
		T.E.	4	Intimal dissection or deep femoral artery stenosis	2
				embolism	2
Early	3	by-pass	1	embolism	1
		T.E.	2	Iliac rethrombosis	2
Late	72	by-pass	56	deep femoral artery obliteration	52
				rotation	1
				compression	3
		T.E.	16	deep femoral artery obliteration	9
				Iliac rethrombosis	7

Fig. 3. Reoperations after alloplastic by-pass implantations in aorto-iliac region

Number of thromboses	Cause	Number	Reoperation	Number	Success
68	deep femoral artery obliteration	60	Deep femoral artery T.E. + prosthesis desoblit.	44	40
			Deep femoral artery T.E. + new by-pass	10	10
			Superficial femoral artery reconstr. + prosthesis desoblit.	6	3
	prosthesis compression	4	decompression	1	1
			Resection + new by-pass	3	2
	Embolism	3	embolectomy	3	2
	Prosthesis rotation	1	new ilico-femoral by-pass	1	1

thrombosis, new arteriosclerotic thrombosis of previously desobliterated segments also played an important role.

The prevention of late thromboses may be achieved, as follows, from these observations through simultaneous reconstruction of the deep femoral artery, when stenoses are discovered during the primary operation. The common femoral artery arteriotomy is extended upon the deep femoral artery and endarterectomy is performed under visual control. After endarterectomy of the aorto-iliac region, the deep femoral artery arteriotomy is then closed by means of a venous patch. After arterial artificial prosthesis implantation, the same procedure can be followed or deep femoral artery plasty is performed by means of prosthesis. More extensive deep femoral artery changes can be by-passed with the saphenous vein.

Simultaneous reconstructions of the deep femoral artery have been performed since 1969 and up to the end of 1977 were used 173 times in 219 reconstructive operations of the aorto-iliac region. Late thrombosis after this preventive procedure was observed in only four patients (2.3%).

The treatment of these thromboses depends primarily on the cause of thrombosis and on the kind of primary operation.

After the *implantation of the artifical prosthesis* (Fig. 3) deep femoral artery obliteration was found to be the cause of thrombosis in 60 patients and in 44 of them the method recommended by us in

Fig. 4. Reoperations after aorto-iliac thromboendarterectomy

Number of thromboses	Cause	Number	Reoperation	Number	Success
22	deep femoral artery obliteration	11	Allopl. bifurc. by-pass + deep femoral artery T.E.	4	4
			Iliaco-prof. vein by-pass	1	1
			Deep femor. artery T.E. + thrombus extraction	3	3
			Deep femoral artery T.E. + redesoblit. of iliac arteries	2	2
			Iliaco-prof. by-pass + deep femor. artery T.E.	1	1
	Iliac rethrombosis	9	Allopl. bifurcated by-pass	5	5
			Redesobliteration (non operated 2)	2	0
	embolism	2	embolectomy	2	0

1968 was used: deep femoral artery endarterectomy and prosthesis desobliteration. In another 10 patients, a new artificial vascular prosthesis was implanted after deep femoral artery endarterectomy and in 6 the outflow from the desobliterated prosthesis was attempted. During reoperation, the deep femoral arteriotomy, prolonged over the distal pole of the anastomosis, is performed. Deep femoral artery endarterectomy under visual control and retrograde prosthesis desobliteration follows. The second branch of the prosthesis or the common iliac artery is used by minor laparotomy, to prevent retrograde embolism. The reoperation is terminated by means of deep femoral artery vein plasty.

Advantages of our method are as follows:

1. Relatively simple procedure. 2. High percentage of success (90%). 3. Rare repeated reconstruction thrombosis — 4 times (9.9%). 4. Renewal of the primary postoperative state and its frequent improvement as a result of the deep femoral artery endarterectomy.

After *thromboendarterectomy* of the aorto-iliac region, in addition to deep femoral artery obliteration, reconstruction thrombosis is often caused by arteriosclerotic changes in the previously desobliterated region. (Fig. 4). Remaining parts of the endarterium may also play a role in peroperative and even late thrombosis. Implantation of an alloplastic bilateral by-pass, combined, if necessary, with deep femoral artery endarterectomy, proved to be the most successfull reoperation.

J. B., 1st Surgical Clinic, U nemocnice 2, 128 08 Prague, Czechoslovakia,

LONG-TERM CHANGES OF CALF BLOOD FLOW AND LOCAL PRESSURE IN PATIENTS WITH AORTOFEMORAL RECONSTRUCTION

LIBUŠE ROMANOVSKÁ, M. KRAJÍČEK and I. PŘEROVSKÝ

Institute for Clinical and Experimental Medicine, Prague, Czechoslovakia

The blood flow in ischemic legs in patients suffering from obliterative atherosclerosis can be improved by surgical treatment. The aim of this study was to quantitate the degree and duration of local circulatory improvement in patients after patent aortofemoral bypass and/or after iliac endarterectomy.

To characterize the hemodynamics of legs both calf blood flow and local systolic pressure were determined by means of strain-gauge plethysmography. As a criterion of the functional capacity of the arterial bed the maximal calf blood flow at reactive hyperemia after five minute ischemia was considered. The local systolic pressure was determined at rest both in the thigh and at the ankle and was expressed as arm-thigh or arm-ankle systolic pressure gradients.

Using this technique, patients were examined a week before surgery and in the 3rd, 6th, 12th, 24th and 36th month of the postoperative period. The effect of operation was described in relation to the patency of vessels distally from recon-

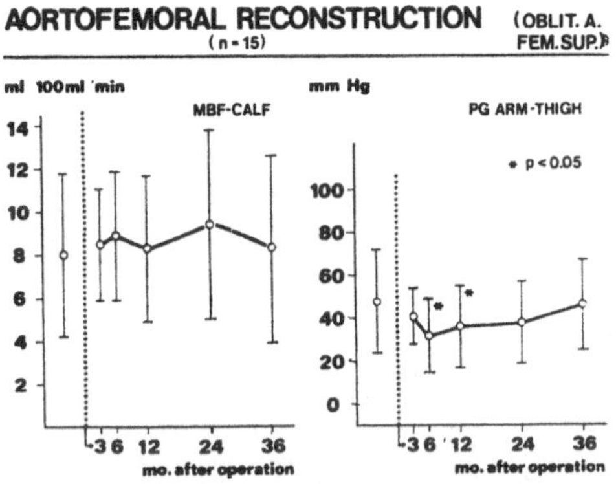

Fig. 2. Maximal calf blood flow (MBF) and pressure gradients (PG) arm-thigh and arm-ankle in the second group of extremities.

struction. 37 of the 46 examined extremities (14 with endarterectomy and 32 with aortofemoral bypass) were therefore divided into three groups according to preoperative arteriograms. The first group included extremities in which only atherosclerotic changes or moderate stenosis of the superficial femoral artery were found. The second group contained cases with a patent superficial femoral artery but with obliterations of the two calf arteries. In the third group were cases with obliteration of the superficial femoral artery and patent calf arteries. The other combinations of obliterative or stenotic processes were excluded because of the small number of cases.

In the extremities of the first group (Fig. 1) the mean postoperative values of maximal blood flow were significantly increased. The mean arm-thigh pressure gradient was positive before the operation; after reconstruction a significant decrease to the normal negative value was found,

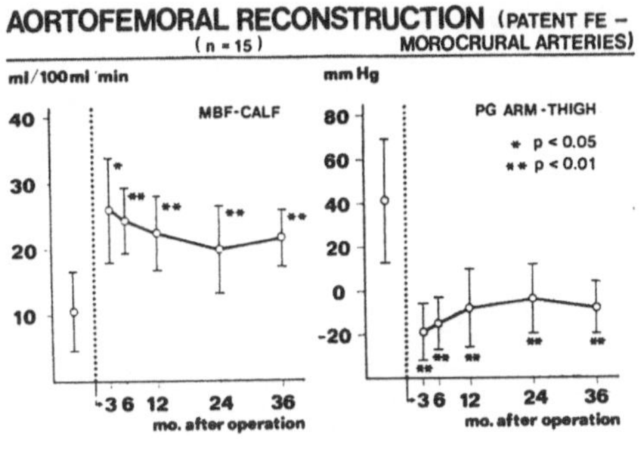

Fig. 1. Maximal calf blood flow (MBF) and pressure gradient (PG) arm-thigh in the first group of extremities.

201

followed by a slight gradual increase. In legs of the second group (Fig. 2) the postoperative maximal blood flow was also significantly increased, but it was less expressed than in the first group. The preoperative value of the arm-thigh pressure was positive because of iliac artery obliteration, the mean postoperative value was normal. The arm-ankle gradient was higher before the operation than the arm-thigh gradient. After the operation

a decrease was also found, but the difference between the two gradients was nearly the same as before operation. In extremities of the third group (Fig. 3), on postoperative increase in maximal calf blood flow was found. A significant decrease in arm-thigh pressure gradient was found only in the course of the first postoperative year. The pressure gradient was, however, permanently positive.

It seems that no differences exist between results found in extremities after endarterectomy and aortofemoral bypass. When reconstruction is patent, the improvement of arterial hemodynamics depends mainly on the degree of atherosclerotic changes in the vascular bed distally from the operation. The decrease in maximal blood flow and the increase in pressure gradients which were observed during the three year period after the operation show that the atherosclerotic process has slowly continued.

It can also be concluded that the noninvasive technique used in this study is appropriate to quantify the long-term changes in blood flow and pressure in the extremities.

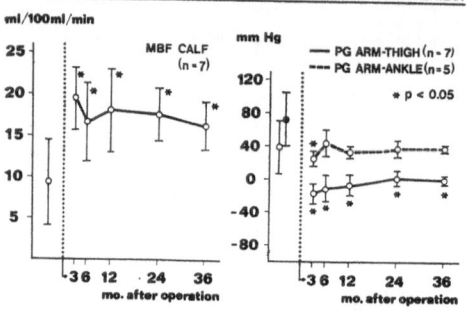

AORTOFEMORAL RECONSTRUCTION (OBLIT. CALF ARTERIES)

Fig. 3. Maximal calf blood flow (MBF) and pressure gradient (PG) arm-thigh in the third group of extremities.

L. R., Institute for Clinical and Experimental Medicine, Vídeňská 800, 146 22 Praha 4, Czechoslovakia

RESULTS OF FEMOROPOPLITEAL VENOUS BYPASS OPERATION IN CHRONIC ARTERIAL OCCLUSION

M. BARTEL, W. WAGNER and I. MARZOLL

Department of Surgery, Friedrich Schiller University, Jena, G.D.R.

After thrombendarterectomy (3) and autologous venous bypass (6) had been introduced for the correction of chronic arterial vascular occlusions in the femoropopliteal region, these methods, for the first time, have been considered as competing procedures. Meanwhile, from literature (1, 2, 4, 7, 8, 9) as well as from our own experience are aware of the advantages and disadvantages of the various corrective interventions. On the basis of this fact, the alternative procedures have developed during the past years into equivalent and complementary reconstructive interventions. Each method can lead to remarkable results, if it is applied on the basis of

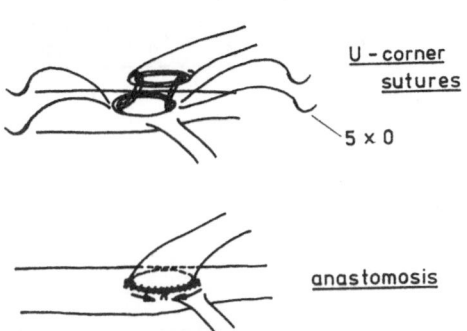

Oval excision of the prox. arteriotomy

Preparation of the vein for anastomosis

U - corner sutures

5 x 0

anastomosis

Fig. 1. Operating technique of the side-to-end anastomosis between artery and vein.

differentiated and critical indication adapted to the morphological substrate of the vessels.

We, too, have adjusted our attitude towards these two procedures and, in the last years, have abandoned the enucleation procedure which, with few exceptions, we practised formerly and instead now, under certain circumstances, prefer venous bypass.

From 1969–1977, 141 autologous venous bypass operations were been performed on 133 patients as primary reconstruction using the free angioplasty according to the operative technique in Figure 1 and not the in situ bypass in the femoropopliteal area. Because of an insufficient "run in", in 15 cases the vascular system set had to be included in the reconstruction. Among postoperative complications, the lymphatic fistulae, which, however, stopped spontaneously after 8–14 days, were of primary importance. In no case could deterioration of the peripheral arterial circulation be observed after the intervention. In the postoperative phase, 2 patients (1.5%) died from myocardial infarction.

Of the 133 patients (141 bypass operations), 117 (123 venous grafts) could be investigated with regard to their late results. Of the remaining 16 operated patients (18 bypass operations), 13 had died in the meantime, follow-up investigations do not exist for 3 patients. Among the 141 venous grafts were 23 occlusions (Table I) including 2 immediate, 14 early and 7 late occlusions. The immediate and early occlusions were obviously caused by suitable venous grafts, considerable differences in the calibers between transplant

Table I. Causes of immediate, early, and late occlusions of a venous bypass (VBP).

Causes	n	techn. defects	unsui-table vein	angiographic vein off		no angio-graph.	diabet. mellit.	disturbed fat meta-bolism
				idem	worse			
Immediate occlusion (48 h postop.)	2		2	2				
Early occlusion (14 d postop.)	14			2	12		3	1
Late occlusion	7				5	2	3	

and artery, stenoses at the distal anastomosis or an insufficient "run off".

The results of our investigations (Table II) based on angiographic control examinations can be summarized as follows:

From half a year to 6 years, of 141 venous grafts 77.2% are patent, 70.7% of the operated patients are free of pain and 25.2% show an improvement in walking distance. They belong to stage II according to *Fontaine*; The angiographically established occlusion rate was 1.5% immediate, 9.9% early (up to the first postoperative year) and 4.9% late occlusions. The number of early occlusions could be reduced by means of critical indication und use of appropriate grafts with an average lumen of more than 4 mm.

According to the literature data (7, 9, 10) and on the basis of our own experience, the autologous saphenous vein bypass is an adequate principle for reconstruction in:

1. all occlusion processes of the a. femoralis superficialis and poplitea during simultaneously existing stenoses or partial occlusions in the arteries of the lower leg,
2. far-reaching occlusions of the a. femoralis superficialis and partial involvement of the a. poplitea,
3. progressing arteriosclerosis of the a. femoralis superficialis and/or po-

Table II. Results of follow-up investigation in a venous bypass (VBP). Classification in stages according to Fontaine.

Follow — up Results of the Saphenous Vein Bypasses in Stages

Stage		1/2	1	2	3	years 4	5	6	7	8	Compared to preop. stage
I	0	34	21	16	8	—	1	2	3	2	0
	*	—	—	—	—	—	—	—	—	—	
II	0	1	3	6	2	—	1	—	3	—	65
	*	7	2	3	—	—	—	1	2	—	
III	0	—	—	—	—	—	—	—	—	—	
	*	1	2	2	—	—	—	—	—	—	
IV	0	—	—	—	—	—	—	—	—	—	
	*	—	—	—	—	—	—	—	—	—	

0 Bypass patent, * Bypass occluded.

plitea, i.e. if the calcification is not limited to only one layer of the vascular wall and

4. recurrent occlusions in the femoro-popliteal vascular region after a previous thrombendarterectomy.

REFERENCES

1. *Conolly, J. E. and E. A. Stemmer (1970):* The nonreversed saphenous vein bypass for femoral-popliteal occlusive disease, Surgery 68, 602—609.
2. *Cutler, B. S., J. E. Thompson, L. J. Kleinsasser and G. K. Hempel (1976):* Autologous saphenous vein femoropopliteal bypass. Analysis of 298 cases. Surgery 79, 325—331.
3. *Dos Santos, J. C. (1947):* Sur la desobstruction des thromboses artérielles anciennes. Mem. Acad. Chir. 73, 409.
4. *Gall, F. (1968):* Venentransplantation zur Rekonstruktion beim Femoralisverschluß. Erfassungen bei 200 Eingriffen. Thoraxchirurgie 16, 7—14.
5. *Krüger, B. J.; H. G. Berger und M. Nasseri (1971):* Die chirurgische Therapie der chronischen Verschlußkrankheiten in der A. fem. superfic. Langenbeck's Arch. Chir. 330, 79—94.
6. *Kunlin, J. (1949):* Le traitment de l'artérite obliterante par la greffe veineuse. Arch. Mal Coeur 42, 371.
7. *Müller-Wiefel, H., D. Borm, H.-D. Bruhn, P. Ilipp, J. Schellmann und J. Sedlmeyer (1971):* Spätergebnisse rekonstruierender Operationen bei chron. aortoiliacalen und femoropoplitealen Arterienverschlüssen. Thoraxchirurgie 19, 488—493.
8. *Schulz, U., K. Lambach und W. Saggau (1976):* Thrombendarterieekotmie oder Venenbypass bei chronischen femoro-poplitealen Verschlüssen. Langenbeck's Arch. Chir. 343, 59—67.
9. *Schwilden, E. D. und H. R. Willem (1973):* Die rekonstruktive Chirurgie des langstreckigen femoropoplitealen Arterienverschlusses. Thoraxchirurgie 21, 177—185.
10. *Vollmar, J.:* Rekonstruktive Chirurgie der Arterien Thieme-Verlag Stuttgart 1975.

M. B., Dept. of Surgery, Friederich Schiller University, Bach Str. 18., Jena 69, G.D.R.

OUR EXPERIENCE WITH THE IN-SITU BYPASS IN CHRONIC OCCLUSIVE DISEASE OF THE FEMOROPOPLITEAL ARTERY

J. D. GRUSS, S. KAWAI and C. KARADEDOS

Dept. of Vasc. Surg., Kurhess. Diakonissenhaus, Kassel, F.R.G.

Out of total of 3389 reconstructive operations on the vascular system we performed at our hospital since July 1, 1971, 1335 were obliterations of the superficial femoral artery. Until 1974, the semi-closed thrombendarterectomy was the primary reconstructive procedure. After a discussion with *Hall*, we used more and more the femoropopliteal or femorocrural in-situ by pass for femoropopliteal occlusions. In the period between January 1, 1975, and December 31, 1977, we have carried out 191 in-situ bypasses; for the time being, shall describe operations. Before going into detail and describing special technical problems, and before giving our results, I would like to specify the therapeutical approach we use today in treating occlusions of the superficial femoral artery.

We use thrombendarterectomy only in exceptionally rare cases such as circumscript occlusions in poor risk patients where larger procedures carry too high a risk. Occlusions of the superficial femoral artery between the inguinal ligament and the Hunter's canal where the distal lumen to it is open, are being reconstructed by interposition of an 8 mm-double-velour-dacron graft. All other forms of femoropopliteal occlusions such as occlusions with restricted outflow, or occlusions reaching beyond the joint are now an indication for the in-situ by pass. This procedure is especially qualified for the revascularization of a single crural artery, and here in particular with an anastomosis to the posterior tibial artery. In approximately 10% of our patients, we cannot find suitable autotransplants. In these cases we use P.T.F.E.-grafts.

For anatomical reasons, the proximal anastomosis must be made transverse end-to-end to the superficial femoral artery. If possible, we try to avoid the thrombendarterectomy of the proximal

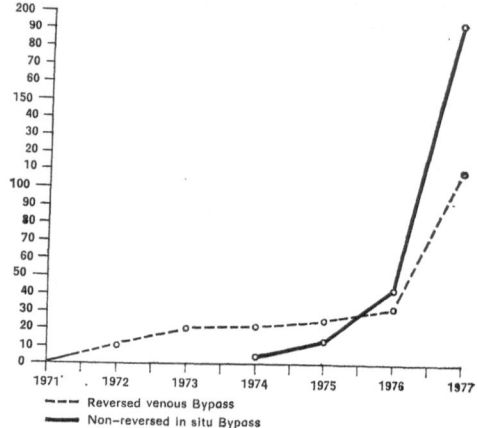

Fig. 1. Our experience with the in-situ bypass in chronic occlusive disease of the femoropopliteal artery.

Tab. I. Our experience with the in-situ bypasin chronic occlusive disease of the femoropospliteal artery.

Reconstructive Procedure in 1335 cases of Superficial Femoral Artery Occlusions 1.7. 1971 – 31.12.1977

Semiclosed Thrombendarteriectomy (TEA)	675
TEA with intraoperative Angiography	192
Reversed venous bypass	109
Non-reversed, in-situ venous graft	191
Homologeous venous bypass	14
Alloplastic bypass	81
Profundaplasty	73
Total	1335

206

Tab. II. Our experience with the in-situ bypass in chronic occlusive disease of the femorpopliteal artery.

1.1.1975 - 31.12.1977

191 in - situ - bypasses	— distal anastomosis
first popliteal segment	53
third popliteal segment	113
tibial arteries	25

Tab. III. Our experience with the in-situ bypass in chronic occlusive disease of the femoropopliteal artery.

1.1.1975 - 31.12.1977

191 in - situ - bypasses

Stage IIb	78
Stage III	74
Stage IV	39

Tab. IV. Our experience with the in-situ bypass in chronic occlusive disease of the femoropopliteal artery.

1.1.1975 - 31.12.1977

191 in - situ - bypasses

1 patent tibial artery	65
2 patent tibial arteries	122
3 patent tibial arteries	4

superficial femoral artery, since we observed two cases which after several months developed high degree stenosis at the anastomosis which had to be corrected. In cases where it is necessary to disobliterate the common femoral artery, or the deep femoral artery, it is sometimes possible to split the inferior epigastric vein dorsally, and use it as a ventral patch for the prolongation of the saphenous vein to close the arteriotomy, thereby creating an end-to-side anastomosis. The distal transplant connection can be accomplished either end-to-end or end-to-side, de-

pending upon the condition of the outflow. In our own series, we used 53 times the I. popliteal segment, 113 times the III. popliteal segment, and 25 times a single crural artery as distal connection. Only in four cases of all our patients were three crural arteries permeable. In 122 cases, there were two, and in 65 cases, there was only one crural artery permeable. Before proceeding with the anastomoses, we destroy the venous valves from the distal side with the stripper mentioned by *Hall*. This stripper is available in several sizes on the market. At the beginning of our experiences with the in-situ bypass, we saw two cases where the greater saphenous vein had been torn by strippers which had been too big. It proved to be advisable to distend carefully the dissected distal saphenous segment with a heparin-saline-solution before inserting the stripper. The destruction of the valves has to be accomplished on the extended leg. After the completion of the anastomoses, intraoperative angiography must be made. By doing so, one can judge the caliber as well as the length of the transplant. One can visualize the anastomoses, and the localization of venous branches. With this method, one can see precisely all efferent branches, especially the perforating veins. Afferent branches of the veins are only filled up to the first valve, and are often only recognizable as small plumb widenings of the transplant. If the valves of the afferent branches are not leaking, they will not fill with contrast medium. These branches are only perceptible after several days or weeks by the appearance of a red, painful spot in the area of the graft as well as by loud, machine-like bruit. These visualized branches are being dissected through additional incisions, and clipped with silver clips. To make sure that the interruption ist complete, we use intra-operative flow measurements near both anastomoses with the Nycotron before and after clipping.

We operated 78 times in stage II, 74 times in stage III, and 39 times in stage IV. Because of the short period of time for the follow-up, it is not possible to compare the results. Of the 191 in-situ bypasses which have been performed until December 31, 1977, 176 grafts are still functioning. Our permeability rate after two years is 85%. According to our observations, a forecast about the permeability to be expected can be better made by the preoperative ultrasonic pressure measurement rahter than the morphology of the vessels as seen by the angiogram. It is relatively unimportant whether one, two or three crural arteries are open, if the preoperative delta-p is over 0.3. Independently of the morphology, we saw always immediate or early occlusions in patients whose preoperative delta-p was below 0.3. In these patients, the intraoperative flow measurements showed values below $60-70$ ml/min.

J. D. G., Kurhess. Diakonissenhaus, Dept. of Vascular Surgery, Goethestrasse 85, D-3500 Kassel, F.R.G.

RECONSTRUCTIVE SURGERY IN ISCHEMIC DISEASES OF LOWER LIMBS

CL. OLIVIER, R. RETTORI and J. B. LEVY

Department of Surgery and Vascular Pathology, Hôtel-Dieu, Paris, France

Acute ischemias are always serious accidents in all vascular patients.

Materials

Our series is composed of 307 ischemic accidents in 273 patients: 102 (1/3) in patients free from any arterial disease and 2/3 in patients with arteriopathy. We did not include ischemia occurring in patients previously operated on for arteriopathy of the limbs. There were 113 women (41.4%). This percentage is slightly higher than in chronic arteriopathy. This is due, in part, to the fact that ischemia in healthy arteries occurs slightly more often in women than in men. However, we found that a little more than 1/3 (36.4%) of the women had ischemia of pathologic arteries.

Exact mechanism of ischemia is often difficult to specify, because it is not easy to know if it is an embolism on pathologic arteries or an in situ thrombosis occurring suddenly or after general hemodynamic trouble. Moreover, this mechanism is less important that the previous arterial state, because we can hope to restore a normal arterial bed by mere embolectomy in a patient with healthy arteries, but it is more often illusory if the arteries are pathologic.

In our series, embolisms are due in 73% of cases to cardiopathies, but in 6% of cases the cause is an aortic or iliac lesion, aneurysm or atheroma. One third of our patients had healthy arteries; only 10% had medically treated arteriopathy and 38% unknown or totally neglected arteriopathy.

The frequency of acute ischemia of pathologic arteries is difficult to evaluate. In the same period (1960—1976) about one operation out of 6 was performed for acute ischemia. Cases with high risk of ischemia (serrated stenoses, aortic plaques or ectasias) are more readily operated on nowadays and we can hope to see this emergency rate lowered significantly.

Treatment

Without reverting to preoperative explorations, we must insist on some points:

transfer of the patient to a specialized unit, under heparin, which is done in only half of the cases;

the difficulty of knowings the exact anterior arterial state;

interest in Doppler velocimetry; arteriography, on the other hand, does not seem to us obligatory and only thin needle femoral arteriography will justify later use of fibrinolytics.

In 30 cases of subacute distal ischemia in 26 patients, we performed only a sympathectomy (1 death, 21 successes): we performed an amputation 8 times in 7 patients; but sympathectomy permitted us to keep the knee in 5 cases.

Results of arterial flow restorations

This restoration was performed in 197 cases (61% of the observed ischemias): 95 times for ischemia on healthy arteries in 82 patients and 102 times for ischemia on pathologic arteries in 94 patients. In 133 cases, thrombectomy was performed, 95 times in 82 patients with healthy arteries and 38 times in 36 patients with chronic arteriopathies.

The results (table I) show that embolectomy succeeded in 2 cases out of 3 on healthy arteries, but only in 1 case out of 3 on pathologic arteries, because restoration of the arterial existent bed just before the accident is revealed deficient in most cases. This embolectomy is the only treatment for a patient for whom nothing else can be suggested because of his arterial or general state.

Associated sympathectomy can be useful. Principally in pathologic arteries it permits improving the capacity of the peripheral bed to obtain an increased flow so as to limit the risk of thrombosis: this result was obtained in 9 out of 14 cases.

Table I. Results of Thrombectomies

Operations	Normal arteries				Pathologic arteries			
	N	S	A	D	N	S	A	D
Thrombectomies	92	60	17	15	24	9	8	7
Thrombectomies + lumbar sympathectomies	3	2	1	0	14	9	2	3
Total	95	62	18	15	38	18	10	10

N = number of operations, S = success, A = amputation in surviving patients, D = death

The percentage of deaths can appear important: 17% in healthy arteries (15).

The percentage of deaths can appear: 26% (10 patients out of 38) in pathologic arteries. This reflects the percentage of aged patients, with poor general state, with limited cardiac, renal or respiratory function, unbalanced both by the accident and its treatment. Most of these deaths are due to renal or cardiac causes.

Amputations in nearly same rate are due to the late of reccurrent character of this act more than to technical failure itself (exceeded ischemias with distal and venous thrombosis).

In fact, success of a too late desobstruction often leads to irreversible renal insufficiency: this is true of massive embolisms of the aortic arch or of the two limbs simultaneously in cardiac patients and in ischemias seen too late.

Some operations have been associated with one venous desobstruction for phlegmasia coerulea and 3 arteriotomies using patch. More interesting are the 17 tibial aponeurotomies performed immedia-tely or secondarily, generally 12 to 24 hours after revascularization. They aim at limiting edematous venous compresion. This act can permit amelioration of the circulatory state.

Results of arterial reconstructions by by-pass are summarized in table II. They were all performed for acute ischemia on pathologic arteries.

We performed 34 by-passes in 30 patients for aorto-illiac thrombosis, with 8 deaths and 30 by-passes on 28 patients for femoro-popliteal or tibial thrombosis, with 5 deaths. In more than half the cases, the operation was successful. The vital risk is great with the abdominal approach. This has lead us for 3 years to perform 13 atypical by-passes in 12 patients with nearly half the vital risk for nearly same amputation rate (a little less than 20%).

At the femoro-popliteal level and at the femoro-tibial level, risk of failure leading to amputation prevails over vital risk: 8 amputations among 30 revas-cularizations at this level, of which 4 were

Table II. Arterial by-pass: 64 (58 patients)

By-pass	Success	Amputation	Death
Aorto or ilio-femoral: 21	11 (52.4%)	4 (19%)	6 (28.6%)
Axillo-femoral: 11	7	2	2
Crossed femoro-femoral: 2	2 (69.2%)	0 (15.4%)	0 (15.4%)
Femoro-popliteal and femoro-tibial 30	17 (56.7%)	8 (26.6%)	5 (16.7%)

among the 10 more distal revascularizations.

These especially distal and late revascularizations of antero-external and posterior tibial aponeurotomies are interesting. On the other hand, associated lumbar sympathectomy has been performed only 3 times: it increases the vital risk without changing, directly at least, the chances of success, which depend particularly on the possibilities of tissue recovery.

Half of the 38 post-operative deaths after ischemias on healthy arteries is due to renal insufficiency or to toxemic shock; the rate is lightly lower (30%) in case of pathologic arteries. This is explained by the better tissue tolerance to ischemia and by the lower number of complete massive ischemias. The other deaths are generally due to heart failure, myocardial infarction or pulmonary embolism.

Conclusion

Delay between beginning of ischemia and the therapeutic act is the chief factor in prognosis. In patients with arteriopathy, chances of success are near 75% if the patient is operated on during 12 hours after the advent of symptoms and are 50% if the patient is treated from 12 hours to 48 hours after; they fall to 20% if the patient is treated on the third day.

In embolism on healthy arteries, delay is perceptibly less important that the proximal centre or than the reccurrent obliterative character of embolism (5 deaths among 15 cases). The present attitude pertmitted a perceptible improvement of the results and non-operable patients often profit by thrombolysis which permits a success rate of nearly 54%.

The use, since 1973, of atypical by-passes for high ischemias improved our results, reducing the total mortality rate to under 18%.

REFERENCES

Cormier J. M., Devin R. (1969): Traitement des oblitérations artérielles aigues des membres. Rapport au 71e Congrès Français de Chirurgie Paris, 29—2 octobre 1969, Paris, P.U.F., 1969, p. 391—635.

Eriksson I., Holmberg J. T. (1977): Analysis of factors affecting limb salvage and mortality after embolectomy. Acta Chir. Scand. 143, 237—240.

Fogarty T. J., Daily P. O., Shumway N. E. et Krippaehne W. (1971): Experience with balloon catheter technics for arterial embolectomy. Amer. J. Surg. 122, 231—237.

Freund U., Romanoff H. et Floman Y. (1975): Mortality rate following lower limb arterial embolectomy: causative factors. Surgery 77, 201—207.

Kim M., Ott C., Bayle J., Airault C. et Brutus P. (1975): Les paramètres de l'urgence dans l'ischémie aigue des membres. Ann Med Reims 12, no spécial, 81—83.

Levy J. B., Gedeon A. (1977): Artériopathies des membres inférieurs au stade de claudication intermittente. Report au 79e Congrès Français de Chirurgie, Paris, 19 septembre 1977, Paris, Masson et Cie.

MacGowan W. A. L., Mooneram R. (1973): A review of 174 patients with arterial embolism. Brit. J. Surg. 60 ,894—898.

Olivier Cl. (1974): Conduite à tenir devant l'ischémie aigue d'un membre inférieur. J. Chir (Paris) 107, 71—78.

Olivier Cl., Rettori R. et Levy J. B. (1977): Traitement chirurgical des ischémies aigues des membres par embolies sur artères présumées saines. J Mal Vasc 2, 67—72.

Olivier Cl., Rettori R. et Levy J. B. (1977): Ischémies aigues des membres inférieurs sur artères pathologiques. A propos de 205 cas survenus chez 197 malades. Chirurgie 103, 544—551.

Cl. O., Department of Surgery and Vascular Pathology, Hôtel-Dieu, Paris, France

INDICATIONS AND RESULTS OF THE DIRECT SURGICAL TREATMENT OF CHRONIC ARTERIAL OCCLUSIVE DISEASES

G. ZANNINI and G. C. BRACALE

2nd Medical School University of Naples, Department of General Surgery, Naples, Italy

The indication for surgery and the choice of techniques are derived from three criteria: clinical, instrumental and arteriographic evaluations.

From the clinical point of view we consider the stage of the illness; generally in the most serious forms there are only minor possibilities of medical treatment and therefore surgery is necessary.

We suggest sympathectomy in a mild form of claudication intermittent if the results of medical therapy is unsatisfactory. In those forms of medium intensity tending to evolution, direct surgery is suggested, associated or not associated with sympathectomy. As far as localization of the obstructions is concerned, the direct operation is indicated in proximal occlusions of large and medium size vessels, while in distal localizations indirect surgery is indicated. When more districts are involved, an associated operation is indicated, but there is a priority problem. If there is a functional factor the patient will be improved more by sympathectomy, if there is an organic factor, by direct operation.

Instrumental examination is important to make a quantitative analysis of the defect, for the prognosis and to evalute the surgical treatment.

Arteriography is always the principal test for the surgeon, as it determines the level of the vascular obstruction, the extent of collateral circulation and the presence of multiple lesions.

There are three sorts of surgery: sympathectomy alone, direct operation (thromboendoarteriectomy with angioplastic, or graft) and associated operations. In our experience, the general criteria in choosing an operation are: selective indications separated by indications of necessity and by associative indications.

Selective indications for direct operations are based on clinical data (age of the patient, working capacity, general condition) and on some angiographic elements (level and length of the obstruction, conditions of collateral circulation). It is, therefore, important to determine the segmentary characteristics of the obstruction. Indications for necessary operation have to be employed when the segmentary characteristics is missing because of an extended distal obstructions. Angioplasty is indicated only in limited lesions. We suggest it rarely, not only because segmentary obstructions are rare but because the angiographic picuture does not often correspond to the anatomo-pathologic situation of the artery wall during the operation. For all segmentary obstructions of the large artery, thromboendarteriectomy is suggested. The TEA is a more limited operation and is shorter and less difficult than by-pass and graft, and it is suggested also according to the general conditions of the patient and the local conditions of vascular circulation below the obstruction.

Contraindications are: alterations of the arterial wall, tortuosities, aneurysms, calcifications, vascular hypoplasia and inflammation of the arterial wall. These operations are rapid and very satisfactory for the surgeon but they may also be dangerous. However, caution must be taken to avoid serious ischemia of the limbs during the operation or soon after.

A good cleavage plan has to be found, wall fragments should not be left, the vessels should not be thinned, the thrombus has to be entirely removed, the endoarterium has to be distally fixed with

Kunlin points; using the ring stripper we must make direct control with another distal arteriotomy and another distal angioplasty. An angiographic check during the operation is indispensable. The figures help to demonstrate the need for using anticoagulants and antiaggregants to prevent the formation of thrombus on the internal wall of the artery.

It is difficult to formulate a rigid scheme to choose between by-pass and graft. We feel that by-pass is better in very long obstruction compared to TEA and grafts as it offers the advantage of saving the collateral circulation. Generally it is more useful for arteries of small diameters or when there is a minor flow for proximal alterations.

The substitution assures a laminar type flow which is similar to physiological flow; at the level of the anastomosis in the by-pass graft it can produce a turbulent movement because of small technical defects. Thus the risk of thrombosis is increased. In addition, we have frequently seen a decreased incidence of dehiscence in grafts rather than in by-passes.

Among complications the first is thrombosis; it is present much more frequently in operations below the inguinal ligament and less frequently in vessels of larger diameter. The vascular surgeon must find the best technical solutions, to try the most suitable materials and to bear in mind the greatest number of details.

The successes of all these operations are immediate. Evaluation of these results indicates that the reduced success is present in operations on arteries of minor caliber and in TEA.

REFERENCES

Zannini G. et alt. (1969): Cinq années d'experience avec l'implantation de prothèses vasculaires. Buenos Aires.

Zannini G. et alt. (1970): L'implantation des greffons tubulaires de dacron sur les artères jambieres.

G. Z., 2nd Medical School University, Naples, Italy

CAUSES OF FAILURE AFTER RECONSTRUCTIVE ARTERIAL OPERATION IN PATIENTS WITH CHRONIC ISCHEMIC DISEASE OF THE LEGS

V. KOŘÍSTEK, J. ČERNÝ and P. ŠIMEK

Second Surgical Clinic, Faculty of Medicine, J. E. Purkyně, Brno, Czechoslovakia

Perhaps in no other branch of surgery is the success of an operation dependent to such a degree correct indication of the operation, selection of an optimum operational method and a perfect operation technique as in reconstructive arterial surgery.

In this paper we shall deal with the most frequent causes of operational failures after surgical treatment of chronic occlusive disease of the lower legs. Our results were obtained in a group of 312 patients with the aforementioned disease, mostly operated on at the 2nd surgical clinic in Brno from 1970 to 1976. In these patients, altogether 469 operations were carried out in different parts of the arterial bed of the lower legs.

The reconstructive arterial operation in aorto-iliac, femoro-popliteo-crural and combined the in aorto-iliac and femoro-popliteal regions were carried out in 61, 172 an 79 patients, respectively.

Numbers of operational methods carried out in these patients are in Table I.

Venous by-pass	210
Endarterectomy	135
Prosthesis aorto-femoralis	92
Profundoplasty	32

Local complications encountered during the early and/or late post-operative period are as follows (Tab. No 2).

Thromboses	early	11.85%
	late	18.58%
Infection		2.24%
Pseudoaneurysma		1.60%
Haemorrhage		1.28%

The most frequent causes of immediate or early thrombosis in the reconstructed arterial region were:

a) incorrect indication of the operation on the basis of incorrect evaluation of the angiographic finding (incorrect evaluation of the run-in and, especially, run-off status) or of the general condition of the patient. This means that the patient should not be operated on.

b) selection of an improper operational method

c) technical mistakes

Wrong evaluation of the angiographic

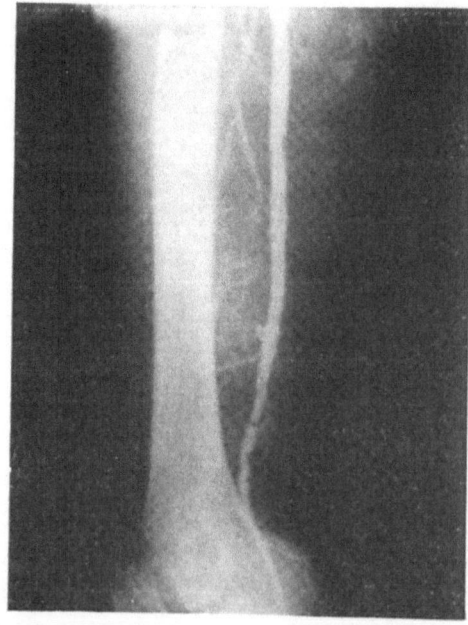

Fig. 1. The step of intima in the distal section of the endarteriectomed popliteal artery.

214

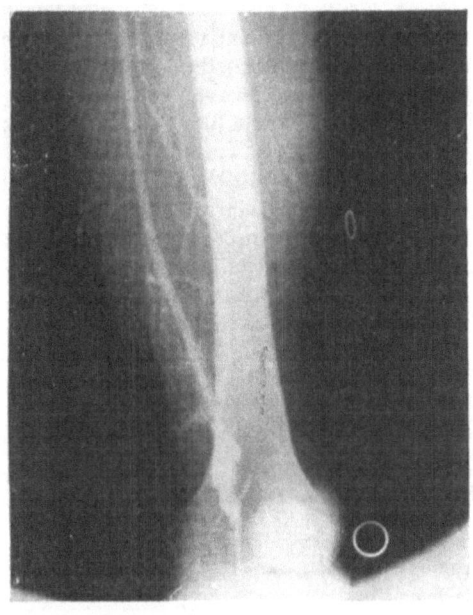

Fig. 2. The perforation of the popliteal artery by the striptor.

cause of immediate or early thrombosis in the reconstructed region. It is very probable that we are not able to avoid this potential hazard in some cases, in spite of the fact that it is taken into account during every operation. An immense number of possible technical mistakes can be made in reconstructive arterial surgery and even the smallest of them may result in total operational failure. The highest number of technical mistakes can be made by the surgeon himself, e.g. a stenosis in an anastomosis, wrong estimation of the length of the venous graft or prosthesis, torsion of the implant, wrong localization of the venous graft in a tunnel between muscles, omission of a residual plate within the arterial lumen after endarterectomy, perforation of arteries, dissection of the arterial wall, insufficient fixation of the distal part of endarterium, etc. (Figrs. 1 – 3).

The peroperative angiography is usually a reliable indicator of technical mistakes finding may occur in patients examined angiographically in only one anteroposterior projection. In such cases, much more serious arteriosclerotic changes are found during the operation, especially in a. profunda femoris and a. poplitea and its branches.

At present, when there is a wider choice of possible operations, the selection of the best operative procedure is not easy. Even then it is necessary to realize that only one of all possible operative methods is the most suitable or optimal. However, the selection of the best procedure must be based on many years of experience obtained on the basis of previous operative failures. The postoperative complications, e.g. uremia, heart attack, bronchopneumonia, embolism of a pulmonary artery etc., can result from incorrect evaluation of the patient's general condition before the operation, imperfect preparation for the operation, selection of an unsuitable method of anesthesia, or worng postoperative care.

A technical mistake is the most frequent

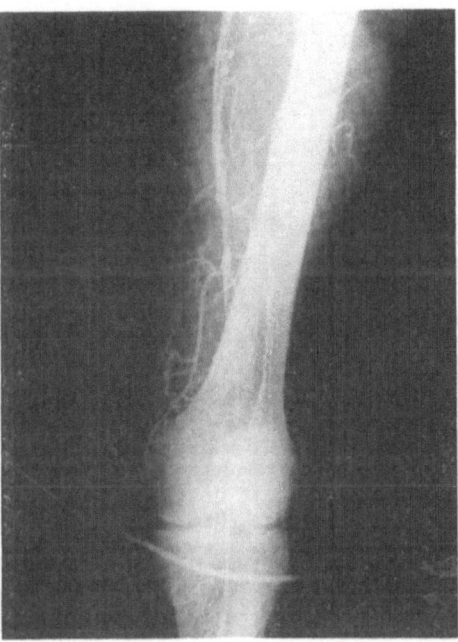

Fig. 3. Released residual plate of endarterium in the femoral artery after semiclosed endarteriectomy.

which would result in an immediate or early obliteration of reconstructed arterial regions. Peroperative angiography is therefore carried out during all operations performed in the femoro-popliteo-crural region.

The highest number of early thromboses was found in patients after endarteriectomy and in those with simultaneous reconstruction of the aortoiliac and femoropopliteal regions. In this group of patients, the highest number of complications occured in those with "blind" orthograde endarteriectomy of the femoral artery. A lower number of complications was observed after semi-closed endarteriectomies and the lowest after open endarteriectomies.

It may be concluded that wrong indication or technical mistakes are the most frequent causes of immediate or early failures of arterial reconstructions. As the highest number of complications was found in patients treated by endarteriectomy, the routine use of this method was abandoned and it is used only in cases of segmentary obliterations and when no venous graft of the necessary quality is available.

K. V., Second Surgical Clinic, Faculty of Medicine J. E. Purkyně, Brno, Czechoslovakia

OUR EXPERIENCE WITH FEMORO-FEMORAL CROSS-OVER

F. BRESADOLA, C. GUERRERA and J. L. OROZCO

*Institute of General Clinical Surgery and Surgical Therapy,
University of Ferrara, Ferrara, Italy*

Alloplastic prosthesis and endoarteriectomy are at this time considered to be the most logical approach to the revascularization of the lower limbs in the therapy of chronic obliteration of the aortic illiac axis.

They involve, however, still a considerable incidence of morbidity and mortality and if the systematic nature of the arteriosclerotic illness and the average age of the patients are considered, it can be understood that they are not always practicable.

The femoro-femoral cross-over proposed by Vetto in 1962 could be an alternative operation in high risk patients with a monolateral involvement of the femoral iliac axis who cannot tolerate an operation of direct revascularisation.

Due to the good results obtained and the minimal surgical risk one tends to extend at this time indications for this procedure also to young patients, who are in a good general condition, not only as an operation in alternative but also as an elective choice.

We carried out a femoro-femoral cross-over on 14 patients: 13 males and 1 female of an average age of 59 years. Seven patients had thrombosis of a branch of a previous aortic bifemoral transplant. The other seven patients were in cardiorespiratory conditions of such character

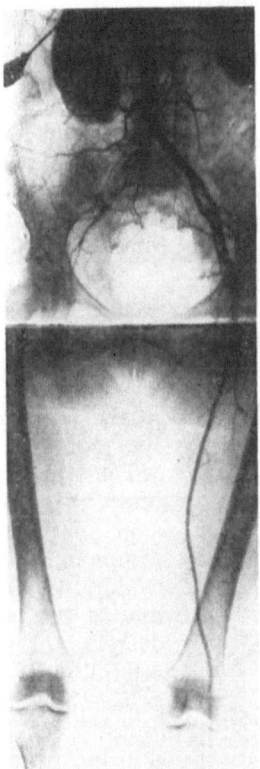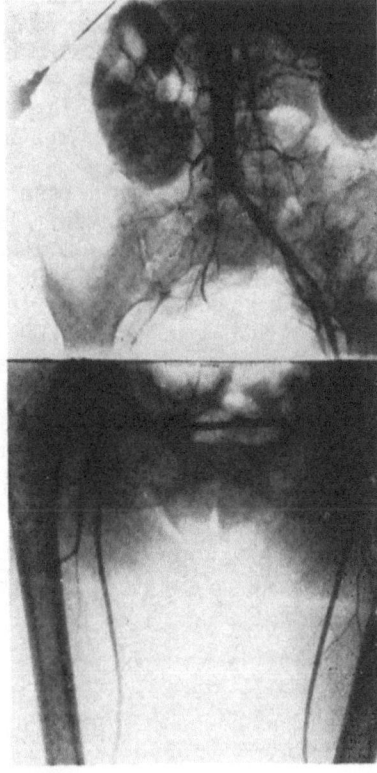

Fig. 1. Schematic drawin of the characteristic velo city patterns recorded afte the walk test, with indica tion of the mode of calcu lation for cfi.

that a direct intervention was not advisable.

In 6 cases there were gangreneous lesions in the toes; 4 cases suffered from resting pains and the other 4 cases had a disabling claudication.

The cross-over was carried out also in the absence of peripheric pulses but with a good pulsation of donor's limbs in the femoral. A reduction of the oscillographic index to 50% in the donor's limb did not contra-indicate the intervention. Aortography had always been carried out and the indication for the intervention was given in the presence of stenosis up to 60% (2 cases).

Principal times of intervention

Exploration of the inguinal region affected and evaluation of the possibility of a downflow. We are not interested in the superficial femoral but we are particularly occupied with the deep one: in 10 cases the prosthesis had been set at its origin after endoarteriectomy, in other cases it was applied on the normal femoral.

Exploration of the donor's femoral axis. Formation of a subcutaneous, overpubic tunnel.

Taking of the saphena magna of the donor's limb whenever it is possible to carry out a by-pass in the vein. We had, however, good results with a synthetic prosthesis, too. The femoral donor artery is opened at the medial anterior wall taking a triangle of the lower part, a latero-terminal anastomosis is carried out between the artery and the vein which is dissected like a mouthpiece of a clarinet with a continous suture with yarn 50 and, an atraumatized needle. On the receiving femoral the anastomasis is carried out in the same way. In order to put the prosthesis in the right position and to control the haemostatis in the tunnel we carry out a suplementary vertical superpubical incision.

Results

There was no case of mortality and no postoperative complication. One patient died after 8 months due to other reasons. Another patient had a thrombosis after 12 months but as he had not shown any ischemic symptom the by-pass perhaps helped to build up a sufficient collateral circle. Another patient had thrombosis of the deep femoral below the prosthesis; a by-pass between superpubical prosthesis and deep femoral was carried out below the obstruction. The other cross-over are patent and function at a distance of 7 to 46 months.

The resting pains have disappeared and the disabling claudications, too.

The amputation stumps and the trophic lesions always healed. Two patients at a distance of time from the intervention (18 − 25 m) showed a phenomenon of "theft" of the donor's limbs with claudication of 250 − 300 m, therefore it was not necessary to re-intervene.

Conclusions

According to us the evaluation of the donor's arterial axis is fundamentally. Parsonnet showed that a sane limb can increase up to 10 times its capacity after the opening of the by-pass. Therefore, it can deliver a good flux of both the limbs. But the circulation is compromised; the revascularization takes place with the possibility of ischaemia in the donors limb. Trimble showed that there is only ischaemia in the presence of a 80% stenosis in the donor or if the peripheric resistences are higher in the donor's axis than in the receiver's.

We had both phenomenons of the theft in the patients having a 50% stenosis in the donor's axis. These phenomenons which appeared at a distance from the intervention depend on the illness progression of the donor's limb. Vetto and Mannock, however, sustained that the evolution of the illness can be slowed down due to the increase of the flux and the decrease of the lateral pression on the arterial walls.

We think that the progression of the illness is inevitable and that it can condition the result of the intervention in the time. The treatment of the aortoiliac lesions must be the most radical possible as in those seats where the evolution is slowlier.

The cross-over, however, represents the best alternative if the clinical and instrumental study of the donor's axis permits to forsee good results for a sufficiently long time.

REFERENCES

Baker R. (1972): Femoro-femoral cross-over grafts Brit. J. surg. 59,9: 701.

Brief D. D. Alpert J. Parsonnet V. (1972): Cross-over femoro-femoral grafts: compromise or preference Arch. surg. 105: 889.

Davis R. C. (1972): Broadened indications for femoro-femoral grafts Surgery 72, 6, 990.

Mannick J. A., Nabseth D. C. (1968): Axillo-femoral by-pass graft. N. Engl. J. Med. 278:461.

Parsonnet V., Alpert J. (1970): Femoro-femoral and axillofemoral grafts compromise or preference; Surgery 67: 26.

Trimble I. R. Stonesifer G. L. (1972): Criterial for femoro-femoral by-pass Ann. Surg. 175: 985.

Vetto R. M. (1966): The femoro-femoral shunt; an appraisal. Amer. J. Surg. 112: 162.

F. B. Institute of General Clinic Surgery and Surgical Therapy University of Ferrara, Ferrara, Italy

REVASCULARIZATION OF THE PROFUNDA FEMORIS ARTERY — LONG TERM RESULTS

E. A. KOKKINOPOULOS, M. SECHAS, N. EXARCHOS
and G. SKALKEAS

*2nd Department of Propedeutic Surgery, Athens
University, Athens, Greece*

Arteriosclerotic occlusive disease of the lower extremities is characteristically segmental in nature, although the locations and patterns of involvement may be multiple and varied. Combined disease of the aortoiliac femoropopliteal arteries is frequently seen in patients with vascular insufficiency of the lower extremities. In recent years the important role of the deep femoral artery in providing blood flow to the leg especially with a completely occluded superficial femoral artery has slowly become appreciated. Bilateral aortofemoral by-pass has proved satisfactory to profunda femoris vessels alone. However, this vessel itself is not immune to the arteriosclerotic process and may be a common cause for late failure in aortoiliac surgery. There appear to be three indications for profundoplasty:

1) To provide an adequate run off vessel for a proximal by pass;
2) As a limited procedure in poor risk patients;
3) As an alternative to distal by pass. During the past five years, surgery on the profunda femoris artery for arteriosclerosis obliterans was performed on thirty-nine (39) limbs, in thirty-two (32) patients at the Second Department of Propedeutic Surgery. A single limb was revascularized in each of 25 patients. In five patients, two limbs were repaired simultaneously. One patient had two limbs revascularized two years apart. In one patient, one limb was reoperated on for a second procedure on the profunda femoris artery three years after the initial repair.

The patients ranged from forty to eighty one years of age, the average being sixty-

two. There were twenty five male and seven female patients. Thirty percent of the patients 10 (ten) had diabetes melitus, 57 percent (eighteen) had coronary artery disease, and 58 percent (nineteen) had hypertension. The presenting symptom was severe claudication in ten limbs (25.8%). Rest

Table I.

During the past five years	
Number of patients	32
Surgery Profunda F. Artery	39 limbs
Single limb revascularized	25 patients
Two limbs revascularized	5 patients
One pt. two limbs two years apart,	
In one pt. one limb revascularized 3 years later	

pain, ischemic ulcers or distal gangrene requiring vascular repair for salvage of the limb was the primary indication in 29 limbs (74,2%). Angioplasty was performed on 39 limbs. The superficial femoral artery was occluded in 27 limbs and was stenotic in five. The popliteal — tibial run off was graded according to the following criteria:

1 — Good: patent popliteal artery with two or three vessels open to the foot;
2 — Fair: popliteal artery open (or) stenotic, and at least one tibial artery open to the foot with the other at least partially filled by collaterals;
3 — Poor: occlusion of the popliteal and all three tibial arteries, with or without collateral refill of thv tibial vessels at the mid calf (or) ankle.

Run off was graded as good in ten limbs, fair in eleven and poor in eighteen. The type of operative procedure performed in association with profundoplasty dependent on the status of inflow to the common femoral level, the degree of arteriosclerotic involvement of the profunda, and the status of run off. Three techniques for profunda femoris artery repair were employed:

1 — In twelve limbs, a tongue of an aortofemoral by pass graft was extended as a patch to relieve stenosis of the proximal profunda.

2 — In seven limbs, in which the obstructing lesions were limited to the profunda orifice and the proximal 1 to 2 cm of the artery, simple endarterectomy with tack down of the distal intima was sufficient to restore flow.

3 — In twenty limbs, patch angioplasty was employed. The saphenous vein was utilized in twelve patients, patch velour graft in five patients and an endarterectomized segment of the occluded superficial femoral artery was employed in three patients.

Claudication was the primary indication for surgery in eight (8) limbs. In seven (7) limbs were markedly improved and one was moderately improved. Limb salvage was the presenting problem in thirty-one

Table II.

		Results:	
For claudication —	8 limbs	7 limbs improved	
		1 limb moderate	
Limb salvage	— 31 limbs —	In 26 limbs rest pain relieved (79,6%)	
		Ischemic necrosis healed — (69 %)	
		In 5 limbs amputation — (16%)	

(31) limbs. In twenty-one (21) patients (79.6%), the rest pain was relieved and ischemic necrosis and minor amputations healed, permitting salvage of twenty-six limbs, (69%). One patient required a subsequent proximal inflow procedure, after profundoplasty alone failed to relieve his problem completely. There was no improvement in five (5) limbs in the salvage category (16%) and all 5 limbs required amputation. Two repairs became thrombosed in the immediate postoperative period. One repair remained patent with relief of rest pain initially; however, it became occluded after three months because of decreased cardiac output associated with severe heart failure.

The overall amputation rate was (14.5%) six limbs were directly related to popliteal tibial run off. In all of these limbs the run off was classified as poor. Two patients (6%) died in the immediate postoperative period. All were high risk patients, operated on for limb salvage and in each instance repair of the profunda artery was carried out in association with aortofemoral by pass. The causes of death were

Table III.

1. Profundoplasty alone	in 23 limbs
2. Profundoplasty as run off vessel for a proximal by pass	in 10 limbs
3. Profundoplasty as an alternative to distal by pass	in 6 limbs

renal failure in association with pulmonary complications, heart failure and infected graft in one. Profundoplasty alone was performed in 23 limbs using a vein patch graft or velour graft. This is an ideal procedure for poor risk patients. Profundoplasty was used in 10 limbs as the run off vessel for a proximal by pass. The grafts remained open in 100% of those with claudication and in 70% of those operated on for limb salvage. Profundoplasty was used in six limbs, which had been operated on unsuccessfully for a distal by pass. (Femoral-popliteal bypass).

Conclusion

Restoration of circulation in an obstructed profunda femoris artery is an effective technique for relieving claudication and for salvaging the end stage ischemic limb when the superficial femoral segment is occluded. When the surgeon has the option of revascularization by either femoral-profunda repair or femoro-popliteal by pass, femoral-profunda repair may be the procedure of choice, since it is less traumatic, is easier to perform, and will relieve ischemia effectively.

REFERENCES

Martin P., Franley J. E. et al., (1972): On the surgery of atherosclerosis of the profunda femoris artery — Surg. 71: 182.
Morris G. C., Edwards W., Colley D. A.,

Crawford E. S., De Bakey M. D., (1961): Surgical importance of the profunda femoris artery — Surg. 82: 32.

K. E., Dimocharous 9, Athens T 601 Greece

FEMORO-TIBIAL BYPASS: AN 8-YEAR EXPERIENCE

A. CAVALLARO, V. SCIACCA, A. ALESSANDRINI and S. STIPA

University of Rome, Rome, Italy

In 1969 we performed our first femoro-tibial reconstruction: it was a femoral-to-peroneal by-pass which made if possible to save a very ischemic limb: the by-pass is still patent, and the patient, who was also submitted to transmetatarsal amputation of a gangrenous first toe, has been fully asymptomatic through the entire follow-up. Since then 74 patients were considered for femoro-tibial reconstruction; 13 of them were finally judged unsuitable for a surgical reconstructive procedure; in 10, exploration of leg arteries was the only surgical procedure as no artery suitable to be the termination of a by-pass was found; a femoro-tibial reconstruction was performed in 51 patients.

They were aged from 28 to 85 years (mean 56); 45 were males.

Associated diseases were present in most patients, as follows:
diabetes 35%
heart disease 33%
lung disease 23%
kidney disease 15%
cerebrovascular insufficiency 10%
other 10%

62 reconstructive procedures were performed on 51 limbs (2 limbs were operated on three times and 7 limbs twice).

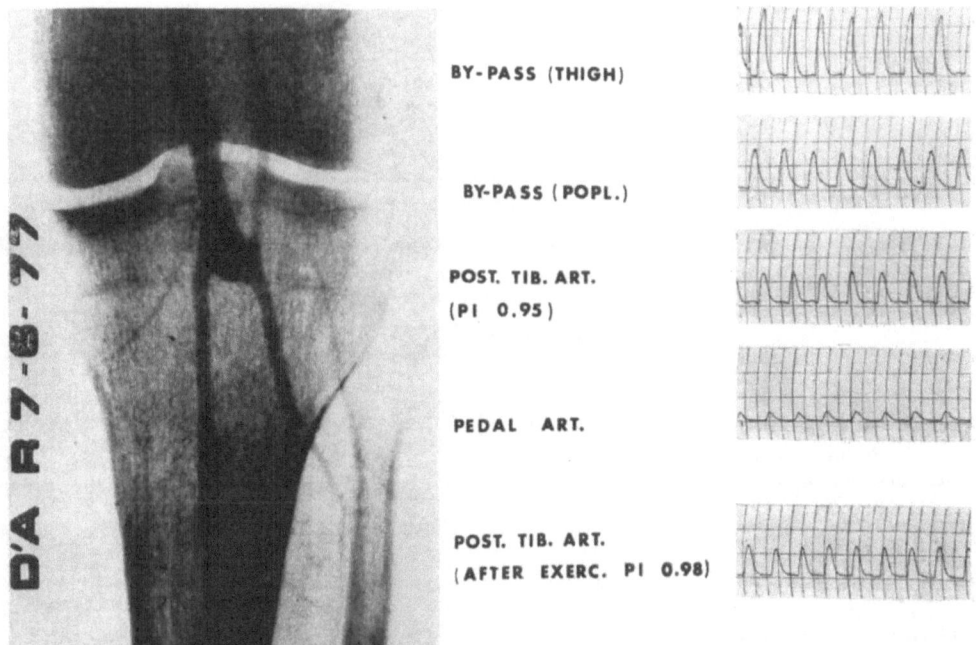

BY-PASS (THIGH)

BY-PASS (POPL.)

POST. TIB. ART.
(PI 0.95)

PEDAL ART.

POST. TIB. ART.
(AFTER EXERC. PI 0.98)

Fig. 1. Angiographic and Doppler control, 30 months after by-pass operation from the common femoral to the popliteal artery with a side branch to the low posterior tibial (an autologous vein was used for the reconstruction).

223

The underlying disease was in general of degenerative type (atherosclerosis), but in in 5 patient the final diagnosis of segmental arteritis was established: they were under forty years of age, and three of them had a positive serological assay against Q 18 Rickettsia.

The chief clinical indication for surgery was a threatened limb (rest pain 14, gangrene 32): in only 5 patients it was a heavy and truly invalidating claudication

A careful Doppler investigation was the main basis of the preoperative evaluation: very frequently we could not rely on angiographic visualization of peripheral leg arteries (the post-ischemic hyperaemia angiographic technique could be performed seldom).

Consequently, a definite surgical program was often determined only at the surgical desk, when a "suitable" segment of the tibial or peroneal artery was found and its out flow directly assayed by angiography.

The termination of the by-pass was as follows:
tibioperoneal trunk 5
peroneal 5
posterior tibial (upper third) 4
posterior tibial (middle third) 6
posterior tibial (lower third) 21
anterior tibial (popliteal space, above the interosseous membrane) 9
anterior tibial (anterior leg compartment) 9

A reversed autologous vein (saphenous, basilic, cephalic or segments of them sutured end-to-end to form a convenient graft) was used almost in every instance; a PTFE prosthesis was used in two limbs.

In 5 patients both the popliteal artery and one tibial vessel were revascularized using the jump-by-pass technique (Fig. 1); the sequential by-pass technique was used in another patient.

Two patients died in the p. o. period: both were diabetic and presented several significant associated diseases.

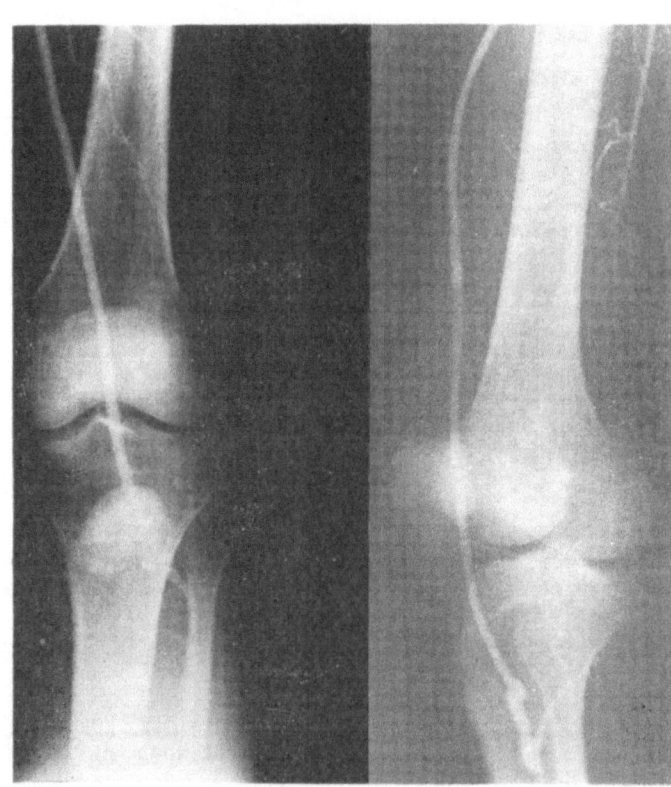

Fig. 2. Pseudoaneurysm at the anastomotic site between a reversed autologous vein and the anterior tibial artery at its origin. After excision of the pseudo-aneurysm, the by-pass was transposed subcutaneously, lengthened by means of an additional piece of vein and the anastomosis was placed on the anterior tibial artery in the upper third of the anterior leg compartment.

At the end of the follow-up, 33 reconstructions were patent and a high percentage of limb salvage was achieved: A minor (transmetatarsal or digital) amputation was successfully added to the reconstruction in 12 patients.

Follow-up 6 – 102 months (mean 36)
patients 49
by-pass patent 33
limb saved 41
no symptoms 20/41
claudication 20/41
restpain –
gangrene 1/41

Graft thrombosis occurred within three months after the operation; only two grafts failed after this time interval.

When early thrombosis occurred, reoperation (performed 9 times on 7 limbs) was never successful, and we argue that in those patients there was a real misjudgement as for the technical feasibility of the femoro-tibial reconstruction.

Apart from thrombosis, the only other significant complication was an anastomotic pseudoaneurysm, which was easily corrected (Fig. 2).

In general, the results are very satisfactory.

We have not observed, after the failure of a femoro-tibial graft, any worsening of leg or foot circulation in comparison with the preoperative status: we feel that, in the next future, we will accept a broadened indication for femoro-tibial reconstruction.

C. A., I Cat. di Semeiotica Chirurg. Policlinico Umberto I, Viale del Policlin, 00161 Roma, Italy

RECONSTRUCTION OF THE POPLITEAL AND CRURAL ARTERIES BASED ON OUR OWN MATERIAL

S. BAK and J. KULIKOWSKI

Department of Vascular Surgery, Biernacki Hospital — Krakow, Poland

Operative treatment of foot and crural advanced ischemia caused by occlusion of the arteries is often dificult, and many questions dealing with this problem are still open for discussion. The small caliber or the crural arteries, the character

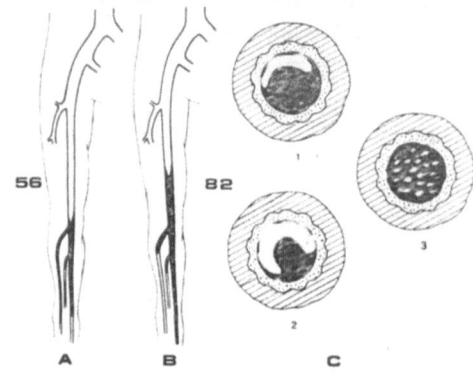

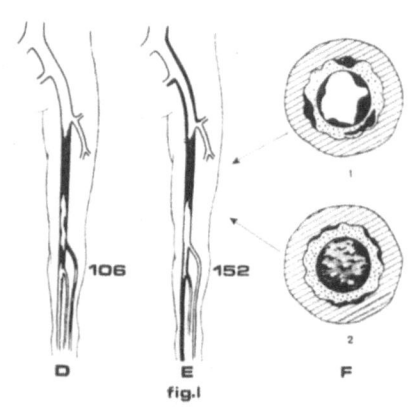

fig.I

Fig. 1. a) occlusion of the bifurcation of the popliteal artery and of the crural arteries. b) occlusion of the popliteal artery and the crural arteries. c) types of occlusion, cutaway view. Arteriosclerotic changes: d) femoral and crural segment e) iliac, femoral and crural segment f) incomplete and complete occlusions of the artery, cutaway view.

and extent of occlusion in the peripheral arteries, all tend to increase the technical difficulties.

During the period 1967–1977, reconstructive operations were performed on 396 patients with changes in these arteries.divided into 3 age groups. Group I included 138 patients up to 40 years of age. These patients had mostly thrombangiopathy, that is, thrombotic changes prevailing in one or both of the crural arteries, and in the bifurcation of the popliteal artery as in Fig. 1a or in the whole popliteal artery as in Fig. 1b. As a result of recanalization we find, as shown on the diagram of the artery, a partial patency of the lumen of the artery or complete occlusion with focal cell infiltration. In the latter case desobliteration is often impossible to achieve. The intima adheres to the elastic membrane and cannot be separated. If desobliteration can be achieved it consists in removal of the organized thrombus and is therefore incomplete (Fig. 1c).

The second group included 106 patients aged 41–50. The changes in the crural arteries were similar to group I, in the femoral artery they had change of arteriosclerotic character (Fig. 1d).

The third group consisted of 152 patients over 50. The changes in this group were an extensive arteriosclerosis in the crural and femoral arteries (Fig. 1d), and sometimes in the iliac segment (Fig. 1e). Desobliteration in these patients consisted in performing a trombendarterectomy (Fig. 1).

The patients came to the department with changes in the lower limb that were in various stages of advancement. 253 patients were admitted with peripheral

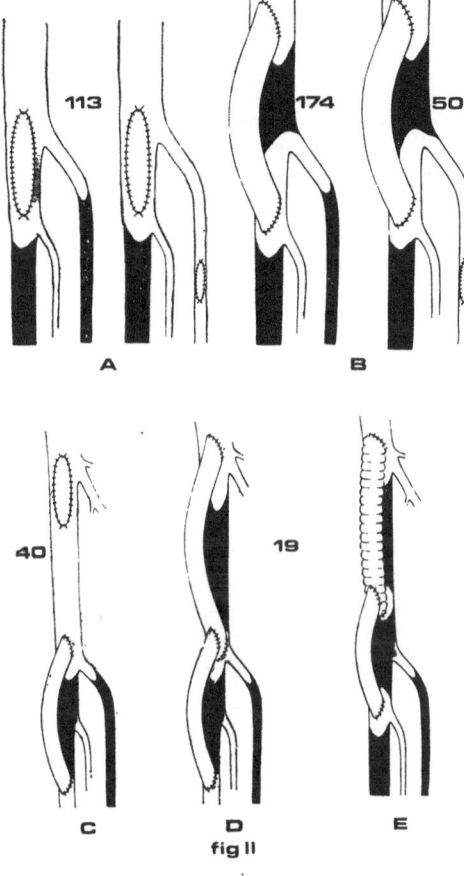

necrosis and rest pain. In a majority of cases primary amputation was indicated. In 57 patients, ischemic ulcerations or purulent processes were found, 86 patients had intermittent claudication on short distances (under 100 m).

The choice of reconstruction was dictated by the type and extensiveness of obliteration in the arteries, peripheral necrosis or ulceration and the general condition of the patient. Complete revascularisation of the limb was impossible to achieve in many patients. The reconstruction was stopped upon achieving circulation of the blood in half the length of the crural arteries or in the total length of one of the tibial arteries (anterior or posterior). In many patients this was achieved by combining various methods of reconstruction. Moreover, in many patients, mainly of the third group, the operation was performed in 2 stages. If reconstruction of the femoral or the iliac segment did not achieve the expected improvement, the treatment was performed in the next few days in the crural or popliteal region.

Types of reconstruction are shown in Fig. 2. In Figs 2a, b the methods were used mostly on patients in group I, in Figs 2c, d, e — mostly on patients in group III. In 182 patients with incomplete reconstruction of the crural arteries, lumbar sympathectomy was additionally performed.

Fig. 2. a, b) methods of reconstruction in thrombangiopathy c, d, e) methods of reconstruction in arteriosclerotic changes.

Table I. Therapy results

		Good	Improvement	lowering of amputation level	Amputation	Death	Total
Necrotic	Gr. I	49	—	23	17	—	89
lesions or	Gr. II	38	3	10	12	1	64
rest pain	Gr. III	59	9	14	12	6	100
Ischemic							
ulceration	Gr. I	21	3	3	4	—	31
or purulent	Gr. II	7	—	3	2	—	12
processes	Gr. III	8	2	1	2	1	14
Intermittent	Gr. I	10	3	3	2	—	18
claudication	Gr. III	22	6	3	6	1	38
Total		234 (59.1%)	31 (7.9%)	63 (15.9%)	59 (14.8%)	9 (2.3%)	396

Table I shows the results obtained. Good results were obtained in 234 cases (59.1%), improvement or lowering of the level of amputation in 94 cases (23.8%), amputation in 59 cases (14.8%), death occurred in 9 cases (2.3%).

It appears that in many patients in whom complete reconstruction was impossible to achieve, the limb was still saved for various lengths of time. The results shown here confirm the view that in persons with indications or diagnosis for primary amputation due to advanced ischemia reconstructive operations should be performed in an attempt to save the lower limb.

S. B., ul. Slawkowska 24a/2, Kraków, Poland.

LONG TERM RESULTS OF SURGICAL TREATMENT IN BUERGER'S DISEASE

Y. MISHIMA and K. ISHIKAWA

Department of Surgery, University of Tokyo, Tokyo, Japan

Although there are some discrepancies concerning the real existence of Buerger's disease, we could confirm that the process might be distinguished from arteriosclerosis obliterans or simple thrombosis in a large number of patients with chronic arterial occlusion of the extremities. (2) In Buerger's disease the small arteries in the distal portion of the extremities are involved much more frequently, whereas atherosclerotic occlusion developed preferably in such major channels as the iliac, femoral and popliteal arteries.

Surgical therapy for arterial diseases of the extremities consists of an indirect procedure for the release of vasospasm and direct arterial surgery for the reesblishment of arterial flow. In Buerger's disease, arterial reconstructive surgery rarely seems to be of value. The long-term results of surgical treatment were poor, especially for intermittent claudication. (4) Though the distal tibial bypass is supposed to be effective in cases with atherosclerotic occlusion, it is not feasible for patients with Buerger's disease because the lessions involved relatively small arteries and are sometimes multiple. For these circumstances, special indirect arterial reconstructive techniques have been introduced by two institutions in Japan. These procedures were mainly applied in patients who were not regarded as suitable candidates for conventional arterial reconstruction.

Drs. Inokuchi and Kusaba, University of Kyushu, introduced a new operative procedure termed popliteal endarterectomy with arteriovenous shunt. (1) The theoretical basis of this procedure is the fact that the genicular network of the artery is able to maintain its patency and collateral

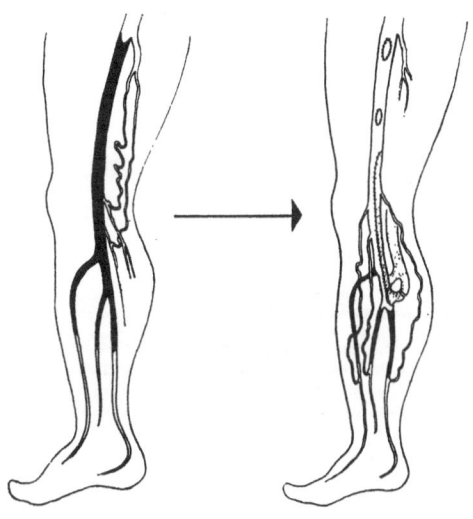

Fig. 1.

vessels originating from it improve the blood flow to the distal ischemic limb if an arteriovenous shunt between the popliteal artery and vein is created after femoropopliteal endarterectomy. (Fig. 1).

On the other hand, Drs. Kasai and Nishimura, University of Hokkaido, developed a new technique of omental transplantation. (5) As shown in Fig. 2, the omentum resected as a free graft by dividing the righ gastroepiploic artery and vein at their origin is transplanted subfascially in the ischemic lower extremity, anastomosing the graft vessels to the femoral vessels using a vascular stapling device. The effective mechanism of this procedure would be biological revascularization through the implanted arteriolar network of the omentum.

Table I shows the long-term results or surgical treatment in 606 cases collected

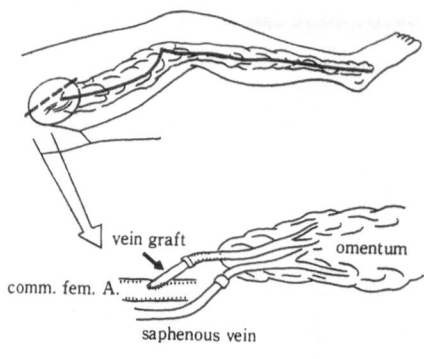

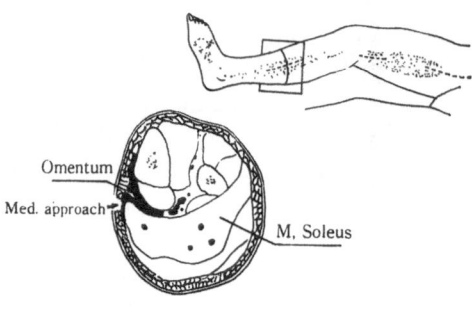

Omental Transplantation

Fig. 2.

by the Ministry of Health and Welfare Japan Buerger's Disease Research Committee for two years from 1973 to 1975, including those of these two techniques. (3)

Table 1. Long term results of surgical treatment

	No. of Limbs	Improvement Discharge	Late
Thromboendarter-			
ectomy	29	62%	21%
Bypass	40	73%	53%
Dotter's Dilatation	5	100%	—
Thrombectomy	5	80%	20%
Resection &			
Grafting	4	100%	100%
Patch angioplasty	4	25%	0%
A—V shunt	59	76%	58%
Omental			
Transplantation	10	70%	—
Sympathectomy	221	83%	52%

Total 606 Cases, Research Committee

Direct arterial reconstrultion was indicated in 109 cases. Of 29 endarterectomized vessels only 3 remained patent after 3 years, whereas the patency of 40 bypass grafts has been maintained in 17 cases after 3 years. Among other procedures, Dotter's dilatation, thrombectomy and resection with grafting showed excellent results on discharge, but the late results were not satisfactory except resection with grafting, performed in cases with occlusions well confined to the femoropopliteal region.

Clinical effects of the arteriovenous shunt procedure were as follows: Improvement was observed in 76% on discharge and in 58% at the time of follow-up. No instance was found with overloading signs after shunt operation, such as enlargement of the heart size, tachycardia or abnormal ECG findings.

As to the result of the omental transplantation, claudication improved in 60% of case, rest pain subsided remarkably in 90% and the ischemic ulceration healed up completely in 7 cases within 3 months after operation.

Follow-up of 221 lumbar sympathectomies showed immediate improvement in 83% and no change in 10% on discharge, although the operation was accompanied by poor results in muscular circulation. There was no operative death. Sympathectomy may not result in an increase of deep or muscular circulation, but is of value for patients with extremely reduced cutaneous circulation by vasoconstriction, because the angiospasm must play a significant role in the development of ischemic changes in Buerger's disease. To expect the improvement of the late results of surgical treatment, it should be emphasized that the long-term postoperative care of the patients including complete abstinence from smoking is mandatory even after healing of the ischemic ulcer took place.

During this period, 17 limbs had to be amputated above the ankle because of massive necrosis, excluding 1 limb amputated the forearm. Sympathectomy was

230

usually helpful to promote wound healing of the stump.

It can be concluded that the treatment for chronic arterial occlusion of the extremities should be planned according to the patient's complaint and to the site and extent of occlusive lesions rather than accordant to the pathological basis of the disease and it is also very important to take care of patients for a long period, even after the complete disappearance of the symptoms.

REFERENCES

1. *Inokuchi, K., & Kusaba, A. (1972):* A—V shunt procedure for the cases with extensive arterial occlusion of the lower extremity. (in Japanese) Geka-Chiryo, 26, 121—129.
2. *Ishikawa, K., Kawase, S., & Mishima, Y. (1962):* Occlusive arterial disease in extremities, with special reference to Buerger's disease. Angiology, 13, 399—411.
3. *Ishikawa, K. (1975):* Annual report of the Ministry of Helath and Welfare Japan Buerger's Disease Research Committee.
4. *Mishima, Y., & Ishikawa, K. (1977):* Buerger's disease; Current status in Japan. J. Malad. Vasc. 2, 121—127.
5. *Nishimura, A., & Kasai, Y. (1974):* Revascularization of the leg with freed omental transplantation. (in Japanese) Shujutsu, 28, 447—453.

Y. M., University of Tokyo, Faculty of Medicine, 7—3 Hongo, Bunkyo-ku, Tokyo Japan

THE TREATMENT OF CHRONIC ARTERIAL OCCLUSION OF THE UPPER- AND LOWER-LEG BLOODFLOW WITH A FEMORO-POPLITEAL AND FEMORO-CRURAL BYPASS. — INDICATIONS, SHORT- AND LONGTERM RESULTS

S. HORSCH, TH. LANDES, A. ZEHLE, H. J. EISENHARDT and H. PICHLMAIER

University Hospital, Surgical Division, Cologne, F.R.G.

In 1949 *Kunlin* introduced the autologous vein bypass as method for the reconstruction of the occluded vessels of the upper leg. Since then, the autologous vein bypass has become a routine operation at most centers for vascular reconstruction, and the follow-up examinations have the best longterm results with this method (*Gall, F.,* 1968, 1969). Even in cases of occluded distal portions of the poplitea, where there is no distal connection for the conventional femoro-popliteal bypass, the femoro-crural bypass has been used increasingly in recent years. Due to its high rate of early complications, this method is still highly problematic and its indication should only be made as an alternative to amputation.

In about 20—25% of the patients, a good autologous saphenous vein cannot be found for the reconstruction of the occluded vessel. In this case, in stages III and IV according to *Fontaine* other materials have to be used for reconstructive surgery (*Schlosser, V.,* 1977).

If the conservative treatment such as kinesitherapy, vasodilators and strict abstaining from nicotine does not bring relief from discomfort and if the patient is obviously hampered in his professional and private activities by a reduced painfree walking distance, we consider the vascular reconstruction to be indicated. Stages III and IV present definite indications for the operation.

Table I. Early results of femoro-popliteal bypass (1. 1. 1968 — 31. 3. 1978)

	Autol. Vein	Impra	Gore-Tex	Solco-graft	Total
n	96	7	2	7	112
good	78	4	2	3	87
improved	8	1	0	2	11
worsened	3	2	0	1	6
Amputation	5	0	0	1	6
died	2	0	0	0	2

Long-term results of femoro-popliteal bypass
Average observation period: 3.8 years

Results	Autol. Vein	Impra 12 Months	Gore-tex 12 Months	Solco-graft	Total
	88	7	2	7	104
good	57	2	2	2	64
improved	19	1	—	1	21
worsened	4	2	—	3	9
died	8	1	—	1	10
Preop. Stage	n				
II	51				
III	36				
IV	25				

Case reports

Femoro-popliteal bypass: (Tab. I)

112 femoro-popliteal (supraglenoid) bypasses with autologous veins were placed in 102 patients.

The average age of the 11 female and 91 male patients was 61 years.

51 interventions were made for stage II b, 36 for stage III and 25 for stage IV.

Results

Good early results were obtained with 87 patients. 2 patients died of cardiac infarction and pulmonary embolism during their stay at the hospital. Early thrombosis of the graft was observed in 11 patients; in 5 cases the reoperation was successful, 6 patients had to be amputated.

After an average observation period of 3.8 years, 64 patients showed good long-term results; the bypass was patent and the walking distance unimpeded. 21 patients felt better compared to the preoperative condition, 9 patients had increased discomfort. 3 patients were reoperated succcesstully, 10 patients had died in the meantime of unknown causes.

Femoro-crural bypass: (Tab. II)

During the same period, 70 patients with combined upper- and lower-leg arterial occlusion were treated.

The average age of the 63 men and 7 women was 61 years.

24 patients were in stage III, 46 patients in stage IV.

Each case showed an extended femoro-popliteal (distal) occlusion, with at least one lower-leg artery occluded. In 13 patients the lumbar sympathectomy had not reduced necrosis and rest pain, 7 patients had been amputated on the other leg for the same disease.

Material and method

In 37 cases the autologous saphenous vein was used for the bypass, one Sparks mandril, 4 Dacron-velours grafts, 7 bovine heterologous protheses (Solcograft), 4 Impra grafts, 2 Gore-Tex grafts, 9 combined bypasses with autologous vein and Gore-Tex. The vein was used for bypassing the knee-joint.

Alloplastic material was used when no suitable autologous vein was available.

Results

44 patients showed improved conditions.

13 cases of early thrombosis led to amputation. In 5 patients with a previous lumbar sympathectomy the early thrombosis of the graft did not jeopardize the limb.

1 patient died of renal failure.

48 of the non-amputated patients are alive after an average of 3.1 years (Tab. III).

In the meantime, 2 patients died of carcinoma with a fully functional transplant. 23 patients have a usable limb which is free of pain, 4 patients had died of

Table II. Early Results of femoro-crural bypass (1. 1. 1968—31. 3. 1978)

Preop. Stage	n
III	24
IV	46

Material	Autol. Vein	Spark's	Impra	Core-Tex	Solco-graft	Dacron-Velours	Vein + Impra	Vein + Gore-Tex
Total: 70	37	1	4	2	7	4	6	9
good	25	0	2	1	3	2	4	7
worsened	3	0	1	1	3	2	1	1
Amputation	8	1	1	0	1	0	1	1
died	1 (renal failure)	0	0	0	0	0	0	0

Table III. Long-Term Results of femoro-crural Bypass (1. 1. 1968—31. 3. 1978)

Average observation period: 3.1 years

Material	Autol. Vein	Impra <8 Months	Gore-Tex <7 Months	Solco-graft	Dacron Velours	Vein + 2—8 Months Impra	Vein + 2—6 Months Gore-Tex
Total 54	28	3	2	6	2	5	8
good (graft patent)	13	1	1	1	0	2	5
graft thrombosed, limb not endangered	7	1	1	2	2	2	3
Amputation	3	1	0	2	0	1	0
died	5	0	0	1	0	0	0

unknown causes. 18 grafts have thrombosed, but due to meanwhile developed collateral systems their limb is not imperiled. 7 patients had to be amputated at the thigh.

In cases of combined upper- and lower-leg occlusion, the reconstruction is to be considered only as alternative to the amputation.

The autologous large saphenous vein has undisputed priority among graft materials. In cases of unavailability of this autologous vein, other prosthetic material must be used. The combined bypass appears to show advantages.

Indication and execution of this technically demanding operation should be left to the experienced vascular surgeon.

REFERENCES

1. Gall, F. 1968: Venentransplantation zur Rekonstruktion beim Femoralisverschluß. — Erfahrungen bei 200 Eingriffen. Thoraxchir. 16, 7,.
2. Gall, 1969F.: Die chirurgische Behandlung der chronischen arteriellen Durchblutungsstörung im Aortoiliacalen und femoro-poplitealen Bereich. Bruns Beitr. Klin. Chir. 217, 18: 691.
3. Kunlin, J., C. Bitry-Boély, M. Volnie, Ch.Beaudry 1951: Le traitement de l'ischémie artéritique par la greffe veineuse longue. Rev. Chir. 89, 206.
4. Schlosser, V., F. Herdter, G. Spillner, A. Ahmadi 1977: Neue Transplantat-Materialien in der rekonstruktiven Arterien-Chirurgie. Fortschr. Med. 95, 15: 1012.

S. H., Clinic of Surgery, Josef-Stelzmann Str. 9, 5. Cologne 41, F.R.G.

MANAGEMENT OF THORACIC OUTLET COMPRESSION SYNDROME

G. TUSCANO, F. ROMANI, G. POMPEI and E. RICCHI

Dept. of Surgery, Modena, Italy

The thoracic outlet syndrome is a group of symptoms in the neck, shoulder, arm or hand due to compression of the subclavian vessels and brachial plexus.

Before reaching the root of the arm, such vascular and nervous structures must cross a series of more or less narrow rigid spaces, thus even a minimal or only dynamic anatomic variation is sufficient for the compression or angulation of one or all structures. In this report our diagnostical experience refers to T.O.S. therapy.

During the last 5 years we have observed and studied 88 patients with T.O.C.S. 47 were hospitalized for surgical therapy, 10 underwent bilateral treatment. In all 57 operations were performed. 55 patients (62.5%) were female, 33 (37.5%) male, their age ranging from 18 to 70 years (average age 38). Prevailing symptoms were neurological in 47 patients, arterial in 25 and venous in 16. In about 50% of cases symptoms were due to the assuming of specific positions of the arm. In 5 cases clinical onset coincided with trauma of the shoulder. 24 patients were engaged in vigorous activities requiring efforts and strain of the upper extremities. 2 patients had already undergone surgery elsewhere (excision of scalenous and cervical ganglionectomy). Postural tests (Adson, standing at attention, abduction and hyperabduction) were positive in about 60% of cases. In 19 patients with unilateral subjective symptoms clinical and instrumental investigations demonstrated that the condition was bilateral. In one patient, thrombosis with total obstruction of the subclavian artery caused by compression of the cervical rib was observed. Clinical onset in one case presented an acute ischaemic condition resulting from embolus of the brachial artery due to post-stenotic aneurysm of the subclavian artery. In 5 cases clinical symptoms began with acute venous thrombosis.

Besides clinical investigation, preoperative diagnostical evaluation was based on x-ray exposure of the cervical vertebral column and of the chest, photopletlysmography and plethysmography in basic or dynamic conditions and ultrasound.

Impedence reography was only employed in cases with venous occlusion. Thermography was used in 14 patients but useful data was not obtained due to difficulties in the estimation of bilateral temperature variations accompanied by changes in position.

A dynamic selective arteriography was performed 19 times, this always proved positive except in 2 cases.

A phlebographic examination was carried out 16 times due to frequent venous symptoms found in our patients, this differing from other series reported. This examination proved positive in 11 cases.

During the past 3 years we also carried out studies of neuro-muscular speed conduction. This investigation was useful as indication for surgery in cases where nervous symptoms prevailed. Out of 88 patients observed and studied, 55 (62.5%) were selected for surgery, 8 however refused surgical therapy. In 33 cases the clinical symptoms, confirmed by instrumental investigations, were mild and physical therapy was considered sufficient We reserved surgical treatment to patient presenting severe nervous symptoms not responsive to treatment, arterial insuficiency with or without organic changes, intermittent or total venous occlusion.

57 operations were performed since in 10 cases, as we have already stated, surgery was bilateral.

We performed the following interventions: (Table I).

Table I. 57 operations in 47 patients with T.O.C.S.

First rib resection	36
+ Thoracic ganglionectomy	4
+ Venous thrombectomy	2
+ Minor pectoral muscle resection	5
Cervical rib resection	15
+ Scalenotomy	15
+ Brachial embolectomy and subclavian aneurysm resection	1
+ Venous graft	1
Venous axis intervention (without osseus resection)	6
+ Venous thrombectomy	1

There were no postoperative deaths and even postoperative morbidity was quite low. (Tab. II).

Table II. Complications in 57 interventions for T.O.C.S.

Lymphorrea	1
Wound infection	3
Hemothorax	1
Transitory brachial plexus lesion	1
Brachial nerve numbness	3

All patients were inspected after surgery, the period varying from two months to five years. Results obtained and classified according to clinical and instrumental examinations were the following: excellent, absence of symptoms; good, considerable improvement with persistence of mild symptoms; fair, good decompression but little improvement of symptoms; negative, no improvement and inadequate decompression. (Tab. III).

Table III. Results of 57 interventions for T.O.C.S.

	First rib resection	Cervical rib resection	Venous axis intervention
EXCELLENT	27 (75.0%)	12 (80.0%)	5 (83.3%)
GOOD	5 (14.0%)	2 (13.3%)	= =
FAIR	3 (8.3%)	= =	= =
FAILURE	1 (2.7%)	1 (6.7%)	= =

Istituto di Patologia Chirurgica e Propedeutica Clinica della Universita' Degli Studi di Modena, Italy

INDICATIONS OF RECONSTRUCTIVE SURGERY IN ANGINA ABDOMINALIS

F. PIRK, L. HEJHAL, I. SKÁLA, J. PIRK, M. HACO,
A. BELÁN and M. KRAJÍČEK

Metabolism and Nutrition Research Centre of the Institute for Clinical and Experimental Medicine, Prague, Czechoslovakia

The first successful aortomesenteric by-pass done in 1961 reawakened interest in the syndrome of abdominal angina. Between 1963 and 1971 we performed eight of these operations. It became evident that, if correctly indicated, the by-pass can lead to complete disappearance of complaints. Therefore we recently focused attention on more detailed indication for operation.

Stenoses and occlusions of the splanchnic arteries are relatively common — in our patients the ratio of stenoses of the renal artery to involvement of the splanchnic region is 4 : 1. However, the clinical syndrome of abdominal angina is not common, since collateral circulation in this area develops fairly readily. During the last year we examined eight patients with evidence of involvement of the splanchnic arteries using abdominal aorto-graphy. Abdominal angina was evident in only two: none had signs of malabsorption. This corroborates previous observations that only a small portion of stenoses and occlusions of the splanchnic arteries is clinically or functionally significant. So far, the view persists that assessed stenoses are functionally significant only when collaterals are also observed on angiography. One of our patients represents a borderline situation where the typical symptoms of abdominal angina were misinterpreted solely because the proved stenoses had no collaterals.

A 63-year-old patient was never seriously ill. In the last 5 months he complained of pain in the umbilical area, starting 10−15 minutes after meals. He observed that the pain subsided if he did not eat. Therefore he reduced his food intake to a minimum and lost 15 kg. Aortography revealed stenoses of the coeliac and superior mesenteric arteries without collateral circulation. Exploratory laparatomy showed only atheromatous changes in the abdominal aorta. After operation his complaints gradually subsided until they disappeared completely: the patient started to eat and his caloric intake amounted to 3.500−4.500 calories/ /day. An overall medical examination revealed normal findings. We attributed his dramatic improvement to the development of collateral circulation. Our hypothesis was confirmed by check-up angio-graphy.

This case merits attention. It demonstrates that the view naintaining that the absence of collaterals implies functional irrelevance of the assessed stenoses is incorrect. Logically, the development of functionally adequate collaterals requires a certain period of time. If the formation of collaterals lags behind the ischaemic process, a clinical picture of severe abdominal angina may develop which, however, need not necessarily be permanent. This was the case with our patient: hitherto this has not been differentiated from classical abdominal angina.

Another point we should consider is when to indicate reconstruction and how long we can wait for spontaneous development of an adequate collateral circulation.

The second patient with abdominal angina was a 50-year-old man with no history of serious disease. At the age of 49 he gradually developed intensifying postprandial pain in the epigastrium. Despite repeated hospitalization the cause of the complaint was not identified. He lost 16 kg within a year as a result of reduced food intake. Aortographic examination confirmed occlusion of the superior mesenteric artery and stenosis of the coeliac artery.

An aortomesenteric by-pass was performed. Immediately after the operation the complaints disappeared. His caloric intake exceeded 3.000 cal/day and he put on 16 kg. Check-up angiography 5 months after the operation revealed a patent by-pass. In the meantime the coeliac artery became completely closed. The blood supply is satisfactorily ensured via the pancreatico-duodenal artery.

We should like to emphasise that the syndrome of abdominal angina is not rare and should be considered in gastro-enterology more frequently. We think that this problem deserves utmost attention since patients with abdominal angina are seriously endangered if they do not receive adequate help.

We have tried to show that there exists a transitory form of abdominal angina which is caused by a temporary disproportion between the progress of the ischaemic process and the formation of collaterals.

The most important indication for a reconstruction operation thus remains the typical clinical picture including stenoses or obstructions of the splanchnic arteries, regardless of the presence of collaterals. The clinical picture determines how long we can wait for the development of spontaneous collaterals. For more objective assessment of the extent of ischaemia of the splanchnic area, it appears promising to measure the flow through the splanchnic area by catheterization of the hepatic veins and to assess the decrease of oxygen after a load, as is done by some authors.

P. F., Institute for Clinical and Experimental Medicine, Vídeňská 800, Praha 4 - Krč, Czechoslovakia

SURGERY OF THE INTESTINAL ARTERIES

H. DENCK and G. KOBINIA

First Surgical Department of the Hospital of the City of Vienna— Lainz, Vienna, Austria

Although today the technical problem of reconstructing the blood flow after acute or chronic occlusions of intestinal arteries or veins is regarded as having been solved, mortality is still very high, especially in case of acute occlusions of intestinal arteries, in which it reaches 80 to 100%. In acute occlusions two facts are apparently responsible for the high mortality rate: on the one hand we think far too seldom of an acute vascular process when we are confronted with acute abdominal symptoms, and on the other the necessary major surgical intervention, such as laparotomy and vascular operation, is simply too much for the patients in question. The clinical picture of an acute occlusion of intestinal arteries presents 3 stages: Stage I is characterised by an acute attack of pain and a state of shock, lasting 6 hours; stage II may last up to 24 hours and may be qualified as silent interval, the abdomen is slightly distended but relatively painless; during stage III enteroparesis, peritonitis and intoxication occur.

It is obvious that successful operations may only be performed during stage I when the intestinal lesion is still reversible, with the exception of such cases of peripheral embolism that can be treated by circumscribed intestinal resection even during stage III.

Consequently, whenever a vascular process is suspected in case of a fibrillating vitium, the suspicion must be immediately examined by angiography nad if confirmed embolectomy must be attempted immediately. If for outside reasons immediate angiography is impossible, it is better to perform an exploratory laparotomy than to lose precious time. If after initially successful embolectomy symptoms reappear, a second look must be carried out promptly and gangrenous intestinal loops must be resected. Some authors perform a second look on principle after 24 to 48 hours. Only if we operate resolutely and in good time, we shall in future be able to improve the still unfavourable prognosis of acute mesenteric occlusions. In 28 of 65 patients under observation an embolectomy was performed, which was successful in 9 cases.

While the surgical indication is very simple in cases of confirmed acute mesenteric arterial occlusions, it is very difficult in chronic occlusions or stenoses of one or more visceral arteries, for we know that even stenoses or occlusions of three vessels may occur without any symptoms. Among our angiographic patients we found in 20% of all routine high lumbar aortographic examinations more or less by chance stenoses or occlusions of one or more visceral arteries. Only one sixth of these patients presented in fact symptoms which could be brought into connection with the angiographic findings. In 3 patients, for instance, we found a high-grade mesenteric stenosis and violent abdominal symptoms apparently caused by it; however upon laparotomy in one case an abscess-forming pancreatitis was identified as cause of the complaints, and in the two other cases deep-lying penetrating duodenal ulcers, which had been overlooked during the ex-ray examination. After treatment of these basic diseases all three patients are symptom free.

The typical clinical picture of chronic intestinal ischemia is described as follows: ischemia upon food intake, ischemic intestinal cramps (intermittent intestinal claudication; *Ortner*), chronic diarrhea, steatorrhea, loss of weight reaching a state of cachexia, deficiency states   such as anemia, tetany, osteomalacia, vitamin deficiency and protein deficiency oedema. However, only in very rare cases the clinical picture is complete enough to permit a tentative diagnosis. The functional disorder is caused by a lesion of the mucous membrane (atrophy of the villi) and by the resulting maldigestion and malabsorption. In cases of high-grade ischemia we find also pain at rest, i.e. a continuous state of abdominal pain and the occurrence of localised inflammatory processes, similar to those in Crohn's disease, which cause secondary strictures (e.g. at the sigmoid flexure after occlusion of the inferior mesenteric artery). Finally, in cases of chronic intestinal circulatory disorders necroses, ulcers, gangrenes, perforation and peritonitis may occur. Thus, Fontaine's system of circulatory disorders I—IV may easily be applied to intestinal circulatory disorders: stage II-intermittent intestinal claudication, stage III-pain at rest with localised intestinal lesions and formation of strictures, stage IV-necrosis and ulcer.

In case of appropriate clinical symtoms and singular stenoses or occlusions the operation is indicated only when the collateral circulation is not sufficient.

The method of choice in stenoses at the branching of the mesenteric artery is the interposition or the aorto-mesenteric bypass, using either a vein or plastic; if the saphenous vein is too thin, the plastic graft should be preferred, promising a wider lumen and good patency. When the indication is correct, success is very good, especially in pronounced cases. The retroperitoneal approach from the left side after resection of the 11th and 12th rib has worked well. We were successful in nine out of twelve cases operated in that way. In cases of transplantation of the aortic bifurcation and simultaneous stenosis of the mesentric artery, the mesenteric stenosis should absolutely be corrected, otherwise the postoperative insufficient perfusion of the superior mesenteric artery may cause complaints.

Acute occlusions due to embolism or a dissecting aneurysm are rather rare in the supply area of the coeliac trunk, while chronic occlusions or stenoses in this area are far more frequent, the effect of the diaphragm being of some pathogenetical importance. While the clinical picture of stenoses or occlusions in the supply area of the superior mesentric artery is fairly typical, this is absolutely not the case when the insufficient perfusion occurs in the area of the coeliac trunk, but we find pain in the upper abdomen which cannot be explained by any other cause. Sometimes deep-seated peptic ulcers or chronic pancreati.is are brought into connection with the existence of a stenosis of the truncus. Therefore the indication for surgical intervention is extremely difficult and the results are not always satisfactory, as the relationship between complaints in the upper abdomen and a stenosis of the truncus does not necessarily exist in all cases.

The relevant literature gives a series of good possibilities of revascularisation in cases of stenoses in the area of the coeliac trunk, their applicability depending on the site and the extension of the stenosed vascular section. When the compression is caused from outside by the diaphragm, we have the possibility of splitting the aortic hiatus. In cases of additional organic stenosing, the desobliteration may be completed with or without a patch graft. If we have a purely organic branching stenosis a re-implantation may be performed under the condition that the peripheral part of the coeliac trunk is sufficiently long and the arterial wall is fit for anastomosis. For all interventions directly at the branching off of the coeliac trunk (with the exception of simple diaphragm splitting), the retroperitoneal approach from the left side used by *Van Dongen* is recommended. Other possibilities of revascularisation are bridge grafts from the aorta to the hepatic artery or to the lienal artery; the bridging may either be performed from the subdiaphragmal section of the aorta (*Piza*), or — which is far less risky — from the infrarenal aorta (*Denck*). These interventions may be performed after median laparotomy, the disadvantages of the difficult access in the subdiaphragmal section are compensated for by the advantages of less arteriosclerotic alterations and better haemodynamics.

The venous bypass from the infrarenal aorta to the often post-stenotically enlarged lienal artery or to the hepatic artery has proved most successful (intraperitoneal operation). In 9 cases operated according to that method we had 2 re-occlusions and

2 re-stenoses. 6 of our patients are still free of symptoms to-day, 5 years after the operation. It is interesting that the two patients with the re-occlusion are also fairly free of complatins, follow-up angiograms showed a major improvement of the collateral circulation. In recent years we have gradually changed to a direct operation at the coeliac artery, using the retroperitoneal approach and the resection of the 11th and 12th rib, and performing either a patch graft or a re-implantation.

Cases in which the crura of the diaphragm cause impression, kinking or stenosing of the coeliac trunk present no surgical problem. In 12 such cases we have performed a simple splitting of the diaphragm, and in ten of the cases the angiogram proved in fact the removal of the kinking. These patients were afterwards free of symptoms. The retroperitoneal approach from the left side has proved successful in these cases.

In conclusion we may say that surgery of symptomatic stenoses of the intestinal arteries may produce excellent results.

Finally a word should be said about iatrogenic lesions in the area of the intestinal arteries.

We had 8 such patients, twice we had to ligate the coeliac trunk in cases of an extensive cardiac carcinoma, which had no consequences. In 4 patients lesions of the hepatic artery occurred during extensive tumor operations, in two of them an attempted reconstruction by suturing was without success, the other cases had to be ligated. 2 of these patients died in hepatic coma, 2 survived and are completely free of symptoms.

The superior mesenteric artery was injured twice in the course of extensive tumor resections of the pancreas, and twice we had to interpose a venous graft. This patient died 12 days after the operation due to rupture of a septic aneurysm. In the second patient the superior mesenteric artery could be sutured, and the postoperative course was without complications. This shows that the coeliac trunk and the proper hepatic artery can be ligated without consequences, however it cannot be predicted in which cases hepatic coma may occur. We believe that in every case reconstruction should at least be attempted. There is no doubt that reconstruction is necessary after operative lesions in the area of the superior mesenteric artery, the most difficult problem being the maintainance of aseptic conditions when simultaneously an operation on the intestines has to be performed.

H. D. Surgical Dept, of the Vienna Lainz City Hospital, Wolkerbergenstr, 1., A-1130, Vienna, Austria

CLINICAL AND EXPERIMENTAL RESULTS OF THE SURGERY OF THE EXTRACRANIAL CEREBRAL VESSELS

H. DENCK, G. S. KOBINIA and G. W. HAGMÜLLER

First Surgical Department of the Vienna Lainz City Hospital, Vienna, Austria

Since 1961 we had to perform 1153 reconstructions of extracranial cerebral arteries. We had to operate only 6 times on the vertebral artery, 11 times an extra-intracranial anastomosis was performed, 93 times stenoses or occlusions in the region of the aortic arch and 1 049 times the carotid artery was operated on. I would like to give you now a very concise presentation of our actual point of view.

It is assumed that in 15−20% of all patients suffering from cerebral occlusive disease stenoses or occlusions in the region of the extracranial vessels are found. The artery the most concerned is the internal carotid artery with 60%, followed by stenoses directly at the aortic arch, those of the vertebral artery and the common carotid artery. Most frequently atherosclerotic plaques or ulcers occur, leading to stenosis, total thrombosis or microembolus. Quite frequently however also looping and kinking can be found. Rarely trauma with intima lesion and consecutive thrombosis, arteriovenous fistula or tumors with vascular compression and aneurysm are found. The surgical therapy consists in open desobliteration with or without patch plastic.

The keystone in the preoperative diagnosis is the preoperative angiogram which we feel should be performed as aortic arch angiography, which, in turn, should be followed by selective catheterisation of one of the carotid or subclavian arteries, if and as necessary. Selective filling by puncture of one carotid artery is not sufficient for an operation indication because of possible stenoses at the aortic arch not visualised by the selective method and it is a well known fact that lesions of

the extracranial cerebral vessels quite often are multiple. In case of carotid artery stenosis open desobliteration followed by patch plastic is the therapy of choice. In a study on 282 patients we could find out that when using the inner shunt strokes happened only very seldom, and therefore we primarily apply the inner shunt as means of security in contrast to those who apply a shunt only in selected cases and those who never use it. Principally now we perform carotid artery operations in local anaesthesia while talking to the patient. After exposure of the carotid artery and i.v. administration of 55 000. I. U. heparin we perform the arteriotomy and then the local desobliteration, which usually lasts not longer than up to 3 minutes. Then the shunt is inserted for the time required for the patch plastic. If the patient however stops counting or talking at the time of clamping his carotid artery then we insert the shunt immediately and perform the desobliteration under the protection of the shunt.

Since performing our operations on the carotid artery in local anaesthesia we never found any intraoperative apoplectic insult. For cases of kinking we usually perform the muscle loop plastic according to Schultze-Bergmann with the sternocleidomastoid muscle , which in most of the cases suffices to guarantee an unobstructed flow. The kinking is rarely that highgraded that reimplantation has to be performed. The results for our muscle loop plastic however are excellent.

For the cases of stenosis of the vertebra artery the open desobliteration via an incision in the subclavian artery is the therapy of choice. Lesions of the vertebral artery have to be operated only when they are bilateral, as one vertebral artery would suffice to nourish the posterior parts of the brain. Acute occlusions of the carotid artery should be operated unrelated to the time delay as long as the patient is conscious.

Out of 12 patients fully conscious, on whom we operated during the first 36 hours after the onset of the progressive stroke we got 9 total remissions and only one death. After 20 operations on unconscious patients we got 2 partial remissions and 8 deaths. We evaluated 420 patients operated on at least 5 years before and we could find that the long term results of stage I and stage II are excellent with a success rate of 89%. The operative mortality was 3%.

Which now are the main reasons for death following carotid artery reconstruction? First of all rethrombosis in the region of the operation can ensue with consecutive cerebral colliquation. This complication is not necessarily fatal, it is however a hazardous situation for the patient. Second danger for those, operated in stage III is that in the stage of fresh colliquation revascularisation of the artery can lead to bleeding into the colliquation, a complication which usually is fatal.

Stenoses of the aortic arch were operated ninetythree times, fourty one times by direct transthoracic approach and 52 times by extraanatomical bypass. The idea reconstruction for these occlusions still is a direct reconstruction as performed with an aortosubclavian bypass or by open desobliteration, which alone is capable to fully restore the normal hemodynamic situation. Naturally a transthoracic direct operation in section I of the subclavian artery is not only a big operation but the artery itself is extremely difficult to handle due to its extreme wall fragility. Desobliteration not always can be performed in the right layer. Therefore the extraanatomical bypass operations have been favoured and especially the carotidosubclavian bypass has been advised for the treatment of the subclavian steel syndrome. We have examined the hemodynamics of these extraanatomical detours and could find that in spite of a considerable flow increase in the common carotid artery there is both a slight decrease of pressure in the internal carotid artery as a certain decrease of flow after opening a carotidosubclavian graft. Under normal circumstances this small pressure and flow reduction might be neglectable, in cases of cerebral sclerosis however it can lead to clinical signs of carotid artery insufficiency. Another question we were interested in was how big the flow in the graft had to be in order to reverse the retrograde vertebral artery flow to its normal orthograde direction. Assuming a normal subclavian artery flow of 200 to 300 ml, the critical flow in the bypass must average about 150 ml to stop the retrograde vertebral flow and should be about 200 to 250 ml to perfuse the vertebral artery sufficiently. Considering the complications among 52 extracranial bypass operations we find one case of persisting steel in spite of a patent graft and another case with ipsilateral vertebral artery thrombosis with lethal issue among the carotidosubclavian grafts. No complications however were found among the subclavio-subclavian grafts, which according to our experimental and postoperative measurements by strain guage plethysmography give better values for the resting flow and flow during reactive hyperemia then the carotidosubclavian grafts. According to these facts we now prefer the subclaviosubclavian bypass with a 8 mm dacron graft performed by two supraclavicular incisions.

H. D., I. Surgical Department of the Vienna Lainz City Hospital, Wolkersbergenstr. 1, A-1130, Vienna, Austria

LUMBAR SYMPATHECTOMY AS AN ALTERNATIVE TREATMENT OF OCCLUSIVE ARTERIOSCLEROTIC DISEASES OF THE LOW EXTREMITIES

G. MESSARIS, A. LIAKOS, N. MAROPOULOS, M. KATIRI
and J. VOULGARIS

1st Surgical Clinic of "Agia Olga", Hospital N. Ionia Athens, Greece

The first lumbar sympathectomy for vascular diseases was performed by *Diez* in 1924 on a patient suffering from occlusive thromboangiitis of the low extremities (Bürger's disease).

This method yielded very satisfactory results. It has been establisted and used for several years till the introduction in surgery of various types of angioplastic operations.

The above operations were considered to be the method of choice for treatment of occlusive arteriosclerotic disease of the low extremities and of its manifestations.

Consequently, due to the overestimated results, they were used almost exclusively in many centers during the last ten years.

With a lapse of time and as a result of experience acquired in the meantime, lumbar sympathectomy started to regain ground. Today we are in a position to say that this operation offers an alternative solution for those patients in whom the direct vascular operation was not successful, as well as for those in whom the angioplastic operation is neither possible

Table I. Indications for lumbar sympathectomy.

1.	Raynaud disease
2.	Acrocyanosis
3.	Causalgia
4.	Erythromelalgia
5.	Occlusive arterial disease of the low extremities:
a.	Coldness, numbness
b.	Intermittent claudication
c.	Rest pain
d.	Ischemic and nutritional disturbances
e.	Impending gagrene
f.	Failure of angioplastic surgical procedures
g.	Contra-indications for angioplastic surgical procedures (atherosclerotic cardiovascular and cerebrovascular aged disease.).

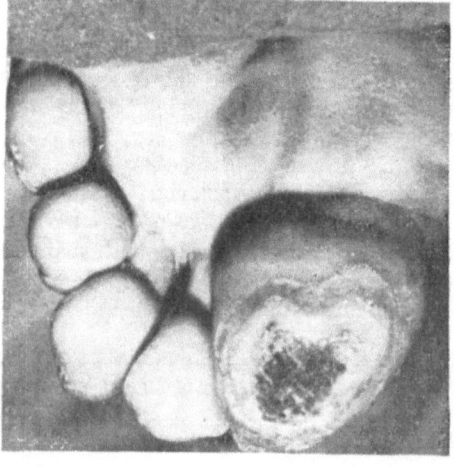

Fig. 1. Before lumbar sympathectomy.

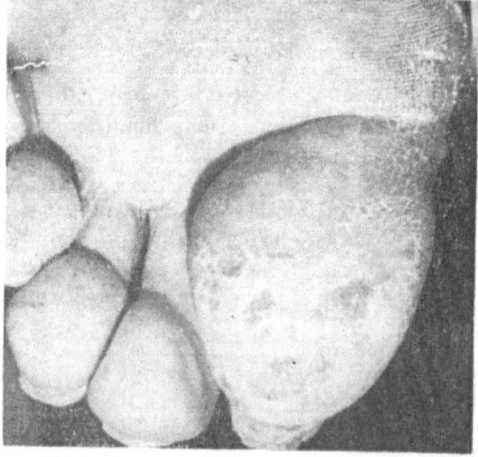

Fig. 2. Ten days after lumbar sympathectomy.

nor desirable (old and weak persons, suffering from a serious arteriosclerotic disease with manifestations from the heart or from the brain).

According to the above mentioned contraindications and unseccesful results of the angioplastic operations, the suggestion for lumbar sympathectomy is strongly indicated. We feel that the indications for performing lumbar sympathectomy are the following: (Table I).

During the last triennial period 1975 to 1977 with criterion the above indications, we performed 11 lumbar sympathectomies

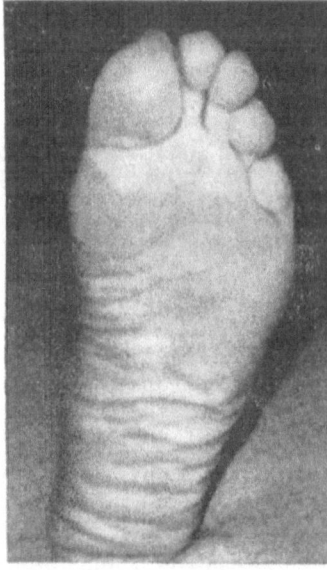

Fig. 3. Complet healing of the ulcer.

on aged persons suffering from occlusive arteriosclerotic disease of the low extremities. In all these cases serious ischemic manifestations from the myocardium or from the brain existed.

The results of lumbar sympathectomy appear satisfactory and in the majority of cases the following results were obtained: Relief of ischemic pain and healing of ischemic alterations of the skin (trophic ulcer).

Also, in those cases where digital gangrene appeared, amputation of the leg was avoided and has been restricted to the afflicted part.

The results were very satisfactory in a case of thrombosed arterial iliofemoral by-pass. The successful percentage of lumbar sympathectomies leading to a) relief to an intermitent claudication, b) restriction or avoiding of amputation and c) improvement of ischemic skin manifestations, fluctuates between 70% and 80%. A successful percentage is around 72.7% Table II.

Table II. Success percentage for lumbar sympathectomy.

Kimmonth	80%
Sailagyius	71%
Smithwick	70%
Our material	72.7%

Taking into consideration a) the advanced age of the patients and b) the existance, in all these cases, of an ischemic heart or brain disease, this percentage can be considered as excellent.

In conclusion, the readaptation of lumbar sympathectomy for an occlusive arteriosclerotic disease of the lower extremities and especially when performed on aged or weak patients with ischemic heart or brain insufficiency constitutes the preferred method for immediate and future results. It is known that the blood supply from the neighbouring circulation is doubled within 48 hours, so that decreasing of this blood supply takes a long time and it remains steady at a proportion of one and a half for a long period.

Therefore, lumbar sympathectomy is considered to be superior to angioplastic operations in the following points:

a) It is a non haemoragic operation (no need for blood transfusion).

b) A low number of immediate postoperative recurrences are found.

c) There are no late postoperative recurrences (thrombosis of by-pass etc.).

d) A few days of hospitalization is sufficient.

EXPERIMENTAL AND CLINICAL EMBOLIZATION OF THE SPLEEN

J. VOSMÍK, K. FORTÝN, M. HACO, J. ČOUPEK and V. RUŽBARSKÝ,
M. VIDLÁKOVÁ

Institute for Clinical and Experimental Medicine, Prague
Institute of Macromolecular Chemistry, Prague, Czechoslovakia

The risk of surgical splenectomy depends largely on the size of the spleen, on the primary disease and particularly on the extent of the blood coagulation defects. Miller et al. give 8.9% hospital mortality after splenectomy in congestive splenomegaly. In some patients, surgical splenectomy cannot be performed at all.

In 1972 we started our experiments on dogs with intraarterial embolization of the spleen by a mixture of 40% glucose, collagen broth and barium sulphide.

Three of 9 animals survived chronically and their spleens practically disappeared. In a group of 37 dogs we used super-hydrophylic metacrylate spheron balls of 25 to 35 microns in diameter.

As an indicator of splenic function depression we used Howell Jolly corpuscles incidence in peripheral blood, which was 100% in the first and more than 50% in the second group. We used splenic artery embolization in 4 patients. In two of them spheron balls of 100 to 200 microns in diameter and in the remaining two spheron balls of only 50 to 60 microns were applied.

Methods and results

By Seldinger method a catheter was introduced via the femoral artery and put forward super-selectively into the splenic artery near the hilum of the spleen. Arteriography was performed. Spheron balls were injected manually at a slow rate by small boluses. After the embolization arteriography was repeated. Before and after the procedure 1/2 gram of cephalosporin was injected via the intraarterial catheter. Broad spectrum antibiotics were given 7 to 10 days after the procedure. Blood and urine amylases, leukocyte and platelet counts were followed.

The first case was a patient 12 years after a gunshot injury of the liver, repeated reconstructions of biliary ducts, with huge splenomegaly and prolonged bleeding from oesophageal varices. Intended splenectomy and splenorenal shunt could not be performed due to complete obliteration of the peritoneal cavity by dense adhesions. Splenic embolization was performed by 100 000 spheron balls of 100 to 200 microns in diameter. The platelet count increased from 40 to 90 000, the serum and urine amylases remained within normal. Abdominal pain in the left upper quadrant appeared on the fifth day after the procedure and persisted for ten days. Two minor episodes of oesophageal varix haemorrhage were controlled conservatively. The patient died of liver failure on the 20th day after embolization. On section the patient showed splenic infarctions up to 8 mm in diameter and partial splenic vein thrombosis.

In the second patient the portocaval end to side shunt got partially occluded by a thrombus on the 3rd postoperative day. Seven days after thrombectomy total occlusion of the portocaval shunt was angiographically confirmed.

Since the patient underwent repeated laparotomies at an other department, further surgical intervention was not considered and splenic embolization was performed by 50 000 spherons of 100 to 200 microns. Amylase levels were within normal, platelet count rose from 90 to 110 000.

The post-embolization course was complicated by the transient left side pleural effusion and abdominal pain in the left upper quadrant. The patient has not regained bleeding from oesophageal varices for one and a half year. The third patient was operated for bleeding from oesophageal varices caused by portal vein thrombosis at another hospital. The inferior mesenteric to left renal vein shunt and ligation of splenic artery were performed. Six months after the operation the patient was admitted to our department with a recurrence of bleeding. Closure of previous portasystemic shunt and renewed arterial supply were demonstrated angiographically. An attempt to perform a mesentericocaval shunt proved unfeasible because of superior mesenteric vein thrombosis and presence of the bridging collaterals with a thin wall and a small diameter. Splenic embolization was performed in two sessions within the interval of 20 days using 50 000 spherons of 60 microns in diameter in each session. The course was uneventfull and the patient has not rebled 8 months after the procedure.

The fourth patient was 72 years old and suffered from repeated oesophageal bleeding and liver cirrhosis. He was considered bad risk for a portacaval shunt because of coeliac artery stenosis and a poor arterial supply to the liver. Splenic embolization was performed by 100 000 spherons of 60 microns in diameter. Slight and transient abdominal pain in the left upper quadrant appeared. He died of liver failure 20 days later. Detailed section did not show any thrombosis in the splanchnic venous bed. Most of 50−60 micron splenic arteries were occluded with one, exceptionally two spheron balls. No spheron particles were found in the liver, pancreas, lung and brain.

Discussion

The contribution of splenic inflow via short gastric veins to the eosophageal varix bed varies widely but in individual cases is the prevailing and even the only source.

According to our and other authors experience splenic artery ligation has not proved to be successful because of the rapid establishment of splenic arterial inflow through collaterals. Chuang and coworkes and Castaneda-Zuniga et al. advocate embolization of the spleen by small emboli and repeated application.

In our first two cases 100 to 200 micron particles caused blockage of numerous arterial branches probably of the same diameter with a limited possibility of collateralization. This was suggested by angiographic appearance after the embolization and confirmed at section in one case. In further 2 cases 60 micron particles did not cause infarctions of recognisable size as evaluated by angiography. At section of one patient no separate infarctions were found but the upper part of the spleen was ischaemic without any adverse reaction. Thrombotic occlusion of the splenic vein in splenic sectorial portal hypertension seems to be ideal for indication of splenic embolization. Our two patients with portal vein thrombosis followed this indication. In both the procedure proved to be successful until present time. The danger of splenic, portal and even mesenteric vein thrombosis resulting from exstirpation of a large spleen has been well known. Also the incidence of pulmonary embolism has been reported to be high (5.12%).

Massive splenic embolization which we observed in the first patient with huge splenomegaly exhibits the same danger. Consumption coagulopathy was not followed in our cases and deserves more attention. Subsequent embolization by small particles at several sessions seems to be worth clinical trial in carefully selected cases of splenomegaly in portal hypertension.

J. V., IKEM, Vídeňská 800, Prague 4, Krč, Czechoslovakia

SURGICAL TREATMENT OF KINKING AND COILING OF THE INTERNAL CAROTID ARTERY

C. BELIAN and J. NEUGEBAUER

Department of Vascular Surgery of the Friederichshain-Hospital, Berlin, G.D.R.

15−20% of the cases of cerebrovascular insufficiency are caused by coiling or kinking of the internal carotid artery.

Morphologically we distinguish, like Herrschaft and Vollmar, three forms:
1. the C- or S-form (elongation)
2. coiling or tortuousity
3. kinking.

Combinations of these three forms are of course possible, and we may observe a simultaneous concomitant carotid artery bifurcation stenosis. Pronounced coiling shows, in most cases, kinking, although this cannot always be angiographically proved. That ist why for an X-ray demonstration of kinking an angiographic examination in various neck-positions, the so-called functional angiography, is often required. Indication for an operation depends on the angiographic result and the degree of cerebrovascular insufficiency. In this context the following guidelines are used by us: At an asymptomatic stage (stage I) coiling is operated by kinking and concomitant carotid artery bifurcation stenoses. Kinking without concomitant carotid artery stenosis is likewise an indication for an operation. Pure coiling is not operated at an asymptomatic stage. At the stage of transient ischemic attacks (stage II), coiling and kinking as well as pure coiling are operated. At the stage of acute and progressive stroke (stage III) we have not so far been faced with taking such a decision.

At the stage of complete stroke (stage IV) we operated on a few patients. After reconstruction, 50% of the patients showed an improved condition.

Among the patients of the Department of Vascular Surgery in Friedrichshain − Berlin, we found among 249 reconstructions of the internal carotid artery, 47 operations of 41 patients which were carried out because of coiling or kinking.

6 patients were operated upon bilaterally. The age of the operated persons ranged between 17 and 68 years. There were 12 men and 29 women. These patients suffered 38 times from kinking which was, in 7 cases, combined with a concomitant internal carotid artery bifurcation stenosis and 9times with coiling.

At the same time, there occurred elongations of the other brachycephalic arteries in 6 cases, constricting changes of other extracranial arteries in 3 cases and arterial insufficiencies of blood circulation of the lower extremities in 5 cases.

According to the degree of cerebrovascular insufficiency, 1 patient was at stage I, 36 patients at stage II, no patient at stage III and 4 patients at stage IV.

The operative correction of coiling and kinking was carried out 31 times by way of resenction of the internal carotid with reinsertion into the common carotid artery and 11 times of resection of the internal carotid with end-to-end-anastomosis, while in 7 cases simultaneously an endarterectomy internal carotid operation was carried out. During the first years of our work, 5 internal carotid transposition operations took place.

Intra-operatively the intravascular pressure was measured according to Michal, Hejnal, Hejhal and Firt. A temporary intraluminar shunt was not required in any subsequent case. All patients were operated upon in general heparinization.

As post-operative complications we observed 2 secondary bleeding, 5 temporary recurrence pareses and 1 hypertonic crisis. After the operation, 22 patients were symptom-free, 17 patients were improved while 2 patients were unchanged. No patient had become deteriorated or had died as a result of the operation.

Demonstrations of pre- and post-operative angiographs. (Figrs. 1 + 2).

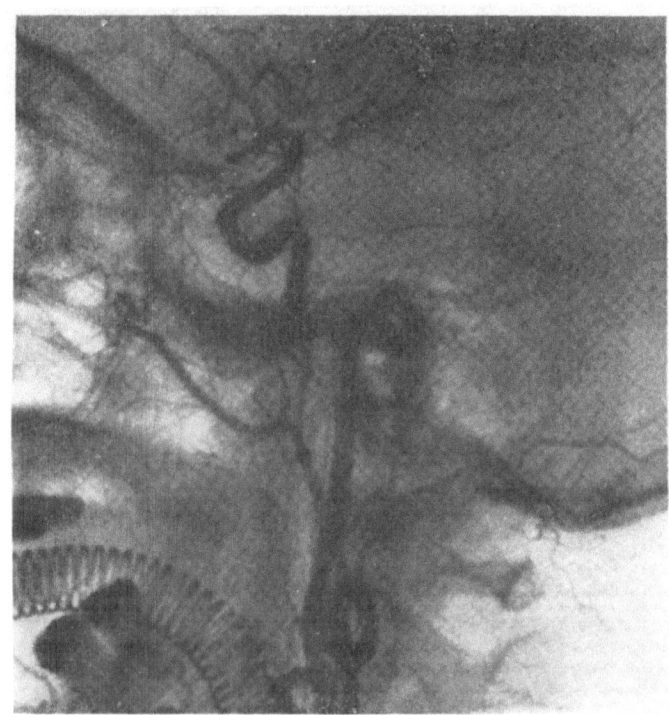

Fig. 1 Pat.: S. H., 54 yrs, coiling of the internal carotid artery on the left: preoperatively on, the right: corrected.

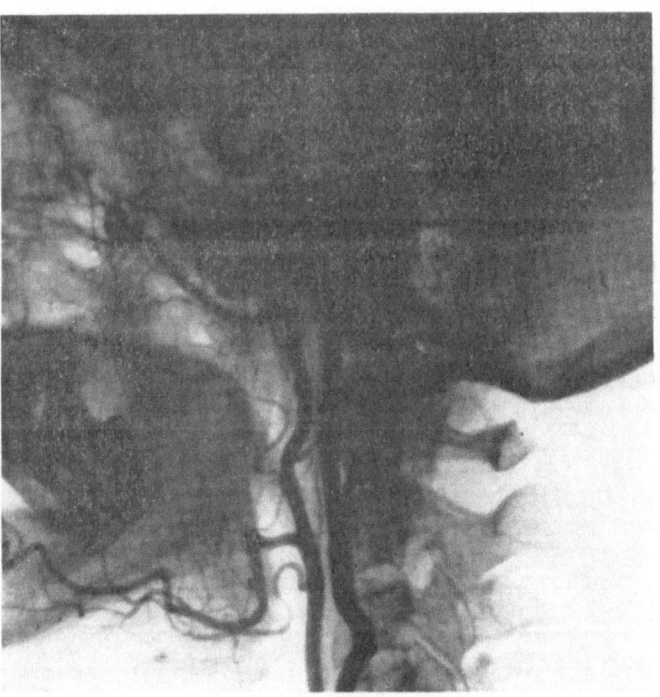

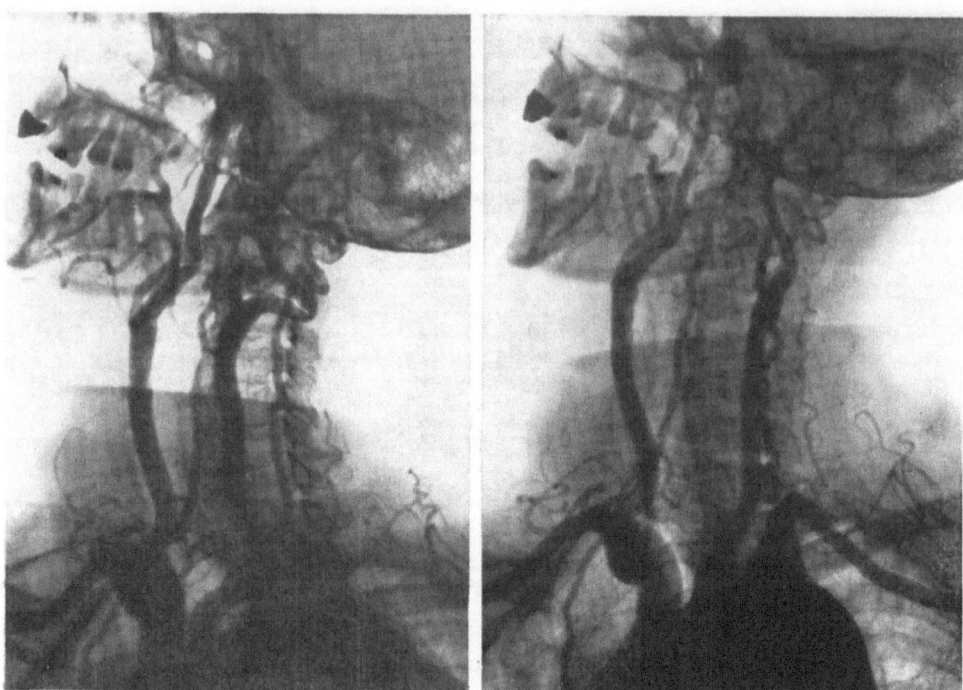

Fig. 2. Pat.: S. G., 58 yrs, kinking of the internal carotid artery on the left: preoperatively on, the right: corrected.

C. B., Baumschulenstr. 92, 1195 Berlin, G.D.R.

EXPERIMENTAL A—V FISTULA: DILATATION OF MUSCULAR TYPE ARTERY AT ELEVATED FLOW RATES

V. SMIEŠKO, V. M. KHAYUTIN, M. GEROVÁ, J. GERO
and A. N. ROGOZA

*Institute of Normal and Pathological Physiology, Slovak Academy
of Sciences, Bratislava, Czechoslovakia
Institute of General Pathology and Pathological Physiology, Academy
of Medical Sciences, Moscow, U.S.S.R.*

Introduction

Increased blood flow (BF) to skeletal muscles during exercise is accompanied by dilatation of the respective conduit arteries. This dilatation was thought to be induced by a process triggered in the muscular tissue, reaching the nerve endings (*Schretzennmayr*, 1933) or the arterioles (*Hilton*, 1959; *Folkow*, 1964) and spreading proximally up to the main conduit artery. The increased BF, however, has been shown to induce dilatation of a large conduit artery which may be disconnected from the consecutive vascular bed (*Lie at al.*, 1970; *Ingebrigtsen et al.*, 1973). The basis of this locally induced dilatation is presumed to be a Bayliss-type response to altered transmural pressure (*Jaffe and Rowe*, 1970) or a mechanism sensitive to the BF increase (*Lie et al.*, 1970; *Ingebrigtsen et al.*, 1973). The aim of the present study has been to demonstrate this dilatation in a small muscular-type artery and to determine the role of the pressure and/or flow in its initiation.

Materials and methods

Using a contact inductive transducer (*Gerová and Gero*, 1969), the external diameter of the artery predominantly supplying the gracilic muscle (GA) was monitored in 9 dogs under thiopental anesthesia during changes of BF through this artery by means of an A—V shunt. After the animal had been heparinized, its right femoral artery was ligated proximally to the origin of GA and distally to the origin of saphenous artery it was connected to the left femoral artery (Fig. 1 A). The peripheral end of GA was connected by a tube to the left femoral

vein. GA inflow and outflow pressure were measured by Statham manometers, BF through GA was monitored by a Statham electromagnetic flowmeter or a photoelectric drop recorder. The resting BF and intravascular pressure were

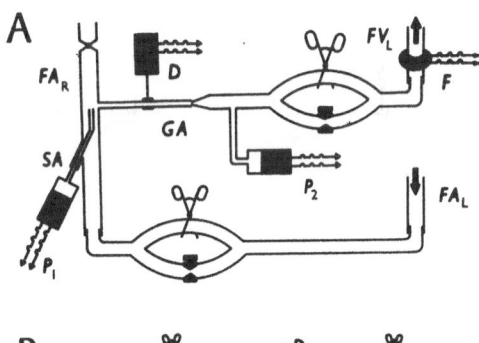

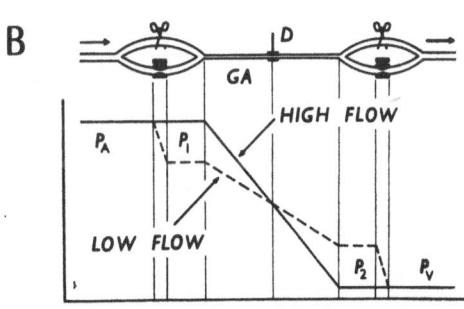

Fig. 1. Scheme of the experimental setup (A) and the respective pressure distribution during blood flow changes (B). GA — gracilis artery. FA_R — right femoral artery, FA_L — left femoral artery. FV_L — left femoral vein, SA — Saphenous artery, D — diameter recorder, P_1 — pressure recorder near central end of gracilis artery, P_2 — pressure recorder near peripheral end of gracilis artery, F — electromagnetic flowmeter, P_A — arterial pressure, P_V — venous pressure. Notice that the intravascular pressure at the point of diameter measurement remains unaltered (B).

251

Fig. 2. Dilatation response of the gracilis artery to a sudden increase in blood flow under varying intravascular pressure at the site of diameter measurement (see text). P_1 — pressure near the central end of GA, P_2 — pressure near the peripheral end of GA, F — blood flow, D — diameter. (In B, flow was recorded with an inserted filter.)

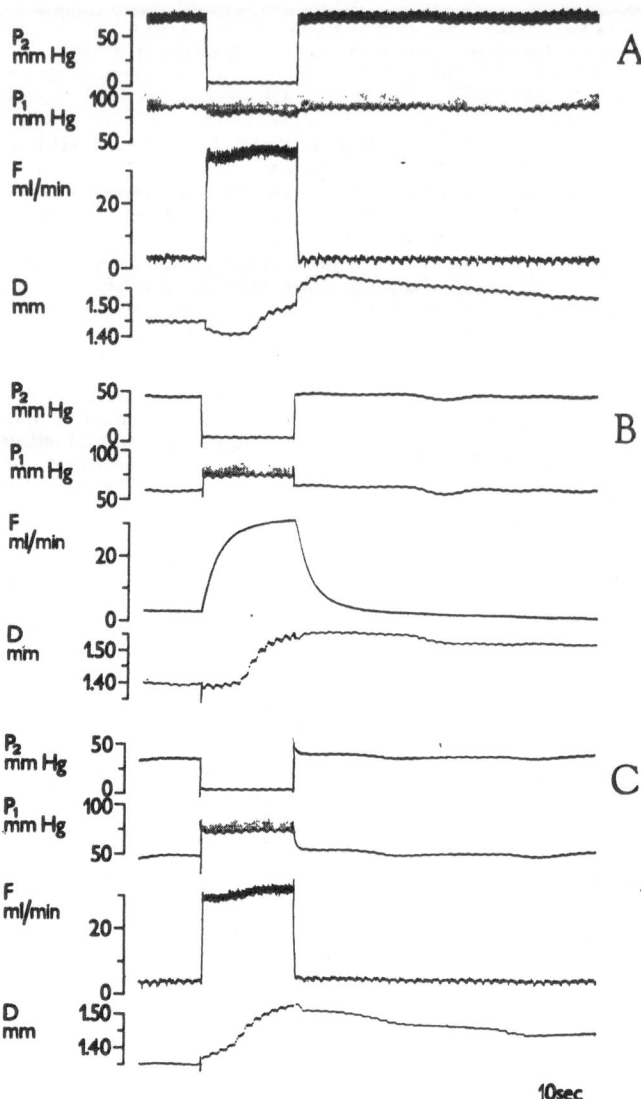

controlled by screw clamps applied to the polyvinyl tubes on the inflow and outflow sites of GA. Opening of a clamp on two shunting tubes enabled an increase in BF through GA either without or with a simultaneous alteration in the intravascular pressure at the point of diameter measurement (Fig. 1 B).

Results

In Figure 2 three responses of the GA diameter to enhanced BF are illustrated. The three records differ in respect of intravascular pressure at the site of the diameter measurement (as inferred from the initial passive change in diameter): in A, the diameter simultaneously with BF increment decreased, in C increased, whereas in B the diameter remained unchanged. As is evident from the figure, in spite of the differences in intravascular pressure and in the respective initial diameter changes, several seconds after the BF was increased a dilation response of GA could be observed in all of the situations.

In a series of similar experiments (n = 18) BF through GA was increased from 4.9 ± 0.7 to 45.5 ± 6.6 ml/min (M ± S.E.M.). The latency period was 11.3 ± 1.3 sec and the time for dilatation to reach its maximum value amounted to 39.0 ± 5 sec. The extent of dilatation (difference between the minimum and maximum diamater during increased BF expressed in percents of the resting diamater) ranging in individual animals from 5.2 to 20.4% was 12.6 ± 1.3%. After restoration of initial BF, the time required for the GA diameter to return to 50% of the maximum dilatation represented 109 ± ± 20 sec.

Discussion

Dilatation with increased BF was also demonstrated in the small artery of the muscular type (external GA diameter was 1.4 ± 0.1 mm). Although data concerning this dilatation were obtained on large arteries of the elastic-muscular type, i.e., on a. illiaca and a. femoralis (*Lie et al.*,

1970; *Ingebrigtsen et al.*, 1973), several relevant characteristics (time course of diameter increase and return, amplitude of dilatation) are comparable. The only parameter differing significantly is the latency period which for large arteries ranged between 10 and 45 sec and for GA between 5 and 28 sec.

On the basis of a vibration-induced relaxation of the vascular muscle, a hypothesis is derived assuming that dilatation during enhanced BF is due to vibrations of the arterial wall caused by turbulence (*Ljung and Silvertsson*, 1975). In the present experiments, however, vasodilatation has been frequently observed at BF increments up to 10 ml/min, when turbulence can hardly be assumed.

Moreover, the experimental setup used here enabled maintenance of the intravascular pressure either constant or increased and decreased during enhanced BF. Since dilatation was invariably present in all these situations, it can be concluded that the triggering stimulus is the BF increase rather than the change in transmural pressure.

REFERENCES

Folkow, B. (1964): Description of myogenic hypothesis. Circul. Res. 14 (Suppl. I), 279—287.

Gerová, M., Gero, J. (1969): Range of the sympathetic control of the dog femoral artery. Circul. Res. 24, 349—359.

Hilton, S. M. (1959): A peripheral arterial conducting mechanisms underlying dilatation of the femoral artery and concerned in functional vasodilatation in skeletal muscle. J. Physiol. (London) 149, 93—111.

Ingebrigtsen, R., Lie, M., Hol, R., Leraad, S., Fönstelien, E. (1973): Dilatation of the ileofemoral artery following the opening of an experimental arterio-venous fistula in the dog. Scand. J. clin. Lab. Invest. 31, 255—262.

Jaffe, M. D., Rowe, P. W. (1970): Mechanism of arterial dilatation following occlusion of femoral artery in dogs. Am. J. Physiol. 218, 1156—1160.

Lie, M., Sejersted, O. M., Kiil, F. (1970): Local regulation of vascular cross section during changes in femoral arterial blood flow in dogs. Circulat. Res. 27, 727—737.

Ljung, B., Sivertsson, R. (1975): Vibration-induced inhibition of vascular smooth muscle contraction. Blood Vessels 12, 38—52.

Schretzenmayr, A. (1933): Über kreislaufregulatorische Vorgänge an den grossen Arterien bei der Muskelarbeit. Pflügers Arch. 232, 743—748.

V. S., Institute of Normal and Pathological Physiology, Sienkiewiczova 1, 884 23 Bratislava, Czechoslovakia

VALUE OF REVASCULARIZATION OPERATIONS ON THE BIFURCATION OF THE COMMON CAROTID ARTERY IN PATIENTS WITH CHRONIC STROKE

K. TERŠÍP, J. BARTOŠ, J. MEGELA and B. DRUGOVÁ

First Surgical Clinic and Radiological Clinic, Faculty of General Medicine, Charles University, Prague, Czechoslovakia

Endarterectomy at the bifurcation of the common carotid artery is an important preventing operation in cerebrovascular attacks in patients who have stenotizing or ulcerating arteriosclerotic changes in this area. It is yet not clear whether these operations are of value in patients who have already developed chronic ischaemic cerebral changes. At present rather a negative attitude towards these operations predominates, although it may be assumed that a revascularization operation at the bifurcation of the common carotid artery in the case of extracranial occlusion

Table I. Number and Type of Operations in Patients with Stable Stroke

Type of Occlusion of ICA	Number of Patients	R - ICA	R - ECA	CSE	Total
Unilateral Stenosis	7	7	0	2	9
Bilateral Stenosis	6	10	2	4	16
Stenosis and Occlusion	13	13	5	9	27
Unilateral Occlusion	24	0	4	22	26
Bilateral Occlusion	2	2	2	4	
Total	52	30	13	39	82

R - ICA ... Reconstruction of Internal Carotid Artery
R - ECA ... Reconstruction of External Carotid Artery
CSE ... Cervical Sympathectomy

Table II. Functional Results Surgically Treated Patients with Stable Stroke

Operation	Number of Patients	Normal	Improved	Unchanged	Worse	Deaths
R - ICA	11	0	7	4	0	0
R - ECA	3	0	3	0	0	0
CSE	21	0	10	6	2	3
Combination of Reconstruction and CSE	17	0	7	7	2	1
Total	52 100%	0	27 52%	17 32,6%	4 7.7%	4 7.7%

R - ICA ... Reconstruction of Internal Carotid Artery
R - ECA ... Reconstruction of External Carotid Artery
CSE ... Cervical Sympathectomy

can influence the ischaemic (11) intracerebral foci.

It is known that, after ischaemic cerebrovascular attacks, the condition of some patients markedly improves after conservative treatment and rehabilitation. It seems, however, that these results are more rapid in some patients where it was possible to perform a revascularization operation on the bifurcation of the common carotid artery.

We indicated these operations in our patients with persisting neurological findings after terminated cerebrovascular attacks (described further as chronic stroke) and assume that at least some of them benefitted from these operations. We wanted to know whether a revascularisation operation can also improve the fate of patients where conservative treatment was not very successful or where a long interval had elapsed since the cerebrovascular attack and the neurological finding was already stationary (stable stroke).

During the past 15 years at the First Surgical Clinic of the Faculty of General Medicine in Prague surgical treatment has been provided for 110 patients with obliterating arteriosclerosis at the bifurcation of the common carotid artery. Chronic stroke was present in 62 patients (47.3%).

Reconstruction of the internal carotid artery possibly with concomitant reconstruction of the external carotid artery was performed in 11 patients, reconstruction of the external carotid artery in 3, cervical sympathectomy (CSE) with resection of the obliterated internal carotid artery in 21 and a combined recon — struction of the carotid arteries and CSE in 17. In patients where the operation was bilateral it was performed in two sessions (Table 1).

The results are given in detail in Table II. Regardless of the type of operation favourable results were achieved in about 52% of cases, 32.6% did not improve and 14.4% of the results were unfavourable (deterioration or death).

In general, it may be said that the results of surgical treatment depend on the patient condition, on the size of the ischaemic focus and on the type of obliteration.

Patients with chronic stroke who are operated on in a generally poor conditions with plegias and severe phatic disorders have only a slight chance that their condition will improve substantially. In some life is threatened. After CSE alone three of our patients died, the cause of death being extensive cerebral oedema.

Very favourable results were recorded in patients with ophthalmological disorders of the type of amaurosis fugax; reconstruction of the external carotid artery in cases with occlusion of the internal carotid artery led to disappearance of complaints.

In about half the patients their condition improved after CSE alone and it seems that this operation is justified.

For patients operated in the stage of stable stroke, reconstructions of the stenotic carotid artery are best as, after these operations, the blood supply to the brain increases immediately. The results in these patients also depend on the size and condition of the ischaemic focus in the brain. In some paretic patients early favourable results were achieved.

Evaluation of the improved condition of patients after operation is very difficult. We used as a basis notably comparison of neurological findings before and after operation, subjective complaints of the patients and data from their environment. In some it was possible to provide evidence of an improved cerebral circulation by ophthalmodynamometry, pletysmography and oscillography. All these objective methods, however, provide evidence of more filling of collaterals.

It must be emphasized that the grade of improvement was very invariable and depended only in some cases on the locomotor, phatic or opthalmological disorder.

To obtain more detailed information we separately evaluated patients who were operated on during the early months after the stroke and a group of patients who were operated on after an interval of one year or more following an acute stroke. (9 times after a 1 year interval, twice after 2 years, twice after 3 years and one after 5 years). Ten patients were subjected to reconstruction of the internal or external carotid artery and four to CSE alone. In seven patients the condition improved, six did not improve substantially after operation and one died on the 13th day after operation from ischaemic heart disease (Table III).

Table III. Comparison of Functional Results Surgically Treated Patients with Stable Stroke

Time between Acute Stroke and Operation	Number of Patients	Normal	Improved	RESULTS Un- changed	Worse	Deaths
1 to 6 months	38 (100%)	0	20 (52.6%)	11 (29%)	4 (10.5%)	3 (7.9%)
after 12 months and more	14 (100%)	0	7 (50%)	6 (43%)	0	1 (7%)
Total	52 (100%)	0	27 (51.5%)	17 (32.7%)	4 (7.4%)	4 (7.4%)

K. T., First Surgical Clinic, U nemocnice 2, 128 08 Prague 2, Czechoslovakia

VENOUS HOMOGRAFT IN ADVANCED ARTERITIS OF THE LEGS. REPORT OF 30 CASES

G. DALCHER, P. PRESSEL, A. BUEMI, M. BIETIGER
and G. de HAYNIN

Centre Hospitalier, Mulhouse, France

In the absence of the autologous vein, there are situations (gangrene, rest pain or infection) where a choice must be made: immediate amputation or implantation of allografts.

With the presently available materials, Dacron and Teflon, patency is difficult to maintain for vessels of less than 5 mm in diameter or during passage of joints and they cannot be used in case of infection. Bovine heterograft is a very expensive material and its advantages are not clearly established. Arterial homografts were abandoned because of frequent late aneurysmal failure.

Fresh or stored venous homografts reported by Carrel in 1911 have again been used for about 20 years, mostly for vascular access in chronic renal failure, but also for arterial and even coronary by-passes.

In our treatment of 40 homologous venous loops implanted for hemodialysis, we have used venous homografts in 30 by-passes for arterial disease.

No important data with a development period of over 5 years have been published and therefore we have limited our utilization of homografts to eliminate operations in cases of trophic ulceration, rest pain or infection and in 4 cases of severe limping after failure of previous surgery.

Table I. Report of 30 cases.

16 male
11 female
 3 patients with bilateral bypass
Median age 61 years (range from 49 to 86), 24 had 1 to 3 arterial operations before homograft

Clinical situation

Gangrene or ulceration (Stade IV de Fontaine)	16
Rest pain (Stade III de Fontaine)	6
Intermittent claudication (Stade II de Fontaine) <50 m	4
Infection after previous arterial surgery	4
Total	30

We have used stripped varicose veins. These veins are stored at 4° less than 1 month in a 9% saline solution with 1M penicillin and 1M colimycin added.

Where possible, we used only varicose veins without defects and with a diameter

Table II. Different types of operations performed

Ileo-popliteal bypass through obturator foramen		3
Femoro-popliteal bypass proximal	5	
distal	9	14
Femoro-tibial bypass proximal	5	
distal	2	7
Ileo-profunda femoris bypass		2
Popliteo-popliteal bypass		2
Ileo-tibial proximal bypass		1
Saphenous arterialization		1
Total		30

257

between 5 and 10 mm, but, if neccessary, we also used very poor homografts.

Some patients had composite grafts: homograft and autograft, homograft and Dacron or different segments of homograft from different donors.

We have not taken into account the major blood group compatibilities and never gave immunosuppressor treatment; antibiotherapy was not usually given.

This table shows the different types of by-passes performed. All the cases were salvage operations, where for reasons of infection, of the small diameter of the run-off arteries or of very distal by-pass, we preferred venous homograft to Dacron which was the only other available material.

Our results are reported in Table III, where it can be seen that the principal factor which influences long term patency is the quality of the run-off; graft quality

and the previous clinical situation are less important.

We had 4 cases of death in our series: 1 from post-surgical hemorrhage, 2 from renal insufficiency and 1 from myocardial infarction. The 3 last complications occurred some time after the operation.

We observed no clinical immunological repercussion in the desribed present cases, but more recently had an acute rejection on the 15th day.

In conclusion, thanks to certain improvements of the homograft quality by cadaveric samples of wholesome veins, stored in dimethyl sulfoxide in order to preserve the endothelium, amelioration of the immunological problem taking in account the major blood group compatibilities, it seems that venous homografts can compete with other materials and, moreover, their cost is 24 times less than bovine heterograft and 16 times less than Teflon.

Table III. Importance of run-off quality, graft quality and previous clinical situation for the results

		Nr.	Patency	Follow-up time
Run-off quality	Good	2	100%	27—36 months
	Fair	12	75%	7—27 months
	Poor	16	12.5%	6—10 months
Graft quality	Good	14	57%	7—27 months
	Fair	11	9%	10—13 months
	Poor	5	40%	13—36 months
Clinical situation	Gangrene or ulceration	16	44%	9—27 months
	Rest pain	6	50%	7—36 months
	Intermittent claudication	4	66%	13—26 months
	Infection	4	50%	at the death of the patient (6th and 2nd months after surgery)

REFERENCES

Gottlob R., Donas P., Elnashef B.: Untersuchungen am Endothel arterialisierter Venen. III. Unterschiede zwischen autologen und homologen Transplantaten. VASA 1976, 5: 313—318.

Ochsner J. L. De Camp P. T., Leonard G. L.: Experience with fresh venous allografts as an arterial substitute. Ann. Surg. 1971, 173: 933—939.

Perloff L. J., Reckard R. R., Rowlands D. T., Barker C. F.: The venous homograft; an immunological question. Surg. 1972, 72: 961—970

Staudacher M.: Die homologe Transplantation des gefriergetrockneten Vene. Ein experimenteller Beitrag zum Problem Gefässersatz. VASA 1974, Supp. 2: 1—20.

G. D., Centre Hospitalier de Mulhouse avenue d'Altkirch 68051 — Mulhouse— Cedex, France

THE EFFECT OF BLOOD FLOW ON VEIN GRAFTS IN THE ARTERIAL BED

J. PIRK, B. RADEVIČ, V. RUŽBARSKÝ, P. FIRT and L. HEJHAL

Institute for Clinical and Experimental Medicine, Prague, Czechoslovakia

Long-term follow-up studies of aorto-coronary bypasses have shown in some narrowing of the lumen and late occlusions (*Johnson*, 1970). In contrast, control angiography of autovenous aortorenal reconstructions showed the vein grafts in the aortorenal area to dilate (*Dean*, 1974). We have found no satisfactory explanation in the literature for the different behaviour of vein autografts. Analysis of haemodynamic relations prevailing in these bypasses led us to infer that blood flow may be the causal factor in this processs. We therefore decided to test the validity of this hypothesis by experiment on dogs.

In the first group of dogs we bypassed the abdominal aorta between the origin of the renal and iliac arteries by a simple aortoaortic bypass using the jugular vein and ligated the aorta. In the second group we constructed a bilateral aortoiliac bypass. To decrease blood flow, we narrowed the lumen by ligature. We measured the blood flow, blood pressure and diameter of the bypass (see Fig. 1.). The experiment was terminated after six

months. We dissected the whole reconstruction and measured the same quantities as at the start of the experiment (see Fig. 2.). To assess the effect of flow rate on the altered bypass lumen, we put all reconstructions in one group, ordered them by flow from the lowest to the highest and calculated the regression line equations. A direct, statistically highly significant relationship was found between the flow rate and change of the lumen.

Our findings indicate that flow rate is the principal mechanical factor affecting the fate of vein grafts under physiological conditions. The mechanism by which the rate of flow affects these processes is still speculative. In view of the close relationship between macroscopic and microscopic changes it seems possible that the flow rate is affected by these changes. In the second part of the study we concentrated on this hypothesis.

Dilatation is the morphological hallmark of high-flow grafts. Their walls are much thinner. The intima has segmentary or circular proliferation not more than

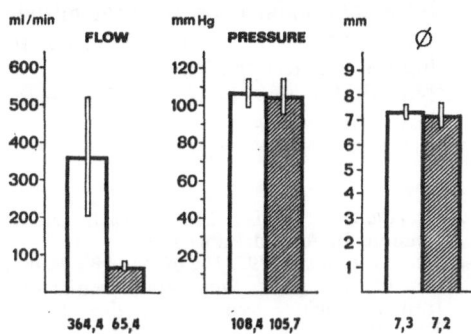

Fig. 1. Graphical comparison of the initial values in Group I (empty columns) and Group II (hatched columns).

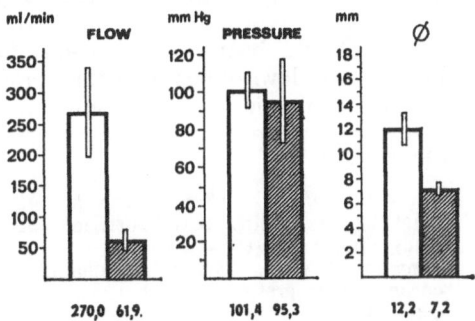

Fig. 2. Comparison of values after 6 months in Group I (empty columns) and Group II (hatched columns).

259

150 μ in thickness. The most characteristic morphological feature of low-flow by-passes are proliferative changes of varied thickness leading to near complete occlusion of the lumen. This subendothelial proliferation consists of a network of collagen fibres containing smooth muscle cells. Some are oriented down-stream.

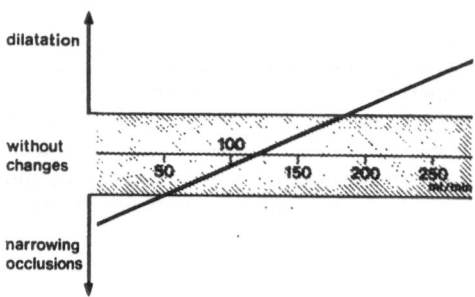

Fig. 3. Graphical representation of the long-term fate of vein grafts in relation to flow rate.

The results confirmed our hypothesis. After six months, high-flow grafts showed diffuse dilatation, increasing the initial lumen by an average of 70%. The outer diameters of low-flow veins were unaltered, their lumina, however, exhibiting different degrees of narrowing. Analysis of the fates of individual grafts demonstrated a highly significant statistical relationship between flow and diameter changes. Comparison of histological and clinical findings showed agreement of the findings between high-flow grafts and aortorenal bypasses, and between low-flow bypasses and aortocoronary bypasses.

To explain the mechanism underlying the changes of vein grafts in the arterial bed, we should bear in mind that, in addition to the laws of hemodynamics, the biological properties of the venous wall

and blood are also important, particulary the damage caused to the vein on surgery (*Stanley*, 1975). Endothelial injury completely changes the properties of the vein inner surface.

On the basis of our experimental results, reports in the literature and application of the laws of haemodynamics, we propose that the following mechanism is involved in the changes of vein grafts in the arterial system. A vein damaged by surgery is placed in the high-pressure system of the arterial bed. Its wall is thus exposed to a higher than physiological tangential force. At low blood flow, platelets and fibrin tend to aggregate on the altered inner surface and mural trombus develops (*McDonald*, 1962). The vein lumen narrows and the tangential force dilating the vein decreases. Moreover, progressive organisation of mural thrombosis and proliferation of medial elements reinforce the wall. The vein is incapable of dilating. At high blood flow the mural thrombus cannot grow since its particles are carried away by the blood stream. The lumen of the vein is wide, its wall is exposed to high tangential force and the vein dilates. The following conclusions can be drawn for the clinical use of vein autografts:

1. Veins are not suited for bypasses with low flow rates of less than 50 ml/min. and for high flow rates exceeding 150 ml/min.
2. Veins are suited for medium flow rate bypasses ranging from 50 to 150 ml/min.
3. Porous prostheses are recommended for high flow rate bypasses.
4. No suitable material is available for low flow rate bypasses.

REFERENCES

Dean, R. H. et al. (1974): Saphenous vein aorto-renal by-pass grafts: Serial arteriographic study. Ann. Surg. 180, 469—478.
Johnson, w. D. et al. (1970): Late changes in coronary vein grafts. Amer. J. Cardiol., 26, 640—646.

McDonald D. A. (1962): Blood flow in arteries. London, E. Arnold Publ. 306.
Stanley, J. C. et al. (1975): Comparative evaluation of vein graft. Preparation media: Electron and light microscopic studies. J. Surg. Res. 18, 235—246.

J. P. Department of Surgery, Institute for Clinical and Experimental Medicine, Vídeňská 800, 146 22 Prague 4, Czechoslovakia

DOES THE GRAFTED FEMORAL VEIN "ARTERIALIZE"?

J. CSENGÖDY and E. MONOS

*3rd Department of Surgery and Experimental Research Institute,
Semmelweis Medical University, Budapest, Hungary*

Introduction

Surgical correction of blood supply disturbances in the lower extremities is frequently applied and amounts to approximately 80 per cent of total vascular reconstructive operations. About two thirds of them involve surgical treatment of segmental femoral artery obstructions. Although several operative methods have been suggested, the best results can be expected from a femoro-popliteal bypass with autogenous vein and thus this procedure is chosen in most cases. Vein grafts usually ensure a fairly lasting improvement in femoral blood supply and their histological structure tends to become "arterialized" gradually (*Csengödy et al.*, 1976; *Szilágyi et al.*, 1964; *De Weese et al.*, 1966). Some weeks following the grafting all three layers in the venous wall are thickened markedly: the intima proliferation is accompanied by fibroblast and collagen accumulation; the amount of collagenic, elastic and muscular elements

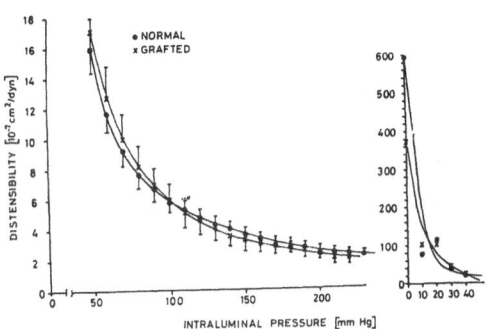

Fig. 2. Incremental distensibilities of normal and grafted femoral veins (relaxed smooth muscle) as functions of intraluminal pressure. The distensibility is inversely proportional to the elastic modulus and to the wall thickness/radius ratio.

is increased in the media; an increase in collagen content can be found in the adventitia as well.

To properly evaluate the function of the grafted veins, it is necessary to know whether or not this histological "arterialization" leads to a hemodynamic "arterialization" of the vessel. The purpose of the present work was to elucidate this problem in a canine experimental model.

Methods

Four to five cm sections of autogenous femoral veins were grafted end-to-end into the contralateral femoral arteries of 9 anaesthetized dogs of 19—25 kg body weight. Three to seven months after the surgical operation a 2 cm cylindrical segment of the "arterialized" vein was transected for testing its passive and active incremental mechanical properties *in vitro*. Ten normal, nongrafted canine veins served as controls.

Large-deformation mechanical test (*Cox*, 1974; *Monos et al.* 1978) was applied by continuously changing (100 mmHg/min) the intraluminal pressure in a 0—250 mmHg range at fixed *in vivo* length of the vein segment. The outer diameter and axial extending force were registered as functions of pressure. The curves were

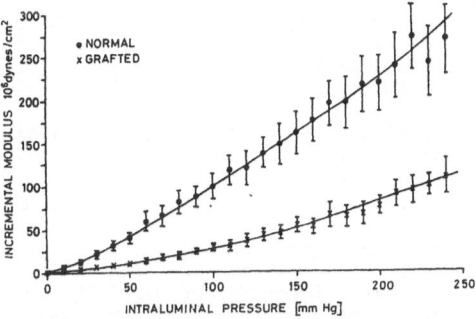

Fig. 1. Incremental elastic moduli of normal and grafted veins (relaxed smooth muscle) as a function of intraluminal pressure. These moduli characterize the specific stiffness of the passive vessel wall elements for 10 mmHg pressure increments.

261

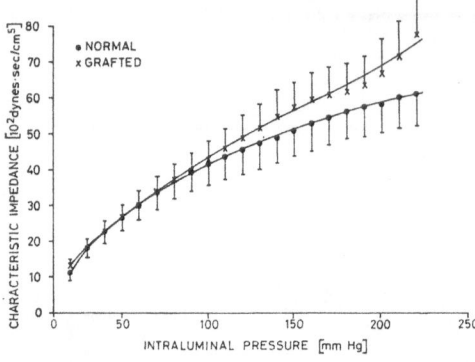

Fig. 3. Characteristic impedances of normal and grafted femoral veins (relaxed smooth muscle) as functions of intraluminal pressure. The vascular impedance, being a ratio of Fourieramplitudes of oscillating pressure and flow, can also be calculated from elastic and geometric parameters of the vessel.

digitalized by 10 mmHg pressure increments, then using these data and the wall volume the following biomechanical variables were computed: normal mechanical stresses (tangential, radial, axial), strain-energy density (SED), incremental tangential elastic modulus (E), incremental distensibility (D), characteristic impedance (Z), strains, and radius to wall thickness ratio (R/h).

Results and conclusions

Three to seven months following implantation normal passive stresses, SED

E and R/h of the grafted veins were by 70–80 per cent lower than those of the controls in the whole pressure range studied. The increased elasticity (= decreased E) of the grafted venous wall material (Fig. 1.) suggests a tendency for hemodynamic "arterialization", as it is known that arteries are more elastic at arterial pressure loadings then normal veins (*Attinger*, 1973). However, wall thickening, i.e. a decrease in R/h, compensates for the decreased elasticity with respect to D (Fig. 2.) and thus values of Z also remain practically the same as in normal veins (Fig. 3.). Norepinephrine (5 µg/ml) induced an active strain only in the grafted veins with a maximum of 5–7 per cent in the 0–10 mmHg intraluminal pressure range. The response was negligible in the arterial pressure range; thus smooth muscle tone probably does not substantially modify the mechanical properties (*Cox*, 1976) of veins grafted into arteries.

It was concluded in accordance with *Wesly et al.*, (1975) that canine femoral veins exposed to permanent arterial conditions behave like rigid tubes at arterial pressure levels, similarly to normal veins. Only a virtual tendency to hemodynamic "arterialization" can be demonstrated in the grafted veins.

REFERENCES

Attinger, E. O. (1973): Structure and function of the peripheral circulation. In: Engineering Principles in Physiology, edited by J. H. U. Brown and D. S. Gann. New York: Academic Press., vol. II., pp. 3–47.

Csengödy, J., Zájer, J., Jánossa, M. (1976): Metabolic properties of veins functioned as femoropopliteal arterial bypass. Congress of Hungarian Society of Surgeons, Debrecen. In Hungarian.

Cox, R. H. (1976): Effects of norepinephrine on mechanics of arteries in vitro. Am. J. Physiol. 231, 420–425.

Monos E. (1977): Biomechanical properties of the arterial wall. In: Actual Problems of Biology, edited by G. Csaba. Budapest: Medicina, vol. 9, pp. 73–131. (In Hungarian).

Monos, E., Cox, R. H., Peterson, L. H. (1978): Relationship between biomechanical factors and vascular reactions during activation by physiological doses of norepinephrine and vasopressin in vitro. Acta physiol. Acad. Sci. hung. In Press.

Szilágyi, D. E., Smith, R. F., Elliot, J. P. (1964): Venous autografts in femoropopliteal arterioplasty. Arch. Surg. 89, 113–125.

De Weese, J. A., Terry, R., Barner, B., Rob, Ch. G. (1966): Autogenous venous femoropopliteal bypass grafts. Surgery, 59, 28–36.

Wesly, R. L. R., Vaishnav, R. N., Fuchs, J. A. C., Patel, D. J., Greenfield, J. C. Jr. (1975): Static linear and nonlinear elastic properties of normal and arterialized venous tissue in dog and man. Circ. Res. 37, 509–520.

J. C., 3rd Department of Surgery Semmelweis Medical University, Nagyvárad tér 1., 1096 Budapest, Hungary

ULTRASTRUCTURAL INVESTIGATIONS OF EXPERIMENTAL VENOUS GRAFTS

MARGIT JÁNOSSA, J. CSENGÖDY, ANNA KÁDÁR and J. ZÁJER

2nd Department of Pathology, Central Electron Micrscopic Laboratory, Semmelweis Medical University and 3rd Department of Surgery, Budapest, Hungary

Introduction

There has been a renewed interest in recent years in the use of autogenous veins as graft material for arterial by-pass in peripheral arterial obstructions. The results of these types of replacement or by-pass vary and are to a certain extent unpredictable. Thus veins implanted into the arterial circulation have an "arterial role" in transmission of arterial blood with considerably higher pressure. This new task can presumably be fulfilled only by reorganization of the venous wall. After an initial inflammatory response, thickening and fibrosis of the venous wall occurred (*McCabe et al.*, 1967).

Our interest was focused on structural changes of the venous wall under the new functional conditions. Intimal thickening and proliferation occurring in the implants were evaluated as "arterialization".

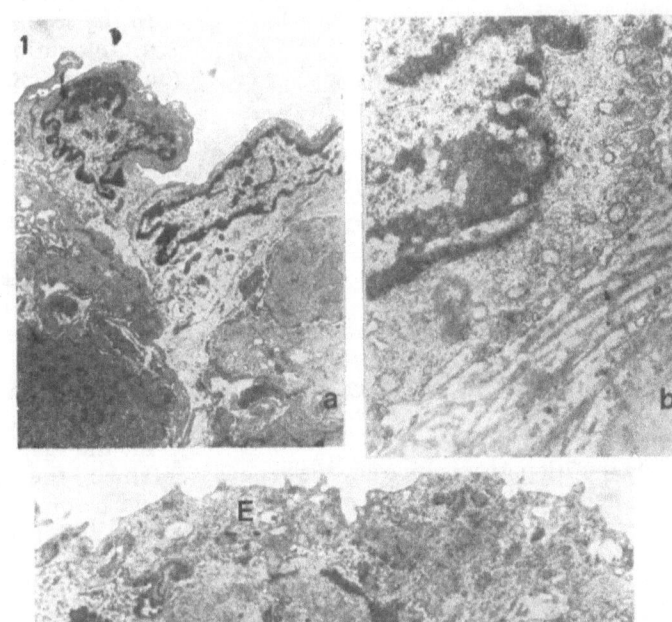

1.a. Normal control femoral dog vein TEM $\times$ 5 920 UA + Pb

b. Normal control femoral dog artery. TEM $\times$ 16 800 UA + Pb

c. One-week venous graft. Intimal proliferation.
E = endothelial cell
S = smooth muscle cell
B = basal membranlike material
TEM $\times$ 12 600 UA + Pb

2.a. Two-week venous graft. Intimal proliferation.
E = endothelial cell
S = smooth muscle cell
El = elastic fiber
C = collagen fiber
TEM × 12 600
UA + Pb

b. Two-week venous graft. Within the widened subendothelial space are some cells originating from the circulating blood.
TEM × 8 400
UA + Pb.

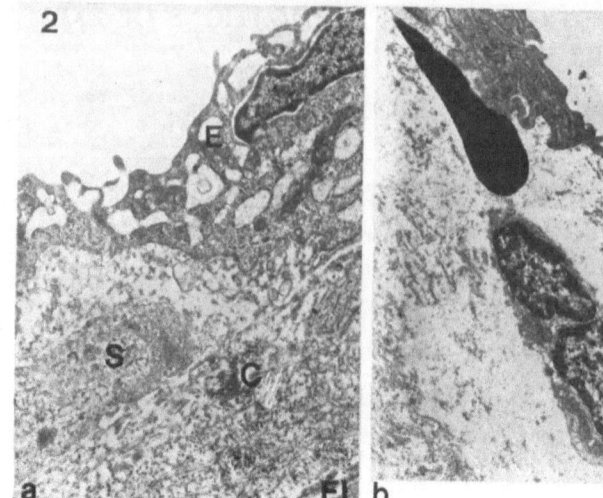

Material and method

The experiments were carried out on 27 dogs. Preparations for anastomoses were made using an "end to side" technique on the femoral artery, using the femoral vein as an autogenous graft. The lengths of the anastomoses were about 3 cm. The morphological changes were studied from the first week of implantations up to 8 months following implantation.

For ultrastructural investigations conventional electron microscopical methods were used.

Only 3 venous grafts of 27 were unable to function because thrombotic obliteration developed during the first days.

Results

Striking intimal proliferation has been found in each graft from the 7th day up to 8 months following the operation. This intimal thickening was covered by a smooth endothelial layer.

On the 7th postoperative day the venous graft had a cell-rich intimal proliferation covered with an endothelial layer (Fig. 1. c.). Increased activity of the endothelial cells was found, e.g. many surface processes and an increased number of dilated pinocytotic vessicles. A widening of the subendothelial layer could be seen. Basal membranelike material and fibrin deposits could be distinguished. The smooth muscle cells in this intimal proliferation exhibited some degenerative changes. A basal

membrane thickening around each smooth muscle cells and electron dense and electron lucent mitochondrial alterations could be detected.

In the second postoperative week (Fig. 2. a.) alterations were similar to those found at the end of the first week: however, elastic fibers and some collagen fibers could be distinguished in the thickened intimal layer of the venous grafts. Subendothelially multilayered basement membranes were visible. Some cells originating from the circulating blood could be observed within the widened subendothelial space (Fig. 2. a.) and intensive elastic fiber production was noted in the 8th month after implantation in the venous graft (Fig. 3. a.). In the subendothelial space a leukocyte could be detected (Fig. 3. b.).

In the gap of the laminae elastica internae, smooth muscle cell migration could be observed in the arterial segment at the proximal part of the venous graft (Fig. 3. c.).

Discussion

In the autogenous veins, implanted into the femoral artery of dogs as by-pass, the following observations were made.

A structural transformation occurs from the 7th postoperative day. This reveals

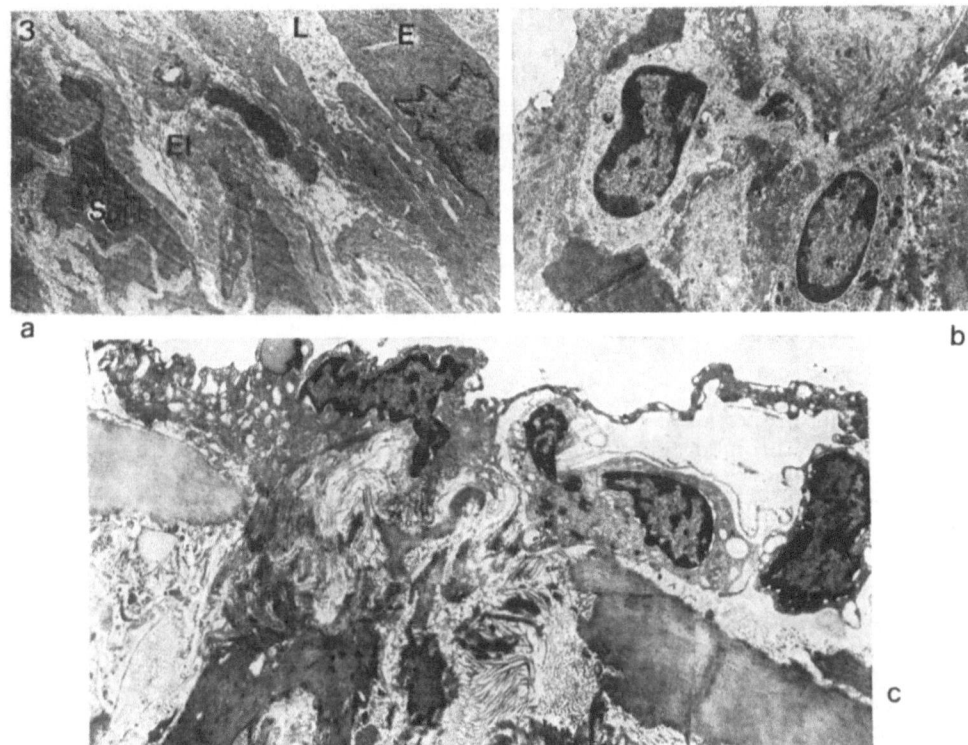

3.a. Eigth-month venous graft. Intimal proliferation.
     L = lumen
     E = endothelial cell
     S = smooth muscle cell
     El = elastic fiber
   TEM × 5 040 UA + Pb
  b. Eigth-month venous graft. In the subendothelial space is a leukocyte-like cell. TEM × 8 400 UA + Pb
  c. Arterial segment at the proximal part of the venous graft. Smooth muscle cell migration in the gap of laminae elasticae internae. TEM × 8 400 UA + Pb.

intimal proliferation and an enhanced production of extracellular material including elastic fibres. In the first weeks the intimal proliferation has a cell-rich appearance, later it becomes "cell-poor".

The arterialization of the venous wall could be explained by endothelial activity involving occurrence of a multilayered basal membrane, by proliferation of the smooth muscle cells and by the striking fibre production, including elastic tissue.

The transformation can develop from the arterial side from which the migration and proliferation of the smooth muscle cells may originate. The cellular elements of the circulating blood may also play an important role in this process.

M. J., 2nd Department of Pathology, Semmelweis Medical University,
Nagyvárad tér 1, 1096 Budapest, Hungary

ROLE OF CHEMICAL MODIFICATION OF SURFACE PROPERTIES ON THE LONG—TERM PATENCY OF VASCULAR PROSTHESES

H. MATSUMOTO, H. MATSUNAGA, M. AYMAMOTO,
T. TAKAMATSU, E. FUKADA and M. SAIGUSA

Dept. of Thorac. & Cardiovas. Surg., Univ. of Tokyo,
Dept. of Thorac. Surg., Saitama Cancer Center,
and Inst. of Phys. & Chem., Saitama, Japan

Introduction

The surface properties of polymers play a major role in thrombogenic effects at the sites of vascular implants. Among the hydrophobic polymers available for vascular prostheses, the fisrt application of expanded polytetrafluoroethylene (EPTFE) to vascular prostheses was reported by the authors (*Matsumoto*, 1972) and by Soyer (*Soyer*, 1972). Clinically, EPTFE vascular prostheses have been used in 60 000 patients as substitutes for the reconstruction of peripheral arteries and large veins as well as the construction of aorto-pulmonary shunts and blood access, all over the world. In our studies, in which the interaction between the blood and the surfaces of synthetic polymers is taken as an interfacial phenomenon, the surface properties of synthetic polymers are investigated with attention focused on their hydrophobicity and hydrophilicity (*Matsumoto*, 1975). As a result of our extensive research aimed at developing antithrombogenic materials, we believe that the coexistence of both hydrophobicity and hydrophilicity in a definite distribution density is necessary for such materials. This is because it appears unlikely that surface factors do not act on the interface between the blood and the biomaterials, namely, the cardiovascular endothelial lining.

Now the role of chemical modification of surface properties on the long-term patency of vascular prostheses will be discussed.

Methods and materials

Microporous EPTFE and woven Teflon prostheses were chosen as the backbones because of their chemical and mechanical properties and their biological inertness. EPTFE and Teflon prostheses can be easily radiation-grafted with hydrophilic or hydrophobic chemical groups. Polyvinylalcohol, polyvinylacetate, polystyrene and polymethylmethacrylate were chosen because they are easily grafted onto EPTFE and Teflon prostheses with a diameter of 10−12 mm. The grafting reaction was carried out in a glass tube after removal of gas at a low temperature and vaccum sealing. A ^{60}Co gamma irradiation sourse was used. The sample was grafted at different temperatures and different dose rates. Immersed tubes were irradiated and submitted to constant stirring. After irradiation, samples were washed and then vacuum-dried. The graft

Table I.

Materials	Follow up (Days)	Patency Rate (U)
Expanded Polytetrafluoroethylene (n = 16)	$\bar{m} = 124$	93.8
Expanded Polytetrafluoroethylene-Vinylalcohol (n = 7)	$\bar{m} = 71$	85.0
Polytetrafluoroethylene-Methylmethacrylate (n = 6)	$\bar{m} = 62$	66.7
Expanded Polytetrafluoroethylene-Vinylacetate (n = 16)	$\bar{m} = 88$	50.0
Expanded Polytetrafluoroethylene-Styrene (n = 13)	$\bar{m} = 60$	38.5
Polytetrafluoroethylene-Methylmethacrylate-OH (n = 11)	$\bar{m} = 82$	27.5

ing ratio is expressed as: $G\% = (W^* - W)/W \times 100$, where W and W^* are the weights before and after grafting, respectively. Before use, each sample was washed several times and its surface properties determined. All vascular prostheses were inserted into the vena cava superior, vena cava inferior and portal veins of dogs for the purpose of determing the effects of chemical modification on the long-term patency. They were removed from 60 to 124 days after implantation.

Results

The results of the evaluation experiment are summarized in table 1. Synthetic polymers used are indicated on the left and the percentage of the prostheses which remained open is shown on the right. The patency of the prostheses was inversely proportional to the increase of γc. As is obvious from the findings obtained by visual observation, the amount of thrombi formed on the inner surfaces of prostheses varied according to the surface properies of the synthetic polymers, resulting from their chemical structures. In EPTFE vascular prostheses whose surface properties were close to those of the cardio-vascular endothelial lining, the amount of thrombi formed was very small. In addition, a scanning electron microscopic study showed neointimizations, even in 15 — 20 cm long implants.

Conclusions

The results of the present study indicate that the role of hydrophilic groups on surfaces on the long-term patency of vascular prostheses made of a hydrophobic polymer are essential and that there is a limitation to the coexistence of hydrophilicity and hydrophobicity.

REFERENCES

Matsumoto, H., Fuse, K., Yamamoto, M., Hasegawa, T., Saigusa, M., Uei, I. (1972): Studies on the porous polytetrafluoroethylene as the vascular prosthesis. Artificial Organs. 1, 44.

Soyer, T., Lempinen, M., Norton, L., Eiseman, B. (1972): A new venous prosthesis. Surgery. 72, 864.

Matsumoto, H., Kimura, T., Takamatsu, T., Fukada, E. (1975): The mechanical behaviors on nonthrombogenicity. The full manuscript of the 1975 symposium on biomaterials.

H. M., Dept. of Thoracic & Cardiovas. Surg., University of Tokyo, 7-3-1 Hongo, Bunkyo-Ku, Tokyo 113, Japan

ADAPTIVE CHANGES IN THE INTERNAL DIAMETER OF THE CAROTID ARTERY TO PROLONGED SHEAR STRESS LOAD AND ITS RELATIONSHIP TO THE OPTIMALITY PRINCIPLE OF THE VASCULAR TREE

A. KAMIYA

Institute for Medical and Dental Engineering,
Tokyo Medical and Dental University, Tokyo, Japan

Introduction

Recent investigations on atherosclerosis (*Fry*, 1968; *Patel et al.*, 1974.) have demonstrated that the shear stress exerted on the vascular surface by the adjacent blood flow plays an important role, not only in the pathogenesis of this disease, but also in the physiological adaptation of the vascular wall. When very great shear stress was loaded, it caused the erosion of the endothelial cell layer followed by blunt pathological changes in histology similar to those in the early lesion of the atherosclerosis. However, moderately increased shear stress simply resulted in physiological adaptive response, i.e., fibromuscular hyperplasia and dilatation of the vascular wall, probably induced through the increased transendothelial protein permeability and the consequent protein accumulation in the intima.

The fact that the increased shear stress causes vascular dilatation suggests that there may be some autoregulatory mechanism of shear stress in the adaptive response. As shear stress (Ss) for laminar flow is given by $Ss = 4\eta f/(\pi r^3)$ where η is blood viscosity, f is the flow rate and r is the vessel radius, an increase in Ss by a steady increase in f will be, in turn, reduced by the adaptive enlargement of r. If and only if Ss is the predominant regulating factor of the adaptive response, can Ss be regulated by the feedback mechanism to remain constant regardless of flow increase or decrease. This study was designed to experimentally examine the above hypothesis of constant shear stress.

Methods

An arterio-venous shunt was constructed between the common carotid artery and the

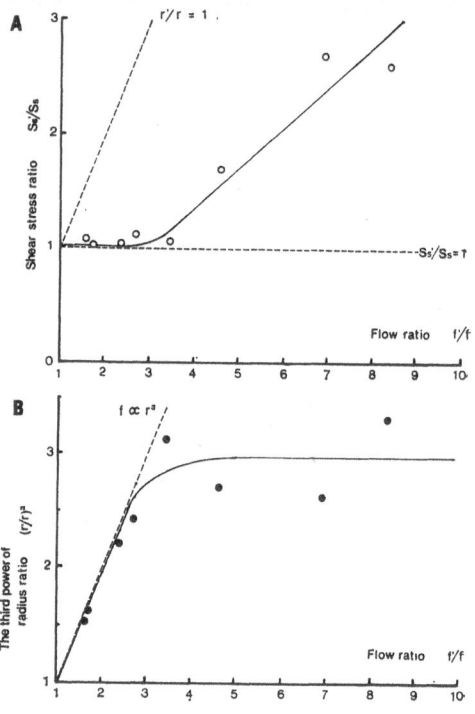

Fig. 1. The upper part: The relationship between the shear stress ratio (Ss'/Ss) and flow ratio (f'/f) obtained in the experiments. The broken line (Ss'/Ss = 1) indicates complete regulation of shear stress by the adaptive response. The broken line (r'/r = 1) indicates the state of no regulation. Notice that when f'/f was less than 4, almost complete regulation was attained.
The lower part: The relationship between the third power of radius ratio and the flow ratio. Notice that when f'/f was larger than 4, the adaptive enlargement of the vascular radius (r'/r) was saturated.

external jugular vein in 8 dogs. Six months after the operation, the blood flow rate, the mean distending pressure and the pressure-volume relationship of the closed segment were measured at the carotid artery proximal to the shunt. The same measurements were carried out at the contralateral control artery sham-operated.

The arterial internal radius was determined from the mean distending pressure during flow measurement and the pressure-radius relationship transformed from the pressure-volume diagram. Using the obtained data of radius r and flow rate f, Reynolds number and shear stress were calculated.

Results

The results showed that the flow rate at the shunted artery f' was, on an average, about 4 times greater than that of the control artery f, while the shear stress at the shunted artery Ss' was only 55% greater than the control Ss due to the compensatory effect of the adaptive enlargement in the shunted arterial radius r' which was 33% greater than the control arterial radius r. Furthermore, as shown in Figure 1, when the flow ratio$\leftrightarrow$f'/f was less than 4 (in 5 animals), the compensatory effect of the adaptive radius enlargement r'/r was so complete that the stress ratio Ss'/Ss became almost equal to unity. This result indicated that, at least for moderate increases in flow rate, shear stress was regulated at a constant level by the local feedback mechanism involved in the adaptive response of the vascular wall. Thus the hypothesis of constant shear stress was verified.

Discussion

When shear stress is regulated constantly as in this experiment a flow-radius relationship $4\,\eta f\,(\pi r^3)$ is valid. The same flow-radius relationship has been predicted by the optimality theory of the vascular tree (*Murray*, 1926). Hence, the regulatory feedback mechanism optimizes the function of the vascular system as the conduit for blood circulation minimalizing the total energy loss, i.e., the sum of the mechanical energy loss due to viscous friction resistance and the chemical energy loss proportional to blood volume necessary to maintain that amount of blood fresh and functional. (If r is too small, the mechanical energy loss becomes too great and if r is too large, the chemical energy loss becomes too great.) Its is concluded that the optimum vascular system can ben actually built up *in vivo* by the local autoregulatory mechanism of shear stress substantiated in this study.

REFERENCES

Fry, D. L. (1968): Acute vascular endothelial changes associated with increased blood velocity gradients. Circ. Res. 22, 165—197.

Murray, C. D. (1926): The physiological principle of minimum work I, Proc. nat. Acad. Sci. 12, 207.

Patel, D. J., Vaishnav, R. N., Gow, B. S., Kot, P. A. (1974): Hemodynamics. Annual Rev. Physiol. 36, 125—154.

A. K., Institute for Medical and Dental Engineering, Tokyo Medical and Dental University, 2-3-10 Surugadai, Kanda, Chiyodaku, Tokyo, Japan

USE OF THE UMBILICAL CORD FOR RECONSTRUCTIVE VASCULAR SURGERY

A. NISHIMURA, Y. SAWADA, Y. NAKANISHI, F. SANO,
Y. KASAI and T. KOMAI

First Department of Surgery and Department of Polymer Science
University of Hokkaido, Sapporo, Japan

In our search for a better vascular substitute for reconstructions below the inguinal ligament we have focused our attention on human umbilical cord veins since 1969. The favorable features of umbilical cord veins as a vascular substitute are uniform internal diameter, sufficient length, valveless and unbranched conduit, tough amniotic covering, ready and unlimited supply and minimal antigenicity.

The umbilical cord vein was first used experimentally in 1951 by Anzola et al. Since his first report on heterologous umbilical cord vessel implants, several investigators have made experimental studies for a new source of vascular graft. These earlier experiments, however, almost all failed due to denaturation of the implanted tissue. In 1969 Sawada, one of the co-authors, employed an umbilical cord chemically modified and preserved using ethyl alcohol and reported very encouraging results in canine experiments of aortic substitution.

Following very favorable experience with these animal implantations the first clinical use of an alcohol-preserved umbilical cord vein was made in 1975 for a femoro-popliteal bypass in a 78 year-old patient with severe disabling ischemia associated with gangrene.

In attempt to obtain more a desirable method of chemical modification, further studies were made on various tissue preparations of the material, that is, grafts treated with saline, alcohol, glutaraldehyde and formaldehyde. The laboratory study includes the pressure tolerance test, the stress-strain profile, the amino-acid analysis and the molecular characterization.

Stress-strain curves were obtained at a constant elongation rate of 1 mm/min, and demonstrated the marked reinforcing effect of alcohol and glutaraldehyde. In alcohol-treated material, however, the mechanical properties deteriorate to the level of the raw material after storage in saline. The materials become correspondingly more rigid and less flexible at higher concentrations of glutaraldehyde. We therefore selected a 1.0% solution of glutaraldehyde which resulted in the best mechanical properties to produce allografts for clinical use. (Fig. 1). It is widely known that the tanning procedure with glutaraldehyde increases the strength of the graft by crosslinking collagen. To identify the number of crosslinks aminoacid analysis was performed. Each amino-acid component was normalized as 100 glycine residues. The component ratios of proline, alanine and glycine did not change. A significant decrease in the content of lysine residue was observed following the glutaraldehyde treatment, regardless of its concentration in a range from 0.3 to 1.5%. On the other hand, alcohol treatment caused no changes et all. (Fig. 2).

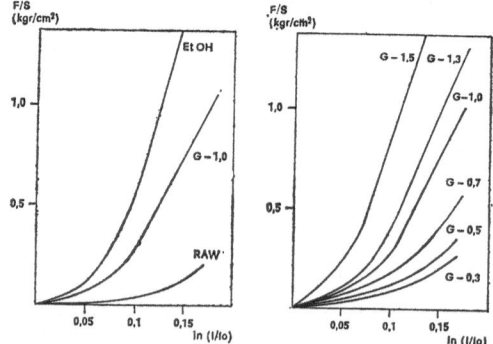

Fig. 1. Stress-strain profile of human umbilical cord vein grafts.

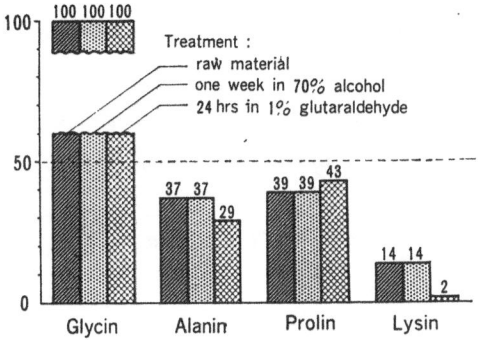

Fig. 2. Amino acid components of umbilical cord (Expressed in ratio vs. Glycin 100).

The stress-strain profiles suggest that the number of crosslinks is proportional to the concentration of glutaraldehyde. Amino acid analysis showed that glutaraldehyde reacted with material independently of its concentration and only part of the reacting glutaraldehyde might be involved in crosslinkage. Free aldehyde residues might therefore be contained in glutaraldehyde-treated material. This free aldehyde residue still remains reactive and could chemically bond with blood protein after the implantation.

In 18 patients the entire umbilical cord with its amniotic covering was utilized after being treated with alcohol or glutaraldehyde. The initial two patients were operated on using the alcohol-treated allograft. In the second case a proximal portion of the graft was found to be slightly ectatic immediately after the implantation. However, it has remained unchanged with an otherwise uneventful postoperative course for 28 months.

As one of the investigators in the international project for FDA approval we implanted 10 Dardik Biografts in a variety of vascular reconstructions. In 4 out of 5 femoro-posterior tibial bypasses

umbilical cord veins were employed as composite grafts with autogenous saphenous veins. In a total of 28 implantations, excluding one case of unrelated death, an over-all patency rate of 82% was achieved. The longest follow-up now extends to 30 months. There was no significant difference in the patency rates between the Biografts and our Biocords. There was only one failure in patients with arterial grafts above the knee-joint. The patency rate of the reconstructions below the knee-joint was 42.8%. With regard to morbidity we had no serious complications in this series. (Table I).

Table I.

	BIO-CORD	BIOGRAFT	Total
BYPASS			
Axillo-Axillary	0	3	3
Ilio-Femoral	1	0	1
Femoro-Femoral	9 (1)	1	10 (1)
Femoro-Popliteal			
Above-Knee	2	1	3
Below-Knee	1	0	1
Femoro-Post. Tibial*	1 (1)	4 (2)	5 (3)
Femoro-Ant. Tibial	1 (1)	0	1 (1)
REPLACEMENT			
Patch, CFA, CIA	2	0	2
Common Femoral A.	1	1	2
	18 (3)	10 (2)	28 (5)

* Composite Graft

In utilizing our grafts it is necessary to trim the ends prior to the anastomosis. It is important to make sure that every suture passes through the intima of the umbilical cord vein. Bearing in mind these technical details, it is easy to perform a smooth anastomosis despite the disparity between the thickness of our grafts and the host arteries.

Finally it should be emphasized that long-term follow-up studies are essential to assess the further durability of these two types of umbilical allograft with quite different coverings; one with polyester net and another with natural amniotic sheath.

REFERENCES

Anzola, J., et al. (1951): Surgical Forum 2: 243.
Dardik, H., et al. (1975): Surgical Forum 26: 286.
Nishimura, A., et al. (1976): Proceed. 10th Intern. Cong. Angiology 496 p.

Sawada, Y., et al. (1970): J. of Japanese College of Angiology 10: 397.
Sawada, Y., et al. (1977): Artificial Organs 6: 316.
Sawada, Y., et al. (1978): Japanese J. of Surgical Society 79: 382.

A. N., 1st Department of Surgery, University of Hokkaido N-15, W-7, Sapporo, Japan

LONG-TERM RESULTS FOLLOWING REPLACEMENT OF THE FEMORAL ARTERY BY PRESERVED DLA-COMPATIBLE FETAL AORTAL GRAFTS IN DOGS

D. A. LOOSE, F. BORCHARD, W. LENZ, P. PFITZER,
H. SCHNAPPAUF and K. KREMER

*Surgical Clinic and Policlinic of Düsseldorf University, Clinic A, and
Institute of Pathology, Düsseldorf University, Düsseldorf,
Ulm University (MNH) Animal Experiments Center, Ulm, F.R.G.*

Experiments were conducted to investigate the function and morphology of fetal aortae transplanted into the femoral arteries of adult beagle dogs to replace stenotic segments of these vessels. By using donor-recipient combinations, which were compatible with the DLA system in the primary histocompatibility complex of the dog, it was attempted to weaken the allograft reaction. We removed eight fetuses on one occasion and nine on a second from three beagle bitches at term. The 26 aortae were removed intact (Fig. 1.) (the lateral branches having been ligated) and subsequently preserved in a nutritional solution (TCM 199 (Difco Lab.), glycerin, antibiotics) at $-80\,°C$ or $-190\,°C$. Studies with cell cultures and DNA cytophotometry showed that some nuclei were still DNA-positive, but with no further capacity for division. Sixteen fetal aortae were transplanted into 13 male and three female beagle dogs with haplotype A 2/B 5. The fetuses had DLA-A 2/ /B 5 homozygotic parents and therefore must also have been homozygotic DLA-A 2/B 5. The recipients had the same haplotype at least once. After preservation periods of one to 89 days segments of the femoral arteries were replaced by the preserved aortae. The nonobliterated grafts were angiographed at approximately one-month intervals (40 to 486 days) and subsequently removed for morphological studies employing light microscopy, scanning and transmission electron microscopy.

On the whole, the aortal grafts tolerated the implantation procedure well, apart from minor haemorrhages from nonligated intercostal arteries. No infection was observed. There was one case of early thrombosis. In five other arteries obliteration occurred in the interim (average duration of perfusion: 130 days). Morphologically, organized thromboses were found at some points in these vessels, with incipient recanalization. In ten animals perfusion was normal up to the time of removal. The control arteriograms revealed four cases of slight vascular tortuosity and in one case a kink in the graft. In one dog a slight dilatation occurred at the aortal arch after transplantation of the thoracic aorta. In the remaining four animals the angiogram showed the form of the aortal graft to be normal (Compare Figs. 2 and 3).

Morphological study of the nonperfused preserved fetal aortae revealed relaxation of the aortal tissue with densely layered elastic lamellae, between which there was

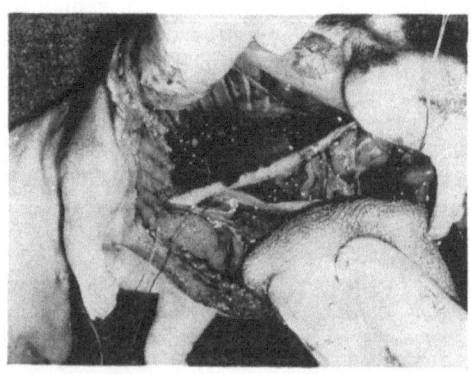

Fig. 1. The situs during removal of the aorta of a beagle fetus.

a large number of minute smoothe embryonal muscle cells with pyknotic nuclei. Electron microscopic studies showed small foci of regressively changed endothelial

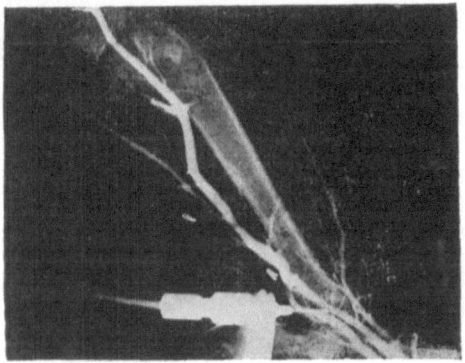

Fig. 2. Angiography of the fetal vascular graft three months after regular circulation. The arrows show the sites of the anastomosis of the interposed vascular graft in the femoral artery of the dog.

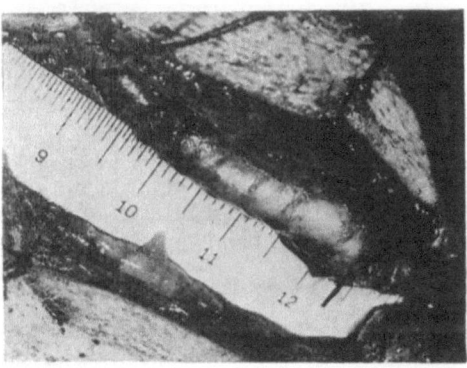

Fig. 3. Same case as in Fig. 2. The situs of the well organized fetal vascular graft three months after implantation.

remnants on the surface. Following perfusion all the vessels were found to have a circumscribed covering of endothelia – some of which were irregularly located – besides fresh, film-like thromboses and very smooth cell-free fibrinous deposits. After several months the smooth muscle cell nuclei disappeared completely and agglomeration and collagenous cicatrization of the elastic lamellae occurred in the media. In two grafts there was a dilatation and in another three there formed a sclerotic pad, caused by recidivous thromboses. Morphologically, there was also evidence of chronic focal inflammation, in particular at the adventitia, in two grafts. These findings make it clear that where the immunological reaction is weak or lacking, increasing degeneration of medial muscle cells and cicatrization at that point will occur. In the lumen, thrombotic processes which contribute to sclerosis of the graft wall are observed at least in the early stage. Later, irregular endothelialization occurs. Whether the dilatations in invididual vessels, described above, should be regarded as the first stage of aneurysms, cannot be stated on the basis of these experiments.

At present the question whether fetal grafts with different tissue antiges are tolerated is still open. It must be answered before a decision can be taken on clinical application. If a weak immune reaction occurs with "nonspecific" homologous transplants, this type of graft, which had an occlusion rate of only 30% in long-term experiments, could play an important role in the replacement of stenotic vessels in the future.

REFERENCES

Borchard, F., Kremer, K., Loose, D. A. (1975): Licht- und elektronenmikroskopische Befunde bei neun autoalloplastischen Arterienprothesen nach Sparks. Thoraxchirurgie 23:83.
Buschard, K., Rygaard, J. (1977): Functional studies of pancreas heterografts in unde mice. Lancet 855.
Weyman, A. K., Plume, S. K., De Weese, J. A. (1975): Bovine heterografts and autogenous veins as canine arterial bypass grafts. Arch. Surg. 110:746.

L. D., Surg. Dept. Univ. of Düsseldorf, Moorenstrasse 5, D-4 Düsseldorf, F.R.G.

HYPEROSTOMY SYNDROME OF THE LEGS, LONG TERM RESULT OF SURGICAL AND MEDICAL TREATMENT

R. C. MAYALL, A. C. D. G. MAYALL, J. C. MAYALL,
U. R. FERRETTI, A. T. BRANDAO and C. M. DUARTE

Hospital da Gamboa, Rio de Janeiro, Brasil

Hyperostomy syndrome was described by Pratesi as an arteriolo-venular disease that simulates an ischemic arterial disease, withcu: evident signs of occlusive arterial disease. More recently this syndrome has been widened and has been observed following some organic venous and lymphatic diseases. Two clinical patterns has been described — first of hyperostomy of unknown origin, and second of hyperostomy appearing together with some organic diseases of the arteries, veins and lymphatics, like obliterative atherosclerosis, post-phlebitic syndrome and diseases with a severe lymphostasis. The most important etiologic factors of this syndrome in the young women is the prolonged use of contraceptive pills, whose hormonal effect produces the venous stasis.

The most important finding of the clinical examination is the disparity between the subjective and objective symptoms and signs. There is always too much complaints and few objective findings in the physician's examination. The oscillometric reading using small cuffs to separate the anterior tibial artery compartment from the calf posterior tibial and fibular artery compartment, helped very much to discover the syndrome in the leg. The skin thermometer is very precise instrument for demonstrating abnormal small shunts below localized areas of the skin at the muscular level due to local hyperostomy.

The serial arteriography under selective conditions of the most affected parts of the legs is the most useful method to confirm the diagnosis. If it is possible to monitor the examination under fluoroscopy using the TV amplifier system the functional diagnostics of this syndrome is much enriched showing, as a rule, the artery stupor and stop page of the blood flow just below the abnormal branching and shunting to the small arteriolo-venular branching.

The most important and pathognomonic findings during arteriography are:
a) first phase arteriography during a simultaneous filling of the arteries and veins, with premature backflow. b) A blurred appearance of the muscle mass around the arteriolar branches during the second or arteriolo-capillar phase, in the places corresponding to the abnormal thermometric and oscillometric findings on the leg. c) Abnormal size, number, extension and direction of arteriolar branches. d) Incomplete or delayed filling of distal arteries of the leg, due to the shunting of the blood flow, as a rule, on the calf. These findings were more common on the posterior tibial and fibular arteries of the leg and on the superficial femoral artery of the thigh. For an accurate mapping of the calf abnormal branching it is advisable to make exposures in different positions of the leg to avoid the superposition of the main trunks of the posterior tibial and fibular arteries and also of the bones.

The conservative treatment is satisfactory at the beginning of the primary process, when there are only functional syndromes. The use of hydrogenated ergotoxine alkaloids is very useful in this stage together with high pressure elastic stockings.

When the hyperostomy syndrome is secondary to an organic pathology, the conservative treatment alone is seldom effective. The surgical interruption of the abnormal branching following the arteriography mapping has very good results in the secondary post-phlebitic and post-lymphedema cases. Some of our patients with severe post-phlebitic syndrome developed suddenly a hyperostomy syndrome. The first case of these series was followed for 14 years without appearance of the symptoms after operation; arteriography performed seven years after surgery has confirmed the success of the precise pre-operative mapping of the abnormal branching.

The surgical treatment of the lymphedemas of the lower legs was completely modified by the interruption of the abnormal arteriolar branching. This complementary operation during Charles operation for dermal-epidermal-lipectomies in the lymphedema patients improved very much the final esthetic appearance and reduced all the per and post operative complications, like hyperkeratosis, acanthosis and hypovolemic shock.

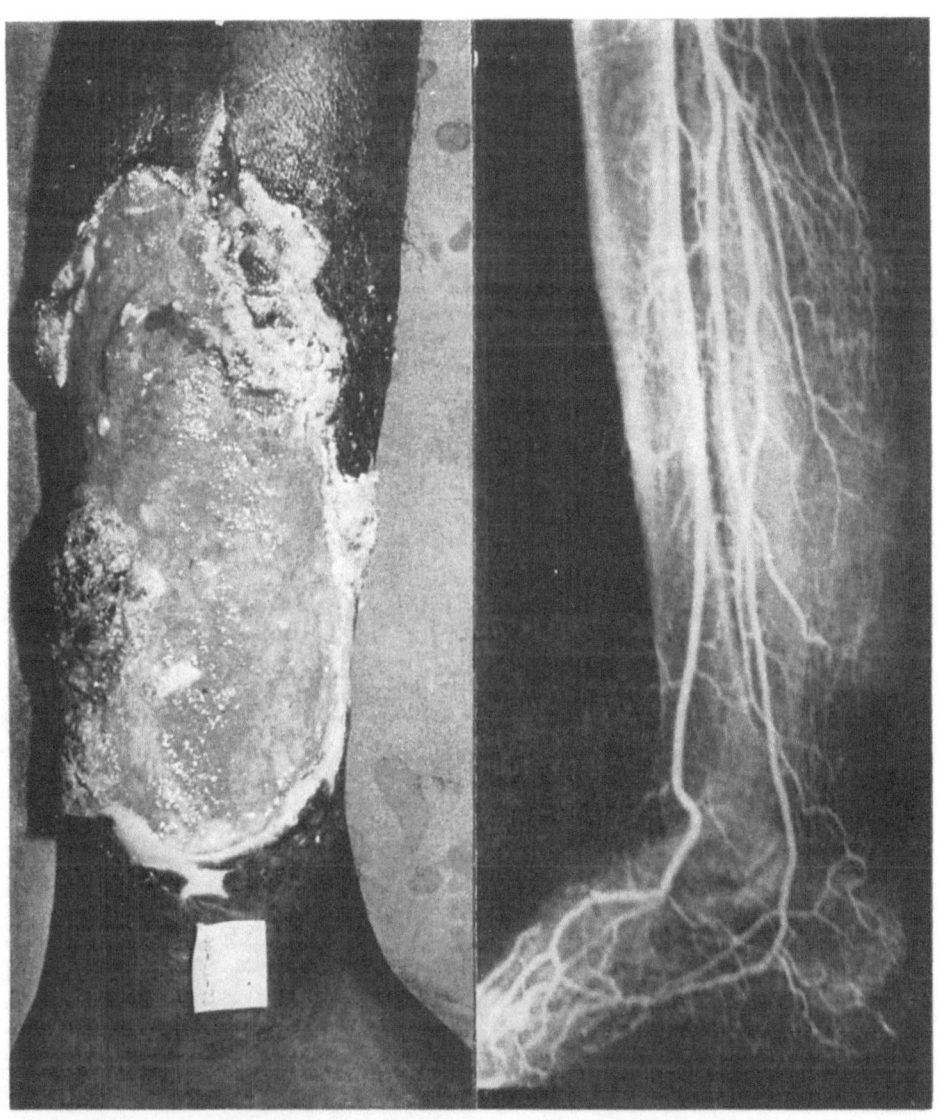

REFERENCES

Amir Jahed, A. K. (1973): Angiodyskinesia, Progress on Angiology. Serv. Ind. Graf. U.F. R.J., Rio de Janeiro, Vol. I: 75—80.

Mayall, R. C. (1976): Sindrome de Hiperostomia— Contribuição ao seu Estudo Clínico e Radiológico. Ed. Graf. Villani Filhos Ltda., Rio de Janeiro.

Mayall, R. C., Mayall, A. C. D. G., Mayall, J. C., Ferreti, U. R., Merhi, E. T., Rojas, J. A., Nobre, J. de C., Villani, M. V.: (1977), Lymphatic malformations and congenital arteriolo-venular abnormalities of the limbs. Hyperostomy syndromes in congenital lymphedemas. In: Progress in Lymphology. Plenum Press, New York.

R. C. M., Caixa Postal 1822 ZC-00, 20.010 Rio de Janeiro — RJ. — Brasil.

EPIDEMIOLOGY AND PREVENTION
OF VASCULAR DISEASES

MEDICAL CARE FOR PATIENTS WITH VASCULAR DISEASES (INDIVIDUAL AND SOCIAL PROBLEMS)

L. GERSON

Neuilly (Paris), France

The prevention of vascular diseases represents at present a big problem for the patient himself as well as for society. The first problem is really a technical and therapeutical one, and the second problem is a problem for humanity and health politics. But both problems are closely linked together, as the solution of the first one depends on the organisation of the second.

A — Therapy for patients with vascular diseases

Such medical care depends upon the diagnostic examination offering data for the therapeutic programme, data on the family and working environment and data on the age of the patient.

I — Patients with atherosclerosis

The examination of patients with atherosclerosis consists of two elements. One determines the stage of the disease and the other depending on risk factors, which may but must not be etiological ones.

a) Initial examination

The medical history is very important, as beside the age of the patient, the duration of the trouble has to be noted, above all temporary lameness, symptoms of brain and motion disorders, heart symptoms and/or digestive troubles. In women, data on the menopausa are of importance.

The examination is only slightly different according to the localisation of the pathological process. The physician has to note the complex of all objective vascular symptoms (of the heart, brain and periphery). The examination is to be completed by an analysis of the risk factors, such as: smoking, obesity, sedentary employment, stress, heredity and arterial hypertension. The metabolism of lipides, glycides, purines, the blood picture, the determination of the number of blood platelets and fibrinogenemia belong to the biological factors. Separate objective indices are the following: changes on the fundus of the eye, changes of the vestibular system and neurological deviations. A part of the functional examination is the Doppler method requiring, however thorough training. Radiology also belongs to the examination methods mentioned above. Although it was a routine examination some years ago, today one has to take into consideration some contraindications. Therefore, it is not suitable in advanced age, in the initial stages of the disease, with suddenly developing forms of the disease and in very weakened patients. This is especially valid for examinations of pharyngeal and vertebral vessels. The radiology serves for the exact demonstration of the collateral circulation.

b) Conclusions of the initial examination

1. Patient with peripheral vascular disorder.

Here, we have to count with disorders of the function of the arteriovenous anastomoses, which are of importance with arterial stenosis. The protection against risk factors and the arrangement of fibrinogenemia should be systematical, even with normal values found. The dispensary examinations depend on three items: on the collaboration of the patient, on the relevance of the vascular disorder and on the collateral circulation and correct therapy. Examinations for checking should be repeated every three years.

The dispensary examination should consist of repeated examinations of the vascular disorders, such as electrocardiographic recording, where the changes may signalize danger to the life of the patient. The basic therapy of atherosclerosis cannot think to cure it, as the characteristics of atheromatosis is generally known. The disappearance of lameness depends rather on the arrangement of the function of arteriovenous anastomoses than on the formation of collateral circulation requiring usually at least two years of treatment. Only after such a period, the dispensary examinations for checking can be less frequent, but should principally be done at least every year. We should not forget, that patients with atherosclerosis most frequently die by heart infarct.

2. Patient with vascular disorder requiring surgical intervention.

This may be e. g. an affection of the aorta bifurcation, a defect of the iliac artery in a young man, a grave affection of the femoral arteries without symptoms of formation of the collateral circulation. Experience shows, that a patient after a surgical intervention for improvement feels healthy. The surgeon as well sees the good result and should agree to the dispensary care for the patient in collaboration with the physician who recommended the operation. It is important for the patients after amputation of a limb and with retarded blood circulation to be further treated by drugs without waiting for the operation wound to scar.

3. Patients with manifestation of atherosclerosis of the carotid and vertebral arteries, who are not treated surgically, should be thoroughly treated by drug therapy, as their condition may become deteriorated suddenly.

4. Patients with coronary atherosclerosis know of the serious nature of their disease, and their dispensary care is regular. It happens frequently, that although the cardiological care is correct, one forgets to care for the arteries of the neck and limbs. Such patients are then examined regularily only with relapses of the disease or with heart complications.

II — Other vascular diseases

a) Raynaud's Disease

Therapeutical difficulties force us to consider carefully, especially with young patients, to think of late scleroderma. We do not think it to be useful to examine such patients, as so far, there is no therapeutic method. A Raynaud's syndrome with collagenoses and hyperglobulias however always requires dispensary care.

b) Aneurysm

After the operation, the therapy depends on the etiology of the disease. Biopsy is therefore essential. Patients, whose aneurysm has not been operated for their age, a reduced resistance capacity, have to rely on drug therapy, which however is only a "defenceless hope".

c) Mega-artery (tumor circulation)

If a surgical intervention is not possible, there remains only to try coagulation.

d) Infectious arteritis and rickettsiosis

The treatment cannot be exactly specified.

e) Periarteritis nodosa and other collagenoses

The treatment of such affections is easier, if the patient has alarming symptoms, and this is to be explained to him.

f) Postphlebitic syndrome

This a special chapter, as the basic disease has not been treated well. Phlebitis represents an entirely different problem than atherosclerosis for the following reasons: Phlebitis are to be found already in young people, and the care for such persons is more difficult, especially if the disease has not been recognized in time. The causes of this disease are different: obesity, statical disorders of the limbs, especially of the feet, arthrosis, standing employment and sometimes also heart and kidney disorders. The patient often comes to the physician already in a progressive stage with an ulcer or extensive hypodermia. The introduction of contraceptives increases the frequency of thromboses. Dispensary care therefore has to be started only after initial drug therapy. especially with segmentary hypertension of swellings, hypodermia and ulcers. The dispensary care should be a longterm one.

B — Social care for patients with vascular diseases

Dispensary Units.

I— Introduction and definitions

As we have already seen, atherosclerosis and the postphlebitic syndrome are dominant among the chronic vascular diseases. Atherosclerosis is a generalized disease with unforeseeable development. The post-phlebitic syndrome is characteristic by the long interval between the primary disease and the consequences appearing unexpected, often after an infection or other intercurrent affections. With these so different diseases, we find cases, where the pathologic occurrences cannot be foreseen, and the physician has to try to prevent permanent effects and deformations. Frequently, we are asked only, if another important affection appears on a terrain, which had to be treated long ago. Now, new problems arise, as well as new expenses for the Social Insurance Office.

Therefore, dispensary care should start for every person, in whom atherosclerosis or thrombosis has been proven. Without doubt, it would be preferable to prevent the atheroma or thrombosis, but a global prevention of such affections, a "check-up" popularly called, derived from the multifactorial genesis of such diseases, is an illusion. In such cases, we have to concentrate upon the systematical dispensary care for everybody, who shows small or great symptoms of premature atherosclerosis or thrombosis, especially early brain symptoms, heart and peripheral atherosclerosis and following thromboses. The social consequences of this secondary prevention are important with regard to financial costs as well as for work disability and/or long-term hospitalisation.

An organisation of dispensary units therefore seems to be less expensive and more profitable. Although we can better imagine specialized hospital units, an out-patient dispensary unit could be enlarged according to need and financial possibilities to a greater organisation unit. Such social institution should be superior to the dispensary units proposed by us.

Concluding, we present a scheme of dispensary units, which doubtless will reduce illness and work disability. We have to take into consideration, that the installation of such units will show useful only after a longer time interval, and therefore, we have to consider short-term financial expenses.

II — Principles of installation of dispensary units

1) A dispensary unit is no therapeutical institution, but an institution for longterm prevention. The following consequences therefore arise:

a) The examination has to be ordered by a physician, and the patient cannot decide upon it himself. It is the physician, who is responsible for the therapy after mutual agreement with the dispensary unit. If the recommending physician is a specialist, e.g. an ophthalmologist, the patient will be called to choose his general practitioner and then to visit a specialist on vascular diseases. The patient will have the possibility to choose his physician, with whom he then remains in permanent connection.

b) The patient will be called for examination once or several times, but he will be hospitalized only if really necessary. Therefore, the connection with the corresponding health center has to be arranged beforehand.

c) The results of the examination will be confirmed in a health certificate stating the health condition of the patient. The procedure has to be economical, taking into consideration previous examinations. The health certificate will be handed to the patient and a copy dispatched to the treating physician.

2) Expenses for the dispensary care will be paid:

a) by the Social Insurance Office, which will check the suitability of the specialized examination. As it is not a research institution, the expenses for a purely scientific examination cannot be paid by the Social Insurance Office. Such expenses will be paid by 100% and/or with partial reduction according to financial possibilities.
b) by participation of the patient, with respect to the regulations of the Social Insurance Office.
c) by an agreement with different social institutions.

III — Procedure at first dispensary examination

a) A medical history will be drafted with every patient, who is called by the unit of dispensary care, and afterwards the patient will be examined by a specialist, an angiologist. The latter will control the data on the troubles which warned the patient or his physician, will write a survey on previous diseases, register all medical and laboratory examinations as well as the therapeutic procedure. All these data will be registered in the basic form in such manner to suit a computer.

b) Then, a second additional form will be written, containing the recommended clinical and laboratory examinations. This form will recommend special examinations by the following branches of medicine: angiology, neurology, ophthalmology, cardiology, gastroenterology, nephrology, haematology, radiology and biochemistry. If needed, the opinions of the surgeon, the orthopedist and above all the vascular surgeon will be noted here.

c) Every specialist adds a special protocol to the additional form. The ophthalmologist adds the finding of the fundus of the eye, the angiologist examines the segmentary pressures and the circulation speed. He also has to examine the pharyngeal arteries (6 arteries at each side), the ophthalmic artery, the limb arteries (5 measurings for every lower limb, 2—6 measurings for every upper limb). The cardiologist, besides the clinical examination, makes an electrocardiogram and an x-ray diagram of the heart. If needed, he adds a phonocardiographic and echocardiographic examination. The dietetian examines for diabetes and gout. He also will look for disorders in the diet and check the patient according to the appertaining questionnaire. The haematologist will be asked to find the exact consequences of thrombosis in order to prevent relapses. The cardiologist then performs the examinations recommended by the previously mentioned specialists. The biochemical laboratory adds the needed metabolic tests and sees to it, that the costs of the examinations do not rise. Therefore, it will perform only such tests which are really necessary to find the exact therapeutical procedure. It also will see to it, that the patient is not transferred unnecessarily.

d) The angiologist collects the various findings and elaborates a synthesis, adding the therapeutical conclusion. He respects the recommendations of the previous specialists, above all those of the dietitians and the surgeons.

e) The form on the diagnostic synthesis will be handed to the patient and to the treating physician. The therapeutical proposal however will be sent to the treating physician only.

f) The patient will be informed of the convenient terms of future examinations and be instructed on the prevention of postoperative, postinjury and/or postlabour incidents.

IV — Procedure at later dispensary examinations

The examinations will be done so, that previous examinations will not be repeated with normal findings. Every specialist marks in the form the procedure of special examinations and underlines the risk factors, against which the patinet should protect himself.

V — Statistical analysis

All medical forms must be suitable for computers. A programme for the statistical evaluation of the results of dispensary care per year will be elaborated. Such results will serve as base for the future activity of the dispensary center.

Conclusion

In the first part we have analysed the importance as well as the technique of the medical care. In the second part we arrived at the conception of dispensary units.

The dispensary unit observes the development of the disease and its incidents and indicates to the general practitioner the procedure of such dispensary care, underlining the most important items, above all regarding the regimen and the work ability. Its activity is different from that of a hospital consulting unit, but it should be in close cooperation with hospitalisation.

The establishment of such dispensary units should considerably reduce the occurrence of infarcts and haemiplegia, which are the most important causes of death as well as the most important kinds of expenses for the Social Insurance Office.

The mutual connection of the units will very rapidly become a necessity for the unification of the technique. Such connection may be established by an organisation similar to a scientific society.

L. G., 3 rue Jacques Dulud, 92 200 Neuilly (Paris), France

ARTERIAL OCCLUSIVE DISSEASE WITH HYPERTENSION AS A POSSIBLE RISK FACTOR?

V. PUCHMAYER, W. SCHOOP, RENATA CÍFKOVÁ, ELLEN JACOB,
J. POKORNÝ, DANA HORÁKOVÁ AND V. BAZIKA.

*IVth Medical Clinic, Charles University Prague, Czechoslovakia, Aggertalklinik,
Engelskirchen, B.R.D.*

From the clinical point of view and epidemiological studies several risk factors of arterial occlusive disease are known. The aim of this study is to evaluate, above all, the possible role of hypertension in this disease.

Methods

▌A total of 982 men and 30 women suffering from arterial occlusive disease and a control group of 411 men and 50 women were examined during a period of one year (Table I). All patients of both groups were thoroughly investigated according to the same crite ia clinically, angiologically and biochemically.The blood pressure was measured in normotonics twice a week, in hypertonics every week day. The systolic pressure of 160—200 torr was considered to be slightly and above 200 torr to be expressively increased; similarly as diastolic pressure of 95—105 torr as slightly and above 105 torr to be expressively elevated. All data were calculated by means of a computer and their statistical significance was evaluated with a chi-square test.

Results

Normal systolic and diastolic blood pressure was found highly significantly more often in all control groups. On the contrary, slightly increased systolic pressure of 160—200 torr and the normal diastolic pressure occurs in obliterations more frequently. In the group of occlusive disease either slightly increased systolic (160—200) and diastolic (95—105) or highly elevated systolic (over 200) and diastolic (over 105) blood pressure occured more often. We received the same

Table I. Division of Patients.

Diagnosis	Number of Patients	Age of Range	Average Age
Atherosclerosis obliterans	908	26—71 years	54.5 years
Thrombangiitis obliterans	59	27—49	39.5
Uncertain etiology	15	35—63	53.5
Total	982	26—71	53.6
Vasoneuroses	74		
Varices	152		
Syndroma postphlebiticum	89		
Syndroma lumboischiadicum	27		
Others	69		
Total	411	26—73	52,7
Number of stenoses and occlusions 2863	Arteriographically proved 1436 = 50.1%		

results if both pressures were increased in various degrees. We have found such significant differences in all age categories of men including the youngest, regardless to the duration of claudications. There were no significant differences between the groups with obliteration and control ones in the occurrence of only elevated diastolic in the combination with normal systolic blood pressure. No difference in systolic or diastolic hypertension was ascertained in women with occlusive atherosclerotic disease. In the same way the differences of both blood pressures in angiitis obliterans did not occur.

No difference appeared between patients with obliterations and the control ones in the occurrence of hypertension as a single factor. In patients with atherosclerotic occlusive disease occurred the systolic-diastolic hypertension significantly more often in the combinations with smoking, blood lipids disorders and positive family history only. In men with the obliterative disease, from the total of 494 hypertonics an increased systolic or diastolic pressure before the onset of this disease in 194, i.e. in 41,1 per cent was ascertained. Only 10 per cent of patients with obturation disease and with slightly increased only systolic pressure (160—200 torr), knew of their elevation of pressure before beginning of their difficulties.

Conclusions

On the whole, 982 men and 30 women with occlusive disease, including 908 men with atherosclerosis obliterans and 411 men and 50 women free from any symptoms of such an illness were investigated. In the control group the normal systolic and diastolic blood pressure occurs significantly more often. Contrarywise in men with obliterative disease, there was significantly more frequent only the systolic hypertension, particularly up to 200 torr, further the increased systolic-diastolic pressure, both slightly and expressively in all age categories including the youngest one. No significant differences of only increased diastolic pressure with normal systolic pressure were found. In women and in patients with thrombangiitis obliterans, we did not find any significant changes of blood pressure. Further, we established that hypertension as a single factor was equally often in obliterations as in controls.

REFERENCES

1. *Büchner, F.:* Chronische Hypertonie als ein Faktor in der Entstehung der Arteriosklerose. Intern. Symp. über Arteriosklerose. Bull. schweiz. Akad. med. Wiss. 1957, 127—138.
2. *Juergens, J. L., Barker, N. W., Hines, E. A.:* Arteriosclerosis obliterans: Review of 520 cases with special reference to pathogenic and prognostic factors. Circulation 21, 1960, 188—193.
3. *Liebegott, G.:* Die intramurale Coronarsklerose bei Hypertonie. Med. klin. 53, 1958, 35, 1465—1466.
4. *Liebegott, K.:* Über. Veränderungen an den peripheren Arm- und Beinarterien bei Hypertonie. Verh. Dtsch. Ges. Kreisl. Forsch. 28, 1962, 221—225.
5. *Nobbe, F.:* Epidemiologie, Ätiologie und Pathogenese der arteriellen Verschlusskrankheiten. Dtsch. med. J. 18, 1967, 285—291.
6. *Pokorný, J., Puchmayer, V.:* Relation of risk factors to the origin of atherosclerosis obliterans followed epidemilogically. Acta VI. int. angiol. congr., Barcelona 1967, 549—552.
7. *Preuss, E., Eder, G., H., Weller, P.:* Risikofaktoren bei peripheren arteriellen Verschlusskrankheiten unerschiedlichen Schweregrades. Z. f. d. ges. inn. Medizin u. ihre Grenzgeb. 25, 1970, 10, 464—468.
8. *Puchmayer, V.:* Beitrag zur Ätiologie und Pathogenese der arteriellen Verschlusskrankheit aus klinischer Sicht. In: Ätiologie u. Pathogenese arterieller Verschlusskrankheiten. Herrenalber angiol. Gespräch 2.—3. 5. 1969. F. K. Schattauer Verlag, Stuttgart—New York 1970, 181—182, 189—190.
9. *Schoop, W.:* Risikofakterenprofil verschiedener Gefässprovinzen. Therapie-woche 26, 1976, 4, 484—488.
10. *Tölle, Gunhild:* Verschlüsse von Extremitätenarterien bei Frauen. Dissertation. Freiburg 1966, 33.
11. *Widmer, L. K.:* Morbidität an Gliedmassen-

arterienverschluss bei 6400 Berufstätigen-Basler Studie. Bibl. cardiol., vol. 13, 1963, 67—114 (Karger, Basel—New York, 1963).

12. *Widmer, L. K.:* Hartmann, G., Duchosal, F., Plechl, S., Ch.: Risikofaktoren und Gliedmassenarterien-Verschluss. Dtsch. med. Wschr. 94, 1969, 21, 1107—1110.

13. *Widmer, L. K., Da Silva, A., Madar, G.:* Hypertonie-Risikofaktor für die periphere arterielle Verschlusskrankheit. In: Zeitler, E.: Hypertonie-Risikofaktor in der Angiologie.

G. Witz-G. Witzstrock Verlag, Baden-Baden—Brüssel—Köln, 1976, 67—70.

14. *Witte, S.:* Ätiologie und Pathogenese peripherer arterieller Verschlusskrankhheiten. Herrenalber angiologisches Gespräch, 2.—3. 5. 1969, F. K. Schattauer Verlag, Stuttgart—New York, 1970.

15. *Zeitler, E.:* Hypertonie-Risikofaktor in der Angiologie. G. Witzstrock Verlag, Baden-Baden—Brüssel—Köln, 1976.

V. P., IV Medical Clinic, U nemocnice 2, 120 00 Prague 2, Czechoslovakia

PROFESSIONAL RISK FACTORS IN ARTERIAL OCCLUSIVE DISEASE

W. SCHOOP, V. PUCHMAYER, E. JACOB, O. VANDERBEKE,
P. BARTŮNĚK and V. ALBRECHT

Aggertalclinic, Engelskirchen, F.R.G. and IVth Medical Clinic,
Faculty of Medicine, Charles University, Prague, Czechoslovakia

From clinical experience, epidemiological studies and also experimental reports, there are at present known several factors supposed to be a possible or certain risk in arterial occlusive disease. We have been interested in whether arterial occlusive disease appears more frequently in certain professions, i.e., whether a certain profession presents an increased risk.

Methods

A total of 982 patients (males) suffering from arterial occlusive disease and a control group of 411 men free from any symptoms of such disease, mostly with varices, vasoneuroses, postphlebitic syndrome and other maladies were examined over a period of one year. All the patients were thoroughly examined, according to the same criteria, clinically, angiologically and biochemically. According to profession, the patients were subdivided into different groups. A possible trauma in the anamnesis on the localisation of the occlusion was followed, especially in grinders using a vibrating machine or pneumatic hammer workers or, as the case may be, the mode of holding the instrument. All data were prorated, calculated by means of a computer and the statistical significance was evaluated with a chi-quadrat test.

Results

When assessing the degree of difficulty of the performed work it became evident that patients whose work is mainly mental belong significantly more frequently to the group of occlusion patients. On the other hand, patients performing light physical work were more frequently found in the control group. With the medium hard and hard work no differences were found. As regards the single professional groups (Table I) among arterial occlusive patients, more frequently scientific work and, generally speaking, mental workers occur. On closer analysis we see that primarily those patients are concerned who performed mental work for over 20 years. Among thrombangoitis patients, forestal and agricultural workers occurred more frequently. Crane men and professional drivers were often established in the group of the occlusion patients. We have come to the same results with this group in all age classes with the exception of the youngest, i.e. up to 39 years. It has been shown that, again, those drivers belong to this category who were active in this profession longer than 15 years. Above 20 years, the significance will again be increased. This also explains the negative results in the youngest age group. Furthermore we examined whether this profession involves any relationship to a certain localization of the occlusion, especially in

Table I.

occupation	after 10 years	after 15 years	after 20 years	total		
white collars			$p<0.05$	$\frac{11}{411}$	$p<0.05$	$\frac{50}{982}$
crane men				$\frac{1}{411}$	$p<0.05$	$\frac{13}{982}$
professional drivers		$p<0.05$	$p<0.025$	$\frac{11}{411}$	$p<0.001$	$\frac{72}{982}$
farmers and foresters - thrombangiitis				$\frac{1}{156}$	$p<0.01$	$\frac{6}{50}$
cutters - digital arteries occlusions	$p<0.05$		$p<0.01$	$\frac{7}{866}$	$p<0.001$	$\frac{15}{73}$

the iliac, femoral and popliteal region. With a statistical comparison to other professional activities, no influence of localisation was sustained. Neither a right-hand nor a left-hand lateralising exists. Grinders using vibrating machines have digital arterial occlusions significantly more often than all other professions. Work for 10 years is decisive and after 20 years of activity the significance continues to rise. Pneumatic hammer workers represent a special class. They are found significantly more frequently among occlusion patients and in the group of obliterating atherosclerosis. The manner of holding the hammer is different. We were interested above all in possible localisation of the influence. Of 31 patients who did not press the pneumatic hammer

pressed with their stomachs directly, were found 100 per cent occlusions and stenoses in the regions of abdominal aorta and pelvic arteries and but in no case was this process found exclusively in the other arteries. 5 of these workers, i.e. 45 per cent, had isolated illnesses in the abdominal-iliacal region. The comparison of this finding with workers free from direct pressure on the stomach and in other professions were highly significant. In all cases the exposure to the pneumatic hammer work has at least 5 years. Contrary to much of the literature data, digital artery occlusions were not found frequently in these workers. In 4 other cases frequently relapsing trauma on the thigh existed and in all the 4 cases a femoralis occlusion occurred.

Table II.	AOD 962	pneumatic hammer	
		direct pressure on abdomen 11	indirect pressure on abdomen 9
AOD of aorto-iliac arteries	418 —— p<0,001 → 11	← p<0,005 —— 3	
AOD of aorto-iliac art only	75 —— p<0,005 → 5	← p<0,025 —— 0	
AOD of aorto-iliac arteries and other localisations	6 —— p<0,025 → 9		
AOD of other localisations only	0 —— p<0,01 → 6		
occlusions of aorto-iliac arteries	4	2	
stenoses of aorto-iliac arteries	0 ← p<0,005 —— 1		

AOD = arterial occlusive disease

directly to their chests, only 3 suffered from subclavia occlusion; consequently, the frequency was the same as in all other workers. One patient with direct pressure on the right thigh had a femoralis occlusion in the right hand side. Among 9 men who did not press the instrument directly with their stomach, nobody had an isolated disease of the aortailiacal sector; 3 had, it is true, localisation, but at the same time also had obliterations in other arteries, and 6 had isolated sclerotic occlusions in other artery sectors (Table II). Such frequencies do not differ statistically from the frequencies in other workers. However, in 11 workers who

In an analysis of risk factors of the mentioned risk professions, the following risk factors were found:
1. All the 11 pneumatic hammer workers with direct pressure on the stomach had 2 or more risk factors, one of them always being smoking.
2. The mental workers after 20 years activity frequently had 3 risk factors, especially hypertension and blood-lipid disturbance.
3. Professional drivers after 10 and particularly after 15 years had more highly elevated blood pressure, i.e. systolic above 200 and diastolic above 105 torr, than in all other professions.

4. The drivers with occlusions differ from those without arterial occlusion disease in that they more frequently have 3 or more risk factors. One of them is aways highly increased blood pressure and the second heavy smoking, i.e. 20 cigarettes daily over more than 20 years or 30 and more cigarettes daily.

REFERENCES

Björkerund, S. (1969): Atherosclerosis Initiated by Mechanical Trauma in Normolipidemic Rabbits. J. Atheroscler. Res. 9, 209—213.
Junghanns, H. (1937): Blutgefässchädigungen durch Dauererschütterungen infolge Arbeit mit Pressluft werkzeugen als Berufskrankheit Langenbecks Arch. klin. Chir. 188, 466.
Mathias, K., Beduhn D., Wenz W. (1976): Angiographische Befunde bei Aortenverletzungen nach stumpfen Thoraxtrauma. Herz/Kreisl., G. Witzstrock Verlag, 8, 9, 525—530.

V. P., IVth Internal Clinic, FVL UK, U nemocnice 2, 120 00 Praha 2, Czechoslovakia.

THE VALUE OF RESCREENING OF SOME RISK FACTORS WITH RESPECT TO THE IMPORTANCE OF INTERVENTION

J. KOLLÁR, M. TAKÁČ, M. ČESNEKOVÁ, H. KLVAŇOVÁ,
D. MOJŽIŠOVÁ, J. POPERNIKOVÁ, J. ORČO and P. ŠEFARA

Ist Dept. Internal Med. of Šafarik University, Košice, Czechoslovakia

According to our experience from 2 100 examinations of subjects in the East Slovakia region aged 35 — 55, we have come to the conclusion that systolic-diastolic hypertension and hypercholesterolemia are closely associated with premature coronary heart disease (CHD). The criteria employed for the diagnosis of CHD and risk factors were those published in the reports of WHO.

In this communication we report the prevalence of only two of the twelve risk factors observed in our survey. Within the 5 years period of observation, systolic-diastolic hypertension and hyper-cholesterolemia have shown the highest prevalence of all the verified risk factors. The marked rise in serum cholesterol and blood pressure are highly and significantly correlated with CHD, and have the highest relative incidence. If, of the total 5.7% of prevalence of definitive CHD, 5.4% occurs in patients with hypertension and 4.5% of the total of patients with CHD have hypercholesterolemia, then it appears justified to concentrate our attention on interpretation of the hypertension and hypercholesterolemia,

If Stamler J. (1973) and other epidemiologists consider values of investigated risk parameters distributed in the lowest quintile as being within the borders of the norm, then our findings are in good agreement with this statement. The lowest quintile of systolic blood pressure in men in the rural and industrial population has levels below 120 Torr. Distribution of blood pressure levels at 90-percentile indicates that, in males aged 35 — 39, the "normal 90-percentile range" is at 148.6 Torr, in females the values are almost identical (146.8 Torr). A disquieting finding in females aged 51 — 55 are blood pressure levels distributed above 177.8 Torr at 90-percentile, and in males above 178.6 Torr. We can conclude that subjects living in the social-economic conditions of the investigated region exhibit a rapid dynamic increase of blood pressure levels during this 15 years, amounting to up to 31 Torr in females and 30 Torr in males.

Subjects aged 35 — 55 have diastolic blood pressure levels in the lowest quintile below 76.6 Torr. Subjects aged 45 — 49 have diastolic blood pressure levels at 90-percentile above 98.4 Torr, and subjects aged 50 — 54 above 104.7 Torr. Diastolic blood pressure levels at 90-percentile in subjects aged 35 — 39 are below 88.8 Torr, which corresponds to "the normal range".

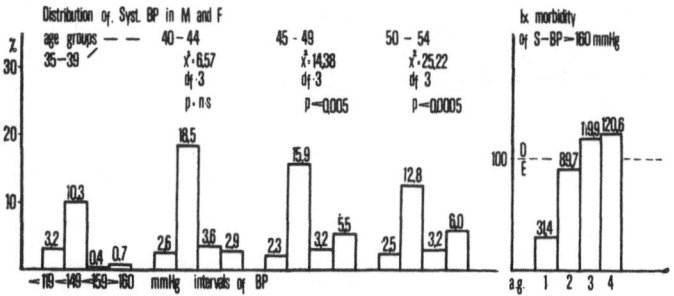

Fig. 1. Distribution of systolic blood pressures in males and females of the 35 — 54 age groups. Explanations: Syst. BP.-systolic blood pressure, M-males F-females, Ix-index, 1, 2, 3, 4- age groups: 35 — 39, 40 — 44, 45 — 49, 50 — 54.

289

It may be stated that increase of blood pressure relation in subjects aged 40—44 is insignificant (Figure 1). From the practical point of view, primary prevention should be indicated at the peak of working performance, i.e. before the age of 40 years at the latest. After 40 years of age the blood pressure situation will grow even more unfavorable. Our hypothesis is confirmed by the high prevalence of CHD in hypertensive subjects and also by the index of morbidity values. Therefore, it is not surprising that subjects with systolic-diastolic hypertension present about a 5-times higher risk for development of CHD, compared with borderline lood pressure levels.

Our attention has also been centred on the dynamics of serum cholesterol levels in the population discussed. It can be the commonly accepted values, the "normal range" of serum cholesterol is within the range of the lowest quintile, that is below 197.3 mg/100 ml in subjects aged 35—39, and 211.6 mg/100 ml in subjects aged 40—45. Distribution of serum cholesterol levels in the 9th decile is over 287.5 mg/100 ml, with the exception of subjects aged 35—39, who have serum cholesterol levels in the venous blood below 254.4 mg/100 ml. The data presented — as illustrated in Figure 2 —

further demonstrate that the risk of hypercholesterolemia in these subjects is 4.8-times higher compared with normocholesterolemic persons for the development of CHD.

Quantile distribution of the investigated parameters convinced us that age in the atherogenetic process represents risk factor "number one", according to the trend of the increase in the blood pressure and cholesterol levels. Is this finding of any practical significance for primary prevention? We suppose, that is not possibile to succeed in the struggle against the natural reactions of the organism and keep the pressure as well as cholesterol level in the lowest quintile. It would be a great success to keep systolic and diastolic blood pressure levels in the observed population below the 5-th decile of pressure levels, i.e. about 128.3/82.3 Torr, and cholesterol levels about 216.7 mg/ /100 ml.

In this report we have emphasized the importance of primary prevention on a mass scale to reduce in an important way the incidence and mortality rate of CHD, hypertension and hypercholesterolemia. The main question is how the major risk factors can be safely modified in the investigated population.

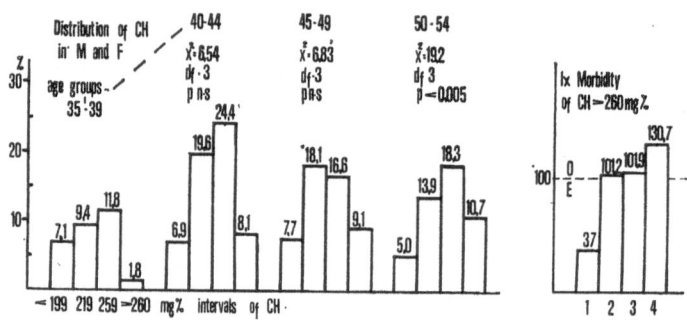

Fig. 2. Distribution of serum cholesterol levels in males and females of age groups 35—54.
Explanations: Ix-index, below 199, 219, 259 mg/100 ml, over 260 mg/100 ml, 1, 2, 3, 4- age groups: 35—39, 40—44, 45—49, 50—54.
Significant increase of serum cholesterol levels in investigated population in the 50—54 age group alone.

J. K., Ist. Dept. Internal Medicine of Šafarik Univ. , 041 00 Košice, Czechoslovakia

EPIDEMIOLOGY OF PERIPHERAL VASCULAR DISEASE BY THE DOPPLER ULTRASONIC TECHNIQUE

M. KORNITZER, M. DRAMAIX, G. De BACKER, J. SOBOLSKI, S. DEGRÉ and M. DE MARNEFFE

School of Public Health and Department of Cardiology, Brussels Free University and Ghent State University, Belgium.

Introduction

The aorta and the arteries of the lower limbs are one of the most common localisations for atherosclerosis. In comparison with coronary heart disease, epidemiological studies of peripheral vascular diseases (PVD) are rare. This can partially be explained by the lack of reproducible and sensitive techniques and partly by the low lethality of this disease alone. However, through clear association with other manifestations of atherosclerosis, subjects with PVD are a high risk for premature death (*Juergens*, 1960; *Gordon*, 1972). In the scarce epidemiological studies of PVD the London School of Hygiene standardised questionnaire of intermittent claudication (*Rose*, 1968) is the most commonly used technique for detecting overt PVD (*Widmer*, 1964; *Kannel*, 1970). Blood pressure measurement of the lower limbs has been used recently (*Hylkema*, 1976). In this paper we will present data on the systolic blood pressure of the lower limbs by the Doppler ultrasonic technique, a middle aged male working population.

Materials and methods

A prospective study was started 12 months ago in order to try to elucidate the relationship between physical activity, physical fitness and the incidence of coronary heart disease. During the screening of men aged 40—55 years at their working place the systolic blood pressures of both ankles and right brachial artery were measured by the Doppler ultrasonic technique (*Hylkema*, 1976). The blood pressure was measured in a standardized way by a single trained technician. The subject was in a recumbent position for 4 minutes, time to take a 12 lead ECG at rest. The cuff was firmly attached to the calf and inflated above 200 mmHg, than slowly deflated till the appearance of the typical Doppler sounds in relation to the circulation of the blood in the ankle behind the malleola (tibialis posterior). The pressures were always measured in the same sequence: right ankle, left ankle and finally right brachial artery. The pressures are expressed as ratios of ankle to brachial pressure. [Doppler pressure index = ankle pressure × 100/brachial pressure (%)]. The lowest of the 2 indices was taken. Here are given preliminary results on 1542 subjects aged 40—55 years representing 79% of the total working population from three factories.

Results

The mean ratio for the right lower limb is 117% compared to 112% for the left lower limb (P ≤.001). As the first measurement was systematically taken at the right ankle we considered this significant difference between the two limbs as reflecting the so called "pressor effect" and not to anatomic differences. The correlation

Table I. Prevalences of peripheral vascular disease

	40—44 (N = 545)	45—49 (N = 503)	50—55 (N = 494)	Total (N = 1542)
I) Int. Claudic. (%)	0.4	0.8	1.8	1 % (15)
II) ABP/BBP (≦90%)	3.9	5.6	6.1	5.1 % (79)
Ratio II/I	9.7	7.0	3.4	5.1

between the right and left ankle is .71. Table I shows prevalences of PVD according to two techniques: the standardised questionnaire on intermittent claudication (IC) and the ankle pressure index $\leq 90\%$. The cut-off point of 90% has been considered following studies of *Carter* (1968) showing that an index of 90% or less is highly suggestive of significant vascular stenosis of the lower limb. The prevalence of IC is 1%, increasing with age, as has already been observed. The prevalence of pathological ankle pressure indices is 5.1% or 5 times the prevalence of IC. Differences according to age are small. The ratios of ankle pressure index on IC are between 3.4 and 9.7, decreasing with age. In Table II the relation of IC to the ankle pressure index is considered. When the population is divided into 4 quartiles (Q) according to the ankle pressure index distribution, 11 out of 15 subjects (73%) with a positive IC history fall into the first quartile. The ratio of the prevalence of IC in Q_1/Q_4 is 5.6. More than half of the subjects with a positive IC history (8 out of 15) have an ankle pressure index $\leq 90\%$. The ratio of the prevalence of IC for this "pathological" group on the rest of the population is 20.2. On the other hand, only 10% (8 out of 79) of the subjects with an ankle pressure index $\leq 90\%$ have a positive IC history. Turning to the relation ship of the ankle pressure index to several other factors we compared the so-called "pathological" group to the rest of the population (Table III). In an univariate analysis we observed that the mean systolic blood pressure and heart rate were significantly higher in the pathological group compared to the rest of the population. Prevalences of cigarette smoking and of ECG abnormalities suggesting ischemic heart disease were also significantly higher in the pathological group. No significant differences were observed for height, weight, serum chol., α chol., triglycerides, blood groups, leisure time activity, physical work capacity and angina. We finally performed a stepwise multiple discriminant function analysis between the 2 groups, introducing 14 variables. Two variables discriminate significantly between the pathological group

Table II. Prevalences of intermittent claudication in relation with ankle/arm pressure

$\leq 90\%$ (N = 79)	Q_1 (N = 339)	Q_2 (N = 362)	Q_3 (N = 375)	Q_4 (N = 406)
10.1 (8)	2.8 (11)	0.6 (2)	0 (0)	0.5 (2)
% (N) ← --------------------------- 0.5 (7) --------------------------- →				
← --------------------------- 1 (15) --------------------------- →				

Ratio: R. Q_1/Q_4 = 2.8/0.5 = 5.6; R. ≤ 90/rest = 10.1/0.5 = 20.2

Table III. Ankle blood pressure/brachial blood pressure
A pathological group versus a normal population

	$\leq 90\%$ (N = 79)	$> 90\%$ (N = 1463)	P
Systolic Blood Pressure (mmHg) $\overline{\text{M}}$	137.7	132.4	$\leq .01$
Heart Rate (BPM) $\overline{\text{M}}$	71.2	68.4	$\leq .05$
Cigarette Smokers (%)	63.3	50.3	$\leq .05$
E.C.G. (IV$_{1-2-3}$) (V$_{1-2-3}$) (%)	10.5	5.1	$\leq .05$

and the rest of the population: SBP and cigarette smoking, which are also cardinal risk factors for IHD.

Discussion

As the development of the athero-sclerotic process is slow, the occurrence of significant atherosclerotic lesions in symptom-free subjects is rather common: according to *Widmer et al.* (1964) 30% of subjects with PVD are symptom-free. This stage is most probably detected by the Doppler ultrasound technique (*Carter*, 1968; *Hylkema*, 1976). Ankle pressure indices $\leq 90\%$ are due to the presence of low blood pressure beyond significant vascular stenosis of the lower limbs. In our study, the great majority of these 79 subjects (90%) gave negative IC results. Cross-sectional (*Hughson*, 1978) as well as prospective surveys (*Gordon*, 1972) have been used to study the relationship of IC to "risk factors". *Gordon and Kannel* (1972) have shown that in the Framingham Study 6 factors predicted IC: cigarette smoking, SBP, serum chol.,

glucose intolerance and LVH on the ECG. In a case-control study *Hughson et al.* (1978) observed that smoking was the factor most strongly associated with IC but systolic and diastolic blood pressures and concentrations of triglycerides, urate and fibrinogen were all significantly higher among patients with IC than in the controls. In our study 3 of the Framingham risk factors (SBP, cigarette smoking and ECG abnorm.) were clearly associated with a pathological ankle pressure index in an univariate analysis, whereas 2 of them remained significant discriminators in a multivariate analysis: SBP and cig. smoking. This observation should be an indirect argument for the relation of low ankle pressure indices with IC, the former being a presymptomatic stage. A prospective approach should confirm the hypothesis that the majority of new cases of IC will come from this small subgroup that is symptomfree at present and would be an incentive for the preventive approach of PVD through screening by the Doppler ultrasound technique.

REFERENCES

Carter, S. A. (1968): Indirect Systolic Pressures and Pulse Waves in Arterial Occlusive Disease of the Lower Extremities. Circ. 37, 624—637.

Gordon, T., Kannel, W. B. (1972): Predisposition to Atherosclerosis in the Head, Heart, and Legs. The Framingham Study. JAMA. 221, 661—666.

Hughson, W. G., Mann, J. I., Garrod, A. (1978): Intermittent claudication: Prevalence and risk factors. Brit. Med. J. 1, 1379—1381.

Hylkema, B. S. (1976): Diagnostiek van arteriële circulatiestoornissen in de benen door bloeddrukmetingen met behulp van ultrageluid. Ned. T. Gen. 120, 733—742.

Juergens, J. L., Barker, N. W., Hines, E. A. (1960): Arteriosclerosis Obliterans: Review of 520 Cases with Special Reference to Pathogenic and Prognostic Factors. Circ. 21, 188—195.

Kannel, W. B., Skinner, J. J., Schwarts, M. J., Shurtleff, D. (1970): Intermittent Claudication. Incidence in the Framingham Study. Circ. 41, 875—883.

Rose, G. A., Blackburn, H. (1969): Méthodes d'Enquête sur les Maladies Cardio-Vasculaires. OMS.

Widmer, L. K., Greensher, A., Kannel, W. B. (1964): Occlusion of Peripheral Arteries. Circ. 30, 836—841.

M. K., Serv. d'Epidémiologie et de Médecine Sociale, Université Libre de Bruxelles, Campus Erasme CP 590, Route de Lennick 808, B. 1070 Bruxelles, Belgique

FIVE YEAR INCIDENCE OF ARTERIAL OCCLUSIVE DISEASE IN NORTH CZECH MEN

V. BAZIKA, VL. PUCHMAYER, Z. REINIŠ, J. POKORNÝ
D. HORÁKOVÁ and F. HRABOVSKÝ

*Angiological Laboratory. IV. Medical Clinic. Faculty of Medicine,
Charles University, Prague. Czechoslovakia*

During the years 1958—1968 we examined representative samples of men and women in the country, in the hills and in the Giant mountains and from 1968 we have examined the men employees of the automobile factory in Mladá Boleslav and in Mnichovo Hradiště. In these workers we followed not only the prevalence but also the incidence of coronary and peripheral disorders.

Methods

We proceeded in the same manner with the inhabitants of the country and the employees of the automobile industry. We recorded the personal and family history, carried out a detailed physical examination with special attention to the heart and blood vessels with repeated measuring of the blood pressure in a recumbent possition. All arteries were palpated and auscultated and then we evaluated the quality of the pulse. In uncertain cases we carried out a rest and loading oscilogram. All the diagnostical cases of ischemic disease of the lower extremities were verified arteriographically. We also evaluated the recording of the 12-lead ECG, registered in quiet and after a three minute load according to the Master two-step-test, completed if necessary by cycloergometric examination.

We also measured the height and weight. In the biochemical analysis we examined the urine chemically, blood serum for the cholesterol level by the Lachema bio-test, the blood serum for the content of triglycerides by the Carlson method and the content of lipoproteins by the method of paper electrophoresis with calculation of the beta/alfa index.

The following factors were chosen as possible risks for the rise of occlusive atherosclerosis: family history, smoking, systolic and diastolic blood pressure, obesitas, diabetes, cholesterolemia and beta/alfa lipoprotein index. As a positive family history we have considered the occurence of hypertension, diabetes, myocardial infarction, cerebral vascular event or a sudden death caused by these diseases in the parents or siblings up to the age of 60.

In considering smoking we divided the examined into non-smokers, smokers of up to 10 cigarettes daily, 11 to 20 cigarettes daily and over 20 cigarettes daily. Systolic blood pressure up to 155 torr was considered normal, over 160 torr increased. Similarly a diastolic pressure up to 90 torr was considered normal and over 95 torr increased. We judged the weight according to Broc's specimen. We considered as a overweight an increase in the body weight of over 10% above tolerance. We did not investigate latent diabetes. A positive finding of suggar in urine served to indicate manifest diabetes. We considered cholesterolemia from 251 mg% to 300 mg% as medium increased, over 300 mg%

Table I. Five year incidence of arterial occlusive disease in north czech men

Age group	Men-country			Men-industry		
	Number examined	After five years		Number examined	After five years	
		Number	%		Number	%
30—39	235	—	—	192	—	—
40—49	117	—	—	855	15	1.75
50—59	192	1	0.5	225	7	3.1
60—69	93	7	7.1	Not examined		
70—	17	5	29.4	Not examined		
Total	554	13	2.3	1272	22	1.7

as clear-cut increased. Similarly, a beta/alfa lipoprotein index between 2,51 and 3.00 was considered as medium increased and above 3.0 as a strongly increased.

In the incidential part of the study we compared the results of our examinations carried out by the same method as in the beginning of the long-term research. After five years we investigated the number of persons suffering from ischemic heart disease and from occlusive disease of the lower extremities.

In Table I are given the number of examined men and the new occurrence of occlusive disease of the lower extremities after five years in the agricultural population and in employees of the automobile industry. In 554 men of a rural population aged 30 to 70 years, a total of 13 new cases of ischemic disease of lower extremities were found after a period of 5 years, i.e. 2.3%, it means $4.6^0/_{00}$ in term of one year incidence. However, in the 40—59. age group, only a single new case of obolitera-

tion out of a total of 309 subjects examined appeared after 5 years, i.e. 0.32%, it means $0.6^0/_{00}$ in terms of one year incidence. In car industry workers (aged 30—59) the disease was seen in 22 men out of a total of 1.272 examined, i.e. 1.72%, it means $3.4^0/_{00}$ in terms of one year incidence. All these men however were in the group aged 40—59, then 22 out of 1.080 i.e. 2%, it means $4.0/_{00}$ in term of one year incidence. In other words there was a striking difference in the incidence of the disease for the two groups under investigation in the age group of 40—59 years. In the rural population the development of new cases was found to lag 10 years behind the industrial group.

The occurrence of the single risk factors for both groups at the beginning of our study and after five years can be seen in Tables II to V.

Table II. Family history and smoking in five year incidence of arterial occlusive disease in north czech men

Number of men		Family history		
		Negative	+	+ +
Country	13	8 = 61.5%	4 = 30.8%	1 = 7.7%
Industry	22	5 = 22.7%	10 = 45.5%	7 = 31.8%

Number of men		Smoking			
		Non-smokers	> 10 cig.	11—20 cig.	>20 cig.
Country	13	1 = 7.7%	2 = 15.4%	6 = 46.1%	4 = 30.8%
Industry	22	1 = 4.5%	4 = 18.0%	11 = 50.0%	6 = 27.5%

Table III. The value of blood pressure in five year incidence of arterial occlusive disease in north czech men

Number of men			Systolic b.p.			Diastolic b.p.		
			<160	160—200	>200	<95	95—110	>110
Country	13	Initial examination	11 = 84.6%	1 = 7.7%	1 = 7.7%	11 = 84.6%	2 = 15.4%	—
		After five years	9 = 69.2%	3 = 23.1%	1 = 7.7%	9 = 69.2%	4 = 30.8%	—
Industry	22	Initial examination	17 = 77.3%	5 = 22.7%	—	16 = 72.5%	6 = 27.5%	—
		After five years	14 = 63.7%	7 = 31.8%	1 = 4.5%	15 = 68.2%	7 = 31.8%	—

Table IV. Weight and diabetes in five year incidence of arterial occlusive disease in north czech men

	Number of men		Weight			Diabetes	
			Normal	Overweight +10—20%	Obesity >20%	Negative	Manifested
Country	13	Initial examination	11 = 84.6%	2 = 15.4%	—	13 = 100%	—
		After five years	11 = 84.6%	2 = 15.4%	—	13 = 100%	—
Industry	22	Initial examination	11 = 50%	7 = 31.8%	4 = 18.2%	21 = 95%	1 = 5%
		After five years	11 = 50%	4 = 18.2%	7 = 31.8%	21 = 95%	1 = 5%

Table V. Cholesterolemia and beta/alfa lipoprotein index of arterial occlusive disease in north czech men

	Number of men		Cholesterolemia			Beta/alfa lipoprot. index		
			<250 mg%	250—300	>300 mg%	<2.5	2.51—3	>3
Country	13	Initial examination	8 = 61.5%	5 = 38.5%	—	7 = 54.0%	3 = 23.0%	3 = 23.0%
		After five years	12 = 92.3%	1 = 7.7%	—	9 = 69.2%	1 = 15.4%	2 = 15.4%
Industry	22	Initial examination	12 = 54.5%	8 = 36.4%	2 = 9.1%	4 = 18.0%	4 = 18.0%	14 = 64.0%
		After five years	7 = 31.8%	8 = 36.4%	7 = 31.8%	6 = 27.3%	3 = 13.7%	13 = 59%

The significance of each factor was evaluated by the relative frequency test. Among the employees of the automobile industry these significance factors were found: smoking, the beta/alfa lipoprotein index and a positive family history. At the agricultural workers smoking is the only significant factor. It is interesting that, in both groups, the significant risk factors also appeared in a combination of two or more factors. Both in men of the country and in the industrial population, we generally found the three mentioned factors, i.e. smoking, an increased beta/ /alfa lipoprotein index and a positive family history.

A striking incidence of the mentioned disease appears in men in the country and in industrial workers at the age of 40 to 59, as follows from Table I. The number of new cases then increases markedly in the agricultural population during the next decade. Therefore, the origin of occlusive arterial disease in men in the country is apparently retarded by 10 years.

It has formerly been stated that men in the country, especially in the mountains have a lower occurrence of ischemic heart disease. These persons had a significantly lower intake of animal fat and calories. Therefore we cannot exclude these factors in playing a certain role.

V. B., IVth Internal Clinic, FVL UK, U nemocnice 2, 120 00 Praha 2, Czechoslovakia

EPIDEMIOLOGY AND NATURAL COURSE
OF ATHEROSCLEROTIC ISCHAEMIA OF LOWER LIMBS

A. PISKORZ and S. ZAPALSKI

Department of Cardiovascular Surgery Academy of Medicine, Poznań, Poland

Although reconstructive surgery for atherosclerotic limbs ischaemia (ALI) has been performed for twenty-five years, our knowledge of the natural history of the disease is scarce. Information on the prevalence and clinical characteristics of ALI has been largely derived from the study of hospitalized patients or those with symptoms severe enough to require medical attention.

The study has yielded data that put the significance of ALI into proper surgical perspective and to allow a more rational approach to the decision of whether to advise surgery.

Methods

All patients with ALI in the city of Poznań were registered and the prevalence of the disease was determined. The morbidity rates at the end of 1966 and 1976 were compared.

Diagnosis of ALI was carried out on the basis of typical symptoms (intermittent claudication) and signs of deficient pulses in the lower limb-vascular murmurs and the measurements of opening pressures on different limb levels with a mercury strain gauge pletysmograph or with an ultrasonic technique.

The natural history of ALI has been studied in an unselected group of 2265 patients, 20—85 years of age (mean age 51 years). The disease in this group was diagnosed between 1964—1967. The patients were examined by the same doctors every three months in the out-patients department or at home. Information about deceased patients was given by family members.

All patients were treated medically and operated on only after signs of considerable ischaemia were observed.

The mortality rate as well as the incidence of considerable limb ischaemia (rest pain or necrosis) were analysed over 10 years.

Results and discussion

The morbidity rate among the inhibitants of Poznań over 20 year of age in 1966 was 2.26%. The morbidity rate in 1976 did not increase significantly and was 2.45% (Table I). The 30% increase in the number of patients resulted from an increase in Poznań's population.

The disease occurred mostly in subjects over 50 years. The morbidity ratio for men compared with that for women was 3.94 : 1 in 1966 and changed to 2.8 : 1 in 1976.

The occlusion started mostly in femoro-popliteal segment (70.77%), then in aorto-

Table I. Morbidity rate of atherosclerotic ischaemia of the lower limbs in the population of Poznań over 20 years of age*

Age	1966				1976			
	popula-tion	%	No. of patients	%	popula-tion	%	No. of patients	%
20—29	83 400	27.62	201	0.24	123 600	31.38	372	0.30
30—39	64 900	21.50	662	1.02	67 600	17.16	812	1.22
40—49	48 700	16.14	1296	2.66	67 000	17.01	1898	2.83
50—59	53 600	17.75	2493	4.65	53 400	13.58	2799	5.24
≧60	51 300	16.99	2172	4.23	82 300	20.89	3790	4.60
Total	301 900	100.00	6824	2.26	393 900	100.00	9676	2.45

*) From the Poznań Statistic Annals.

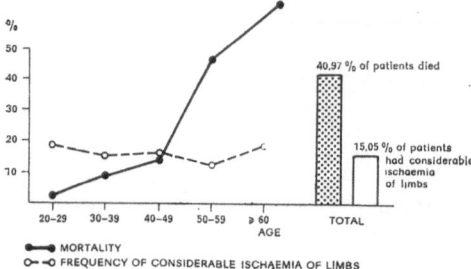

Fig. 1. Mortality and frequency of considerable ischaemia of limbs in 2265 patients related to age (to 10 years follow-up study)

iliac segment (21.02%) and rarely in the peripheral segment (8.21%).

Associated diseases encountered in the group were: coronary heart disease in 50.99% of patients (one third of them had had myocardial infarction); diabetes in 23.97%; occlusion of other arteries in 15.76%; lung diseases in 11.96%; hypertension in 48.96%. The majority of the patients had some of the accompanying diseases and only in 23% of patients, mostly younger, we did not find additional diseases.

Figure 1 shows the mortality rate and frequency of considerable ischaemic signs correlated with age. 21.98% of patients with up to five years disease duration died and in 8.96% considerable limb ischaemia occurred. After up to ten years of disease duration 40.97% of the patients died and in 15.05% considerable limb ischaemia occurred.

The frequency of considerable ischaemia signs was similar in different age groups. The mortality rate was low in younger patients and increased markedly in those over 50 year of age.

The mortality rate and the frequency of considerable ischaemic signs were also correlated with the level of primary arterial occlusion (Fig. 2).

The mortality rate was highest in aorto-iliac occlusion − 28.36% up to 5 years and 54.41% up to 10 years. In peripheral occlusion the mortality rate was 22.58%

up to 5 years and 40.86% up to 10 years. The lowest mortality rate was in the femoro-popliteal occlusion: 20.02% up to 5 years and 36.99% up to 10 years.

The frequency of signs of considerable ischaemia with up to 5 years of disease duration in peripheral occlusion was 11.83%, in aorto-iliac occlusion 9.45% and in femoro-popliteal occlusion 8.48%. Considerable ischaemic signs after up to 10 years of disease duration were most often encountered in patients with aorto-iliac occlusion − 20.59%. In the remaining patients the frequency of marked ischaemic signs was similar (13.54% in femoro-popliteal occlusion and 13.98% in peripheral occlusion).

The high occurrence of atherosclerotic occlusive disease of the lower limbs, high mortality rate and the low number of patients with considerable ischaemic signs seem to indicate in the majority of patients that the medical treatment is quite sufficient. Especially in the age group over 50 years in which the mortality is very high, the operation should be performed only in the presence of signs of advanced ischaemia.

The operation should also be performed on younger patients with intermittent claudication and aorto-iliac occlusion because of the rapid advance of ischaemia in this group.

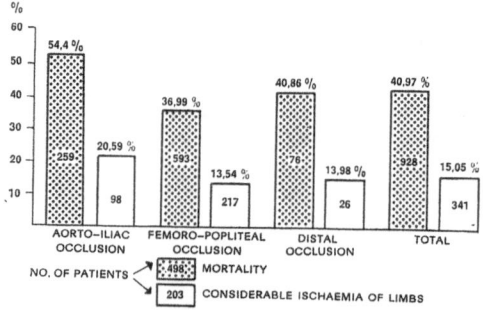

Fig. 2. Mortality and frequency of considerable ischaemia of limbs in 2265 patients related to location of arterial occlusion (to 10 years follow-up study).

A. P., Dept. of Cardiovascular Surgery, Academy of Medicine, Poznań, Dluga 1, Poland

A LONGITUDINAL STUDY OF ARTERIAL BLOOD PRESSURE WITH REGARD TO PRIMARY PREVENTION OF ISCHAEMIC HEART DISEASE

A. SLABÝ, D. HORÁKOVÁ, J. POKORNÝ, R. REISENAUER,
J. TIŠEROVÁ, J. URBÁNEK and Z. REINIŠ

4th Department of Internal Medicine, Charles University, Prague, Czechoslovakia

Many prospective epidemiological studies have conclusively established an association between arterial blood pressure, both systolic and diastolic, and the incidence of ischaemic heart disease (IHD). The prognostic significance of isolated systolic hypertension, however, has been less extensively demonstrated.

We decided to examine some epidemiological features of hypertension related to IHD in employees of two motor works whom we have now been following up for five years. A total of 3.267 men aged 30 to 59 years were examined, 90% of those eligible. Three blood pressure measurements were obtained during the examination at entry, with the subjects supine, diastolic pressure being the fifth phase.

Diastolic hypertension was considered if diastolic pressures recorded on repeated measurements were equal to or higher than 95 mm Hg. Isolated systolic hypertension was defined by systolic pressures of 160 or over and diastolic pressures of less than 95 in each measurement. Comparisons were made with a control group of men with a negative history of hypertension and with blood pressure values not exceeding 140/80[1]

Table I. Some risk factors at entry in male employees of motor works (mean $\pm$ S.D., or %)

Item	Group	30—39 yrs	40—49 yrs	50—59 yrs
Number of subjects	C	637	1027	241
	S	12	37	32
	D	94	309	138
Age (yrs)	C	35.7 $\pm$ 2.7	44.0 $\pm$ 2.9**	52.6 $\pm$ 2.9*
	S	35.2 $\pm$ 3.1	46.0 $\pm$ 2.6**	53.1 $\pm$ 3.0
	D	36.0 $\pm$ 2.6	44.9 $\pm$ 2.7**	53.6 $\pm$ 3.2*
Positive family history hypertension (%)	C	23.8*	18.5*	11.2*
	S	16.7	16.7	6.4*
	D	34.4*	25.5*	23.0**
Weight (kg)	C	78.1 $\pm$ 10.2*	78.2 $\pm$ 10.3*	76.8 $\pm$ 11.9*
	S	80.6 $\pm$ 10.6	77.8 $\pm$ 12.7*	79.0 $\pm$ 10.4*
	D	87.0 $\pm$ 12.4*	84.2 $\pm$ 11.9**	84.2 $\pm$ 12.8**
Resting heart rate (beats per min.)	C	74.8 $\pm$ 4.9**	75.6 $\pm$ 6.4*	76.0 $\pm$ 10.4*
	S	80.2 $\pm$ 15.3*	76.6 $\pm$ 6.1	76.8 $\pm$ 7.7
	D	77.4 $\pm$ 9.3*	77.4 $\pm$ 8.3*	78.4 $\pm$ 7.3*
Serum cholesterol concentration (mmol/l)	C	6.00 $\pm$ 1.25	6.12 $\pm$ 1.16*	6.08 $\pm$ 1.38
	S	6.06 $\pm$ 1.27	6.27 $\pm$ 1.13	6.32 $\pm$ 1.41
	D	6.21 $\pm$ 1.15	6.33 $\pm$ 1.24*	6.22 $\pm$ 1.20
ECG code 3.1 (%)	C	2.2*	5.0*	5.4*
	S	8.3	8.1	12.5
	D	13.8*	17.5*	26.8*

* = $p < 0.05$, C = control group, S = isolated systolic hypertension, D = diastolic hypertension

The prevalence of diastolic hypertension was 10.2% in the age group of 30−39, 17.2% in the age group of 40−49, and 25.1% in the age group of 50−59. The prevalence of isolated systolic hypertension was 1.3%, 2.1%, and 5.8% respectively.

Table I shows some risk factors at entry. Positive family history of hypertension and ECG signs of left ventricular hypertrophy occurred significantly more frequently in the diastolic hypertension group than in the control group, also mean values of body weight and resting heart rate were significantly higher in the diastolic hypertension group. We could not prove similar differences between the control and the systolic hypertension groups, with the exception of the resting heart rate in men aged 30−39. Serum cholesterol concentration was higher in diastolic hypertensive men aged 40−49 compared with the control group. The differences in mean age, though significant, could not explain these findings.

The prevalence of risk factors in the systolic hypertension group being low, we wondered what would be the incidence of manifest IHD in this group. The following events were classified as manifestations of IHD: a new occurrence of angina pectoris definite, of an acute transmural myocardial infarction or coronary death. The incidence was evaluated in those subjects who had the five-year follow-up examinations performed by March of this year. In the age group of 30−39, no case of manifest IHD occurred in five years. For the age groups of 40−49 and 50−59, the five-year incidence of manifest IHD is shown in Table II, together with the standardized incidence ratios. In both age groups, the incidence of manifest IHD was significantly higher in men with systolic hypertension than in the control group. It was of the same magnitude as in the diastolic hypertension group even higher, though not significantly.

During the last three years, a proportion of subjects have been examined on a bicycle ergometer. Exaggerated increases in blood pressure during exercise might represent a risk factor for the development of IHD, as suggested by a recent study. In 179 healthy normotensive men examined by our group, blood pressure values recorded at the sub-maximal age-predicted heart rates were distributed in quartiles and the cutoff points of the upper quartiles in the age groups 40−49 (220/105 mm Hg) and 50−59 (230/110 mm Hg) were chosen as arbitrary critical values for "exercise hypertension". Plasma renin activity (PRA) stimulated by upright posture was determined by a radioimmunological method, as an indirect indicator of adrenergic activity, in two groups of healthy normotensive men, with and without "exercise hypertension", matched for age and weight. Mean values of PRA did not differ (Table III), but − to our surprise − we found a significantly higher percentage of low renin values (<0.5 ng/ml.h) in normotensives with "exercise hypertension".

Table II. Five-year follow-up incidence of manifest ischaemic heart disease (%) and standardized incidence ratio (O/E)

Group	n	40−49 yrs incidence	O/E	n	50−59 yrs incidence	O/E
C	471	4.2* *	0.70* *	84	8.3* *	0.64* *
S	27	18.5*	3.12*	17	29.4*	2.27*
D	116	10.3 *	1.71 *	36	16.7 *	1.28 *

* = p < 0.05, C = control group, S = isolated systolic hypertension, D = diastolic hypertension

Table III. Plasma renin activity stimulated by upright posture (ng/ml . h) in healthy normotensive subjects with and without "exercise hypertension"

Group	40—49 yrs			50—59 yrs		
	n	mean ± S.D.	% of low PRA	n	mean ± S.D.	% of low PRA
C	24	1.160 ± 0.726	4.2*	20	1.366 ± 0.851	10.0*
EH	24	1.158 ± 0.914	29.2*	20	0.948 ± 0.673	35.0*

* = p < 0.05, C = control group, EH = "exercise hypertension" group, low PRA = lower than 0.5 ng/ml . h

A. S., 4th Clinic of Medicine, U nemocnice 2, 128 08 Prague 2, Czechoslovakia

PREDICTION OF THE RISK OF STROKE MYOCARDIAL INFARCTION IN PATIENTS WITH MANIFEST ARTERIOSCLEROSIS

L. HEINEMANN, H. HEINE, C. NORDEN and G. HEINEMANN

Central Institute for Heart and Blood Circulation Research of the Academy of Sciences of the G.D.R., Berlin, G.D.R.

We analysed the prognosis quo ad vitam and the prognosis with regard to acute cardiovascular complications in 1 800 patients suffering from atherosclerosis obliterans in a long-term study (average time 7 years). We concluded that the prognosis depends primarily on age, atherosclerotic localisation and the type and number of additional cardiovascular illnesses.

Our experience leads us to the hypothesis that the longterm prognosis can be predicted with mathematical methods. Mathematical prognostic indices are already being used to predict the course after acute myocardial infarction. These indices are connected with names like *Stupelis, Norris, Gallitz, Oxman, Helmers.*

Individual predictions have been made with the help of risk factors patterns.

The results of the mathematical predictions of complications must be interpreted with caution.

LONG-TERM PROGNOSTIC VARIABLES

IHD (AMI)

HYPERTENSION

HEART FAILURE

PERIPHERAL ARTERIAL DISEASE

CVD (STROKE)

Smoking

Overweight

Cholesterol

Fat disturbance

(Pro-) Diabetes

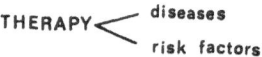

THERAPY diseases / risk factors

Fig. 2.

Our methods: We have analysed model groups of manifest atherosclerosis patients. Using discriminant analysis we discovered why some patients have a good prognosis and others a bad one. This prognostic model allows us to predict an individual prognosis using only the initial data.

The variables which we used were multiplied by their coefficients and added to the prognostic index (Fig. 1). We used 30 variables (Fig. 2). These were simply registered anamnestic data about cardiovascular disease, its complications, risk factors and therapy. The age and time relationships play an important role.

To what extent does our computed

Model of computer-longterm-prognosis
AMJ ● STROKE ● SURVIVAL ●

Variables — age of manifestation / clinical stage — IHD / HYP / CVD / As.obl. / risk f.

complications, therapy

Multiply by
their coefficients of discriminant function

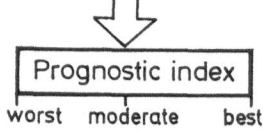

Prognostic index

Fig. 1.   worst   moderate   best

prognosis represent the actual survival rate?

When the prognostic index for each person is compared with the actual development of the disease we found quo ad vitam that our prognosis was correct in CVD 84%, in PAD 81%, in IHD 71%.

The figure shows that the number of survivers increases when the computed prognostic index is positive (Fig. 3). In contrast, the possibility of dying increased when the prognostic index was negative.

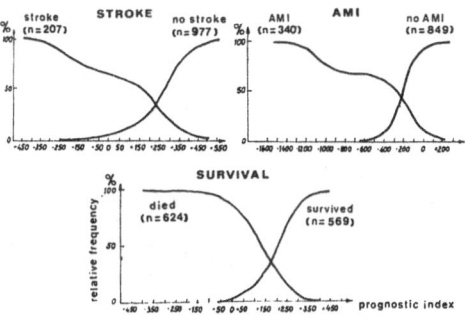

Fig. 3.

15 to 30% of the prognosis were wrong, i.e. patients survived despite a prognosis for death and, or the other hand, patients died despite a prognosis for life.

We examined the patient more closely:
— 5% of those who died although their prognosis was positive died as a result of neoplasma, bleedings, suicide, operation-incident. (The prognosis was only made in regard to cardiovascular death causes).
— approximately 10% of the living who had a negative prognosis were very sick: 70% of them had three to four different cardiovascular diseases, 80% a myocardial infarction and/or a stroke and half of these patients had a clinical manifest heart failure at the beginning of our observation period.

Predictability of acute myocardial infarction and stroke:

For scientific purposes prognosis is possible inspite of the need for caution.

In 70 to 80% of cases the computer prediction of myocardial infarction and stroke was correct.

On the basis of the prognostic indices we recommended five stages for the development of cardiovascular complications: In the first degree of severity there is a 10% risk and in the fifth stage more than a 90% risk.

These stages are the basis of possible practical consequences in the planning of preventing measures. The individual therapeutic necessity should be decided according to the risk regarding myocardial infarction, stroke and death. Studies which we began show that a bad prognosis can be avoided through an intensive programme of control and therapy, i.e. prevention.

We want to emphasize that our results are still in the preliminary stage based on our experience with over 2 000 patients with atherosclerosis obliterans.

The test shows that it is possible to predict the umber of complication-risks in three quarters of the patients with severe atherosclerosis.

Present studies will indicate whether these results are also applicable for mild atherosclerosis groups, risk groups without proven atherosclerosis or even in cardiovascularly healthy persons.

We cannot presently decide whether this model can be used as a screening method in population studies and risk groups.

We believe, however, that prediction of the development of clinically manifest atherosclerosis regarding the complication-risk is possible and that the suggested model can be used in pilot-studies as a decision criteria for prevention.

H. H., Akademie der Wissenschaft, Inst. für Herz und Kreislauf, Wildbergstr. 50, 1115 Berlin-Buch, G.D.R.

MULTIFACTORIAL PREVENTION OF CORONARY HEART DISEASE IN THE MALE INDUSTRIAL POPULATION

Z. REINIŠ, J. POKORNÝ, V. BAZIKA, J. TIŠEROVÁ,
D. HORÁKOVÁ and E. STUCHLÍKOVÁ

Laboratory of Angiology, Charles University, Prague, Czechoslovakia

The principles of multifactorial prevention of coronary heart disease (CHD) consist in discovering major risk factors related to etiology and pathogenesis of the disease. Many international epidemiological studies have shown that geographic differences in the frequency of CHD result from various nutritional and living habits correlated to risk factors. This evidence from epidemiological investigations is supported by clinical, pathological and experimental observations. (*Keys*, 1970, *Stamler*, 1967).

It is generally accepted that major risks of atherogenesis are represented by lipid metabolic errors. On the other hand haemodynamic stress and a low capacity for oxygen transport to the myocardium play the most important role in infarctogenesis. For this reason, the primary prevention of CHD is focused on lowering atherogenic lipoproteins in circulation, on stopping cigarette smoking, on increasing physical activity and on medical prophylaxis of hypertension. (*Reiniš*, 1977).

These basic principles were inbeded in the long-term educational preventive program dealing with the male industrial population of North Bohemia. An intervention group of 2 325 men, 30—59 years of age, employees of the AZNP automobile factory and a control group of 942 men of the same age, employees of the LIAZ automobile factory, were examined at entry using methods of the international epidemiological study in Seven Countries. (*Keys*, 1970).

The prevalence of manifest CHD in men 30—59 years of age in the intervention group was found to be 3.7% compared with 3.2% in men of the same age in the control. Differences in the prevalence data were not significant. (Fig. 1).

In the period of a 5-year follow-up the effect of multifactorial prevention on CHD incidence in 937 men of the intervention group and in 343 men of the control group was evaluated. Incidence of angina pectoris definite, myocardial infarction definite and coronary sudden death was found to be substantially lower in

GROUP	MEN N	PREVALENCE % OF CHD
INTERVENTION	2 325	3,7
CONTROL	942	3,2
TOTAL	3 267	3,5

PREVALENCE OF CORONARY HEART DISEASE (CHD) IN MEN 30-59 OF AGE

INTERVENTION GROUP — SKODA AUTOMOBILE FACTORY
CONTROL GROUP — LIAZ AUTOMOBILE FACTORY
CHD — ANGINA PECTORIS DEFINITE,
MYOCARDIAL INFARCTION DEFINITE

Fig. 1.

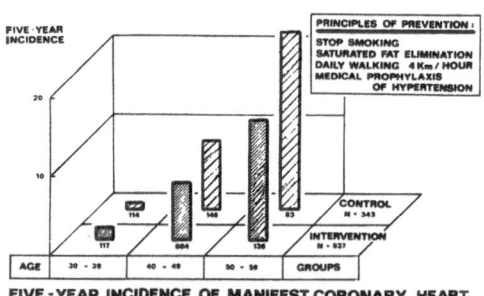

FIVE-YEAR INCIDENCE OF MANIFEST CORONARY HEART DISEASE (CHD) IN MEN FREE OF THE DISEASE AT INITIAL EXAMINATION

Fig. 2.

men of the intervention group than in men of the control group, both without CHD at entry (13 persons, per 1000, per year in the intervention group vs 20 persons, per 1000, per year in the control group (Fig. 2).

These findings were in good correlation with lower CHD incidence in non-smokers $(7.9^o/_{oo})$, in normotensive men $(10.4^o/_{oo})$ and in men with lower cholesterolemia $(12.4^o/_{oo})$ in the intervention group and with higher CHD incidence in smokers $(21.8^o/_{oo})$, in untreated hypertensive men $(38.7^o/_{oo})$ and in men with hypercholesterolemia $(25.5^o/_{oo})$ of control group. (Fig. 3).

The effect of multifactorial preventive procedures was demonstrated in the 5-year CHD mortality, which was found to be significantly lower in men of the intervention group (1.5%) than in men of the control group (3.5%). (Fig. 4).

The results of the first period of our educational coronary preventive program in male industrial population have shown that primary prevention of CHD is effective if the following intervention measures are carried out: 1. cholesterol-lowering diet, 2. stopping cigarette smoking, 3. regular physical activity, 4. therapeutical control of hypertension. It seems to be very useful for future human generations to incorporate the above mentioned principles into the regular educational program of young people.

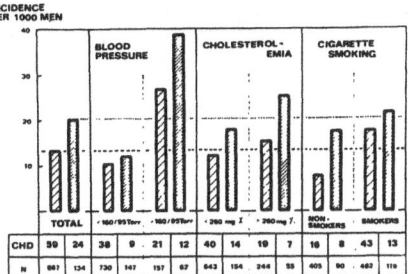

INCIDENCE OF MANIFEST CORONARY HEART DISEASE IN MIDDLE-AGED MEN OF INTERVENTION AND CONTROL GROUP IN RELATION TO MAJOR RISK FACTORS

▨ INTERVENTION   ▨ CONTROL

Fig. 3.

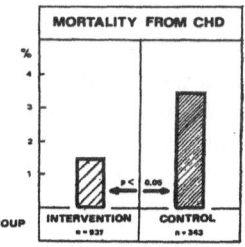

FIVE-YEAR MORTALITY FROM CORONARY HEART DISEASE IN INTERVENTION AND CONTROL GROUP OF MEN 30-59 YEARS OF AGE

Fig. 4.

REFERENCES

Keys, A. (1970): Coronary Heart Disease in Seven Countries. Circulation Suppl. No I. Vol. XLI/4.
Reiniš, Z. (1977): Epidemiologie ischemické choroby srdce u zemědělské a průmyslové populace. Thomayer. Sb. 476.
Stamler, J. (1967): Lectures on Preventive Cardiology. Grune and Stratton, New York.

Z. R., Laboratory of Angiology, Charles. Univ., U nemocnice 2, 128 08 Prague 2, Czechoslovakia

MULTIFACTORIAL PRIMARY PREVENTION STUDY ON MYOCARDIAL INFARCTION AND STROKE

H. GEIZEROVÁ, J. WIDIMSKÝ, H. PISTULKOVÁ, J. JANDA, Z. HEJL,
J. JANOUCH, D. GRAFNETTER, E. KOUDELKOVÁ, M. DOKULILOVÁ,
O. BALCAROVÁ and M. ŠANTRŮČEK

Inst. for Clinical and Experimental Medicine, Prague, Czechoslovakia

In 1976 the National Multifactorial Primary Prevention Study on Ischaemic Heart Disease (IHD), Hypertension and their complications was started in Czechoslovakia.

The objectives of the study are: 1. to detect the risk factors of IHD and hypertension in males 40 – 50 years of age and 2. to test the possibility of risk factor intervention and its effect on total cardiovascular morbidity and mortality in longitudinal follow-up. The principal goal of our study is to work out optimal methods of primary prevention on a popultion basis through existing health care organisations in our country.

In the Prague centre 2.556 men were invited for the 1st screening and 1.240 had already been examined. (I. m. respondence rate about 46%).

The overall frequency of risk factors is given in Figure 1. Figure 2 demonstrates the distribution of highest educational levels attained by our participants. Education is expressed in four categories:

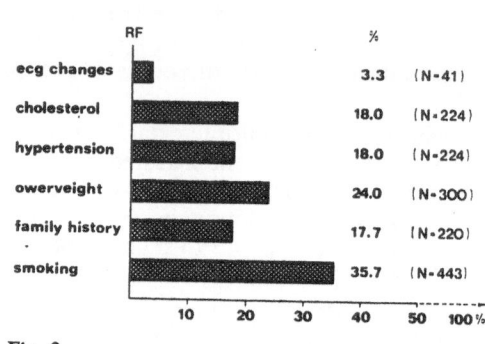

Fig. 2.

1. high school education (HSE) (32%).
2. secondary school education (SE) (36%).
3. Skilled men plus elementary education (ES) (24%).
4. elementary education only or less (EO) (8%).

We found statistically significant less men with hypertension (13% v. 18% – – $p < 0.01$), overweight (18% v. 24% – – $p < 0.01$), smoking (27% v. 36% – – $p < 0.05$), hypercholesterolemia (16% v. 18% n. s.*) and positive family history (13% v. 18% – $p < 0.01$) in the group with high school education (HSE) compared with all the others.

On the other hand, the group of men with secondary school education (SE) contained the highest number of men with hypertension (21% v. 18% – $p < 0.05$). The other risk factors did not reach the level of statistical significance, but the trend was similar as in the HSE group.

In a further group of skilled men (ES)

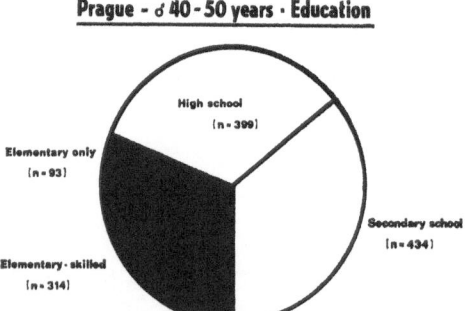

Prague - ♂ 40 - 50 years · Education

Fig .1.

* n. s. – non stat. significant.

306

there were statistically significantly more men who were overweight (33% v. 24% $p < 0.01$), who had hypercholesterolaemia (22% v. 18% $p < 0.05$) and who were smokers (43% v. 30% $p < 0.01$) in comparison with the others.

In the last group of men with elementary education only (EO) were significantly more smokers (53% v. 36% $p < 0.001$) and men with hypercholesterolaemia (27% v. 18% $p < 0.01$).

In our sample, the frequency of some cardinal risk factors was inversely related to the level of education. (Fig. 3). In the group with high school education there

EDUCATION · Prague ♂ 40 · 50 years (N=1240).

	Eo	ES	SE	HSE
HT	−	−	+ ↑	+ ↓
S	+↑	+ ↓	−	+ ↓
CH	+↑	+ ↑	−	−
OW	−	+ ↑	−	+ ↓
FH	−	−	−	+ ↓
N	7.8	25.0	35.0	32.2
%	97	310	434	399

Fig. 3.

was the lowest number of men with hypertension, smokers and overweight men compared to the others. Also hypercholesterolaemia was less frequent, but did not reach statistical significance. An explanation for this finding is not yet available. Our results are in agreement with similar facts from other parts throughout the world (U.S.S.R. and U.S.A.).

Hypothetical interpretation of our data depends on dissimilar living and eating habits (non-smoking, change of diet and daily physical activity, etc.) in various population groups with different educational levels, hopefully the results of successful health education. The finding that less men with a positive family history were found in the group with HSE might indicate some not yet completely understood genetical variable, which may play some role. Further search is desirable. The contribution of these facts is in two areas

1. our facts detect the "high risk" groups in the population.
2. the interesting observation that the lowest frequency of risk factors (obesity, smoking, hypercholesterolaemia in HSE men) is associated with the lowest frequency of hypertension.

REFERENCES

H. Blackburn (1974): Progress in The Epidemiology and Prevention of Coronary Heart Disease. Progress in Cardiology — 3 Edited by Paul N. Yu and John F. Goodwin Copyright (c) by Lea & Febiger 1—36.

C. D. Jenkins (1971): Psychologic and social precursors of coronary disease. (First of Two Parts). Medical Progress, New Engl. J. Med. Feb. 4. 244—255.

J. Stamler, R. Stamler, P. Rhomberg, A. Dyer, D. M. Berkson, W. Reedus, J. Wannamaker (1975): Multivariate analysis of the Relationship of six variables to Blood Pressure: Findings from Chicago Community Surveys, 1965—1971. J. Chron. Dis., Vol. 28, pp. 499—525. Pergamon Press, Printed in Great Britain, 499—525.

H. G., Inst. for Clinical and Experimental Medicine, Vídeňská 800, 14622 Praha 4, Czechoslovakia

THE NEED FOR PRIMARY PREVENTION OF ATHEROSCLEROSIS IN CHILDHOOD

J. HURYCH, F. BRZOBOHATÝ, Z. PETRŽILKOVÁ, Z. PÍŠA and J. HOUŠTĚK

Institute for Clinical and Experimental Medicine and Pediatric Faculty, Charles University, Prague, Czechoslovakia

Prospective epidemiological studies have shown that a number of factors promote the extension of atherosclerosis in the coronary arteries and therefore increase the risk of suffering from coronary heart disease. But the majority of these studies was carried out almost exclusively amongst adult individuals and populations.

The current data strongly suggest that coronary artery disease and hypertension originate early in life, probably in childhood. Although clinical symptoms may not appear until late adulthood, the precursors of atherosclerosis may already be present during early childhood. Of primary interest is the need to understand the early natural history of atherosclerosis so that preventive measures can be instituted early in life.

It is natural therefore that new research and community programmes should be directed increasingly towards younger populations.

A study on precursors of atherosclerosis in an representative sample of 288 schoolchildren (134 boys and 154 girls) aged 9–13 years was carried out in the central Bohemia region.

As a general goal the study should produce information on factors assumed to be related to the development of the earliest stages of atherosclerosis.

The intermediate objective is to explore the ways of reducing known risk factors in early childhood. The main risk factors chosen for this study are: blood pressure, serum cholesterol and glucose tolerance.

Screening was done as a part of regular preventive examinations in schoolchildren. Prior to the first screening, the parents received a personal letter about the purpose of the study and a questionnaire on the family history of cardiovascular diseases, child history (nutrition, illness, smoking, physical activity) and social factors.

The medical examination included weight and height measurements, two estimations of blood pressure, the determination of serum cholesterol and a glucose tolerance test.

Table I gives the mean values and standard deviations (SD) obtained by physical examinations and chemical determinations. No significant differences were found between boys and girls.

Figure 1 shows the frequency of abnormal values (outside the mean + 1 and 2 SD limit) of cholesterol, GTT, systolic and diastolic blood pressure.

We found that 35% of boys and 27% of girls in the total representative sample were over the standard weight for height

Table 1. The mean values and standard deviations for boys and girls.

STUDY OF ATHEROSCLEROSIS PRECURSORS IN CZECH SCHOOLCHILDREN 9-13 years

	MEAN		SD	
	B	G	B	G
No. of children	134	154	134	154
age	10.9	10.8	0.93	0.92
height (cm)	147	147	8.36	9.30
body - wt (kg)	37.9	37.8	7.45	8.77
BP systolic (mmHg)	107	107	8.98	11.96
diastolic (mmHg)	58	59	9.78	10.67
cholesterol (mg%)	153	152	25.79	21.30
glucosa (mg%)	88	90	13.72	16.89

and sex; 30% of boys and 24% of girls were more than 10% above the standard. We found differences especially in blood pressure values between overweight and standard weight children.

There is an urgent and imperative need for preventing the inception of the atherosclerotic process in individuals and in the entire population.

To this end there is a need for more knowledge of the distribution and trend over time of determinants of the disease and risk factors in childhood.

We succeeded in gathering data on some risk factor distribution in schoolchildren; repeated examinations enabled us to follow their natural history.

One of the important observations was the fact that overweight boys and girls tended to have higher blood pressure values than the remainder of the total representative sample of schoolchildren.

As long as these findings are confirmed in further a follow-up study and in larger population samples, then it seems that one of the most important factors in primary prevention should be obesity control starting early in life.

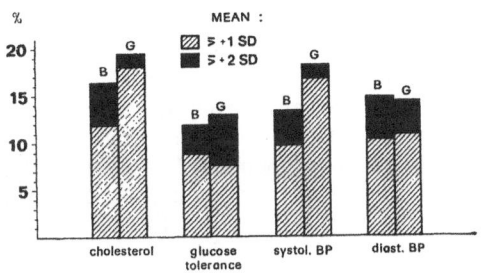

Abnormal values in children 9 - 13 years of age.
(B = 134, G = 154)

Fig. 1. The frequency of abnormal values (outside the mean plus 1 and 2 SD limit) of cholesterol, glucose tolerance, systolic and diastolic blood pressure.

J. H., IKEM, Vídeňská 800, 146 22 Prague 4, Czechoslovakia

309

SMOKING — AN IMPORTANT RISK FACTOR IN ARTERIAL OCCLUSIVE DISEASE

V. PUCHMAYER, W. SCHOOP, E. JACOB and O. VANDERBEKE

IVth Medical Clinic, Faculty of Medicine, Charles University,
Prague, Czechoslovakia — Aggertalclinic, Engelskirchen, F.R.G.

We have followed the influence of smoking in etiopathogenesis of occlusion disease with the same group of patients. We were interested in whether smoking plays a role as an independent factor or only if used in various combinations together with the other risk factors. In addition, we considered the role of various, divergent smokers' habits.

Results

Nonsmokers and occasional smokers occurred significantly more often in control groups with the exception of women and endangiitics (Table I). The differences be-

Table I.

	AOD	control	statistical significance
men total	982	411	
non-smokers	7	46	p<0,001 - control
occasional smokers	5	13	p<0,001 - control (women and endangiitis NS)
smoking	21	13	NS
cigarette smoking	16	10	NS
heavy smoking + severe hyperlipidemia	44	9	p<0,05
S + L + FH	108	27	p<0,025
S + H + FH	25	3	p<0,05
S + L + H	66	13	p<0,01
S + L + H + FH	78	10	p<0,001

(cigarette smoking and smoking marked "as a single risk factor")

AOD - arterial occlusive disease
NS - not significant
S - smoking
H - hypertension
L - hyperlipidemia
FH - posit. family history

tween those patients who had smoking as the only risk factor was not significant in the probands and in the control group, whatever the kind or quantity of cigarettes or total duration of smoking. Among the occlusion disease patients, more frequently smokers with some additional risk factors: in double combination, these were heavy smokers with an expressive lipid disorder, in triple and four-fold combination, smokers with lipid disorders, with hypertension and with a positive family anamnesis.

As far as general smoking habits are concerned, occlusion disease occurred significantly more frequently in smokers who started smoking before their 20th year; this factor was important even in those who had smoked for over 30 years. An important role is played by regular smoking during the day.

The smoking time decisive for obliterating disease and obliterating atherosclerosis is $31-40$ years; however, for endangiitis obliterans it is as short as 5 years. With a closer analysis of ex-smokers, it was shown that occlusion patients cease, as a rule, smoking till after a period of inconvenience longer than one year, the endangiitis stopping smoking completely over 40 years of age and patients with atherosclerosis obliterans older than 60 years. In addition, we have established that patients with obliterating disease stop smoking significantly more often for a period shorter than 5 years whereas the control patients for a period longer than 5 years. From our results it seams that the limit of 5 years of not-smoking plays a certain important role.

We have more closely analysed cigar and pipe smokers where less inhalation is assumed, and compared them with cigarette smokers who inhale. In cigar smokers we did not find any significant differences, whatever the amount they smoked for whatever period of time, even if they started before or after their 20th year, indifferent to proportional or relief smoking. We also came to similar results with pipe smokers, with an exception: mixed smokers, especially combined pipe with cigarettes, consuming more than 1 packet of tobacco per week for a time of $31-40$ years proportionally during the day occurred more frequently in the occlusive disease group.

310

Table II.

Cigarette smoking

	-39	40-49	50-59	>60 years	total	women
Cigarette only Cigarette + mixed smokers	NS	S	S	S	p<0,005 p<0,001	p<0,005 p<0,001

	<16		16-20		>20 years of age	
Beginning of smoking	S		S		NS	

	-5	6-10	11-15	16-20	21-25	26-30	31-40	>40 years
Smoking exposure	NS	SC	SC	SC	NS	NS	S, p<0,001	S - AO

	-5	6-10	11-15	16-20	21-30	31-40	>40	>30
Number of cigarettes	SC	SC women p<0,025	NS women p<0,01	p<0,005 women p<0,01	p<0,005	p<0,005	p<0,05	p<0,001

	proportional		disproportional	
Proportionality of smoking during the day	p<0,001		NS	

	<6 min	7-8 min	<8 min	>8 min
Time of 1 cigarette smoking	S	S	S	NS

S - significant   NS - not significant   SC - significant in the control group

Cigarette smokers (Table II) whether pure or mixed appeared in all the age groups with the exception of the youngest and generally also in all the localisations of occlusion significantly more frequently in probands. As far as the quantity of cigarettes smoked is concerned, a limit of 16–20 cigarettes a day proved to be significant. With women, an amount of 6–10 cigarettes proved to be critical.

In addition, it was studied whether patients smoked proportionally throughout the day or smoked a dominant part of their smokeload during the forenoons, afternoons or evenings. In all the categories of occlusive disease, smokers with regular consumption throughout the day occurred highly significantly. Similarly, in these groups was also included a highly significant occurrence of smokers taking one cigarette within 6 minutes. The limit of 8 minutes proved significant while above 8 minutes the differences were insignificant. In contrast patients in the control group more frequently smoked cigarettes with a filter.

When we simultaneously followed the number of cigarettes smoked daily and the total smoking duration (Fig. 1), we arrived at the conclusion that with 11–15

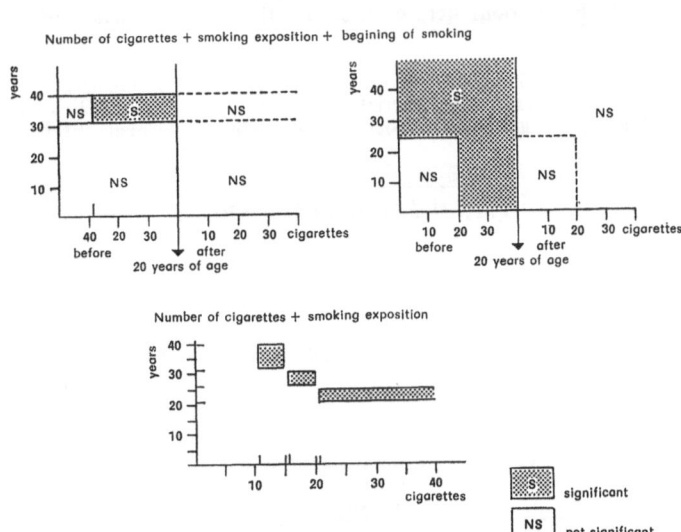

Fig. 1.

cigarettes the critical time is 31—40 years, with 16—20 cigarettes 26—30 years and above 20 cigarettes 21—25 years. The 11 to 20 cigarettes smokers consume an average of 150—200.000 cigarettes over the given time. In addition, the age at which the patient started smoking was followed. If the period of 31—40 years is critical, significant results were found for smokers of 11 and more cigarettes daily, when the patient started smoking before his 20th year. With a start between the 21st — and 30th year and after the 30th year of age the differences in such smokers were insignificant.

The probands group more frequently included smokers who increased the number of cigarettes smoked by 10 per day 5—10 years before the onset of symptoms (Fig. 2).

In endangiitics, the critical exposure time is 5 to 15 years, whatever the type of smoker. Thus they are highly sensitive to tobacco in all forms. In addition proportional smoking throughout the day is very important. In women, the decisive smoking time is the same as that in men, i.e. 31—40 years; however, the critical amount is 6 to 10 cigarettes daily. We obtained highly significant results, whether the women

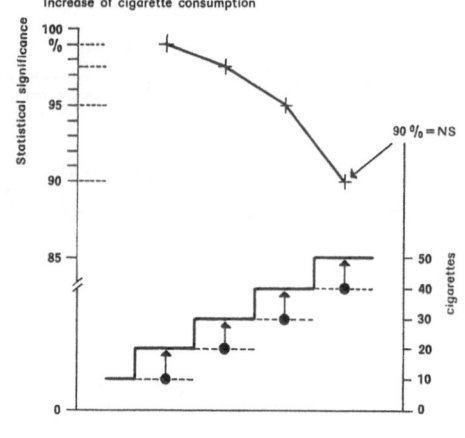

− 39 . p < 0,05	40−49 p < 0,001	50−59 p < 0,025	> 60 years p < 0,05	total p < 0,001

Fig. 2.

smoked proportionally or reliefwise during the day and whether they smoked the cigarette quickly or slowly.

REFERENCES

1. *Lithell, H., H. Hedstrand, R. Karlsson* (1975): The Smokun Habits of Men with Intermittent Claudication. Acta med. scand. 197, 6, 473—476.

2. *Puchmayer, V.* (1970): Beitrag zur Ätiologie und Pathogenese der arteriellen Verschlusskrankheit aus klinischer Sicht. F. K. Schattauer Verlag, Stuttgart—New York, 181—182, 189—190.

3. *Schoop, W.* (1976): Risikofaktorenprofil verschiedener Gefässprovinzen. Therapiewoche 26, 4, 484—488.

4. *Widmer, L. K. et al.* (1969): Risikofaktoren und Gliedmassenarterien-Verschluss. Dtsch. med. Wschr. 94, 21, 1107—1110.

V. P., IVth Internal Clinic, FVL UK, U nemocnice 2, 120 00 Praha 2, Czechoslovakia

ASYMPTOMATIC ISCHEMIC HEART DISEASE IN AN INDUSTRIAL PLANT

J. ŠIMON, L. CAJZL, M. ŠVOJGROVÁ, J. SŮVA, H. GEIZEROVÁ,
B. BŘACH and V. MALOCH

*Medical Department, Medical Faculty in Plzeň, Medical Department
Škoda Works in Plzeň, Institute of Clinical and Experimental Medicine,
Prague, Czechoslovakia*

Some longitudinal studies proved, that the finding of a suspect form of ischemic heart disease (IHD) ascertained by means of an ECG at rest and by the standardized cardiovascular questionnaire has a significant predictive validity. The patients having this form of IHD present an intermediate group between the still healthy but already risk-persons and the ones with a manifest form, i.e. with an acute myocardial infarction or sudden coronary death. It has been referred that at least one half of the total coronary mortality happens even in these asymptomatic patients (*Rose et al.*, 1977). Therefore it is necessary to distinguish which of the known risk factors are in association with the asymptomatic ischemic heart disease (AIHD).

In this study we analyzed a part of our data obtained during the screening phase of a group of about 2500 empolyees in various plants of the Škoda National Enterprise in Plzeň. The study population consists solely of men 40—50 years old. All data have been assessed in a strictly standardized manner in the framework of a larger study: The National Multifactor Primary Prevention Study of Myocardial Infarction and Stroke (*Geizerová et al.*, 1975).

We evaluated by means of the 12 lead ECG record and by the chest pain questionnaire the prevalence of the asymptomatic forms of IHD in various plants. The ECGs were coded by the Minnesota Code (*Rose and Blackburn*, 1968). We observed considerable differences in the prevalence, varying between 8—16 percent. The highest prevalence was observed among employees of the Electrical Engineering Plant and the lowest in the Turbine Plant and the Rolling Mill Machinary Plant. These differences could be observed in spite of the fact that we are dealing actually with a population living and working in the same town and region.

We can see (Fig. 1) that the differences are in good correlation with the frequency of hypertension and hypercholesterolemia. In the plant with the lowest prevalence of AIHD we could ascertain also the lowest prevalence of hypertension and hypercholesterolemia. We were also interested whether smoking of cigarettes would be reflected in the different frequency of the disease. We did not manage to find any statistical significant relationship of asymptomatic ECG changes between smokers and non-smokers. A similar find-

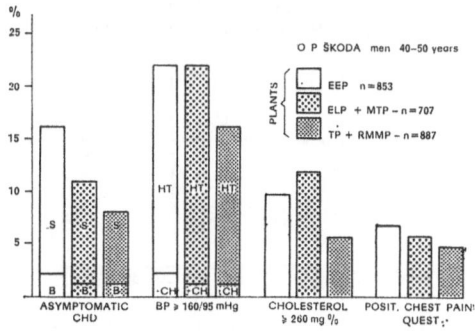

Fig. 1. Asymptomatic coronary heart disease in different plants.
EEP, ELP, MTP, TP, RMMP mean abbreviations of various industrial plants. S means "small" ECG changes (Min. Code 4—1, 2, 3; 5—1, 2, 3; 6—1, 2, 3; 7—2; 8—1, 3 —1,3) B means "big" ECG changes (Min. Code 1—1, 2; 7—1)

ing was recently reported (*Heliövaara et al.*, 1978). Smokers at the same time mostly prevailed in the group of employees effecting a higher physical activity at work than the non-smokers and were less frequently overweighted.

We followed up also an other factor in the whole study, namely the occupational activity in various types of employment. We were able to prove in the white-collar group a higher prevalence of ECG changes than in the blue-collar group (Fig. 2), especially more severe changes comprising the broad and deep Q waves or the left bundle branch block were more prevalent. Occupational activity includes both physical activity and responsibility. We are not yet able to answer definitely the question what is more important for this type of affection, whether it is low physical activity, high responsibility or the behaviour pattern.

Blood pressure is without doubt one of the most important predisposing factors for AIHD. We observed a statistically significant difference between men with and without ischemic ECG changes. The

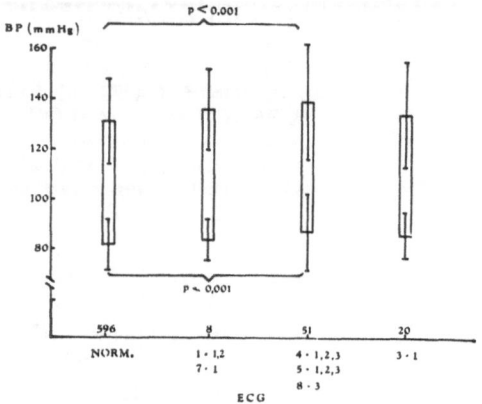

Fig. 3. Blood pressure and ECG changes by Min. Code in men 40—50 years in plants ELP and MTP.

blood pressure in the affected persons was on the average higher (Fig. 3). We noticed, however, that this value remained still within the borderline range. This means that already a moderate elevation of blood pressure brings about a high risk (*Evans*, 1971). According to our experience, hypercholesterolemia correlates better with the more severe changes comprising the large and deep Q wave and the left bundle branch block that with the changes on the ST segment and the T wave and with some other less specific ECG patterns.

In the forefront as a risk for AIHD are the following factors: elevated blood pressure, hypercholesterolemia and the occupational activity. For primary prevention of this type of IHD a multifactor intervention in a large scale of life habits seems to be important (*Council on Rehabilitaion*, 1976). The asymptomatic patients with a high risk of severe coronary events represent an intermediate group with a good chance to comply with preventive advice and intervention as regards smoking, hypertension, hypercholesterolemia and physical activity.

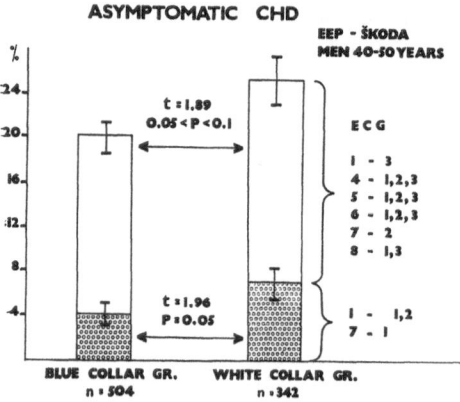

Fig. 2. Asymptomatic coronary heart disease by occupational groups.

REFERENCES

Council on Rehabilitation of the ISC, Report of a Working Group, (1976): Psychological Problems in Cardiac Rehabilitation, König, K., Denolin, H. (eds.), Zürich, 1976.

Evans, J. G., Rose, G. (1971): Hypertension. Brit. med. Bull. 27, 37—42.

Geizerová, H. and Study Group (1975): Manual of Preventive Multifactor Study of Myocardial Infarction and Stroke, Praha.

Heliövaara, M., Karvonen, M. J., Vilhunen, R., Punsar, S. (1978): Smoking, carbon monoxide, and atherosclerotic diseases. Brit. Med. J. 1, 268—270.

Rose, G., Blackburn, H. (1968): Cardiovascular Survey Methods, Monograph Ser. W.H.O. Geneva 1968, no. 56.

Rose, G., Reid, D. D., Hamilton, P. J. S., McCartney, P., Keen, H., Jarrett, R. J. (1977): Myocardial ischemia, risk factors and death from coronary heart- disease. Lancet, 1, 105—109.

J. Š., Internal Clinic, Medical Faculty, Marxova 13, 305 99 Plzeň, Czechoslovakia

ARE EXERCISE TESTS USEFUL TOOLS IN THE FUNCTIONAL EVALUATION OF PERIPHERAL ISCHEMIA?

E. LORENTSEN

Department of Internal Medicine, the Deaconess Hospital, Oslo, Norway

The main problem for most patients with peripheral arterial insufficiency is their restricted walking ability. The evaluation of the degree of walking disability is of great clinical importance, but may be difficult on account of history and physical examination. The simplest way to quantify the disabled function is to measure the distance walked on even ground until complaints occur (relative claudication distance) or until forced to stop because of the complaints (absolute claudication distance). Determination of the absolute claudication distance is influenced by several subjective factors and may be characterized as a semiquantitative method. The coefficient of variation has been found to be much lower for measurements of the relative claudication distance than for the absolute (*Hillestad*, 1963). This result is not surprising as determination of the relative claudication distance is more independent of subjective factors.

The amount of exercise required to precipitate pain has been used as an index of the extent to which the blood supply is actually restricted and a positive correlation between walking ability and blood flow capacity in the calf could be expected. However, in most studies a disappointingly low degree of correlation has been found between these two variables. Table I presents the results of our study. Though significant, the correlation obtained was rather poor.

It has been suggested that the subnormal pressure in the nutrient arteries in patients with peripheral arterial insufficiency may be the chief factor responsible for the diminished blood flow during exercise in patients with intermittent claudication (*Walder*, 1958). In an attempt to evaluate the relationship between the blood pressure in the calf and the claudication distance, calf blood pressure measurements performed immediately after exercise on a foot ergometer were compared with the claudication distance. Table II shows the correlation obtained. The relationship between post-ischemic calf blood pressure, ankle blood pressure at rest, the difference between arm and ankle blood pressure at rest and the claudication distance are also shown. The same poor correlation was found as between the blood flow capacity and the claudication distance.

The unsatisfactory relationship between blood flow/blood pressure and claudication distance may be the reason why walking tests are held to be rather unimportant or discouraged. Before dis-

Table I. Relationship between reactive hyperemia flow in the calf and claudication distance in patients with atherosclerosis obliterans of the lower limbs

Variables	No of pat.	Correlation coefficients	
		r	p
Postexercise first flow/claudication distance	67	0.304	<0.05
Postischemic maximal calf blood flow/claudication distance	67	0.332	<0.01

319

Table II. Correlation coefficients between blood pressure and claudication distance in patients with atherosclerosis obliterans of the lower limbs

Correlation coefficients		n	p
$r_{15} =$	0.388	61	<0.01
$r_{25} =$	0.380	54	<0.01
$r_{35} =$	0.341	68	<0.01
$r_{45} =$	-0.322	68	<0.01

Variables: 1) calf blood pressure immediately after exercise; 2) calf blood pressure immediately after circulatory arrest; 3) ankle blood pressure at rest; 4) difference between arm and ankle blood pressure at rest; 5) claudication distance. n: number of patients.

couraging these tests it should be borne in mind that the hemodynamic measurements referred to were not performed during the exercise. Therefore, they may not reflect the true nature of the conditions prevailing during exercise. This suggestion is supported by a study by *Tønnesen* (1968) who found a relative good coefficient of correlation (r = 0.65) between walking ability and blood flow measured during exercise on a foot-ergometer, whereas no significant correlation (r = 0.19) was found between walking ability and "first flow" during postexercise reactive hyperemia. Neither these flow studies were performed during ordinary walking. Several factors have been shown to influence the claudication distance (*Bollinger*, 1973). They may have contributed to the scatter of the values obtained in the correlation studies mentioned. Among these factors are the degree of physical training. Increased training activity may increase the walking ability without simultaneous measurable changes in the blood flow capacity during

exercise (*Dahllöf et al.*, 1974). The body weight, walking rate and step length are non-hemodynamic factors of importance in walking ability.

The reproducibility of exercise tests is found to be best when the patients walk uphill on a treadmill with the highest walking speed each individual can endure (*Petersen*, 1967). However, most of the patients are unaccustomed to this situation and a training period is needed. Bicycle ergometer tests have been shown to give results with a similar degree of reproducibility and may be easier to perform. Good correlation has been obtained between the bicycle working capacity and the claudication distance and blood flow capacity (*Petersen*, 1974).

In daily clinical practice, measurement of the relative claudication distance on level ground gives sufficient information about the individual functional capacity. The local blood flow and pressure are of less interest than the actual complaints of the patient. A walking test is simple to perform, takes place under physiologic conditions, does not require expensive technical devices and may be repeated as often as desired. The test is not useful for the diagnosis of arterial obliterations. Symptoms of intermittent claudication may be precipitated by different structural defects. As an objective diagnostic test blood pressure measurements at different levels are preferable. These two simple tests, blood pressure measurements at rest and determinations of the walking ability supplied with arteriography before eventual operative treatment, are necessary in the evaluation of most patients with intermittent claudication.

REFERENCES

Bollinger, A. (1973): Laufbandergometrie und Muskelfunktion bei Claudicatio intermittens. Schweiz. med. Wschr. 103, 636—641.

Dahllöf, Ann-Gret, Björntorp, P., Holm, J., Schersten, T. (1974): Metabolic activity of skeletal muscle in patients with peripheral arterial insufficiency. Effect of physical training. Europ. J. clin. Invest. 4, 9—15.

Hillestad, L. K. (1963): The peripheral blood flow in intermittent claudication. IV. The significance of the claudication distance. Acta med. scand. 173, 467—478.

Petersen, F. B. (1967): The effects of varying walking speeds when measuring the claudication distance on horizontal and sloping levels. Acta Chir. Scand. 133, 627—630.

Petersen, F. B. (1974): Physical performance capacity in patients with dysbasia arteriosclerotica. Scand. J. Rehab. Med. 6, 31—35.

Tønnesen, K. H. (1968): Muscle blood flow during exercise in intermittent claudication. Validation of the ^{133}Xenon clearance tech-nique: Clinical use by comparison to plethysmography and walking distance. Circulation 37, 402—410.

Walder, D. N. (1958): A technique for investigating the blood supply of muscle during exercise. Brit. med. J. I, 255—258.

L. E., Diakonissehusets Sykehus, Oslo 4, Norway

CONTINUOUS TREADMILL WALKING TEST IN EVALUATION OF MUSCULAR PERFORMANCE OF ISCHEMIC LOWER EXTREMITIES

ALENA BROULÍKOVÁ and J. LINHART

*Institute for Clinical and Experimental Medicine,
Department of Medicine II., Prague, Czechoslovakia*

Intermittent claudication is the most frequent complaint of patients with arterial occlusive disease of the lower extremities It was soon recognized that subjective. evaluation of walking distance is unreliable. Therefore, measurement on a treadmill has become a standard procedure.

Investigation techniques differ in many respects and make it difficult to compare results obtained in various laboratories and to seek relationships to the hemodynamic parameters. The present paper describes a new procedure employed in our department and based upon continuous exercise which we believe might offer some advantages over conventional methods.

With the common discontinuous procedure, the patient walks with a standard speed until ischemic pain develops. In subjects with good exercise tolerance, the slope of the belt is then increased and estimation of walking distance performed again after one or more breaks. The investigation is usually repeated and mean values are calculated. Thus, the dis-

continuous test is a rather time-consuming procedure.

Therefore, we suggest a new test (Fig. 1). The patient walks continuously and the slope of the treadmill is changed if necessary. The total energy expenditure is calculated using a formula based upon measurements of oxygen consumption, which is a common approach in exercise physiology. It is expressed in kcal/kg of body weight.

Repeated estimation of the walking distance in patients with occlusive arterial disease of the lower extremities indicates that the variability of the continuous procedure is less than 5%, while with the

ARTERIAL OCCLUSIONS
ANKLE PRESSURE VS. ENERGY EXPENDITURE

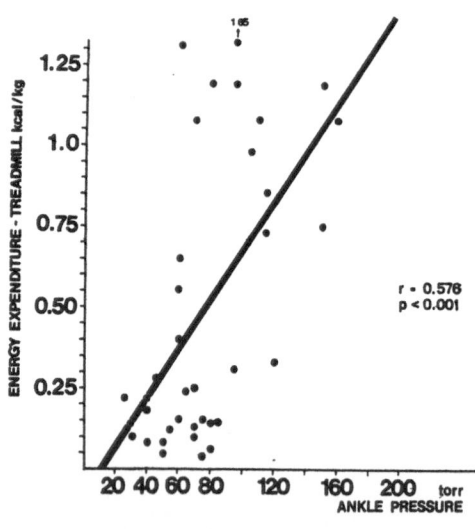

r - 0.576
p < 0.001

Fig. 2. Relationship between systolic ankle blood pressure and treadmill performance (in kcal/kg of body weight).

TREADMILL·CONTINUOUS TEST

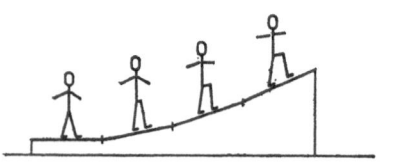

Fig. 1. Scheme of the continuous treadmill walking test for investigation of muscular performance of patient with arterial occlusive disease in the lower extremities.

discontinuous test it is significantly (about four times) higher. The continuous test also requires significantly more work and is consequently more sensitive (*Broulíková, A.*: to be published). Expression of the working capacity in terms of energy expenditure in absolute unit also makes it possible to compare muscular performance in various patients and, eventually, to seek a relationship between muscular work and hemodynamic parameters.

We have found a significant correlation between maximal calf blood flow after 5 minutes ischemia and the treadmill performance and also between ankle blood pressure, as measured by the Doppler technique, and treadmill exercise in kcal/kg of body weight — see Fig. 2.

Thus, it follows from our results that the application of the continuous treadmill test increases the sensitivity of the procedure particularly in patients with less apparent functional lesions, who otherwise might escape diagnosis if a less strenuous test were employed. The test is well reproducible and also requires much less time than the common discontinuous procedure. This is of importance for routine clinical investigations. Expression of muscular performance in quantitative units makes it possible to compare the results for various subjects. This might be of particular value for long-term control of patients with chronic ischemic diseases of the lower extremities.

B. A., IKEM Vídeňská 800, 146 22 Praha 4 - Krč, Czechoslovakia

THE TREADMILL TEST IN CHRONIC ARTERIOPATIC SUBJECTS

A. LIBRETTI, E. ARNOLDI, A. AROSIO, M. CATALANO
and E. BOSISIO

*Dept. of Medicine, University Milan, Hospital L. Sacco,
Milan, Italy*

Proper evaluation of the arterial flow to the inferior limbs is of great importance for early diagnosis of circulatory insufficiency in chronic arteriopathy or diffuse arteriosclerosis. The contemporary determination of systolic arterial pressure in the four limbs after an exercise (*Skinner*, 1967; *Strandness et al.*, 1964), enables discovery of such conditions. This method, firstly proposed by *Strandness* in 1975, was used to study a group of patients with chronic arteriopathy of the inferior limbs and to compare it with a similar group of normal subjects.

Methods

30 subjects were studied, 8 with chronic arteriopathy of the inferior limbs and 22 normal, of which 10 aged less than 30. Diagnosis of chronic arteriopatic disease was made through a clinical examination, oscillographic recording, Doppler investigation (*Franklin et al.* 1961,

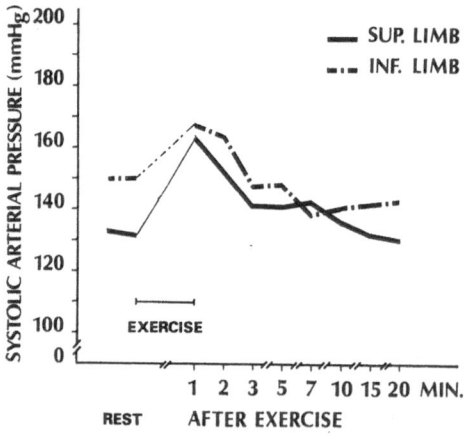

Fig. 1. Mean systolic pressure of superior and inferior limbs in a group of 22 normal subjects before and after exercise on a treadmill.

Kazamias et al. 1971, *Strandness* 1975) and aortic arteriography. All the patients with heart or lung involvement were excluded.

Results

In the normal subjects the mean value of the systolic arterial pressure before exercise resulted in 132 mm Hg in the superior and 150 mm Hg in the inferior limbs. After exercise the mean systolic pressure showed an increase to 168 mm Hg in the superior and to 167 mm Hg in the inferior limbs, and returned to the pre-exercise values after 5 minutes. No significant differences were obverved in the four limbs (Fig. 1). In normal subjects aged over 30 the mean value of the systolic pressure before exercise was 161 mm Hg without differences between superior and inferior limbs. After exercise the mean systolic pressure increased to 197 mm Hg in the four limbs without apparent differences and returned to the pre-exercise values after 5 minutes. In the 8 patients with chronic arteriopatic disease the mean systolic pressure was 155 mm Hg in the superior and 140 mm Hg in the inferior limbs. After the exercise the mean systolic pressure of the superior limbs increased up to 191 mm Hg while in the inferior limbs decreased to 115 mm Hg. The pressure value returned to the pre-exercise levels after more than 10 minutes (Fig. 2). In all the patients the test was repeated after variable periods of time and no significant differences were observed in the behaviour of the post-exercise systolic pressure. In the arteriopatic patients the changes in the systolic pressure after exercise exhibited marked differences in the different subjects. A correlation might be observed between the amount of the systolic decrease after exercise and the degree of arterial involvement demonstrated by arteriography.

Discussion

The results obtained indicate that the exercise test on a treadmill is a useful means for proper evaluation of the degree of arterial involvement in the arteriopatic patients. The hypertensive response, commonly present after exercise, is accompanied in arteriopatic patients by a marked decrease in the systolic pressure in the limbs with arterial lesions, and the amount of systolic pressure decrease appears to be related to the degree of arterial involvement. Since the increase of the systolic pressure during exercise is dependent on an increase of the cardiac output and of muscular blood flow, the hemodynamic condition caused by the muscular exercise may induce a "steal" of blood flow from the vascular district of the involved limb and then a pressure fall. The incapacity to adapt to the hemo-

dynamic changes induced by exercise is obviously proportional to the degree of the arterial lesion. The test proposed is a valid means for the evaluation, through a non-invasive method, of the degree of arterial lesions in early chronic arteriopathy.

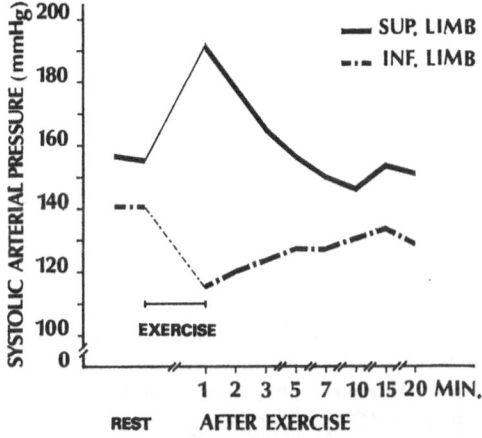

Fig. 2. Mean systolic pressure of superior and inferior limbs in a group of 8 patients with chronic arteriopathy of the lower limbs, before and after exercise on a treadmill.

REFERENCES

Franklin, D. L., Schlegel, W., Rushmer, R. F. (1961): Blood flow measurement by Doppler frequency shift of back scattered ultrasound. Science 134, 564.

Kazamias, T. M., Gander, M. P., Franklin, D. L. and Ross, J. R. (1971): Blood pressure measurement with Doppler ultrasonic flowmeter. J. Appl. Physiol. 30, 585.

Skinner, J. S. and Strandness, D. E. Jr. (1967): Exercise and intermittent claudication. Circulation 36, 15.

Strandness, D. E. Jr. and Bell J. W. (1964): An evaluation of the hemodynamic response of the claudicating extremity to exercise. Surg. Gynec. Obstret. 119, 1237.

Strandness, D. E. Jr. and Sumner, D. S. (1975): Hemodynamics for Surgeons. Grune and Stratton. New York.

Strandness, D. E. Jr. and Sumner, D. S. (1975): Application of ultrasound to the study of arteriosclerosis obliterans. Angiology 26, 187.

A. L., Cattedra di Patologia Medica, Università di Milano, Ospedale L. Sacco, via G. B. Grassi 74, Milano, Italia

HEMODYNAMIC AND METABOLIC CHANGES IN THE LOWER EXTREMITIES DURING ERGOMETRIC EXERCISE AND GLUCOSE INFUSION

H. PODHAISKY, F. E. ULRICH, K. HÄNSGEN, F. NAUNDORF,
G. MÜLLER, E. G. PREUSS and K. SEIGE

*2nd Med. Clinic, Martin-Luther-University, Halle—Wittenberg,
Halle, G.D.R.*

Studies on peripheral circulation and metabolism are important for investigations of pathogenetic connections in patients with occlusive arterial disease (OAD) and diabetic angiopathy (*Alexander et al.*, 1969). We examined the influence of muscle exercise and beta-cell-stimulation on calf blood flow and arterio-femoral venous concentration differences of metabolic parameters. Blood glucose (BG), free fatty acids (FFA), glycerol and immunoreactive insulin (IRI) were determined in the blood samples.

Results

We found increased basic arterial and venous IRI-levels in patients with OAD in agreement with *Stout* (1977). This elevated IRI-concentration decreased after ischemic exercise (for example in the arterial blood from $28.0 \pm 4.1 \,\mu U/ml$ to $13.4 \pm 2.3 \,\mu U/ml$). It is well known that muscle exercise causes a decrease of pancreatic insulin secretion (*Hunter*, 1968) and an improvement of glucose tolerance. The insulin bound peripherally (*Dieterle et al.*, 1973) is released immediately after mus-

cular exercise in the healthy group only, as shown in figure 2.

A significant difference in basic glucose uptake does not occur between OAD-patients and controls. An increase in muscle glucose utilization was absent after ischemic exercise in the OAD-group in contrast to controls. These findings could be connected with a reduced peripheral insulin release. *Berger et al.* (1975) observed the stimulatory effect of exercise on glucose uptake requiring the presence of insulin.

The intravenous glucose load is followed a higher arterio-femoral venous BG-difference. We may explain this effect by a stimulation of glycogen synthesis in muscle. *Nuttal et al.* (1977) recently reported an increase of glycogen synthetase activity in quadriceps femoris muscle after glucose application in normal male subjects. Further, a glucose and insulin induced decrease of FFA and glycerol levels occurs in our examination, as is shown in Fig. 3.

This behaviour of lipid parameters during glucose infusion could be caused by an antilipolytic insulin effect (lipase inhi-

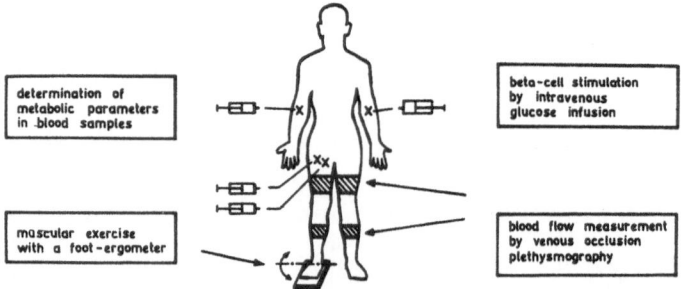

Fig. 1. Experimental methods.

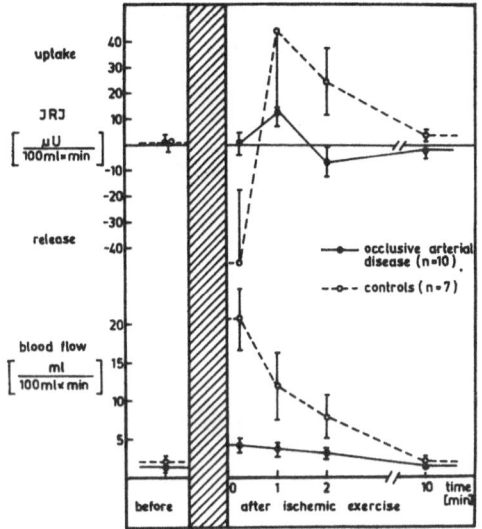

Fig. 2. Calf blood flow and peripheral insulin uptake before and after ischemic muscle exercise in persons with and without occlusive arterial disease.

The hemodynamic, metabolic and hormonal reactions were measured under conditions of limited blood in the phase of reactive hyperemia and during experimental alterations of the substrate supply in the lower extremities and are in agreement with those found by most other authors. An influence of the muscle training state on blood flow and muscle metabolism also appears in our investigations.

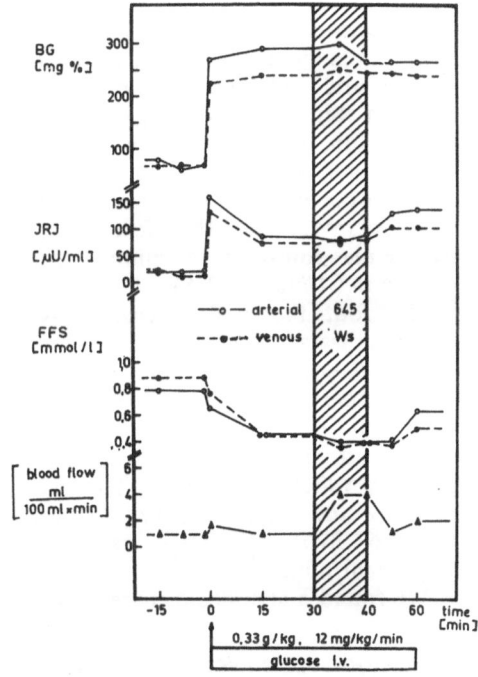

Fig. 3. Calf blood flow behaviour and arterio-femoral venous pattern of BG, IRI and FFA during glucose load in connection with ergometric exercise in a 43 year old healthy male person.

bition and enhancement of reesterfication rate of FFA in fatty tissue (*Bottermann*, 1971)). Additional muscle exercise under glucose infusion does not significantly influence the concentrations of carbohydrate and lipid parameters in blood samples. However, the peripheral glucose utilization increases depending on the blood flow. Considering the amount of muscle blood flow in relation to exercise, reflecting the training state, we observed a tendency to correlation between the topic muscle condition and peripheral glucose uptake. Similar metabolic adaptations of the skeletal muscle after a training period were also found in animal experiments (*Holloszy*, 1977).

REFERENCES

Nuttall, F. Q., Barbosa, J. and Gannon, M. C. (1977): Activation of skeletal muscle glycogen synthase following glucose administration in normal males. Metabolism 26, 719—720.

Stout, R. W. (1977): The relationship of abnormal circulating insulin levels to atherosclerosis 27, 1—13.

H. P., II. Medizinische Klinik und Poliklinik der Martin-Luther-Universität Halle— Wittenberg, Leninallee 2, 402 Halle/S., G.D.R.

FOOT BLOOD FLOW DURING REACTIVE HYPEREMIA IN PATIENTS WITH ISCHEMIC DISEASE OF THE LOWER EXTREMITIES

J. SPÁČIL and J. LINHART

Institute for Clinical and Experimental Medicine, Prague, Czechoslovakia

The main pathophysiological consequence of ischemic disease of the lower extremities is insufficient blood flow. At the beginning of the disease, the blood flow is limited only during vasodilatation. At advanced stage, blood flow is also limited at rest and ischemia of the foot may result in skin necrosis and gangrene. For this reason, foot blood flow should be investigated not only at rest, but also after proper vasodilator stimulus. In this study we investigated the effect of reactive hyperemia following 5 minute arterial occlusion (*Allwood*, 1958).

The foot blood flow was measured using a water-filled (32 °C) plethysmograph (*Barcroft*, 1953; *Abramson*, 1967). The increase in volume during venous occlusion of $40-60$ mm of mercury causes an increase in the hydrostatic pressure which is registred. The average rest flow and maximal (peak) flow during reactive hyperemia was expresed in ml/100 ml/min.

We found a significant increase in foot

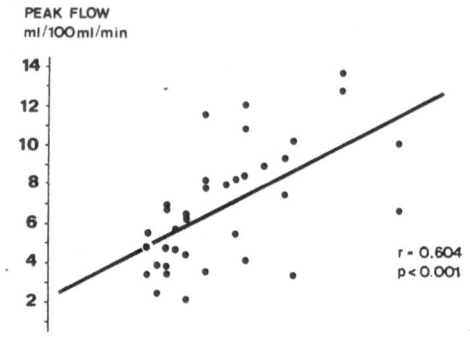

Fig. 2. Correlation of ankle pressure with peak flow during reactive hyperemia in 36 patients.

blood flow during reactive hyperemia in control subjects as well as in patients (Fig. 1). Flows after reactive hyperemia are generally higher than after body heating, which has so far been considered as the maximal vasodilator stimulus (*Linhart et al.*, 1968). Morever, reactive hyperemia is much easier to perform.

Foot blood flows during reactive hyperemia in 36 patients were compared with plethysmographic measurement of ankle blood pressure (*Strandness*, 1969) (Fig. 2). The correlation is not quite close, indicating that ankle blood pressure per se is a poor index of maximal foot blood flow.

From the results obtained we can conclude that measurement of blood flow in the foot during reactive hyperemia may be of considerable practical value. The classical mechanical plethysmograph that we have used so far is more difficult to operate. It is much easier to employ the mercury-strain-gauge plethysmograph (*Whitney*, 1953). However, the cross-section of the foot in the instep is not round and may not meet the theoretical requirements of the strain-gauge system.

FOOT BLOOD FLOW (REST, REACTIVE HYPEREMIA)

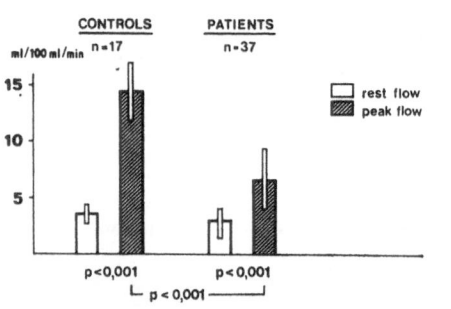

Fig. 1. Foot blood flow at rest and during reactive hyperemia (peak flow) in 17 control subjects and in 37 patients with ischemic disease of the lower extremities.

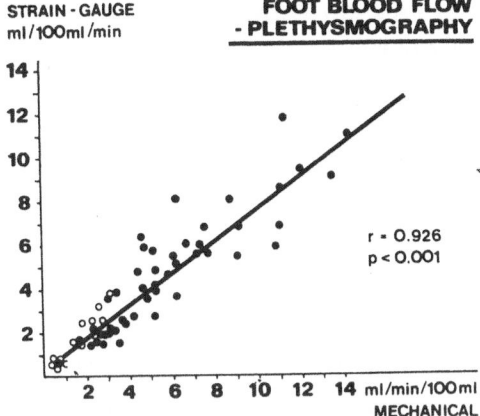

STRAIN - GAUGE
ml/100ml/min

**FOOT BLOOD FLOW
- PLETHYSMOGRAPHY**

r = 0.926
p < 0.001

ml/min/100ml
MECHANICAL

Fig. 3. Correlation of foot blood flow by mechanical and strain-gauge plethysmograph at rest (empty circles) and during reactive hyperemia (full circles) in 13 extremities.

Nevertheless, we made an attempt to compare the two techniques of blood flow measurement in the foot. The mercury-in-silastic tube of the Whitney plethysmograph was placed around the instep. Next, the foot with the tube was inserted into an air-filled mechanical plethysmograph. The results of our measurement after venous occlusions are shown in Fig. 3. Foot blood flows obtained by the mechanical plethysmograph were closely correlated to those obtained by the strain-gauge plethysmograph, although strain-gauge flows were slightly lower.

It has been shown that venous occlusion plethysmography measures total flow and cannot give detailed information on the nutritive fraction of the flow. Nonetheless, plethysmographic measurement of foot blood flow during reactive hyperemia using the simple strain-gauge system is a valuable procedure. It helps to evaluate the actual clinical condition of the patients as well as the effect of therapeutic intervention. We can conclude that this procedure should be one of the standard methods of laboratory investigation in patients with ischemic extremities.

REFERENCES

Abramson, D. I. (1967): Circulation in the extremities. Academic Press, New York and London.

Allwood, M. J. (1958): Blood flow in the foot and calf in the elderly. A comparison with that in young adults. Clin. Sci., 17, 331—338.

Barcroft, H., Swan, H. J. C. (1953): Sympathetic control of human blood vessels. Arnold, London.

Linhart, J., Cachovan, M., Přerovský, I., Hlavová, A. (1968): Measurement of maximal blood flow and arterial elasticity in the course of chronic ischemia of the lower extremities. In: Medical and Surgical Angiological Therapy. Ed. U. Becattini, C.E.P.I., Rome, 271—275.

Strandness, D. E. (1969): Peripheral arterial disease. A physiological approach. Little, Brown and Comp., Boston.

Whitney, R. J. (1953): The measurement of volume changes in human limbs. J. Physiol. (London), 121, 1.

J. S., Institute for Clinical and Experimental Medicine, Prague 4, Vídeňská 800, Czechoslovakia

STRAIN GAGE VENOUS OCCLUSION PLETHYSMOGRAPHY, TECHNICAL POSSIBILITIES AND CLINICAL EXPERIENCES

J. GUTMANN

Laboratory of Physical Medicine, Eurasburg, F.R.G.

The world wide increase of vascular diseases compels doctors to use objective methods of measurement for differential diagnosis and follow up therapy. Venous occlusion plethysmography is a quantitative method for measuring arterial inflow as well as venous outflow segmentally in all limbs. The method using strain gage transducers with mercury-filled tubes has begun to be used in recent years in hospitals and in research, because of its simple application and good reproducibility.

Methods

For measuring the arterial inflow the venous outflow is cut off by an inflatable cuff blown up to subdiastolic pressure while the arterial inflow continues (Fig. 1). The inflow per minute can then be calculated from the increase in the distal volume. Conversely, the rate of the venous outflow can be determined from the decrease in volume after releasing the venous occlusion. For medical purposes it is important whether a certain amount of blood has to supply a larger or smaller area of tissue. The blood flow is therefore given internationally in ml/100 ml tissue per minute. It is mathematically proven that the increase in volume per volume equals twice the change in circumference related to the whole circumference. So the change in circumference

and the circumference must be measured and the quotient calculated. The most important member of the whole plethysmography system is therefore the strain gauge sensor, which has to measure the circumference and the changes in circumference without retroaction on the limb. This sensor looks like an articulated bracelet which has a relatively large contact surface. A very elastic silicone tube filled with mercury is drawn through the plastic links. The sensors are manufactured in different lengths for measurement on fingers and toes as well.

For the use of venous occlusion plethysmography in daily routine and for scientific problems, a complete system of apparatuses and accessories is available. The standard Periquant 3500 equipment contains, in one mobile console, a programmed pneumatic unit, a two-channel measuring bridge and a two-channel compensation recorder with a writing width of about 200 mm. All the operating elements are arranged on the top surface so that it can be operated comfortably while sitting down. The pneumatic control unit has 12 programs for measurement of blood flow at rest, reactive hyperaemia, venous tone and capacity, blood pressure and other factors. For example, to measure reactive hyperaemia the device first produces a suprasystolic pressure for 3 or 5 minutes. When the selected time interval is finished, the suprasystolic pressure is released and the apparatus begins blood flow measurements at 5 sec intervals, so that the subsidence function of the reactive hyperaemia can be traced. The self balancing measuring bridge has a voltage at its output which is proportional to the change in volume in ml/100 ml tissue. This voltage is traced as a plethysmogramme by the calibrated built-in potentiometric recorder. A 10 cm change in the ordinate corresponds to 1 ml/100 ml. The plethysmogramme traced can therefore be evaluated by applying a transparent overlay or a scale. In addition, the voltage can be translated by an analog digital transducer and given directly in figures and printed out.

The modular system of the apparatus is supplemented by various auxilliary devices. For example, a special ergometer for selective loading of individual groups of muscles makes it possible to measure blood flow during muscular work, enabling very many angiological problems to be investigated. Equipment for venous occlusion

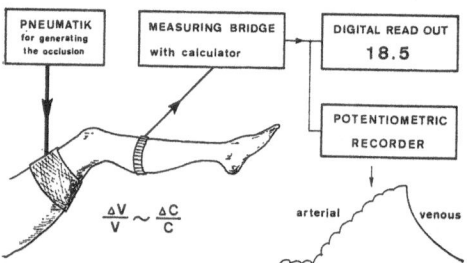

Fig. 1. For quantitative measurement of blood flow the venous outflow is cut off and the change in distal volume is recorded.

plethysmography has attained a very high technical standard, so that the technical errors lie within the limits of ±5%. The errors on the part of the user and physiological errors consist of positional artefact, the error due to too firm or too loose fitting of the strain gauges and wrong adjustment of the correction knob. Experience has shown that fairly careful work will keep the total of all errors below a limit of 10% since the errors also partly compensate each other.

Results

The quantitative measurement of blood flow by venous occlusion plethysmography permits the checking of the functions of the arterial and venous vascular systems by determination of arterial blood flow at rest and the blood flow reserve as well as the rate of venous outflow and the venous capacity. Consequently, it enables recognition of vascular diseases at a very early stage, since alterations in the vascular system are already indicated while they cannot yet be detected by other methods. Only through quantitative measurement of the blood flow can the degree of compensation by the collateral circulation be determined in vascular occlusion. Since it can be repeated as often as necessary, therapy can be controlled at short time intervals.

The blood flow at rest has information value only in special cases. For example the haemodynamic efficiency of arterio-venous fistulas can be investigated by this measurement or the effects of drugs for supervision of therapy. Much more important, however, is measurement of the arterial blood flow reserve which is usually done in a standardized way by measurement of the reactive hyperaemia following three minutes of ischaemia. As Figure 2 shows, the reaction fades very quickly in healthy persons. On the other hand, in sick persons this occurs after some delay or, in severe cases, not at all. For assessment, the peak flow is determined and compared with an internationally recognised table, which was drawn up several years ago, and is based on the work of several recognised angiologists and our own investigations and has proven its value. Another criterion for the assessment of the curves of reactive hyperaemia is the time at which the peak flow appears, which must be within the first 15 sec in healthy subjects. In the dermatological field, measurement of the vascular capacity has a certain importance. The distance from the base line to the horizontal part of the curve gives the vascular capacity, which can sometimes be increased by 50% in venous diseases. But more important than measurement of the venous capacity is measurement of the rate of venous outflow. For this the legs are raised to an angle of 45°. A venous occlusion with a pressure of 80 mm Hg obstructs the outflow, so that the legs

Fig. 2: The reactive hyperaemia after 3 minutes ischaemia shows the blood flow reserve and is a reliable parameter for evaluation of the degree of compensation.

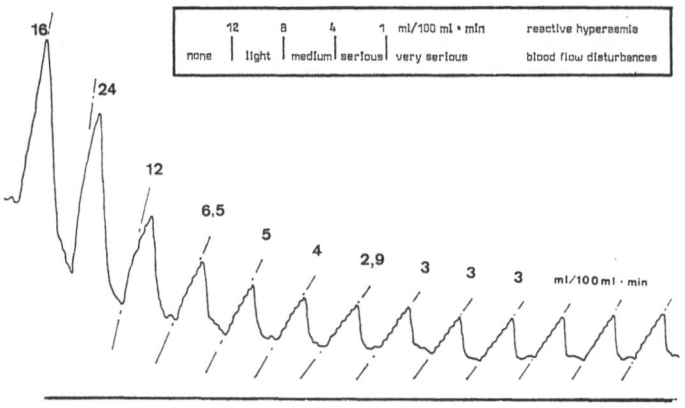

REACTIVE HYPERAEMIA AFTER 3 MIN. ISCHAEMIA

become filled with blood. The venous occlusion is released and blood flows more or less rapidly out according to the condition of the vessels. From the curve the rate of outflow can be determined quantitatively. It is markedly reduced in the presence of thromboses. In addition to the measurement of reactive hyperaemia after ischaemia, it is consequently of interest to measure blood flow in active work. Such measurements play an important role in sports medicine, for instance, but they can also be used clinically, A very simple experiment is testing the function of the muscle pump by standing on tiptoe to the rhythm of a metronome while the plethysmographic curve of the forefoot is recorded. The artefacts of the movement are also recorded, but the envelope curve during the test shows how the filling with blood decreases. From the time the exercise is stopped, the renewed inflow is recorded without artefacts. The difference between the initial level and the deepest point represents the pump output in ml/100 ml (Fig. 3). For measurement of the systolic bood pressure distal to vascular occlusions or stenoses the cuff is blown up to a suprasystolic pressure and then the pressure is slowly released while the plethysmographic curve is registered (Fig. 3). When the systolic blood pressure level si reached the curve increases quite clearly. The pertinent blood pressures are either read off the manometer or else recorded on the second recording channel.

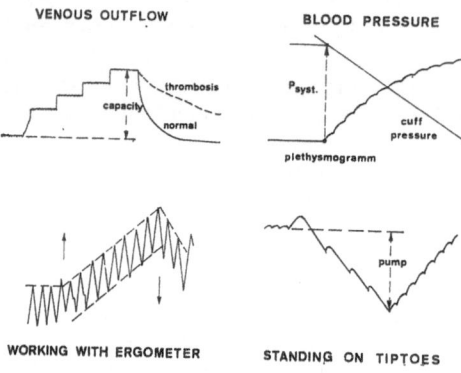

Fig. 3. Different possibilities for use of venous occlusion plethysmography.

REFERENCES

K. Barbey u. P. Barbey: Ein neuer Plethysmograf zur Messung der Extremitätendurchblutung. Zeitschrift Kreislaufforschung 52, S. 1129 (1963)

H. M. Becker u. J. Klemm: Zur Wertigkeit der Dehnungsmeßstreifen-Stauplethysmografie. Herz/Kreisl. 4. Jg., Nr. 7, S. 254—258 (1972).

J. Gutmann: Technical aspects of blood flow measurement. Intern. Congress of testing methods. Clinical Evaluation of Testing Methods of Vasoactive Drug-Effects. Rome 1968.

J. Gutmann u. J. Krötz: Zur Genauigkeit der Dehnungsmeßstreifenmethode bei der venösen Kapazitätsmessung: Folia Angiologica Vol. XX., S. 103 (1972).

G. Rudofsky, F. Nobbe, F.-E. Brock: Venenverschlußplethysmographie, Diagnostik 10, S. 24—26 (1977).

J. G., Labor für Physikalische Medizin, D-8191 Eurasburg, F.R.G.

EVALUATION FOR PARTIAL PROXIMAL RECONSTRUCTION IN PATIENTS WITH SEVERE ISCHAEMIA OF THE FOOT

I. NOER

Department of Clinical Physiological, Bispebjerg Hospital, Copenhagen, Denmark

In chronic severe ischemia in the feet of elderly patients, angiograms often show multiple level obstructions in the arterial system. Evaluation for reconstructive procedures should therefore consider the possibility of partial reconstruction. Which should always include the most proximal lesion with haemodynamic importance; also reconstruction of the large vessels has superior early and late patency. If, for technical reasons, a partial proximal reconstruction is to be prefered, the surgeon must consider whetter partial proximal reconstruction is actually sufficient to relieve the rest pain and to start the ischemic ulcer healing.

Metods

A method of predicting the postreconstructive blood supply to the foot and toes is discussed below.

First the spontaneous prognosis in the patients is evaluated by repeated distal blood pressure measurements (at the toe and ankle) by the strain gauge technique.

According to *Holstein et al.* 1976 a persistent resting blood pressure at the first toe of less than 30 mm Hg implies major or minor amputation in 72% of legs with small skin lesions at the foot (91% of legs with a pressure less than 20 mm Hg). However, a pressure of more than 30 mm Hg is followed by healing in 100% of small skin lesions.

In cases of persistent low toe blood pressure and continuous clinical signs of severe ischaemia (i.e. rest pain in the toes, no healing of ischaemic ulcers) an angiogram including the vessels from the aorta to the ankle is performed. Patients with multiple level obstructions partly proximal to the ligament are further investigated in order to guide the reconstructive procedure.

In the resting supine body position a catheter (outher diameter 1.1 mm) is induced by the Seldinger technique to the brachial artery and to the ipsilateral common femoral artery (in case of absent palpaple pulsation the arterial puncture is partly guided by an ultrasound doppler shift pencil probe). The two intraarterial blood pressures are continuously recorded while the blood pressure at the ankle is measured repeatedly by the indirect strain gauge technique. In many patients a supplementary angiogram through the catheter in the common femoral artery is performed to visualise the arterial system distal to the iliac obstruction, because the translumbal angiogram is often insufficient at this level.

To attain successful reconstruction to the level of the measured pressure in the common femoral artery, postoperative equalization of the brachial and the common femoral artery pressures is suggested. The ankle pressure increase is calculated proportional to the systolic pressure increase in the common femoral artery (viz., measured 160 mm Hg systolic in the brachial artery, 100 mm Hg systolic in the common femoral artery and 50 mm Hg at the ankle, an increase of 60 percent systolic is expected in the leg, i.e. 30 mm Hg at the ankle level.

Results

Twenty one legs (patient mean age 61 ± 9 years) with a constant toe blood pressure below 30 mm Hg underwent the described procedure. Partial reconstruction proximal to ligament was carried out with

Table I. The mean measured preoperative ankle and toe pressure in 21 legs. The effect of the operation is the difference between the postoperative and the preoperative measured pressure. The predicted increase is calculated according to the segmental pressure measurement: = systolic brachial press/systolic femoral press. x ankle press. ÷ ankle pressure.

OPERATIVE RESULTS AND PREDICTION OF POSTOPERATIVE DISTAL PRESSURE (mmHg, n = 21)

	Ankle	I. Toe
preoperative pressure	45.5 ± 10.8	16.6 ± 11.1
postoperative pressure	84.9 ± 22.4	43.7 ± 24.1
increase in pressure	39.4 ± 25.6	27.1 ± 21.5
predicted increase	36.6 ± 16.2	

primary good results judged by palpation of the femoral artery.

In Table I are given the preoperative ankle pressure 45.5 ± 10.8 mm Hg, toe pressure 16.6 ± 11.1 mm Hg and the measured increase postoperatively $39.4 \pm \pm 25.6$ mm Hg and 27.1 ± 21.5 mm Hg, respectively, at the ankle and toe. The correlation between the predicted ankle pressure and the postoperatively measured increase is shown in Figure 1. It can be seen that the ankle pressure following proximal reconstruction is increased in proportion to the common femoral artery systolic increase. However, the most important value is the resulting toe blood pressure. In Figure 2 the measured ankle pressure increase is correlated to the measured toe blood pressure increase. The figure indicates that the toe blood pressure increase is $10-15$ mm Hg less than the increase in the ankle pressure.

By proper measurement of the distal (toe) blood pressure, it is possible to form a prognosis for conservative treatment of ulcers of the foot. Supplementary segmental pressure measurement can foretell the prognosis of the peripheral ischaemic lesion after partial proximal arterial reconstruction.

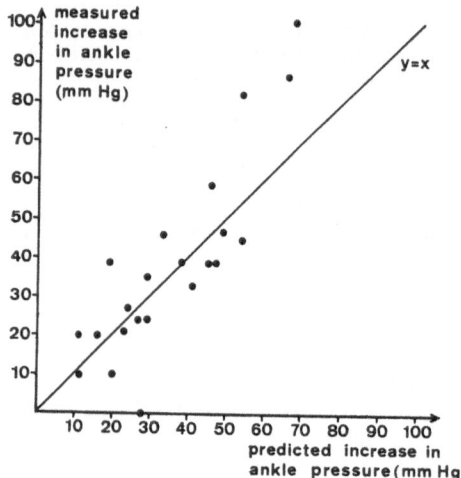

Fig. 1. The effect at the ankle (measured ankle pressure increase) of the reconstruction is compared to the predicted effect. (y = 1.36x ÷ 10.2, r = 0.86).

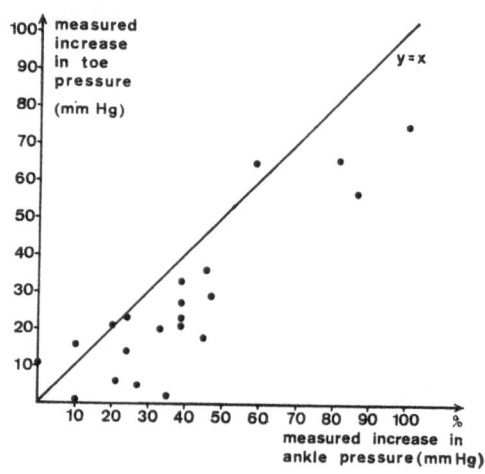

Fig. 2. The effect at the toe (measured toe pressure increase) of the reconstruction is compared to the postoperative measured ankle pressure increase. (y = 0.74x ÷ 2.0, r = 0.88).

REFERENCES

Holstein, P., Krähenbühl, B. and Lassen, N. A.: Induzierte Hypertonie in der Behandlung Peripherer Arterieller Krankheit. In Hypertonie — Risikofaktor in der Angiologie. *Gerhard Witzstoock*, Baden-Baden, Brüssel Köln. p. 157, 1976.

I.N. Department of Clinical Physiology, Bispebjerg Hospital, DK-2400 Copenhagen NV, Denmark

THIRD ORDER WAVES OF PLETHYSMOGRAM (T.O.W.) AND THE DIFFERENTIATION OF ARTERIOSCLEROSIS OBLITERANS FROM THROMBOANGIITIS OBLITERANS

Z. BRASSAI and S. I. CSÖGÖR

2nd Department of Internal Medicine, University of Tirgu Mures, Romanie and Institute for Atherosclerosis Research, University of Münster, F.R.G.

Though there has been some controversy concerning the existence of Buerger's disease as a specific entity, sufficient evidence is available for its recognition. Taking in consideration the sex and age of patients at the start of the process, the location of the occlusion, the characteristic aspect of the skin of the affected extremities, the eyeground, the arteriographic picture, the presence or absence of migratory phlebitis and Raynaud's type of cold sensitivity, differentiation of thrombo-angiitis obliterans and arteriosclerosis obliterans is mostly possible.

The therapeutic importance of this differentiation consists in the good re-activity of Buerger's disease to complete abstinence from tobacco, to admini-stration of vasodilatatory drugs, and to application of anti-inflamatory measures.

The T. O. W. have a frequency of $1-4$ cycle/min and reflect the slow oscillations of vasomotor tonus. In spite of the fact that local factors influence the circulation, the simultaneous recording of T. O. W. coincides with the optimal nervous re-activity indicated by reaction time mea-surement (*Csögör and Brassai*, 1976). There is no compulsory correlation bet-ween the T. O. W. and the variation of cutaneous temperature.

Studying the cold reactivity of the vascular system of patients with obstructive arteriopathies (*Brassai et al.*, 1974) we recorded the T. O. W. and have observed a remarkable difference in the form of T. O. W. in the two groups of patients. Differentiation of arteriosclerosis obli-terans from thromboangiitis obliterans can be a difficult task; therefore we have studied the significance of T. O. W. in the solution of this problem.

Materials and methods

A glass cylinder was secured with putty to the toe of the patients and the volume changes

D.L. dg. = As.o.

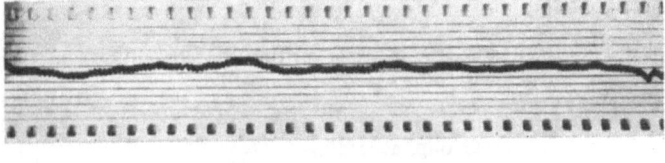

G.J. dg. = As.o.

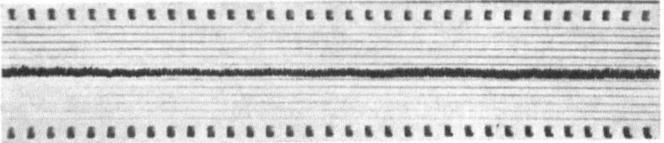

Fig. 1.

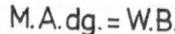

M. A. dg. = W.B.

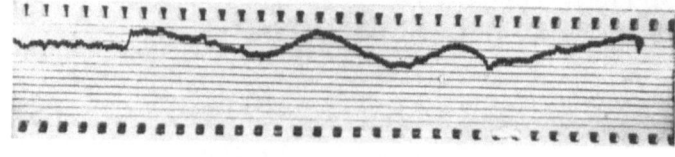

L.C. dg. = W.B.

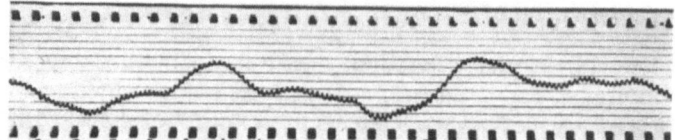

Fig. 2.

of the toe were registered with a Triodyn (Radelkisz, Budapest Hungary) plethysmographic transducer and a two channel oscillograph for at least 15 min. Due to the very low frequency of T.O.W., D. C. amplification and a recording speed of 1.25—2.5 mm/sec were necessary. The examinations were performed in horizontal position after 15 min rest in a comfortably warm room. 105 male patients suffering from arteriosclerosis obliterans or Buerger's disease in stage II—III Fontaine were investigated, avoiding the pervious administration of vasodilatatory drugs or sympathectomy. The patients were hospitalized and the plethysmographic examinations were performed before arteriography. The plethysmograms were evaluated by one of us (S.I.C.) without the knowledge of "clinical diagnosis" (Z.B.). The "clinical diagnosis" was based on anamnesis, clinical, laboratory and angiographic investigations.

In order to render the interpretation of the curves objective, the T.O.W. were considered "flat" when their maximal amplitude was less than three times the amplitude of the first order waves.

Results and discussion

Figure 1 shows two flat curves characteristic for arteriosclerosis obliterans and figure 2 shows curves with ample T. O. W. registered by two patients with Buerger's disease.

Table I summarizes our results and shows that the plethysmographic investigation furnishes valuable data for the differentiation of arteriosclerosis obliterans and thromboangiitis obliterans. In our investigation we used the "clinical diagnosis" as a criterion for the evaluation of the significance of T. O. W. and unfortunately this criterion is quite relative. In some patients the plethysmographic investigation throws new light on the case and stimulates revision of the original diagnosis or confirms it.

Table I. Correlation between clinical and plethysmogaphic diagnosis in patients with obstructive arteriopathies

Groups according to clinical dg.	No.	Concordant	Plethysmogram is Uncharacteristic	Discordant
Arteriosclerosis obliterans	63	54	7	2
Buerger's disease	42	39	2	1
Total	105	93	9	3

Our preliminary studies have shown that the T. O. W. disappear definitely after lumbar sympathectomy and temporarily after the administration of vasodilatatory drugs. In patients with obstructive arteriopathies in stage IV Fontaine the registration of plethysmographic waves is very difficult or imposible and the minor modifications of patients in stage I do not cause significant alterations in the T. O. W.

Therefore, the applicability of the plethysmographic method is limited to patients in stages II and III.

The pathological basis of differentiation of arteriosclerosis obliterans and thromboangiitis obliterans investigating the T. O. W. may be related to the rigidity of arteriosclerotic vessels and to the spastic reactions associated with the inflammatory process, respectively.

REFERENCES

Csögör, S. I., Brassai, Z. (1976): Undele tertiare ale pletismogramei. Centrul de cercetari medicale Tirgu Mures. Sesiunea stiintifica anuala de comunicari. Vol. 1976.
Brassai, Z., Horváth, E., Csögör, S. I., Ferncz, L.,

Benedek, G., Szász, B.: (1974): Efectul bailor carbogazoase in tratamentul arteriopatiilor obliterante periferice cronice. Rev. med.-chir. (Iasi), 68, 603—608.

S. I. C., Institute for Arteriosclerosis Research at the University of Münster, D-4400 Münster, Westring 3, F.R.G.

A STUDY OF THE INFLUENCE OF ACUPUNCTURE ON DIGITAL BLOOD FLOW USING THE STRAIN GAUGE PLETHYSMOGRAPHY TECHNIQUE

A. H. KATSOGIANNIS, P. BALAS and P. NATSIS

Peripheral Vascular Laboratory of the Hellenic Air Force Hospital, Athens, Greece

Acupuncture and its use in anaesthesia has been described by many authors (*Herget and Kalweit*, 1973, *Lowe*, 1973). Even though acupuncture has been used in anaesthesia in China and some other European countries, experience with its influence on the peripheral circulation is very limited. Very few authors have studied the influence of acupuncture on the peripheral circulation (*Laitinen*, 1976, *Celocia*, 1977, *Trnavsky*, 1977). The second author of this study, who has visited China twice, corroborated the use of acupuncture treatment for ischemic conditions of the extremities in the large hospitals of Shanghai and Peking. However the question still exists of whether acupuncture actually influences peripheral circulation of the extremities. In the present study the influence of acupuncture on digital blood flow was investigated by using the strain gauge plethysmography technique.

Material and methods

Sixteen healthy subjects with no clinical evidence of peripheral circulation disturbances were examined. Similarly, four patients with disturbances of peripheral circulation of the upper extremities were examined. The examinations were performed in a room with a temperature of 23—25 °C. Each of the individuals was placed on an examining bed and two mercury strain gauge loops were placed about the distal phalanx of each index digit. Synchronous plethysmograms of both upper extremities were recorded and then a special acupuncture needle was inserted in the right arm in the depression at the lateral end of the transverse cubital crease (Point Quchi, L.I. 11: An Outline on Chinese Acupuncture, 1975). This point was in many instances located by using the special electro-explorer for acupuncture points. Every 5 minutes for a period of 15 minutes synchronous plethysmograms of the two upper extremities were recorded. At the end of this period of time strong stimulation of the point was performed by rotating the needle in a small amplitude and new plethysmograms were recorded. After withdrawal of the needle a five minute time of relaxation was allowed and the reactive hyperaemia test on the left arm was performed (*Stradness* 1965).

Results

In none of the healthy subjects, nor in the patients with vascular disorders, was the volume pulse amplitude of the acupunctured extremity increased. Nor was any change in the morphology of the plethysmographic wave observed. In almost all of the examined cases a significant increase of the amplitude of the plethysmographic wave was observed on the extremity in which the reactive hyperaemia test was performed (Fig. 1). During acupuncture, changes of the amplitude of the plethysmograms were observed in most of the cases, these changes being equal in value on both extremities. In almost all the cases a decrease of the amplitude of the plethysmographic wave was observed during the phase of strong stimulation of the acupunctured right arm; however this decrease was equal in value on both upper extremities (Fig. 2).

Discussion

During the last decade acupuncture has been used extensively mainly in China as well as in European countries for therapy and anesthesia. The second author, during his two recent trips to China, has not

338

Fig. 1. Plethysmograms of the hands after acupuncture of the right arm and reactive hyperaemia test (R. H.T.) of the left arm. Increase of the amplitude of the digital pulse after R.H. T., but no increase after acupuncture.

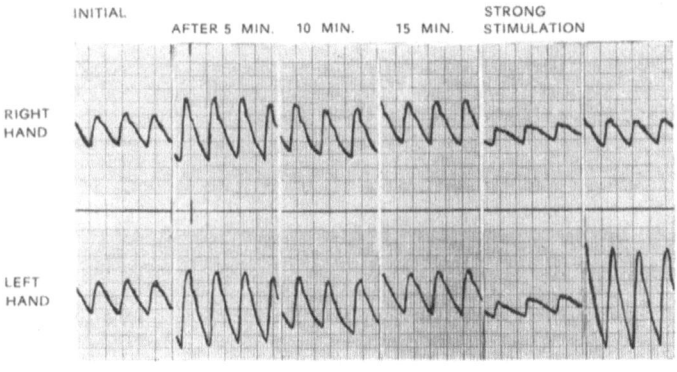

Fig. 2. Decrease of the amplitude of the plethysmographic wave of both hands during the phase of strong stimulation of the acupunctured right arm.

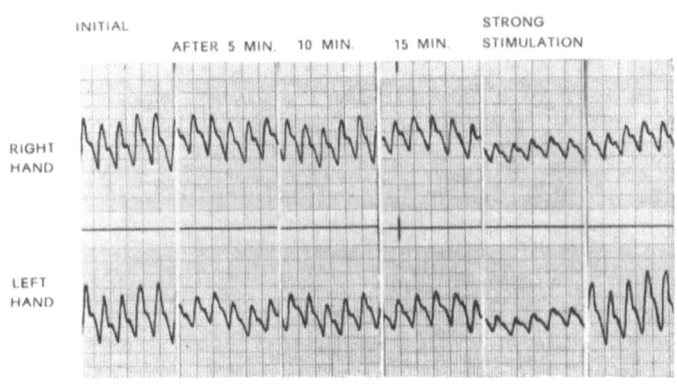

received any positive information concerning the influence of acupuncture on the arterial circulation of the upper extremities. Dr. Ch'en, of the 6th People's Hospital in Shanghai observed an improvement of circulation after acupuncture on a replanted arm. However, other eminent physicians of Traditional Chinese and Western Medicine have stated that acupuncture can result in vasospasm or vasodilation in the hand. *Laitinen* (1975) found some increase of the temperature of the hand skin after acupuncture, as well as a prolongation of the propagation time in the photoelectric plethysmogram. *Trnavsky* also (1977) found an increase of the arterial flow in the lower extremities after electric stimulation of acupuncture points. The acupuncture point Quchi (L. I. 11), which has been used in our study, was described by qualified anaesthesiologists

of Chinese Traditional Medicine to the second author who explained to them his intention to examine the influence of acupuncture on arterial circulation of the hands. During our investigation in a rather small series of healthy volunteers and patients with vascular disorders of the upper extremities no increase of arterial blood flow was observed when checked by strain gauge plethysmography technic.

This result might be explained either by stimulating incorrect acupuncture points not related to arterial circulation of the hand or by failure to produce any influence of acupuncture on the arterial circulation.

In conclusion we recommend further extensive research and stimulation on other acupuncture points in order to find their possible relation to arterial circulation.

REFERENCES

The Academy of Traditional Chineese Medicine (1975): An Outline of Chinese acupuncture, p. 104, Foreign Languages Press, Peking.

Celocia et al. (1977): Changes in the angiographic pictures in Raynaud's disease following acupuncture treatment. Minerva Med. 68, 711—715.

Herget, H. and Kalweit, K. (1973): Anaesthesie-Kongress. Linz.

Laitinen, J. (1976): Temperature measurements and photoelectric plethysmography in the evaluation of acute and long-term effects of acupuncture upon vasomotor activity of hand skin. Am. J. Chin. Med. 4, 169—75.

Lowe, W. (1973): Introduction to acupuncture-analgesia. H. Huber, Bern—Stuttgart—Wien.

Stradness, D. E. (Jr), and Bell, J. W. (1965): Peripheral Vascular Disease: Diagnosis and Objective Evaluation Using A Mercury Strain Gauge. Ann. Surg. 161, 4 (Supplement).

Trnavsky, G. (1977): Rheographic examination of blood flow changes in the lower limbs after electric stimulation of acupuncture points. Wiener Medizinische Wochenschrift. 127, 659—662.

A. H. K., Peripheral Vascular Laboratory, Hellenic Air Force Hospital, Athens, Greece

VENOUS OCCLUSION PLETHYSMOGRAPHIC EXPERIMENTS CONCERNING THE "BORROWING-LENDING-PHENOMENON" UNDER THE INFLUENCE OF PENTOXIFYLLIN AND NAFTIDROFURYL

M. SCHARTL, H. HEIDRICH and S. SCHARTL

Department of Cardiology, Klinikum Charlottenburg, Free University of Berlin West

According to the definition of *De Bakey and co-workers* (1947) and *Gillespie* (1959) the borrowing-lending-phenomenon or hemometakinesia represent a change in blood distribution implying a further decrease in the blood perfusion in the primarily lesser perfused part of the body and a corresponding increase in the blood flow in the primarily better perfused part of the body. Such a borrowing-lending-phenomenon may occur after systemic or intra-arterial application of vasodilating drugs. For many authors, the borrowing-lending-phenomenon is still a basic argument against the use of vasodilators in patients with peripheral arterial vascular disease. We feel that this statement should not be accepted as an unquestionable fact and that all new substances used in the treatment of vascular disease should be examined thoroughly as each has a different vasodilating potency.

Using the venous occlusion plethysmographic technique we therefore tried

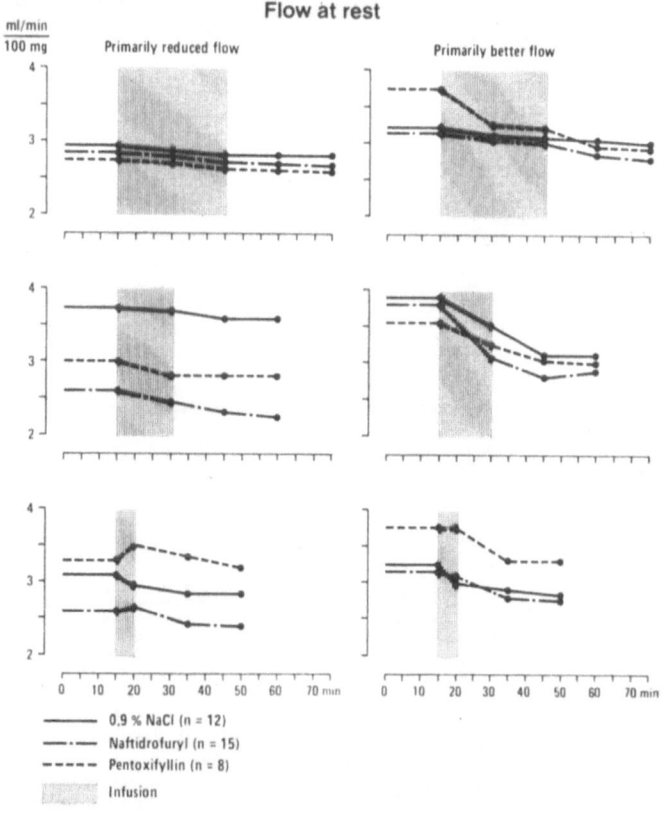

Fig. 1.

341

to discover whether, under clinical conditions and therapeutical doses of Naftidrofuryl and Pentoxifyllin, a borrowing-lending-phenomenon could be observed.

Experiments were performed with 28 patients suffering from peripheral arterial vascular disease, stage II, according to Fontaine. Each patient was randomly placed in one of three groups: 15 patients received intravenously 200 mg Naftidrofuryl, 8 patients 200 mg Pentoxifyllin and 12 patients intravenously 0.9% sodium-chloride. All patients underwent experiments on three successive days with varying infusion times, ranging from 5 to 10 to 30 minutes. Simultaneously, blood perfusion in rest and peak flow were measured by the venous occlusion plethysmographic method with a mercury-strain-gauge at the calves of the lower extremities. Perfusion in rest was determined every minute from 15 minutes before starting infusion and up to 30 minutes after stopping infusion. The peak flow was measured just before starting infusion, at the end of the infusion time and 30 minutes after stopping infusion. For the evaluation of the blood flow at rest, the results of 15 single determinations were averaged for the 15 and 30 minute infusion time period. For the 5 minute infusion time period measurements were averaged. According to the results of the first peak flow determination the extremities were labelled "primarily better" or "primarily less" perfused. The statistical significance was established following the co-variance analysis with a reliability of twice smaller than 0.05.

Results

1. The blood flow at rest was reduced in both the better and lesser perfused extremity after Pentoxifyllin and Naftidro-

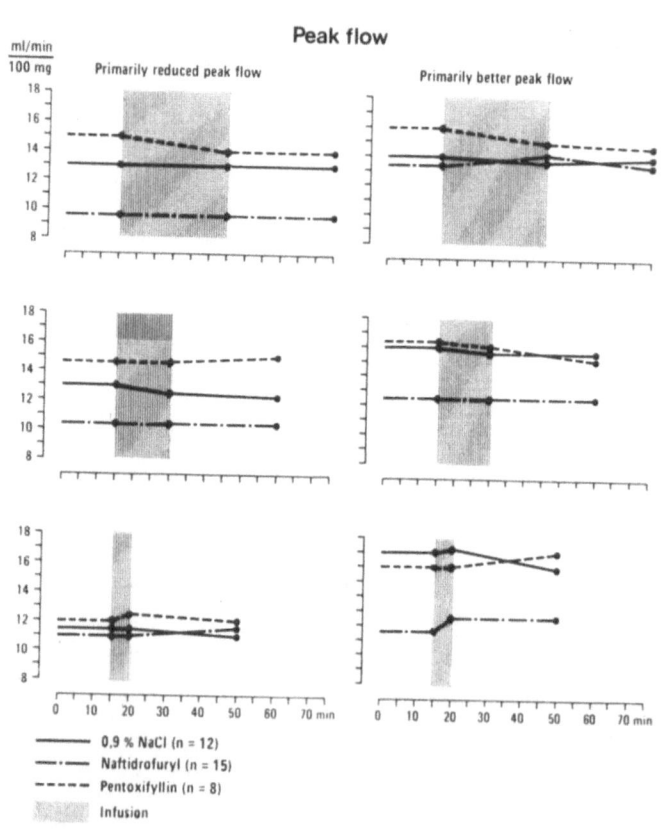

Fig. 2.

furyl in each of the 30 minute, 15 minute and 5 minute infusion period compared with the circulation before starting the infusion. However, the same decrease was observed after sodium-chloride. A statistical difference between Naftidrofuryl and Pentoxifyllin and sodium-chloride group could not be demonstrated.

2. In contrast to the blood flow at rest, the peak flow indicating the degree of reactive hyperemia showed no decrease at the end of the infusion time compared to the rate at the beginning of infusion. There also was no difference compared to the sodium-chloride group.

3. The analysis of the results obtained from the patients showed that, when there was a decrease change of peak flow or blood flow at rest, it was always in the same direction in both the better and less perfused leg. Thus, a borrowing-lending-phenomenon could not be observed.

In our experiments, acute systemic application of Pentoxifyllin and Naftidrofuryl in therapeutical doses with a known effect in long term therapy (*Heidrich et al.*, 1977), did not lead to a borrowing-lending-phenomenon. We therefore feel that this phenomenon should not be an argument against the application of these two substances. This, of course, does not permit us to question in principle the existence of a borrowing-lending-phenomenon following the application of other vasodilating drugs. The decrease of blood flow at rest observed after Pentoxifyllin, Naftidrofuryl and 0.9 NaCl very likely is not a specific drug effect and is of no relevance as the peak flow showed no change.

REFERENCES

De Bakey, M. E., Burch G., Ray, Th. Ochsner A. (1947): The "borrowing-lending" hemodynamic phenomenon (Hemometakinesia) and its therapeutic application in peripheral vascular disturbances. (Ann. Surg., 126, 850.

Gillespie, J. A. (1959): Vasodilator drugs in occlusive vascular disease of the legs. (Lancet, II 995.

Heidrich, H., D. Witt, E. Witt (1977): Periphere Durchblutungsgröße bei arterieller Verschlußkrankheit unter i. v.-Langzeittherapie mit gefäßaktiven Pharmaka. Plethysmographische Vergleichsstudie. (Verh. Dtsch. Ges. Inn. Med. 83, 1750.

M. S., Free University of Berlin, Klinikum Charlottenburg, Department of Cardiology Spandauer Damm 130, 1000 Berlin West 19

EXPERIENCE WITH TRANSVENOUS XEROARTERIOGRAPHY IN VASCULAR SURGERY

P. C. MAURER, B. KRAMANN and J. LANGE

Department of Vascular Surgery and Department of Radiology
Rechts der Isar Medical School, Technical University Munich, F.R.G.

Using the Xeroradiographical technique arteriograms can be performed with a very small quantity of radioopaque fluid, which would not permit opacification of the vessel structures on conventional X-ray-film. This is due to the electrostatic charge pattern and its edge contrast enhancement.

In fact, the contrast material can be diluted to a degree below the threshold of

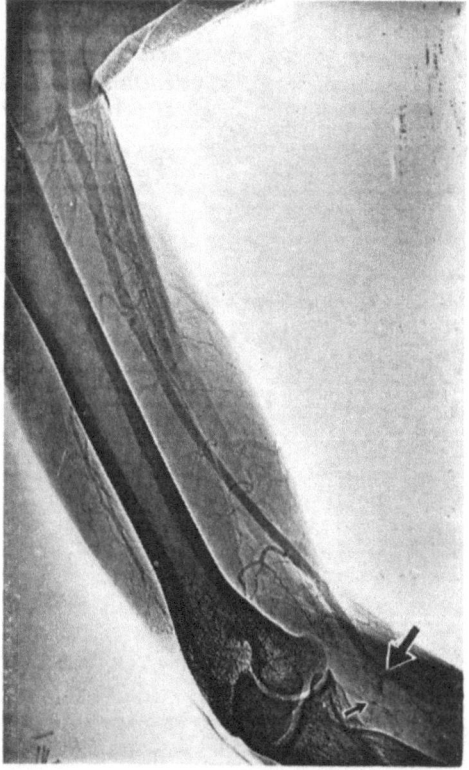

Fig. 1. Fragmented embolisation into the cubital artery and the bifurcation of the radial and ulnar arteries.

pain and thus makes peripheral arteriography a less troublesome procedure for the patient.

Apart from these advantages, vessels of small diameter can be seen in detail. Angiographic visualization of vessels in the trunk, however, has no advantage over the representation on conventional X-ray-film and would be associated with comparatively large radiation doses.

However puncturing the artery Xero-arteriography is — apart from the mentioned advantages — still an invasive method and thus the diagnostic information obtained has to be paid for with a certain risk to the patient.

Our objective was to find a non-invasive and non-traumatic method to opacify peripheral arteries. In order to keep the procedure as simple and sure as possible (in terms of material investment and possible complications) venous catheter methods (normally used for indirect arteriography) were discarded from the beginning.

In "Transvenous Xeroarteriography" — as we have called our method — the contrast material is injected by hand into a cubital vein through a normal injection needle.

A prerequisite for transvenous serial arteriography was the development of a Xerox cassette changer. This device was planned and built by our co-author Dr. Kramann from the Department of Radiology at our Institution in Collaboration with the engineering company Gärtner in Düsseldorf. This Xerox cassette changer has a normal frame speed of one exposure per second and can alternatively be run with size 24/30 film cassettes at a maximum frame speed of two images per second.

Main indications for transvenous Xero-arteriography are: confirmation of pre-operative diagnosis especially in high risk

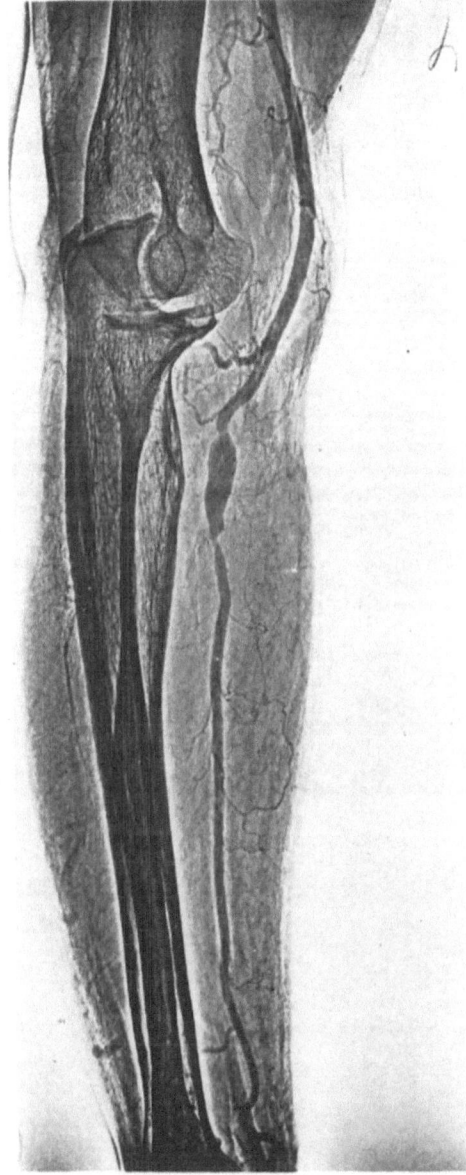

Fig. 2a. Status after automatic saw-injury to the left elbow with large defect of the cubital artery, venous graft between a. brachialis and a. ulnaris; 18 months later aneurysm of the venous graft.

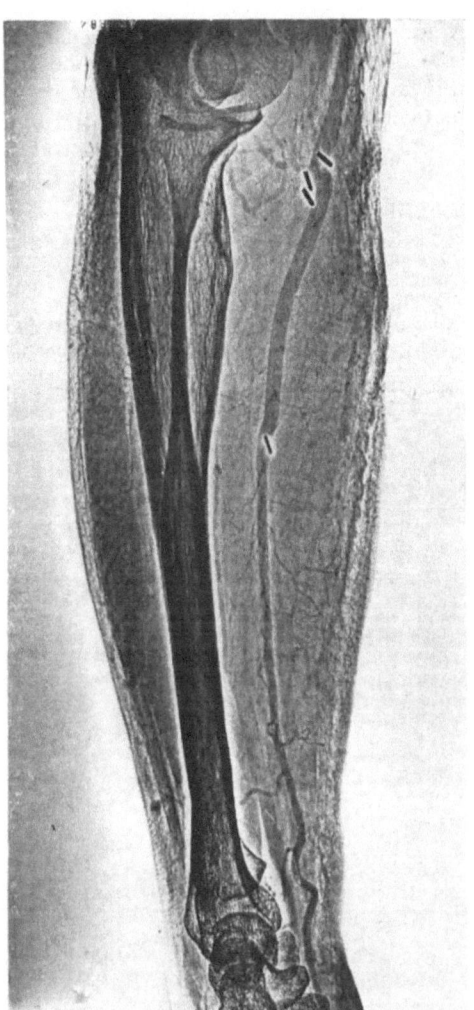

Fig. 2b. Status after resection of the aneurysm and replacement by a new vein graft.

patients and postoperative control of localized vascular lesions of the extremities.

So far 183 patients (mainly from the Department of Vascular Surgery) have been examined by transvenous Xero-arteriography. Only in a very small number of cases were the results not satisfactory. In the beginning, in 9 patients a second series of arteriograms had to be performed. This was, however, not necessary in the last 130 patients examined.

Side effects like headache or nausea were observed only rarely. We hope the following examples demonstrate the practical value of this method.

We hoped that it could be demonstrated that transvenous Xero-arteriography is a practical method for demonstration of peripheral arteries. This really non-invasive technique allows simple and safe visualization of localized vascular lesions.

REFERENCES

Kramann, B., Christen, N.: (1977): Die transvenöse Xeroarteriographie der Extremitäten. Dtsch. med. Wschr. 102, 1031—1033.

Kramann, B., Christen, N., Maurer, P. C. (1978): Transvenous Xeroarteriography of peripheral arteries. Proceedings, International Congress of Cardiovascular Surgery (The M. E. Debakey International Cardiovascular Society) Athens, Greece, June 1977.

Maurer, P. C., B. Kramann, J. Lange (1978): Erfahrungen mit der transvenösen Xero-Arteriographie in der Gefäßchirurgie. Thoraxchirurgie 26, 140—143.

P. C. M., Rechts der Isar Surgical Clinic, Technical University Medical School, 8000 Munich 80, Ismaningerstr. 22, F.R.G.

CONTRIBUTION TO THE ASSESSEMENT OF LYMPHEDEMA BY XERORADIOGRAPHY

J. BRUNA

Radiological Clinic of the Medical Faculty of Hygiene, Charles University, Prague, Czechoslovakia

Introduction

The various methods of lymphedema assessment can be divided into objective and subjective. Of the objective methods, volumetric (*Kuhnke*, 1976), tensometric (*Clodius et al.*, 1976) and others are used. Recently, xeroradiography and xero-radiolymphography (*Bruna, Gravelle*, 1978, *Schertel et al.*, 1975) enabling good visualization of the skin, subcutis and lymphatic vessels, have come into use. Xeroradiography can benefit from the pecularities of this technique, i.e. "edge affect", extent of blackening graduation, simultaneous visualization of soft and hard tissues, visualization of lymphatic vessels even against bone structures. A special possibility is also offered by native xeroradiography of the axilla region (*Kalisher*, 1975). We use xero-radiography, xeroradiotomography and xerolymphography for the assessment of lymphedema (*Bruna, Clodius*, 1978).

Methods

In a group of 30 patients suffering from lymphedema, the possibilities and value of plain xeroradiography, xeroradiotomography and

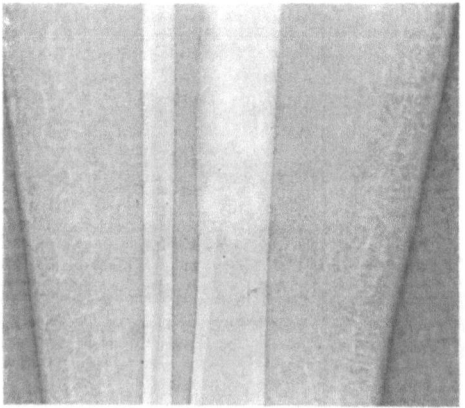

Fig. 1. Plain xeroradiogram of primary lymphedema in negative mode of xerography (115 kV, 35 mAs). There is good visualization of the skin, subcutis and muscle-bone layer.

xerolymphography using Rank-Xerox System 125 were followed. The patients were examined using both techniques i. e. xeroradiography and conventional X-ray film radiography. The examination was focused on soft tissues and lymphatic vessels. Xeroradiograms of extremities were performed in negative and positive modes (115 kV, 15—40 mAs). In the xeroradiograms obtained the skin thickness (C) as well as the thickness of the subcutis (Sc), muscle) bone layer (MB) and transverse diameter (D-

Table I. Assessment of arm lymphedema by xeroradiography

Results Mean ± Dif.	C mm	Sc mm	D mm	MB mm	F 0—2
Normal	1 ± 0.5	9 ± 4	77 ± 7	64 ± 16	0
Lymphedema	3 ± 2	22 ± 14	117 ± 23	70 ± 10	0—2

C = cutis, Sc = subcutis, D = transverse diameter of arm, MB = muscle-bone layer, F = fibrose.

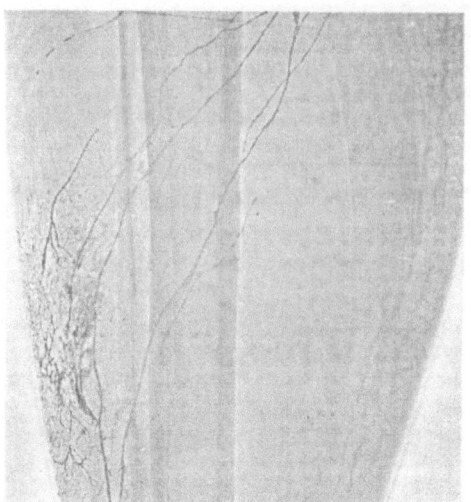

Fig. 2. Xeroradiolymphangiogram of secondary lymphedema (in positive mode of xeroradiography). There is good visualization of the lymphatic vessels with dermal backflow and thicker subcutis.

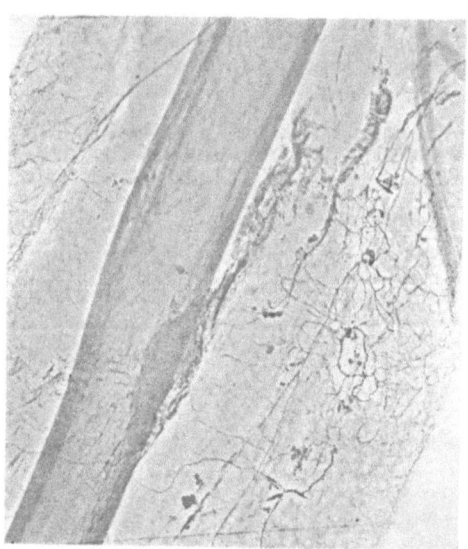

Fig. 3. Xeroradiolymphangiogram of secondary arm lymphedema (in positive mode of xeroradiography). There are good visualized the minute lymphatic vessels in dermal backflow, extravasation of contrast medium and thicker subcutis.

were measured and symptoms of fibrose (F) determined. The lymphography (in the group of 15 patients) was performed by means of direct lymphography consisting of administration of 5—8 ml of Lipiodol Ultrafluid into the lower extremity or 2—4 ml into the upper extremity.

Results and discussion

The results of the assessment of arm lymphedema by xeroradiography are given in Table I. Plain xeroradiography in the negative mode was preferable for the determination of skin (C) and subcutis (Sc) thickness over conventional X-ray examination. Especially good results were obtained using a combination of plain xeroradiography and xeroradiotomography in the negative mode. The muscle-bone layer (MB) is not usually markedly affected, yet in more advanced edemas distinct differences were found even here.

Direct lymphography yields the most exact picture of the character of lymphatic vessel alterations, lymph circulation and lymph node changes. For the examinations we used the technique of pharmaco-dynamic lymphography (*Bruna*, 1974). The positive mode of xeroradiography is better suited for visualization as even minute lymphatic vessels and extravasates are well visualized. The "edge effect" makes possible visualization, of even the dermal capillary network, usually correlated with local dermal back flow. All these alterations are seen by lymphedema and visualized better by xeroradiolymphography than by conventional X-ray film lymphography. But following oil lymphography, worsening of the lymphedema and painfulness of the extremity are sometimes recorded. This is why. Thus we are somewhat wary of using direct oil lymphography in lymphedema. We prefer the plain xeroradiography for the assessement of lymphedema, possibly in combination with xeroradiotomography and coloured lymphography.

The measured extremity circumference values were compared with the values calculated on the basis of xeroradiograms. Simplicity of the plain xeroradiography contributing to the diagnosis and assessment of lymphedema seriousness, permanent documentation and very low radiation doses only one xeroradiograms is usually necessary place this examination among significant objective methods of lymphedema assessement.

REFERENCES

Bruna, J., Gravelle, I. H. (1978): Xeroradiolymphography. Radiol. diagn. (Berl.) 2,

Bruna, J., Clodius, L. (1978): Contribution to the assessment of secondary arm lymphedema by xeroradiography. In Secondary arm lymphedema, edited by L. Clodius, G. Thieme, Stuttgart — in print.

Bruna, J. (1974): Pharmakodynamische Lymphographie. Röntgen-Bl. 32, 262—266.

Clodius, L., Deak, L., Piller, N. B. (1976): A new instrument for the evaluation of tissue tonicity in lymphedema. Lymphology 9, 1—5.

Kalisher, L. (1975): Xeroradiography of axillary lymph node disease. Radiology 115, 67—70.

Kuhnke, E. (1976): Volumbestimmung aus Umfangmessungen. Folia Angiol. 7/8, 228—232.

Schertel, L., Harbst, H., Winkel, K., Lange, S. (1975): Xeroradiography of the lymphatics. Lymphology 8, 94—99.

J. B., Radiological Clinic of Charles Univ., Praha 10, Šrobárova 50, Czechoslovakia

THERMODIAGNOSIS OF CIRCULATORY CHANGES AFTER ARTIFICIALLY CREATED ARTERIOVENOUS SHUNT FOR HAEMODIALYSIS OF PATIENTS WITH CHRONIC RENAL INSUFFICIENCY

F. KADEŘÁVEK, M. KESTLEROVÁ, M. KULHAVÁ and J. POLÁK

Institute for Clinical and Experimental Medicine, Prague, Czechoslovakia

Connection of patients with renal insufficiency to an artificial kidney depends on the patency of arteriovenous shunts upon which the patient's life may, in turn, depend. The patency of a well-functioning shunt can be quite easily examined by palpation or visually. To determine the intensity of blood flow by electromagnetic or ultrasonic techniques, we must know the lumen of the examined vessel. This information can be obtained only by surgical isolation. There are many other techniques that however, provide, only relative data. Of these, thermometry is the least common. Moreover, clinical thermometry is capable of supplying valuable quantitative information. Basically, temperature differences between the shunted and unshunted extremity should correspond to the increase in blood flow.

This study deals with the dynamics of the thermometric picture in shunts during one year from which we can draw conclusions on circulation.

Material and methods

We performed 26 thermometric examinations in patients with arteriovenous shunts and 11 examinations immediately before shunting. The shunts were located in the distal part of the forearm and created by subcutaneous end-to-side anastomosis of the cephalic vein and radial artery.

Of the 26 shunts, 11 were examined one month after shunting, 5 were examined 3 months and ten 12 months after shunting. Four patients examined after 12 months had bilateral shunts, the second shunt was created due to poor functioning of the first one. The remaining patients had unilateral shunts. Of the above patients 4 were studied continually.

Temperatures were measured in unclothed patients at 26 °C room temperature with an Ellab thermoelectric thermometer. The examination was performed after at least 30 minutes of acclimatization under identical conditions.

The results are based on maximum temperatures recorded at the site of the shunt and on the means from 14 sites at the axis of the forearm between the radiocarpal joint and elbow in 4 repeatedly reviewed patients. The sites were 2 cm apart.

We evaluated the intensity of thermoregulatory blood flow which is represented by the quotient of the outer and inner temperature gradient between the skin and room temperatures and sublingual and skin temperatures.

Results

Figure 1 shows the temperature profile of the shunted and unshunted extremity. The temperatures of the shunted extremity were markedly higher, by as much as 2° in the shunt region and decrease with the distance from the shunt. The magnitude and course of the temperature dependence the unshunted extremity were same before and after the operation. The curves show the means in 11 patients one month after surgery.

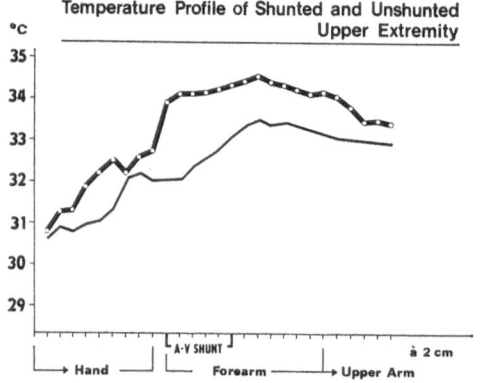

Temperature Profile of Shunted and Unshunted Upper Extremity

Fig. 1.

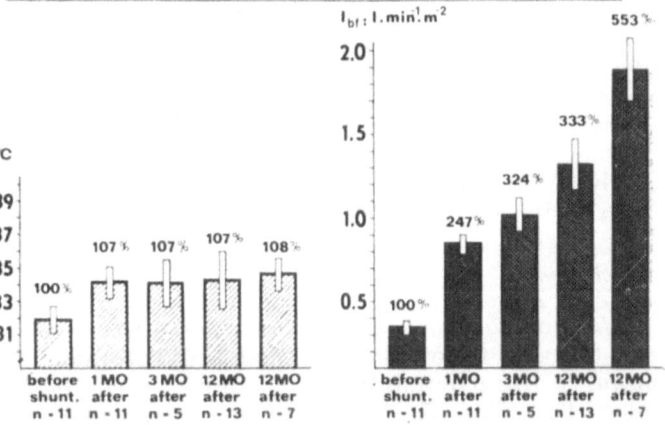

Trend of Maximal Skin Temperatures and Thermoregulatory Blood Flow Intensity after Shunting

Fig. 2.

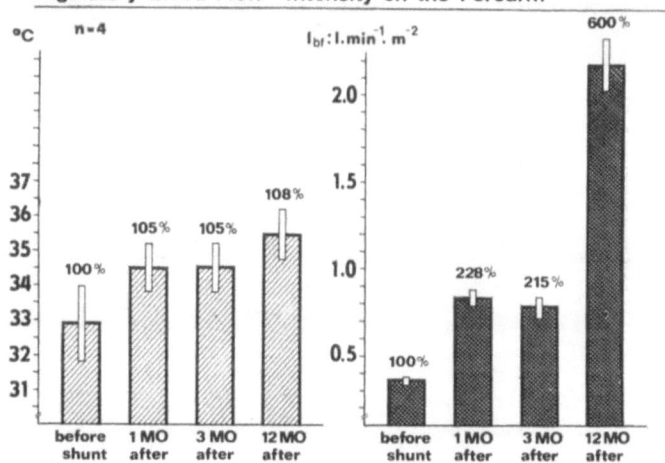

Trend of Skin Temperatures (means of 14 Points) and Thermo-regulatory Blood Flow Intensity on the Forearm

Fig. 3.

Figure 2. shows the trend of temperatures and intensity of thermoregulatory blood flow in all the examined patients. The level of maximum temperatures recorded in the shunt region one and three months after shunting was more than 2° higher than the basic values before shunting. This was true of all shunts after one year; however well-functioning shunts displayed a steady increase in maximum temperature. Relatively minor changes were distinctly more expressed in the derived indicator of the intensity of the thermoregulatory blood flow. The intensity not only doubled but increased steadily; after one year it increased more than five fold over the initial value in well-functioning shunts.

Since the preceding figure does not show the same shunts, the higher value may be due not to the dynamics but to the quality of the shunt. Therefore, the next figure shows a similar changes that occurred in the same shunts during one year. Though the basic data on temperatures before shunting were higher owing to the different procedure used, the dynamics of changes during a one-year follow-up study is comparable with the cumulative data (Fig. 3). The intensity of thermoregulatory blood flow is both absolutely and relatively higher, representing a six fold increase over the initial value.

Discussion

We also studied other skin temperatures and evaluated the overall heat output and intensity of the overall thermoregulatory blood flow. These data inform us on the thermal conditions in the examined patients and thus on the validity of comparisons.

We also monitored the heart rate and arterial pressure in both arms. These values did not change significantly during the examinations.

In conclusion, we have demonstrated a distinct tendency to increased blood flow proportional to the duration of the shunt. The findings agreed with the results of other techniques not specified here. The quantitative data are relative as they are based on comparison with the other extremity. Since the differences in temperatures depend on the presence of the shunt, they provide a basis for determination of the shunt blood flow. The thermodiagnosis is non-invasive and well tolerated by patients. This makes it very suitable for clinical application.

F. K., IKEM, Vídeňská 800, 146 22 Prague 4, Czechoslovakia

COMPARATIVE VALUE OF DOPPLER ULTRASOUND AND SEGMENTAL PLETHYSMOGRAPHY IN THE DIAGNOSIS OF ARTERIAL DISEASES IN THE LOWER LIMBS

D. L. CLEMENT and R. CLAEYS

Department of Cardiology, Section of Hypertension, University Hospital, Gent, Belgium

For years, Doppler ultrasound and segmental plethysmography have been used for diagnosis of peripheral arterial diseases. Although the results obtained with these techniques in normal and abnormal conditions, have been extensively described, data concerning sensitivity and specificity scored by these techniques are scarce. The aim of the present work was to compare the value of these techniques in this respect in a large group of vascular "normal" and "abnormal" limbs.

Methods

In this work the diagnostic performance of the techniques used will be compared to the performance of an experienced clinician using the patient's clinical history, a complete physical examination (*Allen et al.*, 1972; *Clement & Versée* 1975) and oscillography at rest and after exercise. It has been shown that a normal post-exercise oscillogram excludes a clinically significant lesion proximal to the bifurcation of the popliteal artery (*De Weese et al.* 1960; *Schoop* 1975). One hundred vascular "normal" and 100 vascular "abnormal" limbs were investigated.

Systolic blood pressure at the level of the ankle and brachial artery were measured with ultrasound and bidirectional Doppler velocity curves were recorded at the level of the femoral artery (Parks Electronics, type 806). Segmental plethysmography was recorded at the ankle with a cuff inflated at 50 mm Hg (*Winsor et al., 1967*). Part of these results have been presented elsewhere (*Clement et al.*, 1977).

Results and discussion

a) Ankle/brachial artery systolic blood pressure ratio.

In the group with normal limbs (n = = 100) the ratio averaged 1.23 ± 0.20 (mean $\pm$ S. D.) which is significantly greater ($p < 0.001$) than in the group with abnormal limbs (n = 100), averaging 0.72 ± 0.20. Accepting 0.96 as the lowest normal limit, no false positive results were obtained and only 10% false negatives. This is a very favorable score for this technique which is furthermore simple, painless and inexpensive.

b) Doppler velocity curve.

A large number of parameters were derived from this curve. Best performance was scored by the inclination slope, the descending slope and the angle between these slopes. There was a significant difference ($p < 0.001$) for any of these parameters in the groups of normals and abnormals, but unfortunately also a large degree of overlap which cannot be accepted in either screening or hospital conditions.

The morphology of the curve performs much better in the differentiation of normal and abnormal: the negative part of the biphasic curve was absent in 65% of the abnormal cases and in only 12% of the normals.

c) Segmental plethysmography

The same parameters were calculated as for the Doppler velocity curve showing significant differences between both groups. When the three before mentioned parameters are considered together, the total performance of segmental plethysmography is very favorable (only 5% of false negatives with unfortunately 20% false positives).

Thus, the best performance was scored by the measurement of systolic pressure at the ankle. Segmental plethysmography is even more sensitive than the pressure measurement but it yields a large number of false positives. Doppler velocity is least satisfactory, moreover it is technically more difficult and the set is more expensive.

REFERENCES

Allen, Barker, Hines, (1972): Peripheral Vascular Diseases. W. B. Saunders Co. Philadelphia.

Clement D. L., Versee, L. (1975): Klinische diagnose van perifeer vaatlijden. Tijdschr. Geneesk. 31, 244.

Clement, D. L., Clayes, R., Pannier, R. (1977): Detection of atherosclerosis obliterans in the lower limbs in non-invasive cardiovascular diagnosis. Ed. by E. B. Diethrich MTP Press, in press.

De Weese, J. A., Blaisdell, F. W., Foster I. (1960): Pedal pulses disappearing with exercises: a test for intermittent claudication. New Engl. J. Med. 262, 1214.

Schoop, W. (1975): Praktische Angiologie. Georg Thieme Verlag, Stuttgart.

Winsor T., Simmons E. M., Borhani N., Hechter H. H., (1967): A diagnostic aid for determining peripheral arteriosclerosis obliterans. Chest 52, 451.

D. L. C., Dept. of Cardiovascular Diseases, De Pintelaan 135, B-9000 Gent, Belgium

COMPARATIVE RATING OF THREE METHODS (DOPPLER ULTRASOUND) XE — 133 CLEARANCE (RHEOGRAPHY) FOR THE MEASUREMENT OF PERFUSION PRESSURE AND FLOW IN THE LOWER EXTREMITIES OF VASCULAR PATIENTS IN FONTAINE II

P. FARKAS, L. URAI, M. ISTVÁNFFY and M. HALMAGYI

National Institute of Cardiology, Budapest, Hungary

In the present paper we wish to report results obtained by means of the Doppler ultrasound technique, Xe-133 clearance and rheography. The tests were performed on patients in st. Fontaine II. The objective of this work was to establish the relationship between the results of the three tests used regularly in the Angiological Laboratory of our institute and the clinical condition of the patient, on the one hand, and, on the other hand, the correlation between the results of the three tests as well as the specificity and sensitivity of each method. The tests were performed on 71 lower extremities of 49 patients in Fontaine II and 29 healthy extremities of 15 control subjects. The diagnosis of obliterative arterial disease was always verified by angiography. For the measurement of the perfusion pressure 803 Model of Park Electronic Laboratories was used. The ratio of the pressure in the anterior tibial artery to that in the brachial artery was measured in a recumbent position and expressed as the Doppler index. (*Yao*, 1968). The determination of Xe-133 clearance was carried out according to *Lassen's* (1964) original publication in rest and after 2 minutes ischaemic exercise. For the rheographic tests the Schufried type Doppler rheograph was used, the rheogramm of the calf was recorded in the recumbent position at rest, and the calculations were performed with the help of the relative pulse volume given by *Schufried* and *Kaindl* (1967). Walking distance was determined on even ground at a rate of 100 steps per minute. The patients suffering from arterial stenosis were divided into two groups: group I was able to walk less than 150 m without claudication, group II 150 m or more.

Table I shows the group means, the standard deviations and the significance of the differences between the group means. Comparison of the results of two groups with those of the controls by means of analysis of variance shows that there is a statistically highly significant difference between the means in the normal and moderate, i.e. in the moderate and severe group. Thus, all three methods are suitable for classification according to given clinical aspects, as well as for a reliable differentiation between normal and pathologic means. The correlation between the results of tests performed on subjects who have been classified according to their walking distance is shown in Table II. The significance was calculated and these provided unequivocal evidence of a mathematically significant correlation between perfusion and pressure and flow, but only in the group with a walking distance over 150 m and in the controls. The specificity and sensitivity of the methods were also

Table I.

MEAN VALUES, STANDARD DEVIATIONS AND RESULTS OF SIGNIFICANCE TESTS /CLASSIFIED ACCORDING TO WALKING DISTANCE/								
DOPPLER INDEX			133 XE CLEARENCE ml/100g/min			RHEOGRAPHIC. REL. PULZ. VOL.		
CONTROLLS	CLAUD.DIST. 150—500	CLAUD.DIST 25—149	CONTROLLS	CLAUD.DIST. 150—500	CLAUD.DIST 25—149	CONTROLLS	CLAUD.DIST. 150—500	CLAUD.DIST 25—149
n=29	n=17	n=23	n=29	n=17	n=23	n=29	n=17	n=23
x̄ 1,0562	0,700	0,4830	63,78	34,58	24,59	1,0528	0,5741	0,3978
s 0,0642	0,2011	0,1658	10,67	10,09	9,00	0,1648	0,2865	0,1541
t 8,10	4,71		9,55	3,12		7,90	2,78	
p <0,01	<0,001		<0,001	<0,01		<0,001	<0,01	

355

studied (Table III). A nutritive flow of 50 ml/100 g/min or more as determined by Xenon clearance, a rheographically measured relative pulse volume of 1.0 or higher and a Doppler index of 1.0 or higher were accepted as normal values. Thus perfusion pressure measured by the ultrasound technique seems to furnish the most specific and sensitive results.

The clinician wishes to know the meaning of the various pressure and flow values and their relationship the severity of the disease, as well as the correlation between the results. On the basis of our own tests we believe that: 1. all three tests reveal a statistically highly significant difference between the healthy and afflicted extremities. 2. the methods permit dif-

ferentiation between clinically severe and moderate arterial stenosis. 3. there is a mathematically significant correlation both in the healthy extremities and in cases of moderate severity between the values obtained by rheographic results and those obtained by ultrasound measurements. In contrast, no significant correlation was found between the pressure and flow results in the group where the walking distance was less than 150 m. 4. of the three methods, measurements of the perfusion pressure by the ultrasound technique is the most specific and most sensitive and do also quite simple; it is therefore the most favourable for screening tests, that is for the differentiation of the criteria of healthy and sick.

Table II.

Table III.

CORRELATION BETWEEN THE PERFUSION PRESSURE AND FLOW DATA /CLASSIFIED ACCORDING TO WALKING DISTANCE/						
	DOPPLER INDEX	133 XE CLEARENCE ml/100g/min	DOPPLER INDEX	RHEOGRAPHIC REL. PUL.Z.VOL	133 XE CLEARENCE ml/100g/min	RHEOGRAPHIC REL.PUL.Z.VOL
CONTROLLS	r=0,1061 P>0,05		r=0,6357 P<0,01		r=0,3460 P<0,05	
CLAUD.DIST. 150–500m	r=0,2464 P<0,05		r=0,6005 P<0,01		r=0,3403 P<0,05	
CLAUD.DIST. 25–149 m	r=0,015 P>0,05		r=0,2642 P>0,05		r=0,0947 P>0,05	

SPECIFICITY AND SENSITIVITY OF THE TESTS IN THE CONTROLLS n =29 AND IN THE GROUP OF MODERATE SEVERITY n=17			
	133 XE CLEARENCE ml/100g/min	RHEOGRAPHIC PULS. VOL.	DOPPLER INDEX
SPECIFICITY	0,931	0,69	1
SENSITIVITY	0,941	0,941	0,941

REFERENCES

N. A. Lassen, J. Lindbjerg, O. Muuck (1964): Measurement of blood-flow through skeletal muscle by intramuscular injection of Xenon-133. The Lancet 1964, I, 686.

Kaindl F., Polzer K., (1967): Rheografie. Darmstadt: Steinkopff-Verlag 1967, 3.
Yao S. T., J. T. Hobbs, W. T. Irvine (1968): Pulse Examination by an Ultrasonic Method. Brit. Med. Journ. 1968, 4, 555—557.

P. F., Hungarian Institute of Cardiology Budapest, 1450, Hungary

DOPPLER SONOGRAPHY OF FEMORO-POPLITEAL RECONSTRUCTION

J. DÖRRLER and P. C. MAURER

Department of Vascular Surgery
Rechts der Isar Medical School, Technical University, Munich, F.R.G.

Previous studies have furnished evidence that the blood-pressure of the ankle artery in form of the systolic pressure index (ankle systolic pressure/brachial systolic pressure) measured with Doppler Ultrasound allows classification of circulatory disturbances. The systolic pressure is generally accepted as an indirect indication of whether reconstruction by means of a bypass is possible. The complete range of imminent complications can, however, only be kept under control, if it is possible to predict pathological changes and if the angiography is carried out as long as the bypass is still patent.

Of a total number of 65 patients we operated on 30 in stage II and on 28 in stage III and 7 in stage IV. In 52 cases we obtained an improved pressure index immediately after operation, indicating a successful reconstruction.

When comparing the peripheral vascular region with the clinical stage it became evident that these two values do not always correspond. Regular post-operative follow-up was possible in 37 of the 65 patients. In ten cases postoperative measurements showed a falling pressure index.

Angiography was performed on these patients and all ten of them exhibited angiographic changes.

Like other authors we always registered the ankle artery pressure of both legs to eliminate any fluctuations and submitted patients to a strain test in doubtful cases.

In the first case the pressure index of a patient with a left femoropopliteal bypass above the knee-joint was measured in 1975.

One and a half years later the pressure index demonstrated a steady and permanent drop. An angiography carried out subsequently showed severe stenosis in the region of proximal anastomosis, caused by deposits of thrombotic material. At the time of the initial operation this region was free of changes.

In the above mentioned case, we corrected the stenosis by removing the thrombotic material and applying a saphenous vein patch. Postoperatively we again obtained an adequately high and steady pressure index.

In the second case infection developed in the left graft after an aorto-femoral bifurcation with a long profunda plasty

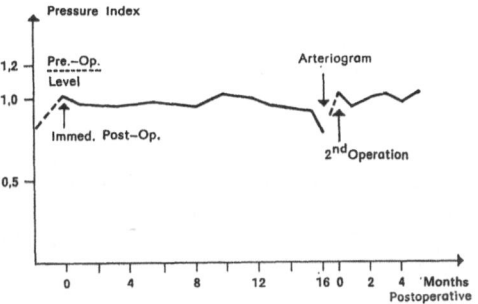

Fig. 1.

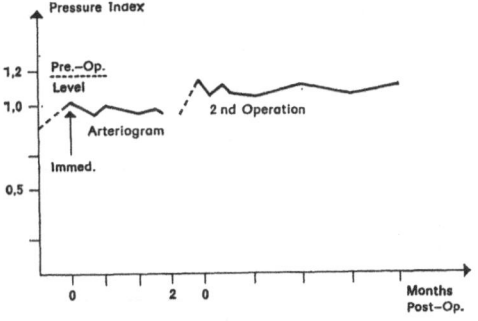

Fig. 2.

357

on the left side. When removing the prosthesis it became evident that a reconstruction of the profound femoral artery was no longer possible. In the absence of a suitable vein we therefore inserted a goretex bypass through the foramen obturatum, connecting it to the superficial femoral artery. Probably on account of the reconstruction of the superficial femoral artery and the simultaneous removal of profound femoral artery, pre-and postoperative measures did not demonstrate any noteworthy difference. As we failed to see any change in the healing of the necrosis of the big toe, we carried out a strain test. During the ischemic provocation achieved by the patient doing fourty toestands, the initial value had not been reached 15 minutes later, which indicated severe stenosis in the region of the bypass.

Accordingly, the subsequent angiography showed stenosis below the distal anastomosis which had not been detectable in the first angiographic exploration. This stenosis was corrected with a jump-graft. The postoperative follow-up showed an increase in the pressure index. Values remained stable during the following check-ups indicating a patent bypass.

In the third case the postoperative pressure index of the anterior tibial artery was measured. We are dealing with a patients, who, failing to appear for the necessary and urgently recommended check-ups, do not return until bypass occlusion occured. The pressure index measured after the first reconstruction furnished values that indicated a patent bypass.

Surprisingly, the bypass proved to be free of changes. In the region of the profound femoral artery, however, the main branch was occluded which obviously caused the deterioration of the pressure index. A profunda plasty was subsequently performed on this patient and the postoperative pressure index attained the initial value.

As a conclusion of our study we are inclined to agree with those authors who do not reject reconstruction attempts even in cases with a systolic pressure index of less than 0.2. We have observed the functioning of a femoro-popliteal bypass over a longer period of time in cases with a low preoperative pressure index (under 0.2). Likewise, an angiographically unfavourable peripheral region has not necessarily proved a reliable indicator of bypass patency.

We therefore feel that reconstruction should be attempted in patients with gangrene and rest pain, as in this group an impending amputation may possibly be avoided. At close intervals follow-ups including serial graphic registration of the systolic pressure index and simultaneous measurement of the other leg as a means of control are essential to ensure and maintain srugical success. Employing this method we were able to detect an impending occlusion in ten of our patients, while in three other cases it played an important part in the planning of the surgical procedure. In doubtful cases with a slight pressure drop ischemic strain through toestands employed together with the simple Doppler-Ultrasonic technique can furnish additional information and ensure that patients receive the necessary angiography and surgical treatment in time.

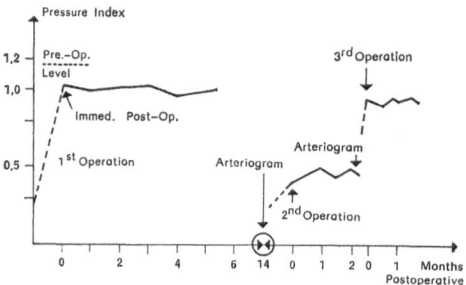

Fig. 3.

D. J., Dept. Vascular Surgery, Ismáningerstr. 22 8000, München F.R.G.

RECORDING THE POST-EXERCISE FEMORAL VELOCITY USING A DOPPLER-VELOCIMETER

M. ZICOT,

Department of Medicine, Liège, Belgium

Introduction

Morphological analysis of the characteristic features of the velocity recorded in the common femoral artery using a directional Doppler meter is helpful for the diagnosis of aorto-iliac obstructions (*Pourcelot*, 1975). The signal is disturbed even at rest when the obstacle to the flow above the common femoral artery is large enough. The pulsatile wave is damped out and a continuous component is often present during the entire period of the cardiac cycle. Nevertheless, by analysing the rest flow we are not always able to exclude the diagnosis of aorto-iliac stenosis. The aim of the present work is to demonstrate systematic recording of the velocity after exercise in order to facilitate such a differentiation.

Material and methods

A constantly emitting directional Doppler flowmeter was used, coupled to a zero-crossing counter producing an analogical curve, which is amplified and recorded by a Siemens-Elema recorder. The common femoral velocity is picked up on the recumbent patient at rest and after a standard walk test (between 2 and 4 minutes after the walk). The patient walks on a treadmill (rate 3.6 km/h, slope 10%) till a disabling ischemic pain appears or till 5 minutes have elapsed.

Morphological analysis is performed to determine the shape of the pulsatile wave. A simplified quantitative analysis is also applied which roughly takes into account the relative importance of the oscillatory and continuous flow components. The ratio CFI = A/B (fig. 1) called the Continuous Flow Index is calculated. A is the amplitude of the positive peak flow and B the amplitude of the total oscillation (fig. 1). When the flow tends to be constant, A/B tends to infinity (B = 0). We consider the results of a preliminary series of 14 normal limbs, 18 limbs with radiological evidence of a superficial femoral obstruction and 15 limbs where the lesions are situated on the aorto-iliac segment (by nagiography).

Results

1) *Morphological analysis*

The pulsatile wave is normal at rest (14/14) and remains so (14/14) after the exercise when the limbs are normal (Fig. 1). An important reduction in the

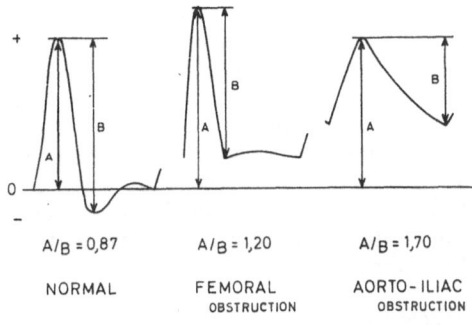

$$CFI = A/B \quad \text{AFTER EXERCISE}$$

| A/B = 0,87 | A/B = 1,20 | A/B = 1,70 |
| NORMAL | FEMORAL OBSTRUCTION | AORTO-ILIAC OBSTRUCTION |

Fig. 1. Schematic drawing of the characteristic velocity patterns recorded after the walk test, with indication of the mode of calculation for CFI.

backflow may be recorded (6/18) in the presence of a superficial femoral blockage but there is no major alteration in the initial "systolic" wave. This is also true in the post-exercise period. The first wave remains narrow (18/18), (Fig. 1) even if the hyperemia is delayed as reflected in the acceleration of the systolic velocity and the presence of a constant flow between the waves.

The presence of an aorto-iliac lesion is

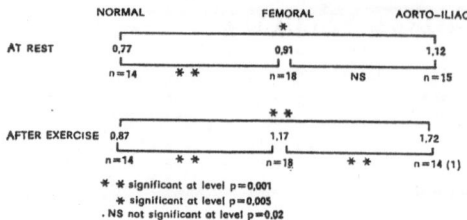

	NORMAL		FEMORAL		AORTO–ILIAC
			*		
AT REST	0.77		0.91		1.12
	n = 14	* *	n = 18	NS	n = 15
			* *		
AFTER EXERCISE	0.87		1.17		1.72
	n = 14	* *	n = 18	* *	n = 14 (1)

* * significant at level p = 0.001
* significant at level p = 0.005
. NS not significant at level p = 0.02

Table I. Determination of the continuous flow index (mean results)
(1) One case is not taken into account for the mean because CFI tended to infinity (heavy turbulences and flat wave)

detected at rest with certainty in 12/15 cases. After the walk test, the situation is objectified in 14/15 cases (14 characteristically damped waves, including 3 cases with heavy turbulence).

2) *CFI Analysis*

The mean results are given in Table I and the details of the data in Figure 2. There is nearly no continuous flow in the normal limbs (CFI < 1) two minutes after the exercise.

A continuous flow component is generally still present in the femoral occlusions within the same interval, due to the delayed hyperemia. The continuous flow is quantitatively very important after the walk test in the presence of aorto-iliac lesions because of the simultaneous damping of the pulsatile wave and the delayed hyperemia.

Discussion

The systematic recording of the flow in the common femoral artery using the Doppler after-the-walk test is useful in order to recognize aorto-iliac stenosis and to differentiate them from more distal lesions.

We missed some of the lesions by looking only at the resting flow. Calculation of

CFI gives a quantitative idea of the importance of the continuous flow components.

Fourier analysis would of course be more accurate but is not strictly necessary for clinical practice. The combination of morphological analysis and consideration of CFI appears very helpful for the diagnosis and the functional assessment.

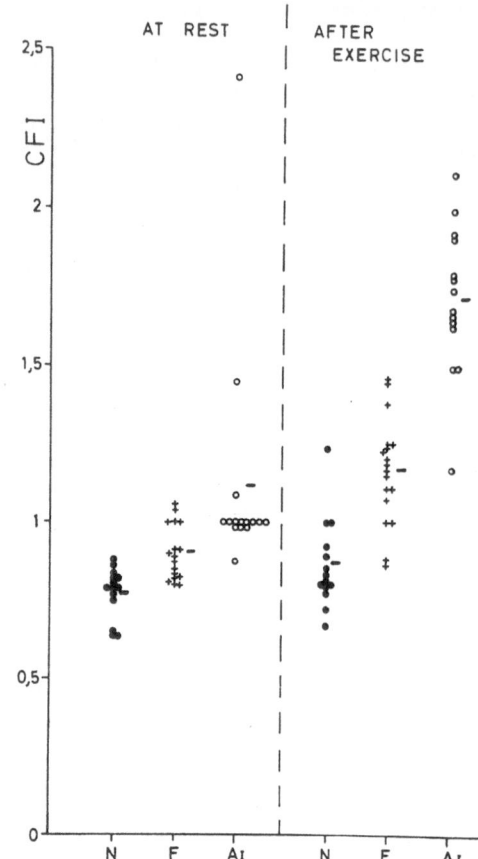

Fig. 2. Values of CFI different situations; the dash present in each column represents the mean. N = normal, F = femoral obstruction, AI = aorto-iliac obstruction

REFERENCE

Pourcelot, L. (1975): Indication de l'ultrasonographie Doppler dans l'étude des vaisseaux périphériques. Rev. Prat. 25, 4671—4680.

M. Z., Dépt. de Clinique et de Pathologie médicales. Hôpital de Bavière B. 4020-Liège, Belgique

ULTRASONIC DUPLEX ECHO-DOPPLER ARTERIOGRAPHY IN DIAGNOSTICS OF ARTERIAL DISEASES

R. KUBÁK and M. NEVRTAL

Dept. of Medical Electronics and Dept. of Pathophysiology,
Technical University and J. Ev. Purkyně University, Brno, Czechoslovakia

The tradition means available for vascular imaging is X-ray angiography, a procedure with a definite risk involving the use of a radiopaque dye injected into the patient's arteries either directly or through a catheter. Procedure cannot be repeated as part of a routine follow up.

The best recent development in the area of non-invasive and repeatedly used methods for evaluation of arterial occlusive disease is the ultrasonic echo-Doppler arteriography (*Barber et al.*, 1974). Digital Duplex Scanner Mark V used in our cardiovascular laboratory for this study involves the integration of real-time B-mode tomographic scanning with the pulsed Doppler technique in one optimum system. This new device is used to visualize atherosclerotic plaques within peripheral vessels especially at branch points and bifurcations where atherosclerotic disease tends to occur first and to detect and quantitate blood flow disturbances resulting from disease processes within these vessels.

Real-time pulse-echo scanning signals develop a dynamic tomographic picture of a cross-section of tissue including arteries and surrounding muscles, veins and other organs whose intensity is proportional to the reflectance of tissue interfaces at the corresponding points in the image plane. Heatlhy artery walls produce large echoes and are clearly visible (Fig. 2). The lumen appears as a dark hole due to about −20 dB lower backscattering of blood measured relative to the 0 dB reflectance level normal artery wall. In contrast, hard calcific shells have a reflectance level a maximum of +20 dB higher. Reflectance of little calcified or soft fatty plaques varies from +10 to −20 dB.

Atherosclerotic plaques accumulating on the interior walls of the vessel tend to restrict the blood flow (Fig. 3). The pulsed

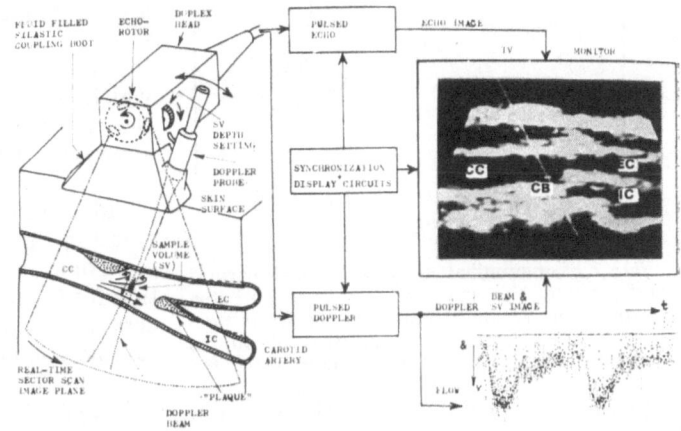

Fig. 1. A block diagram of the Duplex Scanner. The real-time B-mode image is generated by three 5 MHz ultrasound transducers molded into a rotating wheel within the scan head housing. The 5 MHz pulsed Doppler device detects the velocity characteristics of red cells within a small region of space called the sample volume which can be moved along the sound beam axis using a depth setting knob.

361

Doppler concept enables detection of blood flow characteristics in a precisely located position and differentiates between normal blood flow, disturbed flow and non-scattering occlusions.

Our investigation has centered on the carotid arteries which provide most of blood supply to the brain. The overall objectives of this ultrasonic procedure included identifying the lesion, assessing its severity and following the preoperative or postoperative course of the disease process.

A block diagram of the Duplex Scanner specifically designed to provide an image of soft tissue interfaces and simultaneously detect blood flow within vessels 4 cm or closer to the skin surface is given in Figure 1. The pulse -echo rotation head turns at

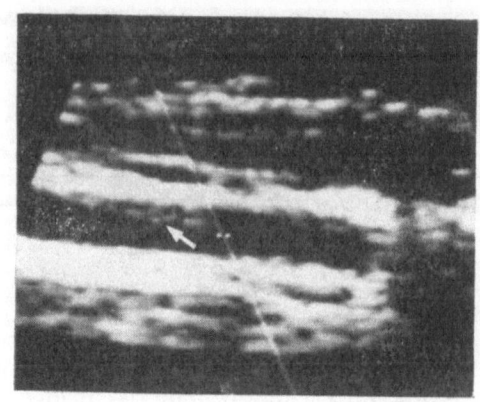

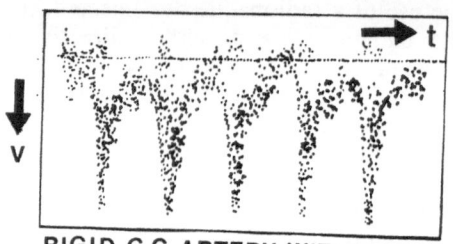

RIGID C.C. ARTERY WITH
ATHEROSCLEROTIC PLAQUES

Fig. 3. Calcified rigid common carotid artery. Intraluminal atherosclerotic plaque (see the arrow) produces the broad-band velocity disturbed flow within and behind the stenotic region.

a rate of $7-10$ revolutions per second to produce a 45 degree scan image at the rate of $21-30$ complete frames per second. The operator can easily angle the scan head along the neck to collect clinically useful information concerning the carotid bifurcation or internal carotid artery. Manual rotation of the Doppler transducer around the pivot point allows the operator to position the sample volume, which is the small region of space where the velocity of red cells is detected, anywhere within the plane of view of the B-mode image.

Pulsed-echo, pulsed-Doppler, synchronization and display position sensing electronics assure proper spatial registration for the tomographic tissue image with superimposed Doppler beam position and sample volume location on the TV screen and simultaneous recording of the blood flow signal from the sample volume space.

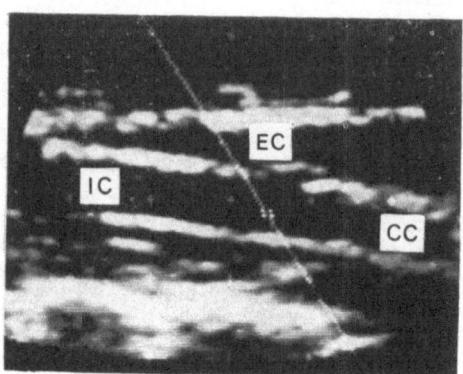

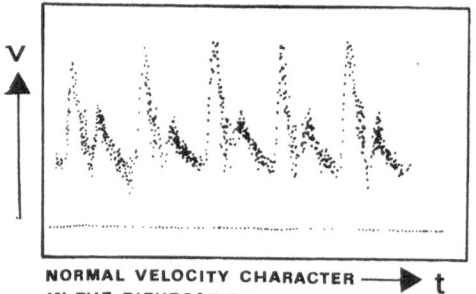

NORMAL VELOCITY CHARACTER ⟶ t
IN THE BIFURCATION

Fig. 2. Longitudinal scan of normal carotid bifurcation. The diagonal line represents the path of the Doppler beam and the white dots on this line represent the position of sample volume. Within the sample volume space the narrow-band tone-like blood flow character was detected. Grid marks are spaced 1 cm × 1 cm.

362

Because of the digitalization of the echo-data which go via the RAM memories, the scan picture can be frozen at any time instant and observed or photographed by an operator on a TV screen.

In a supine position of the patient the scan head is attached to the skin with acoustic gel and the longitudinal section of the common carotid artery with its branches is visualized. In the healthy persons investigated the artery segments do not contain any intraluminal plaque echoes (Fig. 2). Artery walls show elastic smoothly pulsating movements. The transversal tissue cross-section can also be obtained. Locating the sample volume within any space of one of the three carotid arteries enables us to hear and register the typical narrow band normal blood flow character.

If, however, the sample volume is clearly located within the vessel lumen and no flow is detected, the clinician can be reasonably sure that some type of non-reflecting soft plaque structure lies within the vessel.

At the rigid artery a typical finding is the calcified and thickned wall producing specific large echoes with diminished amplitude of volume pulsations. In most cases the intraluminal founded atherosclerotic plaques produce disturbed flow within and behind the stenotic region, Fig. 3.

In a similar manner we are able to locate anatomic and hemodynamic abnormalities in the femoral and other arteries.

Preliminary results of clinical investigations are very encouraging. Use of B-mode dynamic image and the audible Doppler signal yields a high degree of accuracy in the non-invasive detection of intimal arterial disease and occlusions. By additional signal processing we hope to increase our ability to diagnose critical stenoses and make accurate diagnosis of early arterial lesions feasible.

REFERENCE

Barber, F. E. et al. (1974): Ultrasonic duplex echo-Doppler scanner. I.E.E.E. Trans. biomed. Engng, BME-21, 109—13.

R. K., Dept. of Medical Electronics, TU Brno, Purkyňova 95b, 61200 Brno, Czechoslovakia

ARTERIAL NON-INVASIVE METHODS OF INVESTIGATION IN COMPARISON WITH ARTERIOGRAPHY

JITKA ZAPLETALOVÁ, VL. PUCHMAYER, B. DRUGOVÁ,
J. POKORNÝ, J. BARTOŠ and K. TERŠÍP

*IVth Medical Clinic, Radiological Clinic, Ist Surgical Clinic,
Faculty of Medicine, Charles University, Prague, Czechoslovakia*

In an attempt to clarify the diagnostic reliability of some non-invasive methods, we have compared the results of oscillographic and ultrasonic measurements with arteriographic findings.

In 75 men and 6 women within an age range between 23 and 79 years, the mean age being 55.1 years, suffering from ischemic disease of the lower extremities, a direct lumbar aorto-and arteriography of at least one lower extremity was performed. Thus, X-rays of 130 entire lower extremities were obtained (Tab. I).

Oscillographic examination was made using the oscillograph described by Gesenius and Keller. Rest oscillations were registered at particular points on the of lower extremities and then variances above the knuckle after 40 ascents on toes and then 20 squats according to currently used method. The curves were evaluated in accordance with generally known criteria.

In all patients, the systolic blood pressure generally was measured by the ultrasonic method on arteria radialis of the left-forearm using Doppler's instrument (*Vogel*). In two thirds of patients the blood pressure was measured in a similar way on arteria tibialis posterior and arteria dorsalis pedis above the knuckle. In 27 patients on 44 lower extremities, i.e. in one third of the cases, the systolic blood pressure was measured on arteria poplitea above the knee. A difference in the blood pressures between the forearm and thigh, the thigh and knuckle or fore-arm and knuckle of $0-10$ torr was considered to be suspect stenosis, $10-30$ torr definite stenosis and above 30 torr an occlusion in the section between the aorta and the measured point

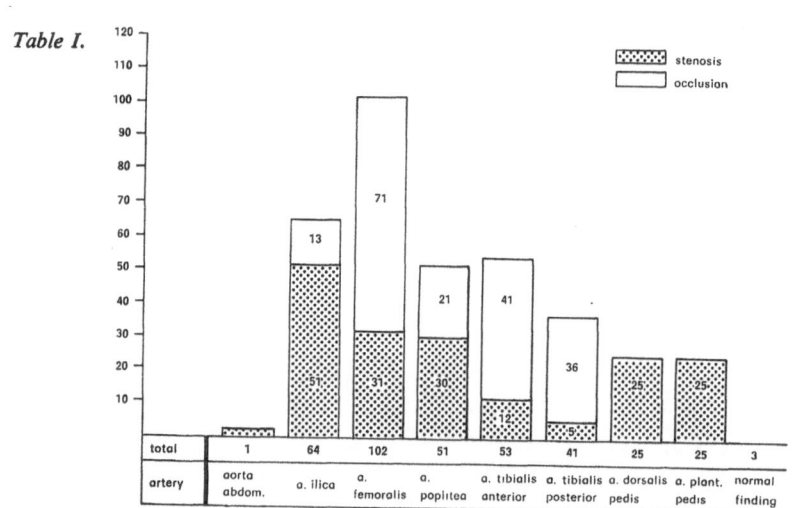

Table I.

Table II.

90 % reliability of methods
(covered by 95% confidence int.)

		oscillography	Doppler ankle	Doppler thigh-ankle	oscillography and Doppler
a. ilica	stenosis	±	−	−	±
	stenosis with a. femoralis - lesion	−	−	−	−
	occlusion	+	+	+	+
a. femoralis	stenosis especially with a. popl. or a. ilica - lesion	+	−	−	+
	occlusion	+	+	+	+
	occlusion with a. ilica - lesion	+	−	−	+
a. poplitea	stenosis	+	−	+	+
	occlusion				
a. tib. ant.	stenosis	−	+	+	+
	occlusion				
a. tib. post.	stenosis	−	−	+	+
	occlusion				

ankle blood pressure, a cuff of a common tonometer, and above the knee a special cuff from an oscillograph were used. Measuring the blood pressure above the knee and above the knuckle makes it possible to discern stenosis or occlusion in the iliacofemoralis section from the fore-arm/thigh gradient and in the popliteal space and tibial arteries section from the thigh/knuckle gradient. A pressure difference above the knee and above the knuckle of 5 up 30 torr reflected stenosis or preobliteration, 30 and more torr an occlusion of the popliteal artery assuming equal pressure on both tibial arteries or if there was a gradient between the thigh and tibial artery with a higher pressure. A pressure difference in the arteria dorsalis pedis and arteria tibialis posterior of 5 torr was not considered in the evaluation, of 5 to 15 torr was considered to be arterial stenosis with lower pressure, above 15 torr to be an occlusion. To distinguish whether lesion of the iliacal or femoral and/or more distal sections was present, oscillography was used.

and/or between 2 points on the lower extremities. A gradient above 100 torr seemed to be a close stenosis and obliteration, or two occlusions in the measured section. For measuring the forearm and

In arteries of 3 lower extremities, a normal finding was established by all methods. The lesions of the arteria dorsalis pedis and arteria plantaris pedis were not found either oscillographically or ultrasonically. One case of abdominal

Table III.

number of lesions	a. ilica	a. femoralis	a. poplitea	a. tib. ant.	a. tib. post	total
1 isolated	100	100	−	100	−	100
1 + 1 in other localisation	78,3	91,9	90,9	94,3	76,9	87,4
1 + 2 in other localisation	73,9	94,4	91,7	85,7	70,6	85,1
1 + 3 in other localisation	87,5	82,4	93,8	81,8	72,7	84,1

90 % reliability of methods
(tested by 95 % confidence interval)

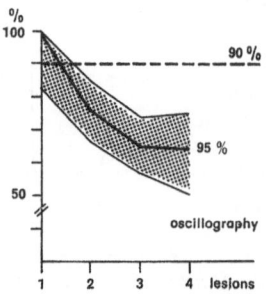

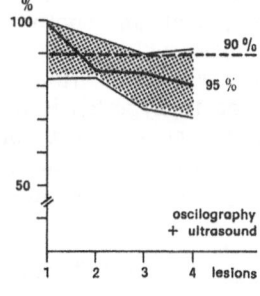

365

aorta stenosis with simultaneous stenosis of both iliacal arteries was not recognized by non-invasive methods. The stenoses of the iliacal artery particularly by ultrasound, especially in combination with lesion of femoral artery, are badly discerned bilateral. Diagnostics of stenosis of the femoral artery with simultaneous affection of the popliteal artery or iliacal occlusion is rather difficult (Table II). As a rule, it cannot be diagnosed by the Doppler method, similarly to femoral occlusion with simultaneous lesion of the pelvic arteries. Stenosis and occlusion of the popliteal artery escape recognition by ultrasound above the knuckle if other sections are simultaneously afflicted. The value of oscillography for occlusions and stenoses of tibial arteries decreases considerably if they are not isolated. Diagnosis of damage to the arteria tibialis posterior, particularly of its stenosis is the most difficult. In isolated stenoses and occlusions non-invasive diagnostics was correct in practically 100 per cent of cases (Table III). With an increasing amount of additional damage, the diagnostic abilities of both methods fall; however, did not an average fall below 84 percent. Detection of additional occlusion or stenosis on the course of the arterial bed in the lower extremity by non-invasive methods was approximately the same, whether the lesion occurred one or two stages higher or lower and the success factor varied around 86 per cent. Oscillography is most useful in the diagnosis of affection of the pelvic down to the popliteal artery, whereas the ultrasonic method is useful mainly for tibial arteries. With the measurement of the blood pressure above knee and knuckle, the diagnosis of the popliteal and both tibial arteries was considerably improved. Both methods fail with bifurcation prothesis and simultaneous hypertension; in one case we did not recognize pre-obliteration of both iliac arteries, in another occlusion of the popliteal artery including trifurcation and

the tibial arteries. Table IV shows false positive findings.

Conclusion

In 81 patients, we arteriographically, ultrasonically and oscillographically examined a total of 130 lower extremities. Through comparison of non- invasive methods with arteriography, we established good diagnostic ability which on an average did not decrease below 84 per cent. Isolated lesions of individual arterial sections were determined in practically 100 per cent of cases. With an increasing number of occlusions, the diagnostic ability falls. The two methods are complementary and form an important functional supplement to arteriography. Used together 90 per cent reliability is attained and this consitutes a sufficient examination method for conservative therapy. For reconstructive intervention, however, an aortography and a perfect arteriography of the whole extremity are necessary.

Table IV.

False positive findings

Doppler

artery	Doppler	arteriography	number
a. tib ant.	stenosis	normal finding	6
	occlusion	stenosis	5
a. tib. post.	occlusion	normal finding	1
total			12

Oscillography

artery	oscillography	arteriography	number
a. poplitea	+ false stenosis	a. fem. - occlusion only	4
		a. iliaca and a. femoralis - occlusion	4
		a. femoralis superf. and prof. - stenosis	1
aa. cruris	occlusion	normal finding	2
total			11

Vl. P., IVth Medical Clinic, U nemocnice 2, 120 00 Praha 2, Czechoslovakia

THE REACTIVE HYPEREMIA TEST ON A LOWER LIMB FOR ASSESSING AN AORTO-ILIAC OBSTRUCTION BY THE DOPPLER EFFECT

J. P. MARCADÉ and F. BECKER

Hospital Saint Louis, La Rochelle, France

The different kinds of morphological alterations of the femoral velocity wave, obtained by directional continuous zero-crossing Doppler testing at rest, were described and classified by *Descotes* in 1975 (Fig. I A). Curves of Type II, III and

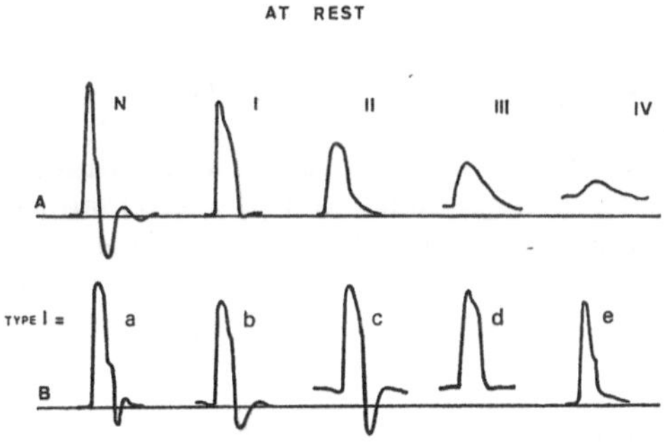

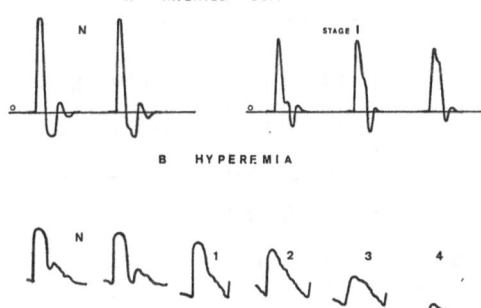

Fig. 1. A: Descotes' classification of the femoral velocity curve obtained by continuous zero-crossing Doppler measurements.
B: Different aspects of minor morphological alterations.

IV appear to be related to major aortoiliac obstructions, whereas curves between normal and type II are very difficult to interpret: permeability is then no longer the principal factor which determines the form of the velocity and the importance of the peripheral resistances plays a significant role here (Fig. I B). We have tried to find out if the role of an eventual aorto iliac obstruction could be determined more precisely by dynamic tests: occlusion of the distal arterial tree by a pneumatic cuff positioned around the upper thigh, reactive hyperemia after one minute of ischemia. The results of comparison with arteriography in 40 arteritic patients are given here.

I — Study of the Doppler femoral velocity waveform during occlusion of the distal arterial tree

When a pneumatic cuff is inflated above the femoral systolic pressure at the upper thigh, the normal femoral velocity wave can be described as follows: sharp positive peak with straight fall of the descending branch under zero baseline; wide, rounded or bifid reversed curve; rounded second positive rise (Type N). In the patients whose femoral velocity curve at rest has minor alterations (waveform situated between normal and type II of the Descotes classification), the curve with inflated cuff can be normal or assume one of the shapes shown in Fig. II A: systolic peak becoming wider on the descending branch more or less close to the top, narrow reversed curve, low second positive rise.

Fig. 2. A: Morphological aspects of the Doppler femoral velocity wave during occlusion of the distal arterial tree by an inflated cuff at the upper thigh (excluding major aortoiliac obstructions).
B: Morphological aspects of the Doppler femoral velocity wave during reactive hyperemia of the lower limb.

II – Study of the Doppler femoral velocity waveform during reactive hyperemia

Reactive hyperemia is a consequence of lowered peripheral resistances; the arterial flow increases in the aorto-iliac axis and becomes more dependent on the permeability of this axis. This must reveal defects which are not obvious at rest. The normal Doppler velocity wave during reactive hyperemia consists of a high systolic curve followed by a low, wide, positive diastolic curve, both very elevated above the zero baseline, sometimes slightly united during the first systoles after the cuff has been deflated. When there is a circulatory brake, the systolic curve is not as high, its descending branch spreads

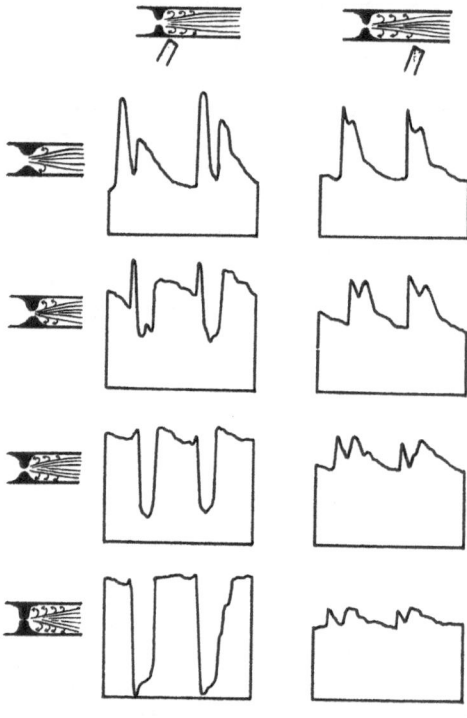

Fig. 3. Morphological aspects of the Doppler femoral velocity wave during reactive hyperemia in cases of external iliac artery stenosis; from left to right: according to the proximity of the probe to the obstruction; from top to bottom: according to the importance of the obstruction and the importance of the hyperemia.

out more or less in the diastolic space and the continuous flow is diminished (Fig. II B). If there is low external iliac stenosis, poststenotic turbulences and systolic reflux induced by hyperemia can be registered. The graphic patterns are then particularly original (Fig. III).

III – Results and conclusions

a) A short, moderate iliac stenosis (50 to 70%) on an otherwise healthy axis may not change the Doppler femoral velocity curve at all, either at rest or under an inflated cuff and becomes visible only during reactive hyperemia. It is therefore essential to perform reactive hyperemia before assessing the normality of a Doppler femoral velocity curve.

b) The most interesting features for diagnosing an eventual aorto-iliac obstruction can then be found during reactive hyperemia. But the circulatory brake becomes more visible as hyperemia becomes more important. This has to be taken into account before interpretation. The importance of hyperemia, for instance, depends on the reactive capacity of the distal arterial tree.

c) The femoral velocity wave under an inflated cuff can be altered by a major aorto-iliac obstruction. In cases of mild aorto-iliac obstruction, however, the wave form reflects the elastic properties of the arterial system.

d) After comparing the importance of the aorto-iliac circulatory brake during hyperemia and the aspect of the femoral velocity curve under an inflated cuff with each patient's arteriography, we came to the following conclusions: the more the Doppler wave is altered by hyperemia while keeping near to normal under an inflated cuff, the greater the chance of finding a moderate localized aorto-iliac stenosis; the more the Doppler wave is altered under inflated cuff while being only slightly changed during hyperemia, the greater the chance of finding a diffuse atherosclerotic iliac axis without significant stenosis.

e) The occurrence of turbulence and systolic reflux during hyperemia permits assessment of the presence of an obstruction located on the external iliac artery.

REFERENCE

Descotes, J., Cathignol, D. (1975): Classification of changes in the ultra-sonic speed pattern in the arteries of the lower limb. Transcutaneous measurement by Doppler effect. Nouv. Presse Med. 29, 2091—2093.

J.-P. M., Chirurgie C, Hôpital Saint-Louis, 60, rue Thiers, 17000 La Rochelle, France

RADIOCIRCULOGRAPHIC MEASUREMENT OF BLOOD FLOW IN OCCLUSIVE ARTERIAL DISEASE OF THE LOWER EXTREMITIES

I. FÖLDES and SUSAN FÉNYES

Korvin Otto Hospital, Budapest, Hungary

Introduction

Since the gamma camera came into general use the radiocirculographic instrument has gradually lost its role in the measurement of central and peripheral blood flow. In our opinion the evaluation of blood supply to the lower extremities is still a field for radiocirculography. If the passage of radioactive bolus is to be registered along the whole extremity simultaneously, separate scintillator probes have to be used. (*Schicha et al.,* 1977).

A fourchannel radiocirculograph has been used since 1969, and more than 800 examinations have been performed. (*Fényes et al.,* 1975). Since the autumn of 1977 we have measure the blood flow in both legs simultaneously with seven detectors.

Methods

The present report is based in radiocirculographic study of 120 patients suffering from arteriosclerosis obliterans and 20 healthy persons. Radiocirculography was associated in every case with an ankle systolic pressure reading, using Doppler's ultrasound apparatus, oscillography and in some instances angiography.

Several variants have been tested for measuring and evaluating methods of radiocirculography. The best results have been achieved by the following method: Fig. 1.

The patient lies on his back in a room of constant temperature. After 20 minutes adaptation seven scintillator probes are placed on both lower extremities. The detector over the abdominal aorta has a slit collimator, and assymetrical collimators developed for nephrography are placed over the common femoral arteries. Blood flow in the popliteal regions is detected from below and in the feet from above with probes of wide-angle collimators. A bolus of 25 µCi ^{169}Yb-EOTA isotope was administered intravenously. The registered signals were stored on magnetic tapes, the time-activity curves were recorded on a compensograph and the area under the ascending line of the curves was integrated electronically with a scaler.

Results

The course of evaluation of flow curves is demonstrated on the case of a patient with left popliteal artery occlusion. Fig. 2 The peak of the time-activity curves for common femoral arteries was reached in 5 seconds. The heart rate was 72 beats/min. so the time interval of 5 seconds corresponds to 6 pulse waves. The impulses obtained in the aortic and popliteal regions were counted for the same interval. As the impulse rate on the feet was low, a 20 second integration period was employed. This is approximately the duration of the first circulation round. After subtraction of the background activity the counts were divided by the quantity of isotope in terms of µCi. Minimal circulation times were also determined from the distance of the starting points of curves.

Experience from 140 examinations show that 10% differences between the respective counts over the two femoral regions and 15% differences over the popliteal or

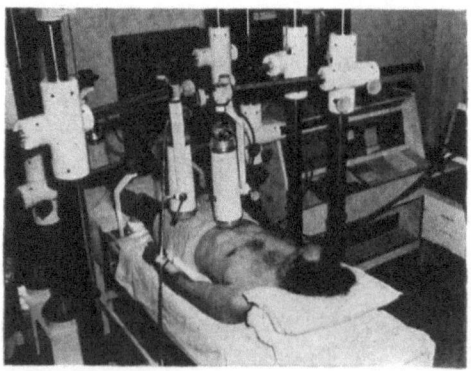

Fig. 1. Positioning of the seven detectors over the lower extremities.

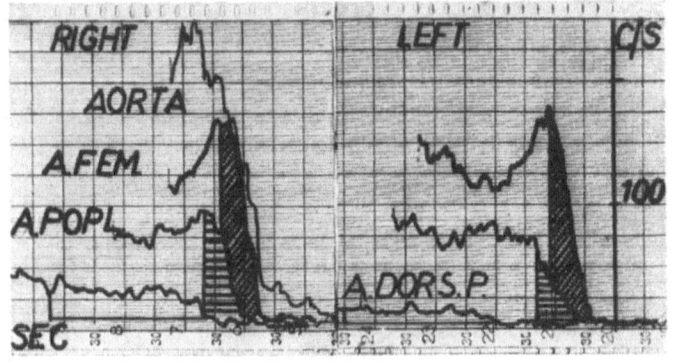

Fig. 2. Time-activity curves registered over different areas of the lower extremities. Areas under the curves are estimated by summing counts until the peak of the common femoral artery curve is reached.

dorsal foot regions can regarded as pathological. In our patient the resting blood flow in the left popliteal region was 25% less and in the foot region 43% less compared with the corresponding regions on the right side. The examination was repeated one week after left lumbar sympathectomy. Left popliteal blood flow increased by 25% of the preoperative value, but was still lower than on the right side. Blood flow in the left foot increased threefold and became twofold greater on the right side. Flow of the left common femoral artery remained unchanged. There was no change in the flow values of the unoperated right leg. This fact supports the good reproducibility of our method. The flow index over the abdominal aorta is variable, as the geometrical position of the abdominal probe is also variable.

The minimal circulation time between the knee and foot decreased to a quarter after lumbar sympathectomy.

Discussion

The impulses detected by the probes over the groin regions come almost completely from blood flowing in the common femoral artery. In the popliteal regions skin blood flow is more important than in the femoral and in the feet skin flow is measured predominantly. There is no significant muscle flow in these areas. The numerical indices developed by here indicate the distribution of the whole isotope bolus. Regional blood flow was estimated by the method reported in a camera study of cerebral circulation. (*Moses et al.* 1973). Under identical

Table I. Effect of left lumbar sympathectomy on blood flow of the lower extremities in a patient with left popliteal occlusion

	Summed Right		Counts Left		
	Before	After	Before	After	
Aorta ABD	12.3	16.1			IMP (5 sec) uCi
A. fem. C	30.3	31.3	31.0	31.3	IMP (5 sec) uCi
A. poplitea	16.9	16.7	12.6	15.7	IMP (5 sec) uCi
A. dors. pedis	17.9	16.8	10.1	30.9	IMP (20 sec) uCi
	Minimal circulation time				
A. O. - A. fem. C	0.4	0.4	0.4	0.	(sec)
A. fem. C. - A. popl.	2.6	3.2	2.6	2.8	(sec)
A. popl. - A. D. P.	4.4	6.0	11.2	2.8	(sec)

371

circumstances we were able to reproduce the results of the measurements.

At present we wish to determine the physiological limits of resting regional blood flow in order to compare the results obtained in a patient with those observed in other cases.

It seems that our radiocirculographic method is suitable for sensitive, non-nivasive measurement of blood flow in the lower extremities and for the localisation of arterial occlusion.

REFERENCES

Fényes, G., Gótzy, G., Fehrentheil, L., (1975): The effect of Prodectin (Pyridinolcarbamate) The effect of Prodectin (Pyridinoldarbamate) treatment on the circulation rate in obliterating arterial diseases of the lower extremities. Therapia Hungarica 2, 64—67.

Moses, D. C., Natarajan, T. K., Previosi, T. J., Udvarhelyi, G. B., Wagner, H. N., (1973): 'Quantitative Cerebral Circulation Studies with Sodium Pertechnetate J. Nucl. Med. 14, 142—148.

Schicha, H., Becker, W., Vosberg, H., Vyska, K., Feinendegen, L. E. (1977): Istopenangiographische Messung der Blutströmungsgeschwindigkeit in Aorta und Arterienstämmen des Menschen I. Nuklearmedizin XVI, 214—217.

I. F., Department of Nuclear Medicine, Korvin Ottó Hospital, Budapest VII., Gorkij fasor 11. Hungary

PHLEBOGRAPHY AND PRESSURE MEASUREMENTS IN THE POSTHROMBOTIC STATE (A COMPARATIVE STUDY)

J. H. A. MÜLLER, J. WAIGAND and D. H. HÖLZER

Diagnostic Department of Cardiovascular Diseases,
Hospital of Friedrichshain, Berlin, G.D.R.

In patients suffering from chronic venous insufficiency of the lower extremities phlebographical examinations were combined with peripheral pressure measurements. A total of 150 extremities were examined according to a standardized ascending limb phlebography, which was succeeded by a phlebography of the pelvic veins if necessary. Immediately before phlebographic examinations the venous pressure measurings were performed in erect posture after puncturing a superficial vein at the ankle. Pressure recordings were made at rest and during exercise (ten times tiptoe-position). In cases of pathological pressure curve further pressure measurings were performed in the same technique fixing distal and proximal tourniquets at various levels of the calf and the thigh. The following aspects were to be examined:

1. To differentiate between primary varicose veins and cases with postthrombotic changes of the deep veins,
2. to evaluate the degree of the postthrombotic state.

Fig. 1 shows the following parameters which are necessary for the evaluation.

P_1 = the hydrostatic pressure in the venous system, mainly depending on the height (normal value: 92.8 ± 6.5 mm Hg)

P_2 = maximal dropping of the venous pressure after exercise (normal value: 26.2 ± 11.0 mm Hg)

Δp = pressure difference $p_1 - p_2$ (normal value: 66.7 ± 9.0 mm Hg)

t_1 = time of pressure decrease and

t_2 = time of pressure increase, mainly depending on the overall pressure decrease and time constant of the

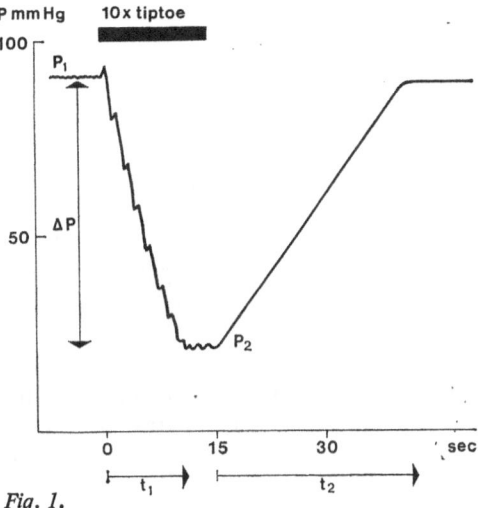

Fig. 1.

pressure transducer and catheter system.

For our evaluations p_1, p_2 and Δp are of main importance.

The next Fig. 2 demonstrated our results of pressure measurements. There are 4 teams of patients: A first normal group, a second group with primary varicosis, a third group with severe varicosis and insufficiency of the saphenous system and incompetent perforating veins, and a fourth group with postthrombotic changes of the deep veins.

There is a statistical highly significant difference between the group I or II compared with group III or IV ($p < 0.01$), where as we could not find a significant difference between group III and IV. Additional recordings after tourniquets show an essential improvement in the third group with severe varicosis, opposite to the postthrombotic syndrome (group IV).

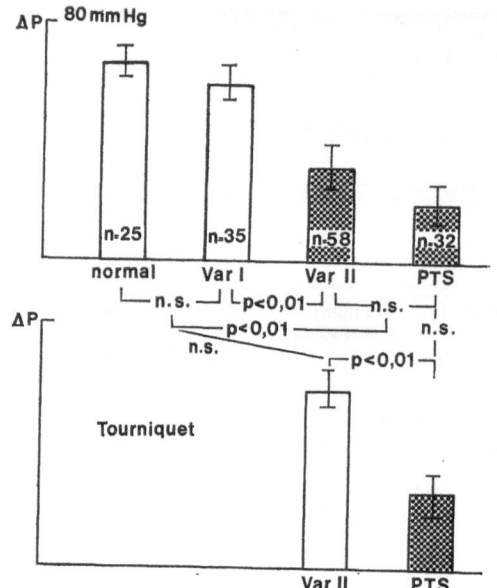

Fig. 2.

functional state of the deep veins of the calf and also of the popliteal veins. Pathological changes of the deep femoral and pelvic veins are recognized not too precisely. An isolated process of the pelvic veins can even show normal pressure measurings.

3. Severe primary varicosis and the postthrombotic state can equally show pathological pressure recordings. Additional measurements after tourniquets in the calf and the thigh permit a differentiation in two groups.

4. Pressure measurements permit an approximate estimation of the grade of postthrombotic changes of the deep veins.

5. Pressure measurements are well suited for control examinations after therapeutical investigations, but don't replace phlebography in all cases.

Now we have a significant difference between group III and IV, too (p < 0.01).

According to May we can divide the postthrombotic state in four stages by phlebography (Fig. 3). The deep veins of the calf and the thigh are evaluated separately. The sum of the grade of postthrombotic changes in the calf and the thigh correlates very closely with the value of Δp by pressure measurements (r = 0.70 and p < 0.001).

Conclusions

1. Normal pressure measurements at rest and during exercise exclude a postthrombotic state of the limb with high certainty.

2. Pressure recordings mainly reveal the

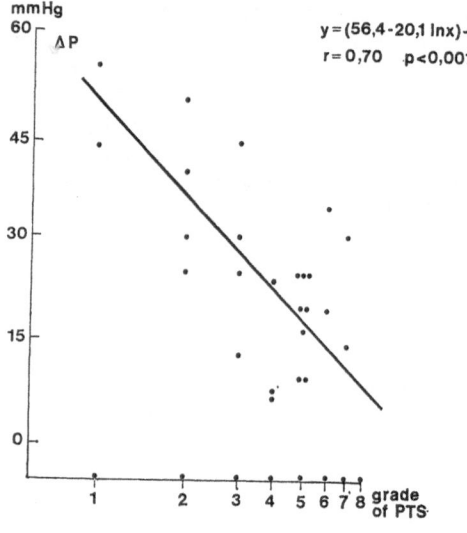

Fig. 3.

J. H. A. M. Cardiovasc Depart., Hospital of Friedrichshain, Berlin, G. D. R.

SEQUENTIAL SCINTIGRAPHY OF THE AORTA AND THE ARTERIES OF THE EXTREMITIES

M. DEGEORGES, J. C. ROUCAYROL, Y. CHAPUIS, J. Y. DEVAUX
and M. HODARA

Hospital Cochin, Dept. of Cardiovascular Diseases, Paris, France

Radio-isotopes are used in the study of large arteries by the method known as sequential angioscintigraphy.

This method consists of the intravenous injection of technetium (99ᵐ Tc): either in the form of sodium pertechnate or affixed to red blood cells. (Type 0, rhesus negative). Theoretically the best images are obtained by using labelled red blood cells, which stay in the vascular compartment, in contrast to the pertechnate ion which rapidly diffuses into the extravascular compartment. In spite of this, the pertechnate ion is most often used because of its convenience:

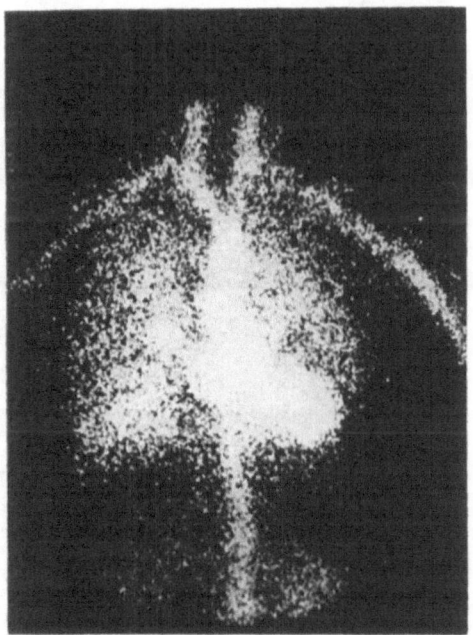

Fig. 1. Normal subclavian and carotid arteries.

- simple and rapid preparation,
- highly specific activity (with bolus effect),
- relatively unimportant extra-vascular diffusion if only first circulatory passage is studied.

Technetium was chosen for the following reasons:

- it is easily obtained (molybdene 99 generator),
- the gamma photons are emitted with an energy of 140 KeV which lies within the most sensitive range of the detector,
- the low irradiation incurred; for only gamma rays are emitted, the period is 6 hours and biological elimination is rapid. For an adult the whole body absorbed dose is 0,17 rad with the activity used (12 mci). Lower doses permit use on children. Only pregnancy constitutes an absolute contra-indication.

The injection is made in an antecubital vein exceptionally in a jugular vein. Technetium in 1 ml of isotonic saline provides a true radioactif bolus. The scintillation data are recorded by a scintillation camera centered on the area to be studied. The results are visualised on the oscilloscope of the camera and pictured on polaroid film. The progression of the radioactif bolus is followed by a second oscilloscope of persistant type which permits the detection of the different phases of vascular filling and allows a regular registration of the images (about every 4 seconds).

The scintigraphic information is simultaneously recorded on the magnetic tape of a data storage system which is coupled to the camera, and thus permits the recreating of the information, this is done either image by image (up to 4 per second) or by lumping the images together on a screen and measuring the radioactivity of a specific zone or, also, by obtaining a representative time-activity curve.

The different components of this system thus provide not only morphological information but kinetic information as well. If the quality of the pictures is inferior to that obtained by X-rays these explorations by radioelements have advantages appreciated by doctors as well as surgeons. In particular: the exam is readily accepted by patients because it is rapid, rarely exceeding 5 minutes; it is not painful since the injections are intravenous without injection pressure and so cause no hemodynamic changes; the product is non-toxic at the low concentrations used; it is non allergenic, and accidental extra-vascular diffusion apparently has no consequences. Dosimetry is low compared with the 2−4 rads of traditional radiological vascular exploration.

All of these characteristics explain why isotopic vascular explorations can be practiced on out-patients, can be practiced repeatedly, can be used soon after surgery, and can replace radiological examinations on patients who are allergic to iodine products or who are too fragile to withstand traumatic intervention.

But this technique also presents some inconveniences. The scintillation camera has a resolution power inferior to that of radiological equipment; the walls of arterial vessels are imprecise and it is impossible to study vessels with a diameter of less than 5 mm. The field explored by the camera is limited and only one area can be studied per exam. Furthermore the exam can only be repeated when the circulating radioactivity due to the first injection has sufficiently decayed, (after at least 24 hours).

The recent use of scintillation cameras of high resolution and large field of view has improved vascular exploration.

Arterial trunks can be examined: aorta (ascending, horizontal, descending, thoracic and abdominal); brachiocephalic artery, carotid arteries, sub-clavian and humeral arteries, iliac, femoral, and popliteal arteries.

Only the vertebral, renal, mesenteric and hypogastric arteries are difficult to visualize. Some of these arteries can also be studied without causing trauma by means of the Doppler effect or by echotomography. However the thoracic aorta can not be studied by ultrasounds and the sub-clavian and iliac arteries can be studied by the Doppler effect only indirectly.

Isotopic angiography permits direct visualisation of these axes and provides a distinction between diffuse and localized stenosis.

The practice of more than 300 sequential angioscintigraphies on arteriopathies at

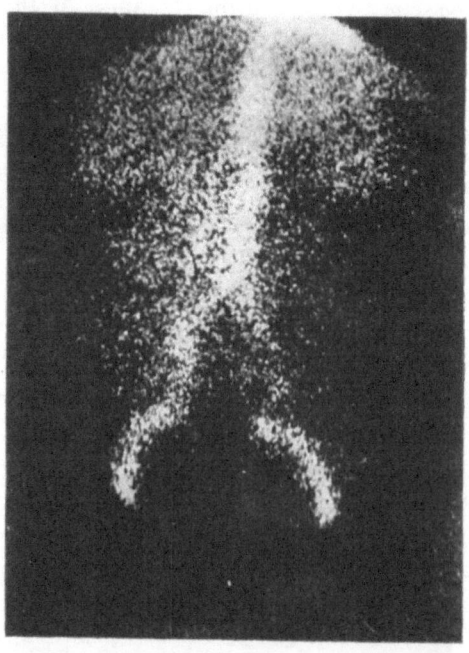

Fig. 2. Stenosis of left iliac artery. The abdominal aorta is of regular dimensions, the two iliac arteries are sinuous. Total stenosis is observed at the middle third of the left iliac artery, repermeability by means of a collateral at the femoral artery.

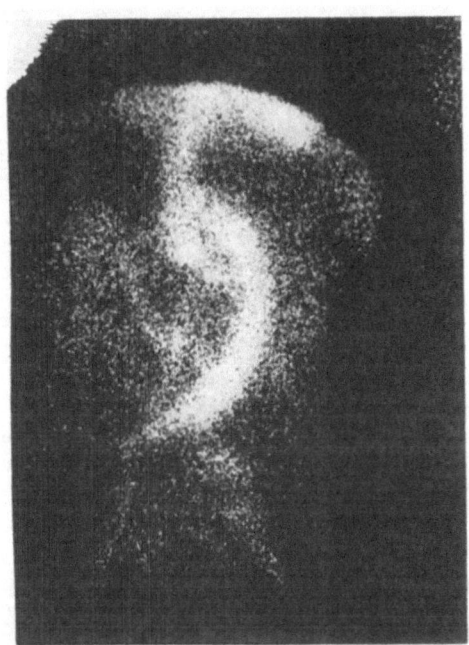

Fig. 3. Aorto-iliac bypass. Intervention short circuiting an aneurysm of the abdominal aorta. Exploration 9 months later.

Cochin Hospital has shown the real interest of this technique. In fact it constitutes a diagnostic aid in determining the indications of radiological opacification, and even, in some cases, which kind: for example the choice between translombar or retrograde method of aortography. The morphological study can show anomalies in arterial diameter, dilatation in the case of aneuıyms, narrowing in the case of extrinsic compression, as well as blocks resulting from thrombi or complete stenosis. The kinetic study permits the evaluation of the functional repercussions of incomplete stenosis, and the extent, localized or diffuse. One restriction must be made concerning dissecting and entirely thrombosed sacciform aneurysms which are more difficult to recognize.

Angioscintigraphy is a convenient method to determine the efficacity of surgical intervention or medical treatment?

Since it can be performed repeatedly, it permits the close surveillance of the evaluation of arteritic lesions under vasodilatators or anticoagulants, and reveals the state of permeability after the removal of obstruction or following graft or bypass. In the absence of aggravation, second interventions can be postponed on particularly fragile patients. Angioscintigraphy is also of great use in emergencies when speed and the innocuousness of the technique can be deciding factors. In particular in the case of acute thrombosis of the lower extremities surgery has been performed solely on the basis of information provided by isotopic exploration.

Sequential angioscintigraphy is thus particularly valuable for the wealth of morphological and kinetic data provided without incurring any trauma. It occupies an important place in the range of exploration for acute and chronic arteriopathy.

M. D., U.E.R. Cochin, 27, rue du Faubourg, Saint Jacques, 75674 Paris Cedex, France

INFLUENCE OF ELEVATED ARTERY PRESSURE ON ALTERATION OF ARTERIAL COLLATERALS IN ANGIOGRAMS

G. NÖLDGE and E. P. STRECKER

Department of Radiology, University of Freiburg i. Br., F.R.G.

Nonsurgical therapy for peripheral chronic occlusive disease is very helpful in its first clinical stages, because the potential formation of collaterals promises good prognosis.

According to the well known fact that the formation of collateral circulation depends on the blood pressure proximal to the occlusion site, the following experiments were carried out on animals to control the stimulation of collateral opening.

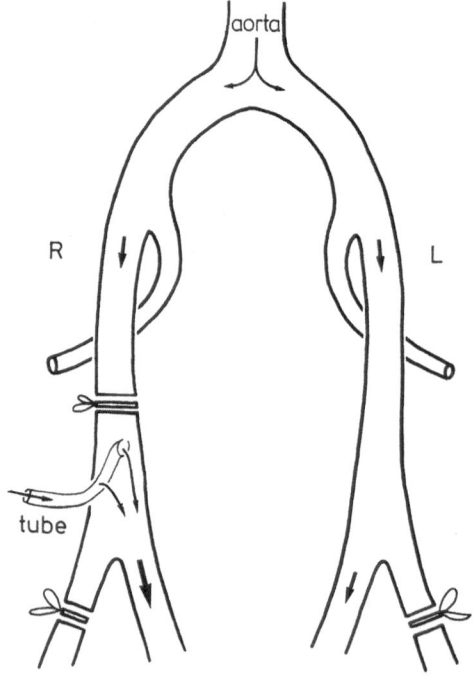

Fig. 1. Part of the experimental arrangement showing the position of the tube with its side hole near the origin of the deep femoral artery for perfusion. Both superficial femoral arteries and the right iliac artery are ligated.

After ligation of the superficial femoral artery in a dog, the influence of increased perfusion pressure on the right deep femoral artery and its potential collaterals should be evaluated.

In ten dogs possible openigs of preformed collaterals were studied at different perfusion pressures by angiograms.

After general anesthesia a teflon tube was inserted through the carotid artery into the thoracic aorta and fixed in this position. Common femoral, superficial and deep femoral arteries were also prepared.

The superficial arteries were ligated distal to the origin of the deep femoral arteries. The left side served as a control.

A teflon tube was inserted with its side hole near the origin of the deep femoral artery.

The right external iliac artery was also ligated, as can be seen in Figure 1, to prevent retrograde flow of the injected blood.

Otherwise it would not be possible to build up a higher perfusion pressure in the deep femoral artery on the right side.

The teflon tube in the aorta and the one in the right common femoral artery was connected with an interposed smoother rubber tube, which was attacted to a peristaltic tube pump.

This experimental set-up was used to show the effect of alteration of the perfusion pressure on open collaterals preformed after ligation of the superficial femoral artery.

The effect of different perfusion pressures was studied by angiograms recorded during the perfusion.

Evaluation of the angiograms of the right and left side yields the following

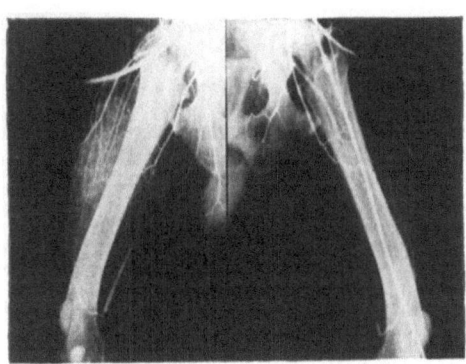

Fig. 2. Marked onset of collateralisation at the perfused right side, no visualization of collaterals on the control side (right side of the figure).

results: An increase of 10−20 mm Hg over normal blood pressure (100−120 mm Hg) shows no significant enlargement of the perfused right femoral artery or any formation of collaterals.

An increase of the perfusion pressure of more than 40−50 mm Hg produces measurable enlargement of the vessel diameter of the deep femoral artery by about 1.0 mm. The control side shows no changes, as expected.

Single collaterals become clearer in their appearances and the number of collaterals increases, not only in the neighbourhood but also in the periphery of larger branches of the right deep femoral artery. The control side does not show marked changes in the vessel pattern, as can be seen in Figure 2.

Step by step elevation of the perfusion pressure shows extravasation at a level of 180−210 mm Hg. Pressures over 210 mm Hg cause heavy extravasation, edema and hematoma in the tissue.

At a perfusion pressure level over 210 mm Hg marked early venous filling was seen in angiograms. A precondition for the existance of this finding is the postulation of arterio-venous shunts, which could not be clearly demonstrated angiographically.

These results demonstrate in our angiograms that increased artificial perfusion pressure opens preformed collaterals. Hypervascularisation in preliminary less perfused tissues can be induced by this experimental arrangement.

These preliminary results can possibly be applied to clinical therapy to accelerate formation of collaterals to treat chronic arterial occlusion disease.

G. N., Department of Radiology University of Freiburg, 7800 Freiburg im Breisgau, F.R.G.

THE SIGNIFICANCE OF EXTENSIVE ANGIOGRAPHIC STUDIES OF PATIENTS WITH KLIPPEL-TRENAUNAY SYNDROME

P. BALAS, D. KELEKIS, K. OECONOMOU and N. XEROMECITIS

First Department of Surgery, Athens University Medical School, Athens, Greece

Introduction

Congenital angiodysplasias of the extremities included in the Klippel-Trenaunay syndrome are characterized by the coexistence of the classical triad: a) venous dysplasia; b) extensive angiomata; c) hypertropy of the bones of the lower extremities.

The progress of the diagnostic methods, especially of vascular examinations and also the haemodynamic study of congenital angiodysplasias has indicated that it is impossible to include many different kinds of vascular malformations in the same category and thus should not be used.

The present study concerns an analysis of the angiographic findings of 4 of a series of 17 patients suffering from a Klippel-Trenaunay syndrome. A further discussion of these findings is also presented.

Materials and methods

Of the 17 patients that were hospitalized between 1969—1977, 10 were selected with extensive dysplasias of the extremities. Four of the above patients were males and six females. The dysplasias occurred in two cases in the upper and in 10 cases in the lower limbs. There was also a coexistence of the classical triad of the syndrome or a combination of symptoms.

Table I.

Examinations	Cases			
	1st ♀ 24 years old	2nd ♂ 27 years old	3rd ♀ 15 years old	4th ♂ 14 years old
Arteriography	Negative	Negative	Negative	Multiple A—V communications concerning all the left tibia, resembling haemangiomata.
Ascending phlebography	*L.L.*: Insufficiency of the perforating veins and varicosities at the tibial region. *R.L.*: Partial insufficiency of the perforated veins with valvular insufficiency at the level of the common femoral vein. The left common iliac vein exhibits high collateral circulation directed to the right common iliac vein. There is no visualization of the I.V.C.	Multiple bilateral varicosities of the superficial veins of the tibial region with hypoplasia of the deep veins. Significant stenosis of the l. common iliac v. with the presence of collateral circulation to the r. iliac vein.	Irregular course of the r. common iliac vein to the l. common iliac vein simulating a subpubic by-pass.	Significant stenosis of the left common femoral vein.

Table I. (Continued)

Examinations	Cases			
Lymphangio-graphy	Negative	Negative	Negative	Negative
Selective arte-riography of the renal and splanchnic arteries	*Renal arteries*: Multiple stenosis of the left renal artery resembling fibro-muscular hyperplasia or polyarteritis nodosa. Multiple cysts of the right kidney. *Splanchnic arteries*: Multiple stenosis of the hepatic artery, with poor hepatic vascularization resembling the cirhotic pattern.	Negative	Negative	Negative

The patients were examined meticulously with detailed clinical and laboratory examinations and were submitted to complete angiographic studies, namely:
1) Arteriography of the affected limb;
2) Ascending phlebography of the affected limb;
3) Lymphangiography;
4) Selective angiography of the splanchnic and renal arteries.

In 4 of these patients, the above detailed angiographic investigation showed the presence of anomalies concerning vessels and organs, apart from the main vascular lesion of the extremity. These anomalies had no relation to the main vascular malformation of the syndrome.

These patients, 2 males and 2 females, had the main angiodysplasia in the lower limb.

These angiographic findings, according to the case and screening, are given in Table I.

Discussion — conclusions

The necessity of further investigation of patients exhibiting the Klippel-Trenaunay syndrome was apparent from the very beginning after the detailed study of congenital angiodysplasias of the limbs. Meanwhile, the angiographic study is the best means of examination for correct diagnosis and study of vascular anomalies as estimation of any possible therapeutic possibilities.

Vascular studies resulted in doubts on the part of many investigators as to whether many kinds of angiodysplasias could be classified under the general entity of the Klippel-Trenaunay syndrome (*De Takats*, 1932; *Lanzara*, 1961; *Malan and Puglionisi*, 1961, *Malan*, 1974), due to the fact that the classification of these angiodysplasias, presenting the classical triad of symptoms of this syndrome, excluding the exact assessment of the anatomo-clinical entity of the main lesion, no longer represents the actually existing abnormality and its use should be discontinued.

In conclusion, the use of multiple angiographic studies is indispensable in any case of angiodysplasia of the limb for precise study of the kind and extent of the abnormality.

Our study is proof that not only vascular examination of the affected limb is necessary, but also further investigation of the splanchnic, renal and eventually the cerebral vessels is required for the discovery of other very important vascular malformations.

REFERENCES

Anagnostou G., Balas P. (1973): Peripheral congenital angiomalformations. Iatriki Epitheorisis Enoplon Dynameon, Athens 7, 901, 1973.

De Takats G. (1932): Vascular anomalies of the extremities. Report of five cases. Surg. Gynec. and Obst. 55, 227.

Klippel M., Trenaunay I. (1900): Du noevus variqueux et ostéohypertrophique. Arch. Gen. Med. 3, 641.

Lanzara A. (1961): Sindromi da comunicazioni arteriovenose congenite degli arti. Progressi di terapia 46, 2.

Malan E. (1974): Vascular malformations (Angiodysplasias). Carlo Erba Foundation, Milan.

Malan E., Puglionisi A. (1964): Congenital angiodysplasias of the extremities. J. Cardiov. Surg. 5, 87.

B. P., Athens University, 1st Surg. Department, 16 Astydanados St., Pagrati — Athens Greece

EVALUATION OF ISOTOPE ANGIOGRAPHY IN VASCULAR SURGERY

Y. MIYAUCHI, I. ADACHI, H. SAITO and K. ITO

First Department of Surgery, Chiba University, School of Medicine, Chiba, Japan

Introduction

Contrast angiography has been used to diagnose vascular diseases and detect the patency of vessels or grafts after reconstructive surgery.

However, this procedure is often associated with significant morbidity among patients who also have diffuse arteriosclerotic disease.

Isotope angiography may be of value in the diagnosis of major to moderate arterial disease and determination of arterial patency, because the method is noninversive and easy to perform. However, the method has not been widely used because it provides poorer resolution than conventional contrast angiography.

In this paper, we would like to evaluate RI angiography from the standpoint of vascular surgery.

Methods and materials

The patient is positioned under the 12 inch circular detector of the Gamma camera with the 6000 hole low energy collimeter in place and with the important area of the arterial tree centered in the field of vision. Twenty millicuries of technetium 99 m pertechnetate in a volume of less than 3 ml are rapidly injected into the antecubital vein. Isotope distribution in the area of interest is visualized on gamma camera oscilloscope and serial 2-second exposures were obtained by manually pulling film from the Polaroid camera throughout the next 20 minutes. About 3 minutes following injection a static scintiphoto is exposed in a majority of the patients.

This technique was used to perform 118 RI angiograms on 80 patients and the conventional contrast angiograms were also obtained on 54 of them. The patients consisted of 75 arterial and 5 venous cases. In this paper, the arterial application of this technique will be mainly discussed.

Results

The disease in which RI angiography was performed were shown in Table I. Aneurysm was the most common disease, followed by arteriosclerosis obliterans, thromboangitis obliterans and A – V malformation.

Table 1. Diseases in which RI angiography was performed.

Aneurysm	
Thoracic aorta	7
Abdominal "	12
Iliac artery	2
Popliteal "	1
Obstructive disease	
Coarctation of aorta	1
Arteriosclerosis obliterans	19
Thromboangitis obliterans	13
Thoracic outlet syndrome	2
A-V Fistula	2
Others	16
	75

At the level of the thoracic aorta, 9 patients were examined using this technique for 8 suspected aneurysms and a coarctation but the results were disappointing in dynamic RI angiography because of the large isotope uptake by the heart and lungs. On the other hand, static imaging gives rather better result according to the degree of abnormality.

At the level of the abdominal aorta, 24 RI angiograms were obtained. Twenty one were suspected as the aortic aneurysm

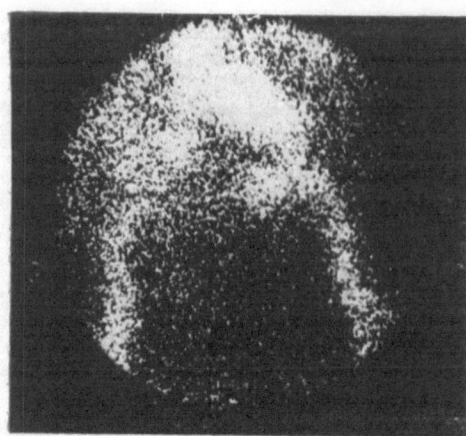

Fig. 1. RI angiogram obtained on a patient with bilateral common iliac and the left internal iliac aneurysms

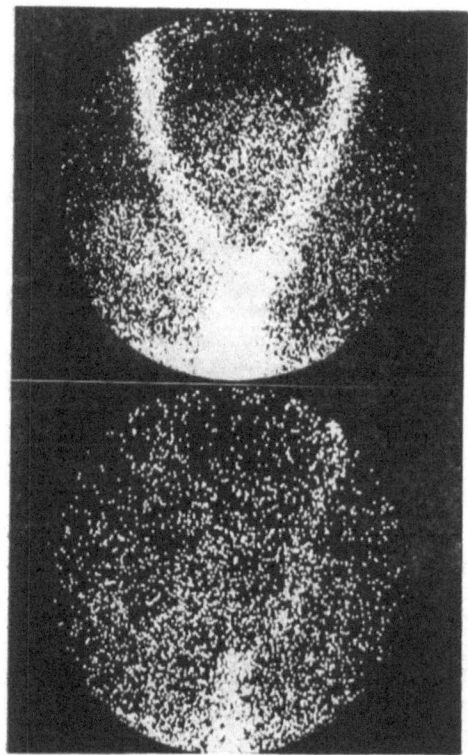

Fig. 2. Preoperative (top) and postoperative (bottom) RI angiograms obtained on a patient with aorto-femoral graft bypass

prior to the examination, 12 were diagnosed as true abdominal aneurysm and the other 10 were diagnosed as aorta tortuosity. Two patients were suspected of aortic occlusions which was confirmed by this technique.

In the patients with abdominal aortic disease, particularly in aortic aneurysm, isotope angiography has it greatest value in assessing the aneurysmal sac, mural thrombus, and the tortuous or stenotic iliac arteries.

At the level of the iliac artery, 17 RI angiograms were obtained on 2 iliac aneurysmal patients, 13 obstructive diseases and 2 other malformations. In 15 out of 17 cases effective information was obtained. Fig. 1 shows a common iliac and the left internal iliac aneurysms. It is slightly difficult to distinguish between a small aneurysm and tortuous iliac artery.

At the level of femoro-popliteal arteries, 17 isotope angiograms were obtained on 14 obstructive, one aneurysmal, 2 A – V malformation cases.

In about 2/3 of the cases useful information was obtained but only poor results were obtained on obese popliteal aneurysmal patients.

In 6 below-the-knee obstructive cases, this technique has no value to visualize obstructive point or collaterals.

This technique has been used to detect the results of reconstructive surgery in 11 patients, proper visualization was obtained in all cases. For example, Fig. 2 shows a typical arterio-sclerotic obstruction of the bilateral iliac arteries and postoperative RI angiogram obtained on the same patient reveals a patent Y-shaped graft bypass.

Discussion and conclusion

RI angiography was introduced by Powell et al. and Rosenthall in 1966 and was used in the diagnosis of arterial aneurysms (*Bergan*, 1974), occlusive arterial diseases (*Dibos*, 1972) and in detection of arterial reconstructions (*Moss*, 1975). However, this technique has not been widely used because it provides poorer resolution than contrast angiography.

From our experience, this technique provides the best result in the diagnosis of aorta-iliac diseases. It could be safely used on severely ill patients and permits multiple follow-up evaluations even in early postoperative stages.

Although isotope angiography is not capable of replacing conventional contrast angiography, it should be used for the screening and evaluation of vascular reconstruction and only those patients with abnormalities identified on isotope angiography need undergo conventional contrast angiography for further delineation.

REFERENCES

Bergan, J. J. et al. (1974): Radionuclide aortography in detection of arterial aneurysms. Arch. Surg. 109, 80—83.
Dibos, P. E. et al. (1972): Intravenous radio-nuclide arteriography in peripheral occlusive arterial disease. Radiology 102, 181—183.
Moss, C. M. et al. (1976): Isotope angiography. Ann. Surg. 184, 116—121.

Y. M. First Dept. of Surg. Chiba University, 1-8-1 Inohana, Chiba, Japan

ARTERIAL INSUFFICIENCY OF THE HAND EVALUATED BY DIGITAL BLOOD PRESSURE AND ARTERIOGRAPHIC FINDINGS

M. HIRAI, S. KAWAI and S. SHIONOYA

Department of Surgery, Nagoya University Branch Hospital, Nagoya, Japan

Introduction

In the evaluation of arterial insufficiency of the upper extremities, all five fingers should be studied separately because the degree of ischemia is often different in each finger.

In the present study, the systolic blood pressure in all five fingers was measured by photoelectric plethysmography in patients with arterial occlusive diseases of the arm and the correlation of these pressures with arteriographic findings was studied.

Materials and methods

Measurement of systolic blood pressure by the photoelectric technique has been described in detail elsewhere (*Hirai and Kawai*, 1977). Systolic blood pressure is determined by slowly deflating the cuff pressure from the suprasystolic values and recording the first inflow with a photocell placed on the finger-tip. A 24 mm wide cuff was used at the proximal phalanx of the 1st finger and a 20 mm wide cuff at the intermediate phalanx of the lateral four fingers. An arm-to-finger pressure gradient of less than -22 mmHg has been chosen as significant from the results of 80 normal subjects.

In the present study, 80 arms from 50 patients with arterial occlusive disease were studied. The arterial occlusion was confirmed by serial brachial arteriography. According to the arteriographic findings, 387 fingers of 80 hands were classified into three groups. The normal finger group consisted of 99 fingers. In this group, no organic abnormality was seen in vessels supplying the fingers. In the uninterrupted flow finger group, consisting of 85 fingers, only one digital artery was supplied by its own metacarpal or common digital arteries through the more proximal arteries without interruption. The interrupted flow finger group consisted of 203 fingers. Occlusion was seen in both digital arteries or more proximal arteries supplying the finger. Therefore, in this group the blood supply to the finger was dependent upon the collateral circulation.

Results and comments

Figures 1, 2 and 3 show the results of correlation of digital blood pressure with arteriographic findings and development of ischemic signs in 387 fingers. Digital blood pressure was recorded as normal in all 184 fingers classified into the normal flow finger group or uninterrupted flow finger group. Therefore, it might be considered that, if there is at least one obstruction-free arterial path to and down the finger, normal digital pressure is obtained.

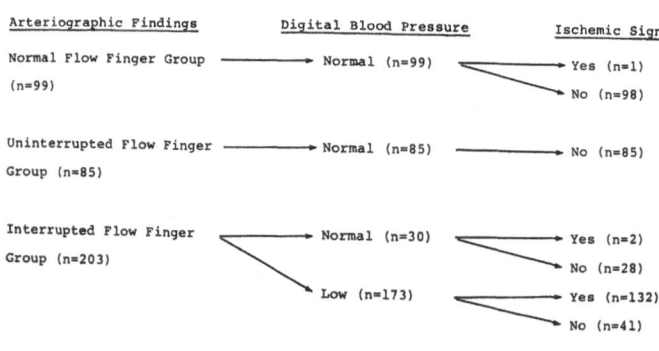

Fig. 1. Correlation of digital blood pressure with arteriographic findings and development of ischemic signs in 387 fingers

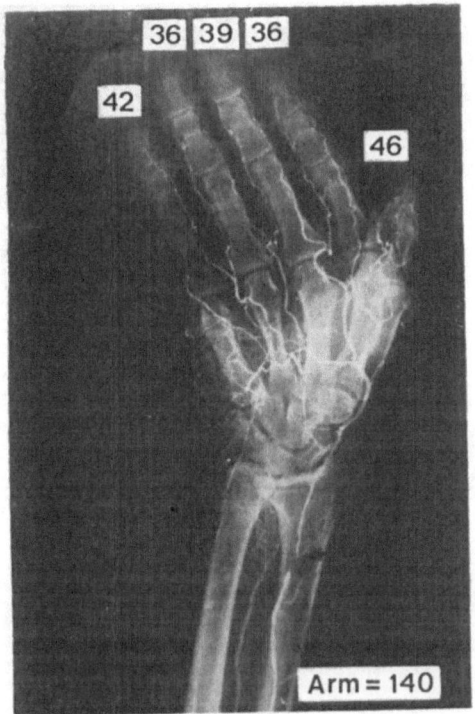

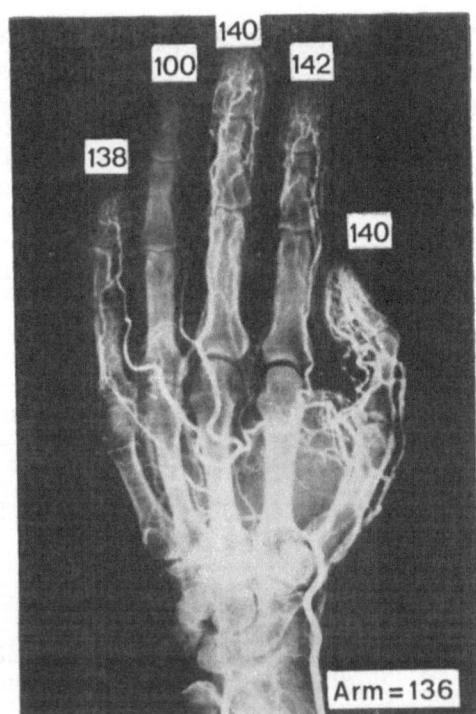

Fig. 2. A 63-year-old male patient with arteriosclerosis obliterans. He complained of cold sensitivity in all fingers. Arteriogram shows occlusion of both radial and ulnar arteries. In the palm and fingers, no occlusive lesions are seen. Blood pressure measurement showed a significantly low digital pressure in all fingers. This case suggests that, if the finger is supplied with blood flow by an interrupted artery, digital ischemia may develop.

Fig. 3. A 47-year-old male patient with Buerger's disease, complaining of cold sensitivity of the IVth finger. Arteriogram shows occlusions of the lateral digital artery of the IInd finger, the medial digital artery of the IIIrd finger and both digital arteries of the IVth finger. Blood pressure measurement revealed decreased blood pressure in the IVth finger and normal pressure in the other fingers. This result suggests that occlusion of only one digital artery does not cause digital ischemia, but occlusion of both digital arteries may cause ischemia.

In all 203 fingers classified into the interrupted flow finger group, a significantly decreased blood pressure was expected, because of occlusion in vessels in or leading to both sides of the finger; 173 of them exhibited an abnormally low blood pressure and 30 had normal blood pressure. In these 30 fingers, well developed collateral circulation was suggested, but it was not always easy to accurately determine the degree of development of collateral vessels on the basis of arteriographic findings. However, only 2 of these 30 fingers showed the development of ischemic symptoms. Therefore, determination of blood pressure is considered to be helpful as a functional diagnostic measure to objectively estimate the flow volume of collateral vessels.

In the correlation between the digital blood pressure and the development of the digital ischemic symptoms in each finger, no ischemic signs were observed in 211 of 214 fingers with a normal digital pressure. Therefore, if digital blood pressure is normal, even though arterial occlusion is shown in arteriograms, digital ischemic signs rarely develop in arterial occlusive disease. Of 173 fingers with a decreased digital blood pressure, ischemic signs in

387

the finger developed in 132. These findings might indicate that the impaired digital circulation due to arterial occlusion in or leading to the finger is a necessary precondition in the development of digital ischemic signs. However, 41 fingers with a decreased blood pressure showed no ischemic symptoms. This finding may indicate that the individual variations in the sensitivity to cold, the environment or working conditions and the degree of disturbance in digital microcirculation due to local trauma or to microemboli influence the development of the ischemic symptoms.

Conclusion

In the present study, systolic blood pressure in all fingers was measured by the photoelectric technique in 80 limbs with arterial occlusive disease and the correlation of such pressures with arteriographic findings was investigated.

Determination of blood pressure might be considered to be of value as a functional diagnostic measure to objectively estimate the flow volume of collateral vessels. If the digital blood pressure is normal, even though arterial occlusion is visible in the arteriograms, digital ischemic signs rarely develop. In development of the digital ischemic signs, impaired digital circulation due to arterial occlusion in or leading to the finger is a necessary precondition.

REFERENCE

Hirai, M., Kawai, S. (1977): The reliability of photoelectric technique for measuring systolic blood pressure of the limbs. VASA 6, 215—219.

M. H., Department of Surgery, Nagoya University Branch Hospital, 2-12-1 Higashisakura Higashiku, Nagoya, Japan

THE COMPARISON OF THE DIAGNOSTIC VALUE IN THE DETECTION OF THE CAUSATIVE LESIONS OF CEREBROVASCULAR INSUFFICIENCY AMONG AORTIC ARCH STUDY, CAROTID AND VERTEBROBASILAR ARTERIOGRAMS

K. KIKKAWA

Department of Radiology, Guthrie Clinic, Robert Packer Hospital, Sayre, Pa., U.S.A.

A total of 116 angiographies which were performed for the evaluation of extracranial cerebrovascular insufficiency during the period of 1968 through 1972, were reviewed: 67 aortic arch studies, 28 common carotid arteriograms, and 21 vertebrobasilar arteriograms.

In the aortic arch study, among 31 patients of the carotid insufficiency, 22 were male and nine female. However, in the vertebrobasilar group 21 were female and 15 male. The diagnosis of extracranial cerebrovascular insufficiency was clinically made on admission, in 25 cases of 31 carotid group, and in 28 cases of the 36 vertebrobasilar patients.

Among 36 patients of vertebrobasilar insufficiency examined by the aortic arch study, eight were found to have abnormal but incidental angiographic findings: 1-with a 50% reduction of the caliber of vertebral artery by osteophyte, 1-less than 50% reduction of the caliber at the origin of a vertebral artery, and 6-slight angulation and stenoses of the vessels by osteophytes. These findings were thought to be of no clinical significance. However, three patients of 36 vertebrobasilar insufficiency were treated in accordance with the angiographic findings: 1-with a tight stenosis of a dominant vertebral artery at origin and ulcerating atheroma of the carotid bifurcation was treated with anticoagulation, 1-with a tight stenosis of the right subclavian artery, and another with a tight stenosis of the left vertebral artery were endarterectomized in each case.

In reference to 31 carotid patients examined by aortic arch study, abnormal but not clinically significant findings were encountered in 14 patients: Most of these were mild stenoses or small atheromas. Seven patients, however, with significant lesions were subjected to endarterectomies because of either ulcerating atheromas or stenoses greater than 75% of the caliber.

In short, among 67 patients who were examined for extracranial cerebrovascular insufficiency, the aortic arch study detected significant lesions in three for vertebrobasilar system (8.3%), and seven for carotid system (22.5%). Among the former, one was treated medically with anticoagulation and two surgically. All of the seven patients of carotid insufficiency were treated surgically.

Common carotid arteriography was employed to evaluate extracranial cerebrovascular insufficiency in 28 patients. Both male and female were almost equally involved. Thirteen of 28 patients were studied for transient ischemic attack and fifteen for the cerebral infarction. Among the former, all but one patient were clinically diagnosed as TIA on admission. In 15 patients of infarction, 10 were diagnosed correctly on admission.

In five of the 13 TIA patients, carotid angiogram showed abnormal findings: 1-localized cerebral edema, 1-occlusion of internal carotid artery at origin, and 3-stenoses greater than 75% at origin of internal carotid arteries. Among 15 patients of cerebral infarction, carotid angiogram demonstrated the abnormal findings in 11 cases: 2-tight stenoses of internal carotid artery, 1-ulcerating atheroma at bifurcation, 1-ulcerating atheroma and occlusion of internal carotid artery, 1-occlusion of middle cerebral artery group, 1-thrombosis of the Sylvian vessels, 2-localized cerebral edemas, 1-generalized cerebral edema, 1-cerebral infarction, and 1-stenosis of the middle cerebral artery. Among the five TIA patients with abnormal findings, three underwent endarterectomies and one was subjected to anticoagulation therapy. Likewise, among 11 infarction patients with abnormal findings, two were endarterectomized, and one anticoagulated. Another patient underwent unsuccessful endarterectomy.

In short, a total of 28 patients were examined by carotid arteriography, 13 for TIA and 15 for cerebral infarction. Five of the former and 11 of the latter demonstrated significant abnormalities (57%).

Vertebrobasilar arteriography was employed in 21 patients of extracranial cerebrovascular insufficiency. Among them, 14 were TIA and seven infarction. In this group, the male were far more frequently affected by the disease process than the female, with a ratio of 17 vs four. In 12 of 14 TIA patients and in five of seven infarctions, the diagnosis was made clinically on admission.

Among 14 of TIA under this category, seven angiograms were abnormal: 1-tight stenosis of left vertebral artery at origin and fibromuscular dysplasia distally and occlusion of the right internal carotid artery and ulcerating atheroma at the left common carotid bifurcation, 1-occlusion of the right vertebral artery at origin and a moderate stenosis of the left vertebral artery at the junction with the right vertebral artery, 1-occlusion of the left vertebral artery at origin and a tight stenosis of the right vertebral artery at origin, 1-stenosis of basilar artery near bifurcation, 2-transient type stenoses of the left vertebral artery by osteophytes with rotation of the head, and 1-thrombosis of the distal right posterior cerebral artery.

In these seven patients, two were anticoagulated because of the angiographic findings, and one was endarterectomized with a vein graft to the right subclavian artery. Among seven cases of infarction of the vertebrobasilar system, three angiograms were abnormal: 1-occlusion of the right posterior cerebral artery, 1-poor visualization of the left posterior cerebral artery and left superior cerebellar artery, and 1-stenosis of both posterior cerebral arteries in the proximal portion. One of these three patients was treated with anticoagulation therapy.

In short, among 21 cases of vertebrobasilar insufficiency, seven of 14 TIA's and three of seven infarctions demonstrated significantly abnormal findings. This represents a 47.6%.

Case presentation

CASE 1: A 45 year old female with a one year history of vertigo and blurring of vision was examined by aortic arch study. A large atheroma in the right subclavian artery was revealed, proximally to the dominant right vertebral artery. The left vertebral artery was small. Endarterectomy was performed, which alleviated her symptoms.

CASE 2: A 49 year old female with two syncopal episodes with transitory right arm paresis during the past two months was studied by aortic arch study. A large ulcerating atheroma of the left common carotid artery bifurcation was revealed. Endarterectomy was performed.

CASE 3: A 64 year old white female with a sudden onset of altitudinal hemianopsia of the right eye was examined in the Ophthalmology Department, and was found to have cholesterol emboli in the superior retinal artery of the right eye with an infarct distal to it. The right common carotid arteriogram depicted a tiny ulcer crater at the bifurcation posteriorly. Endarterectomy was performed.

CASE 4: A 52 year old male patient with a one week history of transient right hemiparesis was examined by a left common carotid arteriography. A tight stenosis of the right internal carotid artery was depicted at the base of the skull. Furthermore, a large elongated ulcerating atheroma was found just below the stenotic lesion. The patient was put on anticoagulation therapy.

CASE 5: A 61 year old male with episodic numbness and weakness of the right arm and right facial weakness, was examined by a left common carotid arteriography. The carotid bifurcation showed a mild stenosis, but tight stenosis was noted in the left middle cerebral artery. He was placed on anticoagulation.

CASE 6: A 68 year old male with a sudden onset of dizziness, ataxia and left hemiplegia was examined by the left vertebral angiogram. It revealed an occlusion of the left posterior cerebral artery.

CASE 7: A 75 year old man was admitted with a one week history of decreased visual acuity with a right lower quadrant visual field defect. The left vertebral arteriogram revealed stenoses at the proximal portion of both posterior cerebral arteries and a decreased perfusion of the territory of the left posterior cerebral artery. Anticoagulation therapy was given.

Conclusion:

Selective arteriography appears to have a much higher yield in detecting causative lesions of extracranial cerebrovascular insufficiency: 57 per cent of abnormal common carotid angiograms compared with 22.5 per cent aortic arch study of the carotid evaluation, and 47.6 per cent of abnormal vertebrobasilar arteriograms in comparison to 8.2 per cent of abnormal aortic arch study in the evaluation of the vertebrobasilar system. Likewise, selective study increases the number of the patients treated accordingly; from 16.4 per cent (10/67) of the aortic arch study to 32 per cent (9/28) of common carotid cases and to 23.8 per cent (5/21) of the cases of vertebrobasilar arteriogram.

Selective angiogram also demonstrates the advantage of revealing the lesions at the base of the skull and within the cranium which have been illustrated by the case presentation.

K. K., Dept. of Radiology, Rob. Packer Hosp., 110 Highland Str., Sayre, Pa 18840, U.S.A.

HEMODYNAMIC ASSESSMENT OF COMMON FEMORAL ENDARTERECTOMY AND PROFUNDAPLASTY

J. FERNANDES E FERNANDES and A. N. NICOLAIDES

Cardiovascular Unit and Academic Surgical Unit, St. Mary's Hospital, London, U.K.

Introduction

Common femoral endarterectomy and profundaplasty became an established procedure for the treatment of lower limb ischaemia in patients with superficial femoral artery occlusion (*Martin et al.,* 1968). The results of this operation have been assessed mainly by the relief of rest pain, by the increase in the walking distance as subjectively evaluated by the patients and also by the return of pedal pulses. Recent work (*Corton,* 1972) using the electromagnetic flowmeter has demonstrated a significant increase in the mean arterial flow through the profunda immediately after profundaplasty. Plethysmographic measurements of foot arterial flow (*Martin,* 1974) were able to detect an increase in foot blood flow two weeks after profundaplasty.

The purpose of this paper was to determine the effect of common femoral endarterectomy and profundaplasty on the distal perfusion pressure before and after exercise measured at the ankle level and also on the walking distance measured on a horizontal treadmill.

Materials and methods

Twenty patients with superficial femoral artery occlusion and severe claudication present for at least six months were studied just before common femoral endarterectomy and profundaplasty, one month later and 16 of them one year later. Eighteen were men and two were women (mean age and S. D.: $60.4 + 10.8$ years). Four have not been studied at one year for the following reasons: one has been lost to follow up; one developed a stroke and was unable to walk on the treadmill; one deteriorated and had an amputation and the fourth has been followed up for less than one year. In 12 patients a femoro-

popliteal bypass was not feasible as judged by the conventional criterion of a poor popliteal run-off on the angiogram. In the remaining eight patients despite a reasonable popliteal run-off, a common femoral endarterectomy and profundaplasty was judged to be an easier and less traumatic operation.

The patients were rested on a couch for 30 minutes; the brachial and ankle pressures were

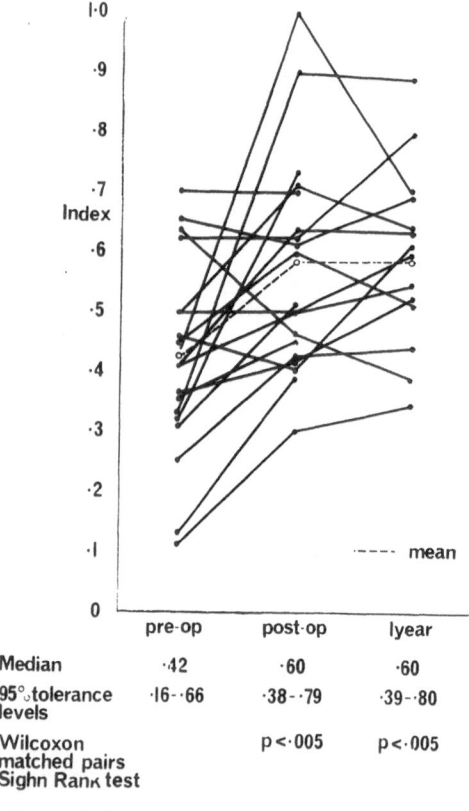

Pressure Index.

	pre-op	post-op	1year
Median	·42	·60	·60
95% tolerance levels	·16–·66	·38–·79	·39–·80
Wilcoxon matched pairs Sighn Rank test		p<·005	p<·005

Fig. 1. Values of the resting pressure index preoperatively and at one month and one year after the operation.

392

measured using a pneumatic cuff and a Doppler ultrasound detector (*Yao*, 1970). The patients walked on a horizontal treadmill at 4 Km/hour until they were stopped by claudication or a maximum of five minutes was reached (333 m). The ankle pressure was measured at the end of the exercise.

Results

The resting Pressure Index, which is the ratio of the ankle systolic pressure over the brachial systolic pressure, was increased in 16 patients, decreased in 3 and remained the same in one at one month after the operation. At one year there was a further increase in the pressure index of 12 patients; in 4 patients there was a slight decrease but the values were lower than the pre-operative levels in only 2 (Fig. 1). The greatest improvement occurred in patients with a pre-operative pressure index of less than 0.5.

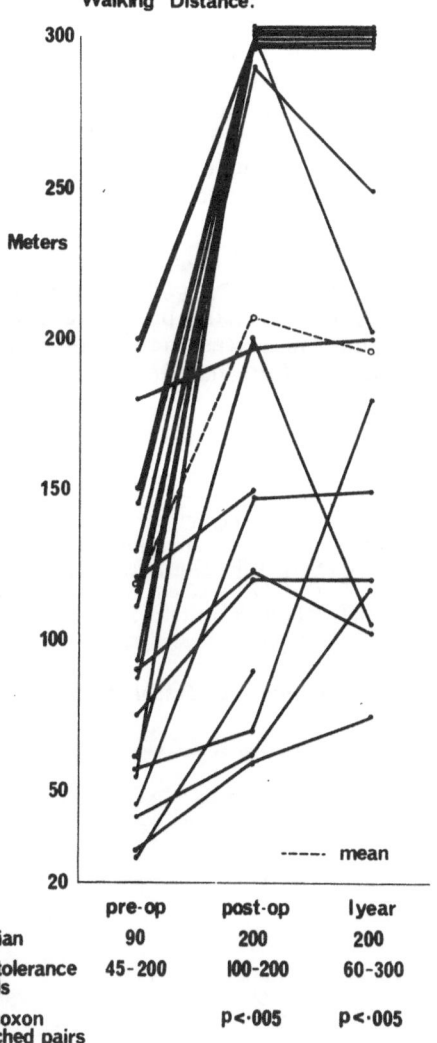

Walking Distance.

	pre-op	post-op	1year
Median	90	200	200
95% tolerance levels	45-200	100-200	60-300
Wilcoxon matched pairs Sighn Rank test		p<·005	p<·005

Fig. 2. Values of the walking distance pre-operatively and at one month and one year after the operation.

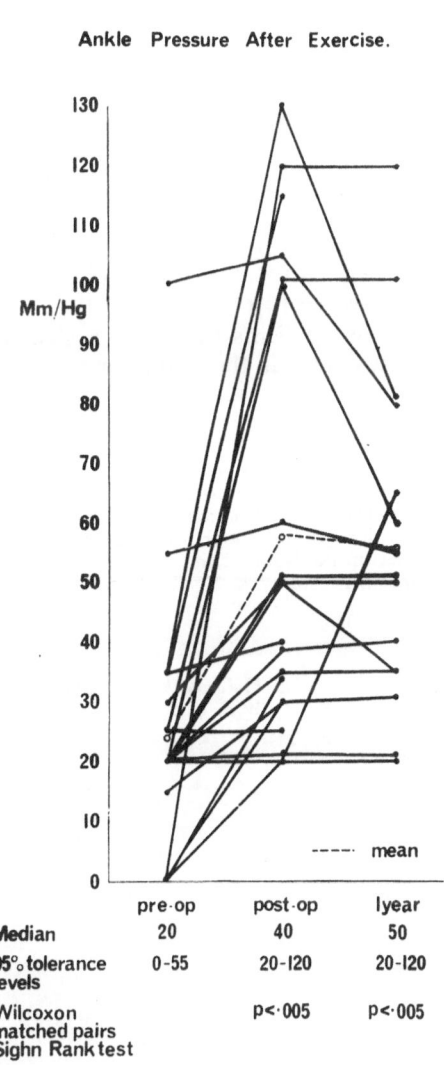

Ankle Pressure After Exercise.

	pre-op	post-op	1year
Median	20	40	50
95% tolerance levels	0-55	20-120	20-120
Wilcoxon matched pairs Sighn Rank test		p<·005	p<·005

Fig. 3. Values of the ankle pressure after the exercise pre-operatively and at one month and one year after the operation.

The walking distance was increased in all patients at one month after operation; in 4 patients there was a decrease in the walking distance at one year, but it was still higher than the pre-operative distance (Fig. 2). At one year 6 patients were able to walk 333 m (5 minutes at 4 Km/hour) without claudication.

The ankle pressure after exercise had increased in all patients at one month after operation; in 3 patients there was a decrease at one year, but the values were markedly higher than the pre-operative levels (Fig. 3).

Discussion

The profunda artery system has a higher resistance to flow; even when a normal driving pressure and flow are restored to the profunda origin, the distal pressures at the calf and ankle were rarely normal (*Strandness*, 1970).

In our patients there was a significant improvement in the resting pressure index but in none of the patients it became normal. Although the higher resistance to flow provided by the profunda system when compared with a normal femoro-popliteal segment, a significant functional improvement can be obtained after this operation.

The ankle pressure after exercise, which represents the distal perfusion pressure at the end of the exercise, was significantly improved in all patients at one month and at one year after the operation. The fact that in 5 of them there was not any fall in the ankle pressure after the exercise suggests that the profunda system was able to provide distal flow and perfusion pressure adequate for the demand of a 5-minute exercise at 4 Km/hour on the treadmill.

These results suggest that common femoral endarterectomy with profunda-plasty is an effective procedure to achieve a significant increase in the distal perfusion pressure before and after exercise.

REFERENCES

Corton, L., Roberts, C., Carse, F. (1972): The value of the electromagnetic flowmeter in arterial reconstruction, in Roberts, V. C., edition: Blood Flow Measurement, London, Secton Publishing Ltd.

Martin, P., Renwick, S., Stephanson, C. (1968): On the surgery of Profunda Femoris Artery. Br. J. Surg. 55: 539.

Martin, P., Jamieson, C. W. (1974): The rationale for and measurement after Profunda-plasty. Surg. Clin. North Am.: 54: 95.

Yao, S. T. (1970): Haemodynamic studies in peripheral arterial disease. Br. J. Surg. 57: 761.

F. J. Cardiovasc. Unit & Vas. Lab. St. Mary's Hosp. Med. School, Praed Str., London W 2, U. K.

HEMODYNAMICS IN THE COLD PRESSOR TEST

M. MIYAZAKI,

Department of Internal Medicine, Kosa-in Hospital Suita City, Osaka, Japan

Introduction

The cold pressor test was introduced by *Hines et al.* as standard for measuring vascular reactivity to could stress.

In the present study, the alterations of blood pressure, heart rate and peripheral and cerebral circulation with the cold pressor test were investigated by means of the on-line Doppler ultrasonic blood flow measurement devised by the author, non-operatively, simultaneously and continuously.

Materials and methods

The subjects were 20 adult males, i. e., 6 normal young males, 7 apparently healthy normotensive males over 70 years of age and 7 male patients with cerebral vascular disease.

The cold pressor test was performed as described by Hines et al. After 10 to 20 minutes of rest, the left hand was immersed up to the wrist in water at 4 °C for about one minute.

The systolic blood pressure, heart rate and cerebral and peripheral circulation were measured in the right side before, during and after the test, simultaneously and continuously.

The alteration of peripheral blood flow (blood flow in the brachial artery) and cerebral blood flow (in the internal carotid artery) was measured by the on-line Doppler ultrasonic technique devised by the author. The alterations of the heart rate and systolic blood pressure were investigated using the Heart Rate Tachometer for heart rate measurement and Shimazu's Continuous Systolic Monitor for systolic blood pressure measurement.

Results and discussion

(I) Normal young males (Fig. 1).

A slight alteration in heart rate and systolic blood pressure was observed.

A biphasic peripheral blood flow pattern was observed, i.e., a decrease of blood flow during and increase of blood flow after the test. On the other hand, no alteration of cerebral blood flow was observed.

(II) Male patients with cerebral vascular disease (Fig. 2).

A slight alteration in heart rate and systolic blood pressure was observed.

No alteration of peripheral blood flow was observed. On the other hand, a

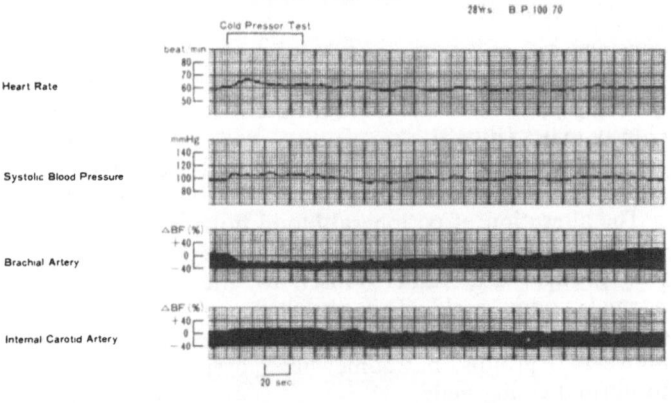

Circulatory Effect of the Cold Pressor Test
(Normal Young Male)

Fig. 1.

395

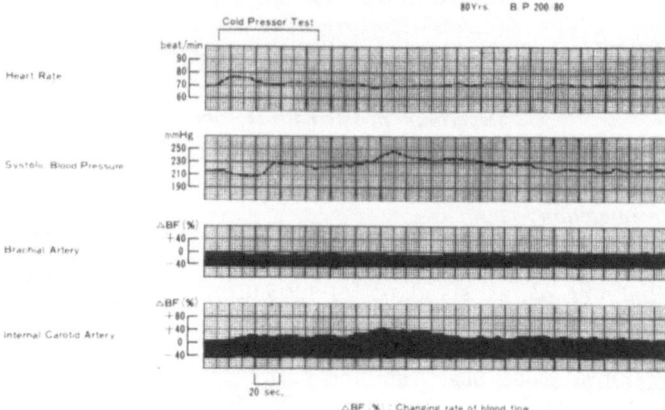

Circulatory Effect of the Cold Pressor Test
(Patient with Cerebral Vascular Disease)

Fig. 2.

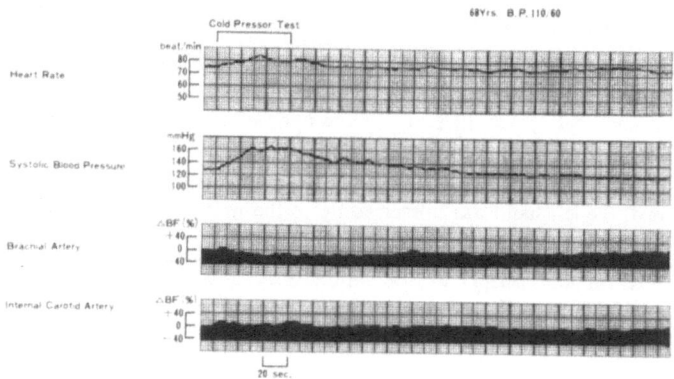

Circulatory Effect of the Cold Pressor Test
(Normal Elderly Male)

Fig. 3.

conspicuous and sustained increase of cerebral blood flow was observed.

(III) Apparently healthy normotensive elderly males (Fig. 3).

A slight alteration in heart rate and systolic blood pressure was observed.

The alteration of peripheral blood flow was between that observed for the above two groups, but rather closer to the normal young male. The alteration of cerebral blood flow also lays between the above two groups, but somewhat closer to normal young male.

The above hemodynamic difference in each group may be due to whether or not dysfunction of the neuroreflective mechanism in peripheral circulation or dysautoregulation in the cerebral circulation was induced by the cold pressor test.

Conclusion

It appears that simultaneous and continuous measurement of blood pressure, heart rate and peripheral and cerebral blood flow may be advantageous in the

396

detection of hemodynamic disorders accompanying dysfunction of the autonomic nervous system, objectively and comprehensively.

REFERENCES

Hines, E. A., Jr. et al.: The cold pressor test for measuring reactivity of blood pressure (data concerning 571 normal and hypertensive subjects). Am. Heart J. 11: 1—9, 1936.

Miyazaki, M.: Multiple and simultaneous blood flow measurement by ultrasonic Doppler technique in man, with special reference to the circulatory effects of induced hypertension on internal, external carotid arteries and brachial artery. Jap. circulation J. 35: 405—412, 1971.

Miyazaki, M.: Effect of undesirable sound (noise) on cerebral circulation. ibid 35: 931—936, 1971.

Miyazaki M.: Effect of cerebral circulatory drugs on cerebral and peripheral circulation, with special reference to aminophylline, papaverine, cyclandelate and isoxsuprine. ibid 35: 1053—1057, 1971.

Miyazaki, M.: Effect of filter-cigarette smoking on cerebral and peripheral circulation. ibid 37: 449—453, 1973.

Miyazaki, M.: Effect of some respiratory maneuvers on cerebral and peripheral circulation, with special reference to maximum breathing, voluntary hyperventilation and the Valsalva maneuver. ibid 37: 455—460, 1973.

Miyazaki, M.: Circulatory effect of ethanol, with special reference to cerebral circulation. ibid 38: 381—385, 1974.

M. M., Department of Internal Medicine, Kosa-in Hospital, Suita City, Osaka, Japan

THERMOGRAPHY IN CONJUNCTION WITH STELLATE GANGLION BLOCK IN THE DIAGNOSTIC INVESTIGATION OF VASCULAR DISORDERS OF THE UPPER EXTREMITIES

A. D. LIAKOS, P. E. BALAS, P. G. IOANNIDIS,
N. XIROMERITIS and E. BASTOUNIS

1st Surgical Department, University of Athens-Medical School, Athens, Greece

Thermography has been extensively used, especially for the study of peripheral vascular diseases.

In the last three years we have used thermography for study of the circulation of the hands in patients with various vasomotor disturbances or arterial occlusive diseases of the upper extremities.

In this work, the circulation of the upper extremities in various vascular disorders is studied using thermography in conjunction with stellate ganglion block.

Materials and methods

Thirty patients with various vasomotor disturbances of the upper extremities, clinically exhibiting Raynaud's syndrome, were subjected among other diagnostic tests to thermography of the hand. Twenty-two of them were females and 8 males, the age ranging between 21—68 years.

Thermographic examination included the following: The patients are initially kept in the examining room for 15 minutes in order to adjust to the room temperature of 20—21°C, and subsequently thermography of both hands is carried out.

Then, stellate ganglion block is performed in the more symptomatic side. (Fig. 2). This block is accomplished by infiltration of the stellate ganglion with local anesthetics through an anterior approach. After successful block of the stellate ganglion, sympathetic tone is abolished on the ipsilateral hand, and the success of the infiltration is evident with the appearance of Horner's syndrome after few minutes. After stellate block serial thermograms were taken on the 5th, 15th and 30th minute.

In a few patients thermograms were taken 15 minutes after stellate ganglion infiltration following immersion of both hands in cold water of 5 °C for 30 seconds.

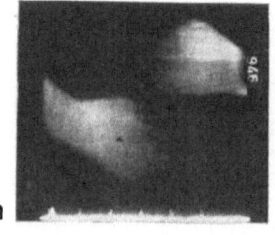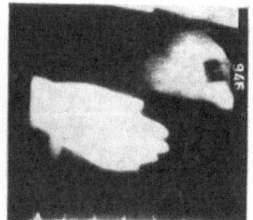

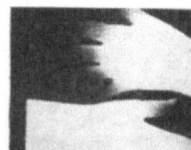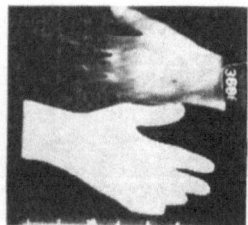

Fig. 1.a—b. Improvement of the thermographic appearance of the right stellate ganglion block.

Results

The improvement in the thermographic appearance of the hand, after abolishment of the sympathetic tone by stellate ganglion block, indicates the existance vasospastic elements on the unerlying condition responsible for Raynaud's phenomenon (Fig. 1).

Thus improvement of the thermographic appearance was noticed, not only in pure vasospastic conditions, but also in scleroderma where an increased sympathetic tone exists, as was shown by our group.

The thermographic picture of the hand after homolateral sympathetic block remained unchanged following immersion of both hands in cold water. This is a characteristic finding while a similar vascular spasm and thermographic amputation of the fingers of the controlateral hand was found (Fig. 2).

In a few cases with distal arteritis no thermographic improvement was observed after stellate ganglion block. In the latter patients Raynaud's phenomenon was present from 3 to 7 years (Fig. 3).

Discussion

It i apparent that vascular diseases are suitable for thermographic investigation, due to the direct dependence between skin temperature and blood perfusion. Especially in the hands, blood vessels occupy the major part of the tissues and thus constitute the main contributing

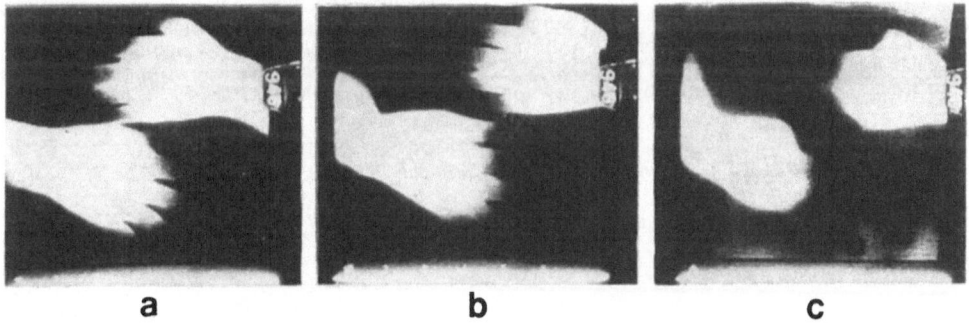

Fig. 2. Thermographic amputation of the fingers of the controlateral hand after immersion of both hands in cold water: a. Before the infiltration, b. 5 min after the infiltration, c. 10 min after the immersion of both hands in cold water.

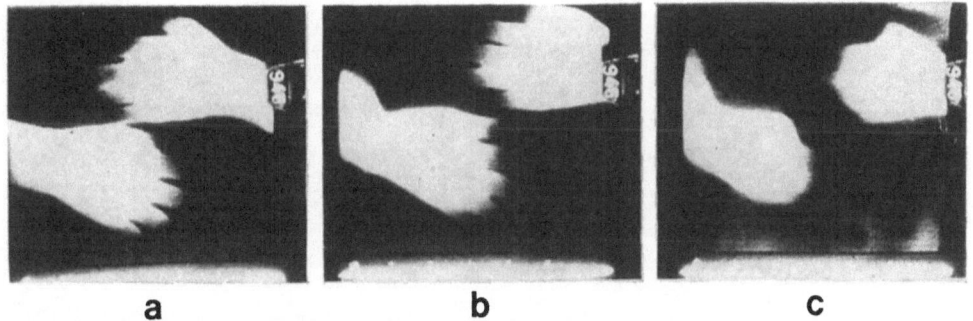

Fig. 3. No thermographic improvement after stellate ganglion block (b). After immersion in cold water, complete thermographic amputation of the fingers (c).

thermoregulating factor. Thermography either alone, or in association with other tests, can provide important information about the organic or functional condition of the vascular system of the upper extremities. Among them, thermography in conjunction with stellate ganglion block was found to be of great diagnostic value.

Based on the thermographic response of the upper extremities after block of the ipsilateral stellate ganglion, important conclusion about the role of sympathetic tone in Raynaud's phenomenon can be derived and the pathogenic mechanism of the underlying disease can be explained.

In conclusion thermography associated with stellate ganglion block is a simple, safe, and very informative method for the diagnostic investigation of vascular diseases of the upper extremities, providing useful criteria for the selection of appropriate treatment.

REFERENCES

Balas P., Kaklamanis F., Tripolitis A., Seitanides V. (1975): Raynaud's phenomenon: Diagnostic investigation and results. Attidi Angiologia, Vol. 2, 330.

Karamanakos P. P., Tripolitis A., Ioannidis P., Delikaris G., and Balas P. (1977): The value of stellate ganglion block in vascular disorders of the upper extremities. Proceedings I International Congress of Cardiovascular Surgery. "M. E. De Bakey International Cardiovascular Society". Athens, June 11—15.

Lawson R. (1957): Thermography — a new tool in investigation of breast lesion. Canad. Serv. Med. J. 13, 517.

Thiers H. et al (1970): Thermographic data in Raynaud's Syndrome. Bull. Soc. Fren. Derm. Syphil. 77: 462—4.

Van Voss Heerma (1969): Thermographic Differentiation of Vascular Diseases of the Arms. Medical Thermography p. 143 S. Kargel-Basel N. York.

Weill F. et al (1969): Semiologie thermographique des ischémies chroniques des membres. Press. Medical 77 No 17, 629—632.

L. A. D., Athens University 1st Surgical Department, 16 Astydanados St. Pagrati, Athens, Greece

ELECTROPHYSIOLOGICAL EXAMINATION OF ISCHAEMIC DISEASES OF THE LOWER LIMBS

V. RAUŠER

Department of Therapeutic Rehabilitation of Institute for Clinical and Experimental Medicine, Praha, Czechoslovakia

Obliterative (vascular) diseases have an adverse effect on the capacity of the neuromuscular system. Its functional deterioration is often more extensive and severe than indicated by histological, morphological and other evidence. It remains unclear which of the structures of the motor system are most commonly and most severely affected. Therefore, we performed electrophysiological functional examination of the neuromuscular system in patients with ischaemic diseases of the legs.

Electrophysiological examination of the functional state of peripheral motor nerves and muscles of the legs was based on electro-diagnostic examination of strength-duration curves for rectangular and progressive impulses used to determine the level of neuromuscular excitability and neuromuscular accommodation. In addition, we examined native electromyograms to validate changes in the action potential of motor units; stimulative electromyography was used for testing the latency of excitability transmission along the peripheral motor nerve. The examination proper was performed at rest and during exercise using the Ratschow ischaemic test lasting not more than 120 seconds. Functional tests proved more capable of detecting mobility disorders.

We examined 68 patients altogether (48 men and 20 women), mean age 44, age range 32–50 years. Diagnostically, the patients were a relatively very homogenous group with ischaemic disease of the legs involving mainly the area of the internal femoral artery. All patients were subjected to thorough angiological investigation, not followed by systematic medical or surgical treatment.

Native electromyograms showed insignificant changes. Even though ischaemic exercise decreased the action potential frequency of the motor units, the changes were not significant. The most significant alterations were displayed by the observed latencies, which lengthened distinctly in the afflicted areas after ischaemic exercise. However, motor-nerve conduction velocity did not change appreciably.

The electromyographic examination was complemented by measurements of strength-duration curves for rectangular and progressive impulses. Ischaemic exercise did not produce conclusive changes at the level of neuromuscular excitability. However, significant changes occurred in the accommodation segments of the curve for progressive impulses. The neuromuscular accommodation decreased in the accommodation area after ischaemic exercise. These changes fully agreed with the hypothesis that neuromuscular accommodation is, to a major degree, influenced by metabolic and biochemical processes in the muscle. This hypothesis was confirmed by the observation of relatively fast normalisation of neuromuscular accommodation once claudication subsided.

The conclusions inferred from the observations may expand our basic knowledge of angiology as well serve the purposes of therapeutical procedures.

Changes that are associated with progressive chronic ischaemia result in diffuse signs in the neuromuscular system. It has been established that the nerve fibre as such is resistant enough to circulatory disorders. The muscle fibre succumbs rather late to degenerative changes; therefore chronic ischaemia manifests itself histologically by a minor finding. But it is becoming increasingly obvious that the neuromuscular end-plate is one of the most sensitive parts. This" site of minor resistance" probably responds most sensitively to functional exercise. Functionally, neuromuscular transmission (capacity) diminishes.

For the time being, electrophysiological examination cannot be used as a diagnostic criterion of ischaemic disease of the legs, but is fit for use as a complementary diagnostic technique. Its findings can be correlated with the results of medical and surgical management especially physical therapy and therapeutic exercise. According to our observations, all exercises should be conducted in a way so that the energy requirements, rhythm and sequence do not excessively drain the energy reserves of neuromuscular transmission. In this way changes in the transmission and decreased neuromuscular accommodation can be prevented. Consequently, therapeutic exercise should be reasonably rationed to stimulate postischaemic hyperaemia and other desirable trophic processes.

REFERENCES

Licht S. (1968): Electrodiagnosis and electromyography. New Haven.
Raušer V. (1976): Elektrophysiologische Studie des ischämischen Muskels, Balneologia Bohemica 5, 2, 33—39.

Řehánek J., Raušer V. (1977): Nervosvalová akomodace jako ukazatel trofiky. Acta chir. ortop. Traumat. Čech. 44, 3, 260—264.

R. V., IKEM, Vídeňská 800, 146 22 Praha 4, Czechoslovakia

THE USE OF POLAROGRAPHY IN VASCULAR DISEASES

A. KRČÍLEK, M. BŘEZINA and L. ŠERÁK

*Medical Faculty, Charles University and J. Heyrovský Institute
of Physical Chemistry and Electrochemistry, Czechoslovak Academy
of Sciences, Prague, Czechoslovakia*

Polarography is an electrochemical method which was invented in 1922 by the Czech scientist, Jaroslav Heyrovský, Nobel Prize winner in 1959. The original polarography consisted of electrolysis of a solution using a dropping mercury electrode. Later on, polarography with solid electrodes, often called voltammetry, was introduced. Using polarography we have determined:

1. the oxygen content of blood,
2. respiration of the vascular wall,
3. the composition of the arterial and venous wall (cystine content),
4. the Brdička protein test
   a) in blood after heparin
   b) in urine

The results of the polarographic determination of oxygen will be discussed. (Fig. 1). We found a decreased oxygen content in venous blood from the anterocubital vein after a cold bath, after compression of the forarm and after excercise of the arm. On the other hand, the oxygen content in venous blood was increased after a hot bath and, when the

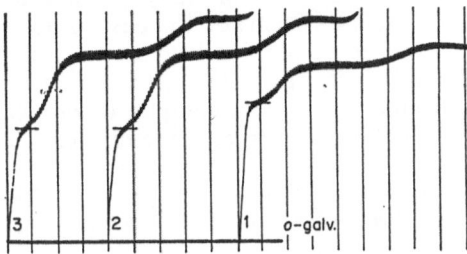

Fig. 1. Polarographic determination of oxygen. Curve 1: supporting electrolyte, curves 2 and 3: arterial blood

hot bath was prolonged, the oxygen saturation of the venous blood was nearly as high as the saturation of arterial blood. In group of patients with varicose veins we compared the oxygen saturation of blood from varicose veins with that from the dorsal vein of the foot. In most cases the oxygen saturation of both samples was at the same level. Our findings contradict the theory of several autors, who see the cause of all varicose veins in arteriovenous anastomoses with high oxygen saturation in varicose veins. After prolonged standing, patients with varicose veins were found to have a decrease of about 25% in the oxygen saturation of blood from the varicose veins.

In all cases the oxygen was determined in the blood after being liberated from oxyhemoglobin with ferricyanide in a polarographic cell under a layer of paraffin oil. Saponin was used as the hemolysing agent.

Respiration of the vascular wall: In order to exclude any toxic effect of mercury on the activity of the biological material, a special arangement for estimation of oxygen consumption of various and human tissue was used by *Šerák:* a physiological nutritive solution flows slowly through an analyser and enters a small flat chamber with the investigated tissue, which rests on a cellophane membrane. After leaving the chamber, in which some oxygen has been consumed by the tissue, the nutritive solution comes into the electrode compartment, where oxygen is determined by a dropping mercury electrode. Using this analyzer, vascular wall respiration was followed. In a group of 40 rabbits experiments, atherosclerosis was produced by feeding cholesterol. The respiration activity of normal aortae was higher than that of atherosclerotic aortae. The respiration activity of aortae with heparin was significantly lower than that of aortae without heparin. Heparin seems to help the utilization of oxygen. These results are in agreement with the good preventive effect of heparin in atherosclerosis.

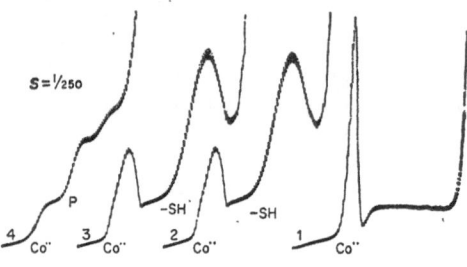

Fig. 2. The catalytic effect of cysteine (curve 2) cystine (curve 3) and protein (curve 4). Curve 1 is supporting cobalt solution.

3. *Cystine content of vascular wall*: The Brdička method of cystine determination was used for dried rabbit vessels aortae and veins (Fig. 2). The cystine content of veins (0.1 – 0.5 g%) was much smaller than that of aortae (1.1 g%). In a group of 10 normal and 20 rabbits with experimental atherosclerosis, the average cystine content was 1.1 g% in healthy and 0.85 g% in atheroclerotic aortae. The cystine content of the vascular wall seems to be proportional to the degree of vascular elesticity.

4. *The Brdička protein test* was applied to the study of patients with vascular diseases (atherosclerosis, venous thrombosis). The test was carried out before and after intravenous injection of heparin. 1 – 2 hours after the heparin injection the height of serum protein double wave decreased, especially the second part of the double wave. This decrease was greater in the above mentioned vascular diseases than in a group of healthy people. This observation can be explained by the suggestion that heparin activates some enzymes, which enable the liberation of fatty acids. These substances are able to bind albumins and to suppress the second part of the polarographic protein double wave.

The Brdička method of protein determination was also used for analysis of plain urine and its filtrates after deproteinization with sulphosalicylic and tungstic acids. Deproteinization with sulphosalicylic acid reduces the number of polarographically active polypeptides with the exception mucoproteins and peptides of lower molecular weight. Deproteinization with tungstic acid also excludes mucoproteins. An increase in the polarographic activity of sulphosalicylic filtrates of urine has been observed in patients with inflamatory diseases, in acute myocardial infarction, acute glomerulonehritis and in patients with cancer. The highest increase was encountered in patients with burns.

The polarographic method can be used for many other types of analyses, for the determination of inorganic substances, enzymes, hormones, vitamins, alkaloids. Polarography has not only analytical advantages, but also provides an understanding of the path of chemical, electrochemical and biochemical reactions. Using polarography we can study complicated biochemical systems on the basis of exact knowledge of physicochemical principles. In this area lies the most important contribution of polarography to medical and biological sciences in the future.

K. A., IVth Clinic of Medicine, Charles University, U nemocnice 2, 128 08 Praha 2, Czechoslovakia

ARTERIAL AND VENOUS BLOOD VISCOSITY IN ISCHEMIC LOWER LIMBS OF PERIPHERAL OBLITERATIVE ARTERIAL DISEASE PATIENTS

S. FORCONI, G. BIASI, M. GUERRINI, P. RAVELLI, C. ROSSI, G. FERROZZI and S. PECCHI

Dept. of Medicine, University of Siena and Dept. of Surgery, University of Milan, Italy

Blood hyperviscosity had been found in ischemic diseases secondary to obliterative arteriopaties (*Dormandy et al.*, 1973; *Ehrly*, 1974; *Dintenfass*, 1976; *Schmid-Schömbein*, 1976; *Chien*, 1976). Some authors have suggested that viscosity on its own may be a prime cause of thrombosis, but decisive evidence is still lacking (*Lancet*, 1975). According to others, hyperviscosity may be a sign or a consequence of the ischemic process.

In our experience, during acutely induced ischemic situations, such as claudicatio intermittens or angina pectoris provoked by exercise, a significant increase of the viscosity was observed in the systemic blood (*Di Perri et al.*, 1977). The question arised whether the increase in the blood viscosity was dependent on the impaired circulation. This working hypothesis led us to study the changes in the blood viscosity and in the determinant variables in the femoral arterial and venous blood of peripheral obliterative arterial disease patients and of normal control subjects compared with the changes observed in the blood flowing in the systemic circulation.

Materials and methods

Thirteen patients, 12 male and 1 female, aged from 42 to 76 years, affected by peripheral obliterative arterial disease of the lower limbs (stage III or IV) were studied. All the patients were hospitalized and awaiting surgery. The diagnosis was confirmed by x-ray aorto or atreriography. We similarly studied nine control subjects, all male, aged from 34 to 69 years, hospitalized and awaiting surgery (5 had inguinal hernia, 1 cholelithiasis, 1 chronic appendicitis and 1 colon diverticulosis), none of whom showed signs of circulatory diseases of the lower limbs, either by clinical or by instrumental measurements.

In all the subjects blood samples were taken simultaneously from: a) the brachial vein, b) the femoral vein and c) the femoral artery.

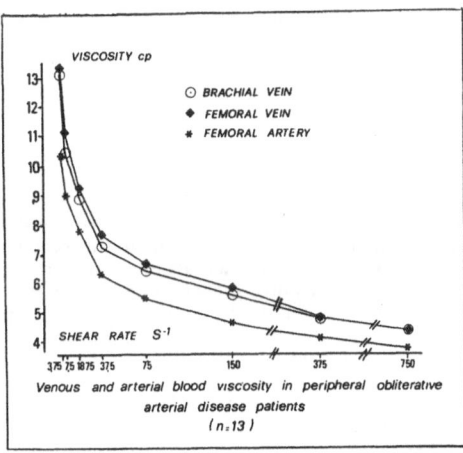

Fig. 1. Mean values of venous and arterial blood viscosity in peripheral obliterative arterial disease patients.

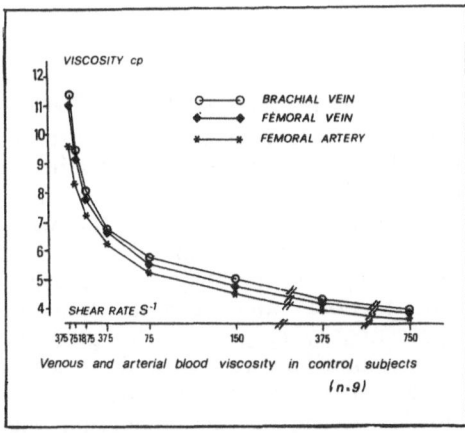

Fig. 2. Mean values of venous and arterial blood viscosity in control subjects.

405

Blood, plasma and serum viscosity were measured with a Wells-Brookfield cone/plate 1/4 RVT microviscometer, at 37 °C, and at a shear rate of 750, 375, 150, 75, 37.5, 18.75, 7.5 and 3.75 s^{-1} for whole blood and at a shear rate of 350 s^{-1} for the plasma and serum. For the whole blood and plasma viscosity, blood samples were anticoagulated with EDTA 10% (0.1 ml in 8 ml of blood). In each sample packed red cell volume and plasma concentration of fibrinogen (M Partigen Immunodiffusion Behringwerke) were also measured.

Results

The average levels of viscosity of blood, plasma and serum, packed red cell volume and plasma fibrinogen concentration of the patients and of the control subjects are shown in the tables.

In the peripheral obliterative arterial disease patients a marked and highly significant increase in the whole blood viscosity was seen in venous blood compared with arterial blood. The increase was present at all the shear rates considered but it was higher at the lowest shear rates. No significant differences were seen between the brachial and the femoral vein but the viscosity in the whole blood coming from the ischemic district was slightly higher. Packed red cell volume was significantly higher in venous than in arterial blood. Similarly an increased viscosity was found in the venous plasma; no differences were seen in serum viscosity and in plasma fibrinogen concentration.

In the control subjects blood viscosity values were decidedly lower than in the patients. The statistical analysis did not exibit any definite differences between various average values, although in the veins there was a slight increase of the whole blood, plasma and serum viscosity and of packed red cell volume, where the plasma fibrinogen concentration was unchanged.

Discussion

These results suggest that the arteriovenous difference in the blood viscosity is higher in vasculopathic patients than in control subjects. The important percentage increase (20% at 150 s^{-1}) of the whole blood viscosity in the femoral vein cannot be explained by the higher venous haematocrit alone and suggests that the hyperviscosity may be locally generated in the blood flowing trough the ischemic tissue, where the local hypoxia and the slowing down of the circulation may provoke an increase in red cell aggregability. The microaggregates persist

Table I. Venous and arterial blood viscosity in peripheral obliterative arterial disease patients. "t" represents statistical analysis (Student's "t" test for paired variables).

Venous and arterial blood viscosity in peripheral obliterative arterial disease patients mean±S.E. n.13 viscosity cp						
S^{-1}	A	B	C	D (t)	E (t)	F (t)
WHOLE BLOOD (SHEAR RATE) 750	4,35±0,27	4,37±0,33	3,78±0,25	0,137 ns	4,736 **	4,976 **
375	4,79±0,31	4,74±0,33	4,10±0,27	0,588 ns	4,259 **	4,261 **
150	5,62±0,39	5,63±0,43	4,71±0,32	0,054 ns	4,562 **	3,900 **
75	6,41±0,45	6,59±0,52	5,48±0,38	0,854 ns	4,272 **	3,860 **
375	7,27±0,49	7,70±0,63	6,37±0,43	1,251 ns	5,448 **	4,046 **
18,75	8,92±0,11	9,25±0,77	7,83±0,51	0,899 ns	5,268 **	3,745 **
7,5	10,49±0,73	11,13±0,94	9,07±0,57	1,400 ns	4,491 **	3,686 **
3,75	13,10±0,97	13,28±1,21	10,41±0,74	0,253 ns	6,140 **	4,247 **
Plasma 375	1,88±0,09	1,87±0,10	1,80±0,09	0,609 ns	5,722 **	5,284 **
Serum 375	1,59±0,03	1,61±0,04	1,57±0,03	1,495 ns	1,141 n.s.	2,151 **
Htc %	43±1	43±1	41±1	1,584 ns	6,161 **	3,866 **
Fibrinogen mg%	372±30	373±30	369±35	0,161 ns	0,327 ns	0,391 ns

A : Brachial vein   B : Femoral vein   C : Femoral artery
D : Brachial vein versus femoral vein
E : Brachial vein versus artery   ** : p < 0,01
F : Femoral vein versus artery

Table II. Venous and arterial blood viscosity in control subjects. "t" represents statistical analysis (Student's "t" test for paired variables).

Venous and arterial blood viscosity in control subjects mean±S.E. n.9 viscosity cp						
S^{-1}	A	B	C	D (t)	E (t)	F (t)
WHOLE BLOOD (SHEAR RATE) 750	4,03±0,15	3,92±0,16	3,83±0,16	2,660 *	2,237 n.s.	1,046 n.s.
375	4,38±0,21	4,22±0,17	4,10±0,17	1,544 n.s.	1,840 n.s.	0,957 n.s.
15	5,05±0,22	4,82±0,24	4,73±0,23	3,729 **	2,026 n.s.	0,627 n.s.
75	5,82±0,29	5,50±0,32	5,39±0,31	2,342 *	3,462 **	0,849 n.s.
37,5	6,84±0,30	6,71±0,36	6,26±0,37	0,808 n.s.	4,271 **	2,629 n.s.
18,75	8,14±0,67	7,85±0,70	7,32±0,45	1,811 n.s.	2,174 n	1,298 n.s.
7,5	9,46±0,90	9,23±0,91	8,30±0,42	1,902 n.s.	1,786 n	1,397 n.s.
37,5	11,43±1,67	11,04±1,70	9,62±0,64	0,730 n.s.	1,482 n	1,100 n.s.
Plasma 375	1,77±0,04	1,75±0,04	1,69±0,05	1,944 n.s.	1,944 n.s.	2,032 n.s.
Serum 375	1,60±0,04	1,61±0,03	1,56±0,03	0,300 n.s.	1,951 n	2,733 *
Htc %	46±1	45±1	44±1	1,818 n.s.	2,075 n	2,031 n.s.
Fibrinogen mg%	364±33	357±38	352±37	0,649 n.s.	0,772 n	0,311 n.s.

A : Brachial vein   B : Femoral vein   C : Femoral artery
D : Brachial vein versus femoral vein   * : p < 0,05
E : Brachial vein versus artery   ** : p < 0,01
F : Femoral vein versus artery

and may lead to an increase in venous blood viscosity (*Schmid-Schömbein*, 1975). Hypoxia, which can change the pH osmolality or the electrolyte content of the erythrocytes, may reduce the red cell deformability (*Braasch*, 1971).

This finding is also in keeping with our observations in some acute ischemic local situations, as in the ischemic phase of Raynaud's phenomenon (*Forconi et al.*, 1978) or in ischemic exercise in arteriopathic patients (*Forconi*, 1977). In these situations, the viscosity increased markedly in the blood from the ischemic area and returned to basal levels after the disappearance of the phenomenon or after rest.

In the studied group of patients, affected by a chronic ischemizing process, the local increase in the blood viscosity also persists in the systemic circulation and, as the viscosity of the arterial blood of the vasculopathic patients was higher than that of the controls, may constitute a further hindrance to flow that, at the microcirculatory level, may worsen the tissue ischemia.

REFERENCES

Braasch, D. (1971): Red Cell Deformability and Capillary Blood Flow. Physiological Reviews, 51, 679.

Chien, S. (1976): Significance of Macrorheology and Microrheology in Atherogenesis. In "Atherogenesis", Ann. N. Y. Acad. Sc. 275, 10.

Dintenfass, L. (1976): Rheology of Blood in Diagnostic and Preventive Medicine. An Introduction to Clinical Haemorheology. Butterworths, London.

Di Perri, T., Forconi, S., Guerrini, M., Rossi, C., Pecchi, S. (1977): Modificazioni della viscosità ematica sistemica in soggetti con vasculopatie croniche distrettuali durante ischemia spontanea o provocata. Boll. S.I.C. in the press.

Dormandy, J. A., Hoare, E., Colley, J., Arrowsmith, D. E., Dormandy, T. L. (1973): Clinical, Haemodynamic, Rheological, and Biochemical Findings in 126 Patients with Intermittent Claudication. Brit. Med. J., 4, 576.

Dormandy, J. A., Hoare, E., Khattab, A. H., Arrowsmith, D. E., Dormandy, T. L. (1973): Prognostic Significance of Rheological and Bochemical Findings in Patients with Intermittent Claudication. Brit. Med. J., 4, 581.

Ehrly, A. M. (1974): Rheological Induced Impairment of the Muscular Microcirculation: a New Pathophysiological Concept of Intermittent Claudication. Proc. IX Internat. Congr Angiol., Firenze, vol. I.

Forconi, S. (1977): Ruolo della viscosità ematica nella ischemia degli arti. Proc. Internat. Sympoium "L'Ischemia", Roma, in the press.

Forconi, S., Guerrini, M., Rossi, C., Pecchi, S. (1978): Local Increase of Blood Viscosity during Cold-induced Raynaud's Phenomenon. Lancet, in the press.

Haemorheology, Blood-flow, and Venous Thrombosis (1975). Lancet, ii, 113.

Schmid-Schömbein, H. (1975): Critical closing pressure or yield stress as the cause of disturbed peripheral circulation? Acta Chir. Scand., suppl. 465, 10.

Schmid-Schömbein, H. (1976): Microrheology of Erythrocytes, Blood Viscosity, and the Distribution of Blood Flow in the Microcirculation. In Cardiovascular Physiology II, Guyton & Cowley eds. University Park Press, Baltimore, pag 1.

S. F., Istituto di Semeiotica Medica, Università di Siena, Nuovo Policlinico, 53100, Siena, Italy

CHANGES IN pH, pO$_2$ AND pCO$_2$ IN THE VENOUS BLOOD OF PATIENTS SUFFERING FROM OBLITERATIVE ARTERIOSCLEROSIS OF THE LOWER EXTREMITIES

MÁRIA SZIRTES, J. SIMONYI, P. SÁRMÁNY, and S. PAPP

Bajcsy-Zsilinszky Hospital, Cardiovascular Surgery, University Budapest, Hungary

In recent years the use of local peripheral blood pressure measurements has proven valuable in estimating the clinical significance of arterial obliterations in the lower limbs. Examinations after exercise are still more sensitive for evaluation of the peripheral hemodynamics. The poststenotic pressures are usually decreased at rest and the postexercise pressures are even lower.

In consequence of the impaired perfusion of the tissues, the metabolism is also damaged. This appears in changes in pO$_2$, pCO$_2$ and pH of the venous blood.

In our study the following problems were examined: Could a difference be demonstrated in pO$_2$, pCO$_2$ and pH between the normal and ischemic leg in venous blood taken from the back of the foot?

How do these parameters change after surgical reconstruction?

How does pO$_2$ change after exercise?

How is the ankle blood pressure related to arm blood pressure change after exercise to pain?

Could a correlation be demonstrated between pressure and metabolic parameters after exercise?

Methods and materials

Group A.) Patients with rest pain due to unilateral obstruction of the femoropopliteal artery were studied before and 2 weeks after reconstructive surgery.

Group B.) Patients with intermittent claudication and normal subjects were studied at rest and after exercise. Patients with venous illnesses were excluded.

In group A. venous blood was drawn by puncture in a supine position without strangulation from the back of both feet at rest.

Blood samples were tested for pH, pO$_2$ and pCO$_2$ using the Astrup method and Siggard Anderson nomogram.

In group B blood samples were drawn at rest and after exercise performed on a bicycle ergometer at a work load of 400 mkp/min to muscle pain.

Systolic blood pressure at the ankle was measured using a "Doppler" ultra-sonic flow detector at rest and after exercise. The ankle pressure was expressed in per cent of the arm blood pressure (Doppler Index, D. I.).

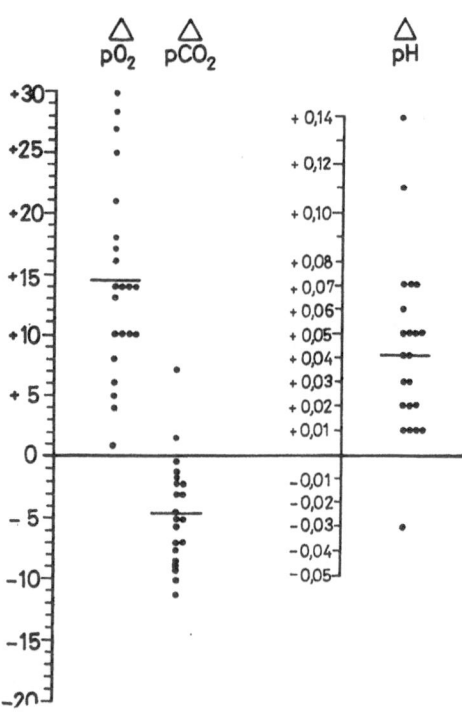

Fig. 1. Differences in venous blood pO$_2$, pCO$_2$ and pH of diseased and normal legs.

Results

The parameters in the venous blood deviated on the diseased side from normal (: pO_2 was lower 50.3 ± 8.6 versus 64.8 ± 5.8, $P < 0.01$; pCO_2 higher 46.6 ± 8.4 versus 42.2 ± 5.5, $P < 0.01$;

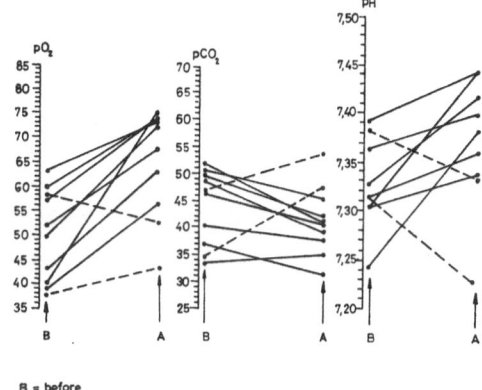

B = before
A = after   surgical reconstruction

Fig. 2. Changes of pO_2, pCO_2 and pH before and after reconstructive surgery.

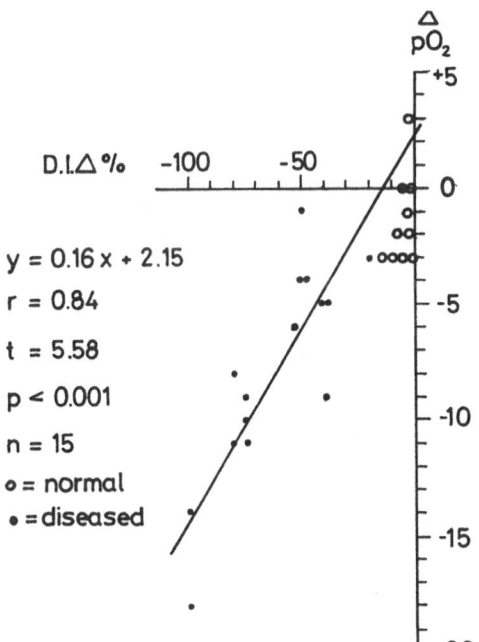

Fig. 3. Correlation between the percentual changes in Doppler Index and venous pO_2 after exercise.

pH lower 7.313 ± 0.046 versus $7.355 \pm \pm 0.042$ $P < 0.01$). Significant diffferences were found between the values for the leg with normal and impaired circulation (Fig. 1).

Fig. 2. demonstrates the effect of successful surgical reconstruction on the venous pO_2, pCO_2 and pH of the extremities with arterial occlusion; the pO_2 of the venous blood increased in every case.

In two cases, plotted with broken lines, where the venous bypass was reobliterated at the time of the second postoperative examination, pO_2 decreased or slightly increased. In a few cases after surgery the pCO_2 values decreased to some extent, but this cannot be considered as a reliable parameter for follow up.

The pH of the venous blood of the limbs with arterial occlusion shifted towards alkaline values following reconstruction; while in cases of reobliteration (plotted by a dotted line) there was no change.

Venous pO_2 was determined in patients with intermittent claudication and in normal subjects at rest and after exercise. The resting values for pO_2 of the venous blood were, in most cases in this group, in the same range as in normal subjects. However the pO_2 of the venous blood of the diseased leg markedly decreased after exercise, while the pO_2 of normal subjects slightly decreased.

Pre- and postexercise measurements of the systolic ankle blood pressure were performed on patients and normal subjects. A marked drop of systolic pressure was found in patients. The post-exercise decrease of ankle blood pressure was more pronounced in legs with low values at rest. A highly significant correlation was found between the systolic pressures at rest and the decrease in the pressure after exercise.

$$(y = -0.9x + 85.4 \qquad r = -0.77 ,$$

$$P < 0.01)$$

Fig. 3 demonstrates the correlation between the percentual decrease in the

Doppler Index (Δ D. I.) and in pO_2 (Δ pO_2) in patients after exercise. A close relationship was found between the two parameters.

These results provide further data on the correlation between hemodynamic and metabolic parameters.

The applied methods can be performed easily and are suited for following up patients with impaired arterial circulation.

REFERENCES

Bollinger, A., Schlump, M., Butti, P., Grüntzig, A. (1973): Measurement of systolic blood pressure with Doppler ultrasound at rest and after exercise in patients with leg artery occlusions. Scand. J. clin. Lab. Invest. 31 Suppl. 128. 123—131.

Bollinger, A. (1975): Kritische Sichtung verschiedener Verfahren zur frühzeitigen Erfassung peripherer arterieller Gefässveränderungen. Vasa 4. 327—333.

Cappelen, Chr., Hall, K. V. (1960): The effect of obstructive arterial disease on the peripheral arterial blood pressure. Surgery 48, 878—893.

Carlson, L. A., Pernow B. S. (1959): Oxygen utilisation and lactic acid formation in the legs at rest and during exercise in normal subjects and in patients with atherosclerosis obliterans. Acta med. scand. 164. 39—52.

Krause, E., Tschirkov, F., Varady, Z., Manegold, K. H. (1974): Tendenzen des Verhaltens von pH-Werten, CO_2-, O_2- Partialdrucken, der LDH-Erhöhung und der Gewebswasserbildung bei mässiger oder extremer Hypoxie der unteren Extremitäten. Thoraxchirurgie 22. 559—563.

Myhre, H. O. (1975): Reactive Hyperaemia of the human lower limb. Vasa 4. 227—234.

Nissen, P., Alexander, K., Wittenborg, A. (1974): Sauerstoffextraktion und Durchblutung unter ergometrischer Belastung bei arterieller Verschlusskrankheit. Vasa 3. 257—262.

Strandness, D. E., Bell, J. W. (1964): An evaluation of the hemodynamic response of the claudicating extremity to exercise. Surg. Gynec Obstet. 119. 1237—1242.

M. S., Bajcsy-Zsilinszky Hospital, Maglódi út 89., Budapest 1475, Hungary

ARTERIOGRAPHY AND DIGITAL PLETHYSMOGRAPHY IN THE STUDY OF DIABETIC MACROARTERIOPATHY OF THE FEET"

J. McCOOK, C. LÓPEZ, N. RODRÍGUEZ, O. OLIÚ,
M. ARIOSA and L. CURBELO

Institute of Angiology; City of Havana, Cuba

Clinical practice is prodigal in examples of diabetic foot that maintain palpable the dorsal pedal and posterior tibial pulses. The existence of an associated micro-angiopathy and the well known tendency of diabetic patients to infections, had served as good arguments in order to give us an explanation of this phenomenon. It has been proved (*Cecile et al.*, 1973 and 1974) by means of arteriographies of the foot, that gangrenous lesions of the toes were a consequence of ischemia and that none of the diabetic patients had normal foot arteries. The fact that arteriography is an invasive method restricts its utilization to hospitalized patients. Thence, the necessity for the appraisal of a method such as the digital plethysmography that, in addition of its innocuousness, offers the possibility of rendering information about the arterial tree in these localizations. The objectives of our study are aimed at the determination of the frequency of cases of diabetic foot with palpable dorsal pedal and posterior tibial pulses, as well as the most frequent arteriographic and plethysmographic patterns and their correlations.

Material and method

For the achievement of such objectives, we analyzed and left included in our study all the cases of diabetic foot admitted during a year in which it was possible to verify the existence of palpable dorsal pedal and posterior tibial pulses and whose studies were completed with the arteriographic and plethysmographic examinations. Arterial lesions were classified into 3 groups: exiguity, stenosis and occlusion. The plethysmographic studies consisted in the reading of a scan at the level of the first toe of the affected foot, before and after alternate manual compression of the dorsal pedal and the posterior tibial

arteries using for this purpose the photoelectric plethysmography method.

Results

A total of 248 patients were admitted to the Institute of Angiology with a diabetic foot, 30 of which, that is, 12.1% had palpable dorsal pedal and posterior tibial pulses. None of the patients had a normal arterial tree. The medial plantar artery was found affected in 100% of the cases, the lateral plantar in 90% and the 1st. dorsal metatarsal in 80%. The dorsal pedal artery was the least affected with only 46.7% of the cases. The detected arteriographic patterns are shown according to their frequency order in Table I.

TABLE I

ARTERIOGRAPHIC PATTERNS IN THE CASES OF DIABETIC FOOT WITH PALPABLES DORSAL PEDAL AND POSTERIOR TIBIAL PULSES. N° AND %. INSTITUTE OF ANGIOLOGY. NOV. 76 - OCT. 77.

ARTERIOGRAPHIC PATTERNS	N°	%
1. Occlusion of the medial and lateral plantar arteries	10	33,3
2. Occlusion of the medial plantar artery	8	26,7
3. Generalized exiguity of the foot arteries	4	13,4
4. Occlusion of the lateral plantar artery	3	10,0
5. Occlusion of the posterior tibial artery	2	6,7
6. Occlusion of the anterior tibial artery	1	3,3
7. Multiple stenoses of the medial and lateral plantar arteries	1	3,3
8. Multiple stenoses of the dorsal pedal and plantar arteries	1	3,3
TOTALS	30	100,0

Source: Arteriographic studies.

Occlusion of the medial and lateral plantar arteries was the most frequent pattern. The plethysmographic study, as planned, was only carried out to a full extent in 5 cases. An analysis of the obtained results (Fig. 1) points out that lessening of the basal plethysmographic

411

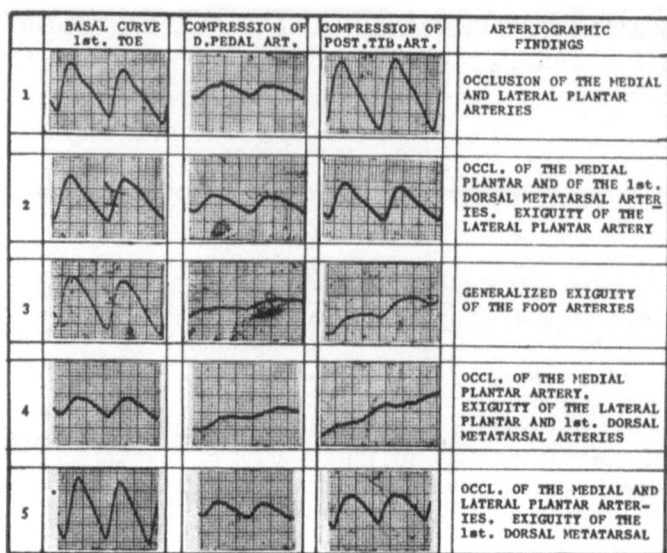

	BASAL CURVE 1st. TOE	COMPRESSION OF D.PEDAL ART.	COMPRESSION OF POST.TIB.ART.	ARTERIOGRAPHIC FINDINGS
1				OCCLUSION OF THE MEDIAL AND LATERAL PLANTAR ARTERIES
2				OCCL. OF THE MEDIAL PLANTAR AND OF THE 1st. DORSAL METATARSAL ARTERIES. EXIGUITY OF THE LATERAL PLANTAR ARTERY
3				GENERALIZED EXIGUITY OF THE FOOT ARTERIES
4				OCCL. OF THE MEDIAL PLANTAR ARTERY. EXIGUITY OF THE LATERAL PLANTAR AND 1st. DORSAL METATARSAL ARTERIES
5				OCCL. OF THE MEDIAL AND LATERAL PLANTAR ARTERIES. EXIGUITY OF THE 1st. DORSAL METATARSAL

Fig. 1.

curve of the 1st toe as a consequence of the compression of the dorsal pedal artery, was present in the cases 1 and 2, both of which had a common lesion, i. e. the occlusion of the medial plantar artery. It was also seen that lessening by compression not only of the dorsal pedal but of the posterior tibial artery as well was present in the cases 3, 4, and 5, which had the lesions in common: the exiguity of the 1st dorsal metatarsal artery and the occlusion of the medial plantar artery.

Discussion

In accordance with Cecile and his coworkers none of our diabetic foot cases had all the foot arteries normal. It is needless to say how small is the diagnostic and prognostic value that should be given to such pulses at the moment of appraising the state of the arterial tree of the foot. Although arteriography deserves improvement, we believe that our attention should be directed to the improvement of the plethysmographic studies. In spite of the small number of cases studied, they permitted to assert the existence of lesions at the level of the medial plantar artery when a 50% reduction or more in the amplitude of the basal plethysmographic register followed manual compression of the dorsal pedal artery and viceversa, the existence of lesions at the level of the dorsal pedal or of the 1st dorsal metatarsal arteries when the lessening of the register followed manual compression of the posterior tibial artery. The double lessening occurred in the cases with lesions in both localizations. Consequently, the study of the arterial tree of the foot in diabetic population, should include similar registers at the level of the remaining toes that would permit to obtain information, especially concerning lesions of the lateral plantar and other metatarsal arteries.

Conclusions

1. The frequency of cases with palpable dorsal pedal and posterior tibial pulses among diabetic feet was 12.1%. The most frequently affected artery was the medial plantar while the dorsal pedal was the least. The principal arterial lesions encountered were: occlusion, exiguity and stenosis, in the order mentioned.

2. The arteriographic patterns most commonly detected (83.4% of the cases) were: occlusion of the medial and lateral plantar arteries, occlusion of the medial plantar artery, generalized exiguity of

the foot arteries and occlusion of the lateral plantar artery. The most evocative plethysmographic patterns were related to the lessening of the basal register in the 1st toe by dorsal pedal compression in cases with occlusion of the medial plantar or by compression of the posterior tibial artery in cases with occlusion or exiguity of the 1st dorsal metatarsal artery. On the basis of the results obtained we feel that it is necessary to improve our plethysmographic studies, the application of which should be made available to the noncomplicated diabetic population.

REFERENCES

Cecile, J. P. et al. (1973): L'arteriographie du pied diabetique. J. Radiol. Electrol. T. 54, 313.

Ibid (1974): Diabetic foot arteriography. J. Cardiov. Surg. 15, 12.

J. McC.: Inst. of Angiology, Calz. del Cerro 1551, City of Havana, Cuba

THE OBJECTIVE ASSESSMENT OF VENOUS INSUFFICIENCY WITH CALF VOLUME PLETHYSMOGRAPHY

J. FERNANDES E FERNANDES, A. N. NICOLAIDES
and T. N. NEEDHAM

Vascular Laboratory, Cardiovascular Unit and Academic Surgical Unit, St. Mary's Hospital, London, U.K.

Introduction

Venous insufficiency can be quantitatively assessed by the measurement of ambulatory venous pressure (*Pollack et al.,* 1949; *De Camp et al.,* 1959; *Lewis et al.,* 1973; *Kriessman,* 1974). However, this is an invasive technique not suitable for routine screening of a large number of patients.

The purpose of the present study was to determine whether calf volume plethysmography, which is non-invasive, could determine the presence of venous insufficiency and objectively measure its severity.

Methods

Ambulatory Calf Volume Plethysmography

Ambulatory calf volume plethysmography was done in all limbs using a mercury in-silastic strain-gauge plethysmograph (*Whitney,* 1953) (Model EC-2 supplied by D. E. Hokanson) connected to a pen recorder (Minograph 34). Two channels were used so that both limbs could be studied simultaneously. The strain-gauge was placed around the thickest part of the calf. The maximum venous outflow (MVO) was first determined with the patient supine and the legs elevated 10° to the horizontal by applying 25 cm wide conical cuffs to the thighs, inflated to 60 mm Hg for 2 minutes and then suddenly released. The MVO was calculated from the recordings of calf volume variation after the cuff was released, and it was expressed in ml/100 ml of tissue/minute.

Subsequently the patient was asked to stand and repeatedly raise himself on his toes (tiptoeing) at a rate of one movement per second for a period of 20 seconds. The ambulatory volume change (AVC) which was the maximum change during exercise was obtained and it was expressed in ml/100 ml of tissue. Exercise was repeated with a 2.5 cm wide cuff just below the knee at 100 mm Hg which occluded the superficial veins.

Ascending venography

Ascending venography was done in all limbs, except the 15 limbs of the normal volunteers, in order to determine the presence or absence of deep venous occlusion (*Craig,* 1977).

Ambulatory venous pressure

The ambulatory venous pressure was measured in all limbs. A 21 G (bore 20 G) 'butterfly' needle was inserted into a vein on the dorsum of the foot and was connected through an Akers transducer (Model 840) and a B.A.P. 001 amplifier to a potentiometric pen recorder (J & J. Instruments, Model CR 552 MK2). Venous pressure was measured with the patient standing still and then doing a tip-toe exercise for 20 seconds at a rate of one heel raising movement per second. This was repeated once after inflating a 2.5 cm pneumatic cuff at the ankle to a pressure of 140 mm Hg and a second time inflating a similar cuff at the thigh to a pressure of 180 mm Hg.

Materials

Fifty limbs of 27 subjects (11 male and 16 female) have been studied. The limbs were classified in the following four groups according to the criteria stated below:

Normal: 15 limbs were classified as normal because the ambulatory venous pressure was less than 35 mm Hg and there was no history or clinical evidence of venous disease.

Superficial venous insufficiency with competent valves in the deep veins (SVI): 14 limbs were included in this group because the high ambulatory venous pressure became less than 35 mm Hg only by applying the venous cuffs during tiptoeing.

Deep venous insufficiency (DVI): 13 limbs were included in this group because the ambulatory venous pressure was high (<45 mm Hg) and was not affected by the venous cuffs.

Deep venous insufficiency and occlusion (DVI + DVO): 8 limbs were included in this group because venography demonstrated occlusion of the ilio-femoral segments and the ambulatory venous pressure was greater than 70 mm Hg even when the venous cuffs were inflated.

Results

The maximum venous outflow was always less than 110 ml/100 ml/min in the presence of deep venous occlusion and more than 125 ml/100 ml/min in the absence of occlusion. There was considerable overlap of the values of the MVO in the remaining three groups (Fig. 1).

The results of the ambulatory volume change are shown in Fig. 2. The mean ambulatory volume change was -2.20 (SD $\pm$ 0.5) ml/100 ml, the negative sign indicating that the calf volume is decreased. The mean ambulatory volume change was -1.3 (SD $\pm$ 0.3) in limbs with SVI, -0.60 (SD $\pm$ 0.1) in limbs with DVI, and -0.06 (SD $\pm$ 0.5) in limbs with DVI

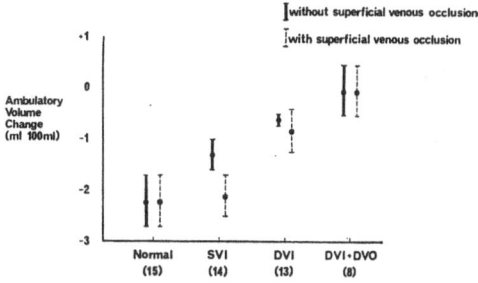

Fig. 2. Results of ambulatory volume change with and without occlusion of the superficial veins.

ambulatory pressure change. The regression line and equation are shown in Fig. 3. In the figure the limbs with DVI, limbs with DVI + DVO, and limbs with onrmal deep venous system (Ambulatory venous pressure and calf volume change measured with venous cuffs occluding the superficial veins) are shown as three completely separate groups.

Discussion

The maximum venous outflow reflects the functional capacity of the venous system to drain the blood collected in the

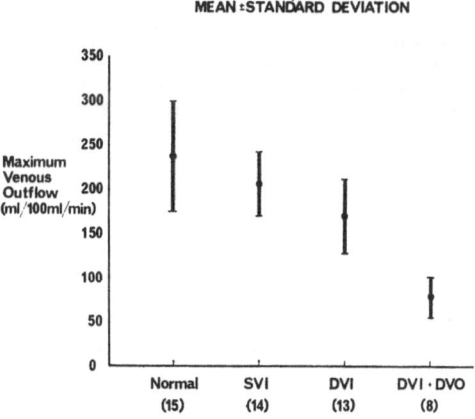

Fig. 1. Results of maximum venous outflow.

and occlusion. In the last group (DVI + + DVO) the ambulatory volume change was negative and small (-0.25 ml/100 ml) in six limbs and positive ($+0.40$ ml/100 ml) (i.e., *calf volume increased*) in two limbs which belonged to patients with pain on walking. The AVC was not significantly affected by the superficial venous occlusion in normal limbs, and limbs with DVI with or without occlusion, but it was brought into the normal range in the limbs with SVI only.

There was a linear relationship between the ambulatory volume change and the

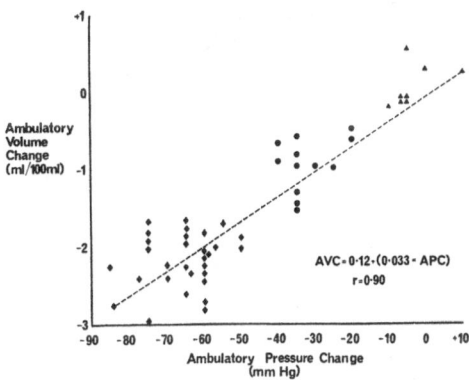

$$AVC = 0.12 - (0.033 \cdot APC)$$
$$r = 0.90$$

Fig. 3. Regression line between ambulatory volume change (AVC) and ambulatory pressure change (APC)

Diamonds: Limbs with normal deep venous system

Closed circles: Limbs with DVI but without DVO

Triangles: Limbs with DVI and DVO

415

lower limbs during the period of venous occlusion, and makes it possible to separate all the limbs with deep venous occlusion.

The AVC without and with superficial venous occlusion provides information about the efficiency of the calf muscle pump, which depends upon the state of the deep venous valves and on the patency of the deep venous system. In the limbs with superficial insufficiency, when the superficial reflux was abolished and the efficacy of the calf muscle pump was restored by a below-knee cuff, the ambulatory volume change became normal. However, if deep reflux was present, the value of the ambulatory volume change did not alter significantly after application of the venous cuffs. The linear relationship (Fig. 3) between ambulatory volume change and ambulatory pressure change suggests that changes in calf volume vary according to changes in pressure, therefore supporting the validity of this test.

This is a useful screening test for limbs with suspected venous insufficiency and an aid to provide an objective diagnosis and quantitative evaluation of the severity of venous insufficiency without an invasive test.

REFERENCES

Craig, J. O. N. C. (1977): Investigations of the leg veins by venography. In: Hobbs, J. T. (Ed.) Treatment of Venous Disorders. Lancaster, Medical and Technical Publishing, pp. 83—95.

DeCamp, P. T., Schramel, R. J., Ray, C. J. et al. (1951): Ambulatory venous pressure determinations in post-phlebitic and related syndromes. Surgery, 29, 44—52.

Kriessman, A. (1974): Peripheral phlebodynamometry. Quantitative method for the differentiation of venous insufficiency in the lower limbs. Deutsch. med. Wschr., 99, 1025—1026.

Lewis, J. D., Parsons, D. C. S., Needham, T. et al. (1973): The use of venous pressure measurements and directional Doppler recordings in distinguishing between superficial and deep valvular incompetence in patients with deep venous insufficiency. Br. J. Surg., 60, 312.

Pollack, A. A., Taylor, B. E. Myers, T. T. et al. (1949): Venous pressure in the saphenous vein at the ankle in man during exercise and changes in posture. J. Appl. Physiol., 1, 649—662.

Whitney, R. J. (1953): Measurement of volume changes in human limbs. J. Physiol. (Lond.), 121, 1—27.

J. F. F., Cardiovasc. Unit & Vas. Lab., St. Mary's Hosp., Med. School, Praed Str. London W. 2, U. K.

INVESTGATIONS OF PERIPHERAL ARTERIAL BLOOD FLOW BY MEASURING THE MINIMAL TRANSIT TIME OF A RADIOACTIVE TRACER

U. ST. MÜLLER, H. VOSBERG, S. HEMMELSKAMP, H. SCHICHA,
W. BECKER and L. E. FEINENDEGEN

*Medical Clinic and Policlinic of Münster, Institute
of Nuclear-Medicine, Jülich, Münster, F.R.G.*

The blood supply of the human body is guaranteed by the function of leading, distributing and smoothing of the arterial system. Radioactive tracers are well suited for the measurement of the function of leading and distributing. The "blood flow" measurement with ^{133}Xenon, in particular, has proved to be useful in brain myocardial muscle and skeletal muscle studies.

The present investigations deal with a method of measuring the velocity of blood flow (function of leading) in the region of the aorta and the arteries of the lower limbs, and the interdependence of the velocity of blood flow and heart rate, with respect to age. The method used is based on measurement of minimal transit times (mtt), measured as the difference of the appearance time of the radioactive tracer, comparable to investigations of the heart function.

Methods

Technetium (99 m — pertechnetat, was used as a radioactive tracer. The investigations were performed in 53 patients of different sex and age. In no case was an obliterative arteriopathy present. Specially designed 8 channel equipment was utilized.

Eight collimators, each with a scintillation counter and a NaI-(TI) crystal were positioned in the following manner: 2nd right intercostal space (vena cava superior, or rather aortic bulb), below of the umbilical region (abdominal aorta), groin on both sides (femoral artery), patella on both sides (popliteal artery) and inner malleolus on both sides (posterior tibial artery).

Two to three mCi of the tracer were injected as a bolus into the right antecubital vein. The impulses of the 8 scintillation counters were accumulated on a magnetic tape with a dissolution time of 100 msec. The results were reproduced for evaluation on a 4 channel recorder with integrated rate meters. During the measurement, an electrocardiogram recorded the actual heart rate (Figure 1).

In the region of the investigated arteries blood velocity was calculated from the time differences

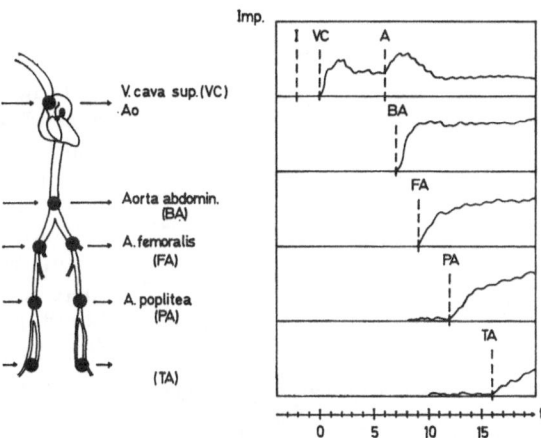

Fig. 1. Left side: Topographical arrangement of the collimators. Right side: Radioactivity recorded over the different arterial regions.

417

of the appearance of the radioactivity and the distance of the collimators. The simultaneous measurement of the total minimal cardiac transit times allowed the selection of patients with heart failure.

Results

1. Dependence of the blood velocity on heart rate.

The velocity of blood increases with increasing heart rate in a linear dependence. The correlation coefficient is significantly different from zero in all the arterial regions which were investigated. There is an increasing difference of the velocity of blood flow in the single regions, when heart rate increases, as can be seen in the different slopes of the regression lines (Figure 2).

2. Dependence of the standardized blood flow velocity on age.

The dependence on heart rate was eliminated by mathematically standardizing the measured velocity of blood flow at a constant heart rate of 80/min.

Figure 3 shows the decrease of standard-

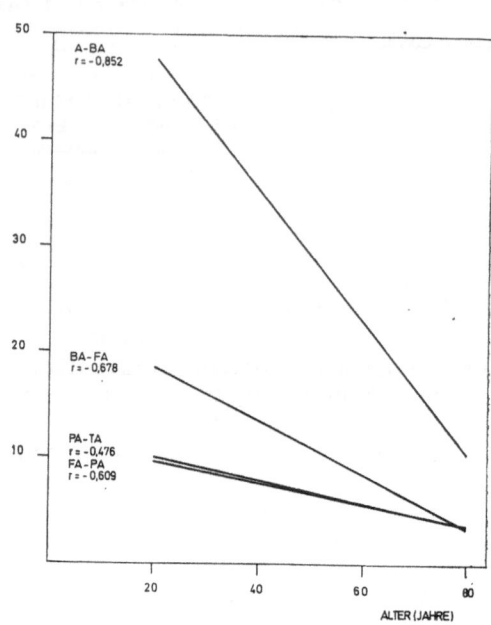

Fig. 3. Dependence of the standardized velocity of blood flow ($\bar{v}_{80}$) on age (Alter). Regions as in Fig. 2.

ized blood velocity with increasing age. At all arterial regions the correlation coefficient of the regression line appears significantly different from zero.

Discussion

The method used seems to be well suited for measuring the velocity of blood flow in the great arteries between the aorta and the tibial artery. There is a linear dependence of the velocity of blood flow and heart rate in a range from 50 to 100/min in the arterial region between the aortic bulb and the tibial artery. The blood velocity decreases from the aorta to the distal arteries. At a heart rate of 50/min there is no difference in the velocity of blood flow distal to the aortic region (Figure 2).

On the other hand, the velocity of arterial blood flow is dependent on age. This was clearly shown when heart rate was

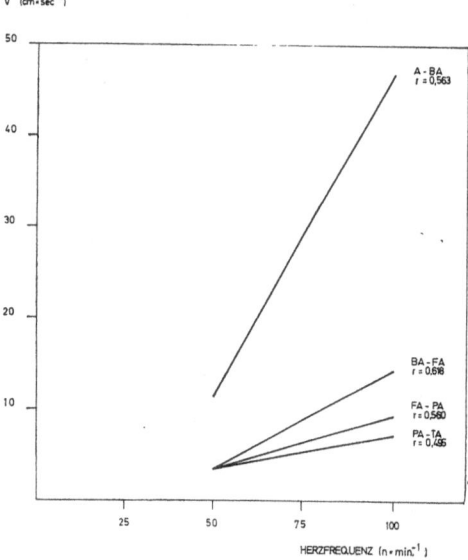

Fig. 2. Dependence of the velocity of blood flow ($\bar{v}$) on heart rate (Herzfrequenz). A — BA: aortic region; BA — FA: pelvic region; FA — PA: region of thigh; PA — TA: region of lower leg.

418

standardized to 80 beats per min. The greatest decrease in the velocity of blood flow with age is found in the aortic region. The diminution of the velocity of blood flow is reduced in distal arterial regions (Figure 3).

REFERENCES

1. *Kappert, A. and Rösler, H.:* Zur nuklearmedizinischen dynamischen Analyse der peripheren Strombahn. In: Zeitler: Diagnostik mit Isotopen. (Bern—Stuttgart—Wien, 1973).
2. *Wagner, H. N. and Rhodes B. A.:* The radiopharmaceutical. In: H. N. Wagner, Principles in nuclear medicine (London—Philadelphia—Toronto, 1969).
3. *Wetterer, E., Bauer R. D. and Pasch Th.:* Arteriensystem. In: E. Schütz: Physiologie des Kreislaufs, Band 1. (Berlin—Heidelberg—New York, 1971).

U. St. M., Medical Clinic and Policlinic of Münster, Westring 3, 4400 Münster, F.R.G.

FUNCTIONAL INVESTIGATION OF OCCLUSIVE ARTERIAL DISEASE OF LOWER EXTREMITIES — ROUND TABLE DISCUSSION

Chairman: W. Schoop (F.R.G.)

Co-chairman: J. Linhart (Czechoslovakia)

Participants: A. Bollinger (Switzerland), D. Clement (Belgium), H. Denck (Austria), H. Ehringer (Austria), J. F. Merlen (France), B. Pernow (Sweden), J. F. Raines (U.S.A.), L. Urai (Hungary).

Raines demonstrated an instrumental system which may detect with reasonable probability the presence of occlusive arterial disease in the extremities. In principle, the technique employs segmental plethysmography with registration of volume pulsations using a pneumatic system, and ultrasonic local measurement of systolic blood pressure. Schoop demonstrated the spontaneous progression of occlusions of the femoral artery. In the majority of patients, there is a strong tendency to femoral occlusions in the contralateral extremity rather than to extension of femoral occlusion proximally beyond the inguinal ligament. Usually, the progression is stepwise rather than gradual, and long periods of stabilization are frequently observed. Femoropopliteal occlusions *per se* are never the cause of gangrene. Careful analysis of a high number of patient reveals that the complication occurs most frequently with diabetes, multiple inflammatory small vessel disease in the foot and calf and improper femoropopliteal reconstructions. Urai pointed out the importance of ultrasound measurements in complete occlusions. Clement commented on the application of Doppler's principle in evaluation of the elastic parameters of the arterial wall with the intention to recognize the asymptomatic form of atherosclerosis prior to obliteration. So far the results have not been conclusive because of considerable overlapping between pathological and normal findings. Linhart pointed out the practical value of body heating which may be used as a measure of vasodilator capacity of vessels supplying the ischemic skin area. Apart from skin temperature measurements before and after the procedure, the effect can also be assessed by an original modification of venous occlusion plethysmography in the foot (Spáčil, J., and Linhart, J.: "Foot blood flow during reactive hyperemia" etc. – see above) employing the strain-gauge system. A surprisingly good correlation can be demonstrated between findings obtained by instrumental devices and some bedside functional test such as positional test; if interpreted properly, the examination may point out the impending danger of necrosis even in patients without corresponding clinical symptoms. – The problems of microcirculation were discussed by Merlen and Bollinger. With full vasodilatation, the capillary pressure in man may be as high as 60 mm Hg (mean pressure) with an obvious difference between the systolic and diastolic value. Pernow and Denck demonstrated favourable results of successful arterial reconstructions from the pathophysiological and surgical point of view. One of the most realiable methods to prove the effect of surgical reconstruction is muscle biopsy at rest and after exercise, which makes it possible to compare the response of tissue lactate and creatinin phosphate before and after operation.

As pointed out by Schoop in the concluding remarks, there has been general agreement that methods of functional investigation, based upon advances of clinical physiology, should be widely employed since they offer important information in addition to the clinical examination.

DYNAMIC METHODS FOR THE CLINICAL INVESTIGATION OF MICROCIRCULATION

A. BOLLINGER

Department of Internal Medicine, Angiology Division, University of Zürich, Switzerland

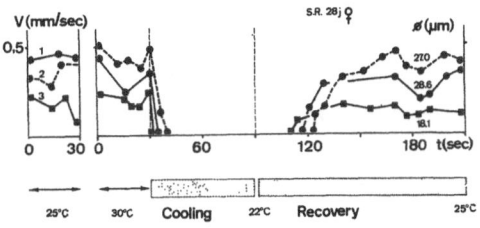

Fig. 1. Flow velocity in three adjacent nailfold capillary loops before, during and after standardized cold exposure. In all the three loops examined the red blood cells stop soon after the beginning of cooling. The diameters of the somewhat enlarged capillaries ($\varnothing$) are given in μm.

Only recently, methods have been introduced to study dynamic phenomena in human skin capillaries. In the nailfold of fingers and toes blood flow velocity is measured by videomicroscopy (*Bollinger et al.*, 1974; *Butti et al.*, 1975, *Anliker and Kubli*, 1975, *Fagrell et al.*, 1977) and pressure by direct micropuncture (*Mahler and Muheim* 1977).

The atraumatic measurement of red cell velocity in nailfold capillaries through the intact skin proved to be a valuable tool for the investigation of physiology and pathophysiology. Mean capillary flow velocity at a controlled nailfod temperature of 30 °C reaches 0.72 ± 0.3 mm/sec. Two physiological flow patterns may be distinguished (*Bollinger et al.*, 1974): a continuous and an intermittent type. In the latter the red cells stop at irregular intervals not related to the respiratory or cardiac cycle. This pattern is probably dependent on the action of the precapillary sphincters.

When several adjacent capillaries are considered, a concordant and a discordant flow pattern may be recognized. Concordant means that acceleration and deceleration occur simultaneously in different capillary loops, discordant, that the speed varies in an opposite direction when compared to adjacent capillaries. The discordant pattern is found as a possible feature in acrocyanosis (*Bollinger et al.*, 1977), where even a reversal of flow may be observed. Other capillaries in this disease exhibit a slow concordant flow.

A standardized cold exposure (insufflation of cold air of about −10° during 1 minute) provokes a standstill of capillary erythrocytes in most patients with primary Raynaud's disease (*Mahler et al.*, 1977). In healthy subjects, however, there is only a decrease in velocity during the test. The rapid recovery contrasts to the behaviour in vasospastic Raynaud's disease. In acrocyanosis no systematic flow stop is

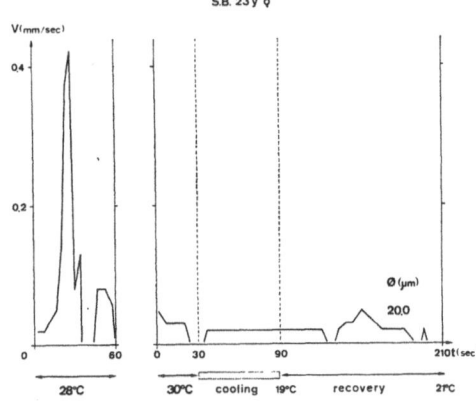

Fig. 2. Intermittent flow pattern in a patient with acrocyanosis. The flow velocities are extremely low. Nevertheless, cooling does not induce a flow stop.

423

induced by cold provocation. Patients with chronic occlusions of hand and finger arteries (secondary Raynaud's disease) show no increased cold sensitivity. The red blood cells do not stop during cold exposure with exception of patients with severe ischemia or with associated vasospasm occurring particularly in collagen vascular disease.

Mean capillar pressure in nailfod loops measured by direct puncture (glass pipettes) averages 30.2 ± 11.5 mm Hg (*Mahler and Muheim*, 1977). The pressure is pulsatile with a mean amplitude of 11 mm Hg. Interesting are spontaneous fluctuations in mean pressure and amplitude which probably go parallel to flow variations. The vasospastic phenomena in acrocyanosis induce low capillary pressures with decreased pulsatility (*Mahler and Muheim*, 1977).

The analysis of capillary dynamics should not only include measurements of velocity and pressure, but also of exchange phenomena at the blood — tissue barrier. Preliminary work in this laboratory indicates that diffusion of fluorescein marked tracers may be quantitated by videomicroscopy and densitometry.

REFERENCES

Anliker M., Kubli R. (1975): A new on- line method of measuring high flow speeds in microscopic vessels by a dual video camera technique, First world congress Microcirc., Toronto.

Bollinger A., Butti P., Barras J. P., Trachsler H., Siegenthaler W. (1974): Red blood cell velocity in nailfold capillaries in man measured by a television microscopy technique, Microvasc. Res. 7, 61—72.

Bollinger A., Mahler F., Meier B. (1977): Velocity patterns in nailfold capillaries of normal subjects and patients with Raynaud's disease and acrocyanosis, Europ. Conf. Microcirc., Bibl. anat. 16, 142—145.

Butti P., Intaglietta M., Reimann H., Holliger C., Bollinger A., Anliker M. (1975): Capillary red blood cell velocity measurements in human nailfod by videodensitometric method, Microvasc. Res. 10, 220—227.

Fagrell B., Fronek A., Intaglietta M. (1977): Capillary blood flow velocity during rest and post- occlusive reactive hyperemia in skin areas of the toes and lower leg, Europ. Conf. Microcirc., Bibl. anat. 16, 159.

Mahler F., Meier B., Frey R., Bollinger A., Anliker M. (1977): Reaction of red blood cell velocity in nailfod capillaries to local cold in patients with vasospastic disease, Europ. Conf. Microcirc., Bibl. anat. 16, 155—158.

Mahler F., Muheim M. (1977): Kontinuierliche Druckmessung in Nagelfalzkapillaren normaler Versuchspersonen und Patienten mit Akrozyanose, in Alexander K., Cachovan M. (ed.), Diabetische Angiopathien, G. Witzstrock, Baden-Baden, 313—315.

A. B., Angiol. Abt., Kanton-Hospital, Rämistr. 100, 8091 Zürich, Switzerland

424

SYNTHESIS AND MIGRATION OF PROTEINS IN JUXTAGLOMERULAR CELLS. AN ULTRASTRUCTURAL RADIOAUTOGRAPHIC STUDY

M. CANTIN, YVON DESORMEAUX and S. BENCHIMOL

Department of Pathology, University of Montreal, Canada

The juxtaglomerular apparatus of complex is made up of the macula densa, the lacis cells and the juxtaglomerular cells (JGC) or epithelioid cells of the afferent glomerular arterioles. Since the synthesis and intracellular transport of proteins have not been investigated in JGC by biochemical techniques for obvious reasons, the present report represents an ultrastructural radioautographic study in JGC of the rat, using L-tyrosine-3,5³H as label.

Materials and methods

Preparation for electron microscopy

Female Sprague-Dawley rats (Madison, Wisc.) with a mean initial body weight of 40 g (range: 35 to 45 g) were fed a sodium-deficient diet (ICN Pharmaceuticals Inc., Cleveland, Ohio) for a period of 30 days with access to deionized water ad libitum. On the 30th day of the experiment (when the rats reached a mean body weight of 101 g (range: 90 to 108 g)), they were injected, under light ether anesthesia, through the jugular vein, with 4 mCi of L-tyrosine-3,5³H (New England Nuclear, Boston, Mass.) specific activity 40—60 Ci/mM) in 0.2 ml of 0.9% NaCl. They were sacrificed in pairs 5 min, 20 min, 1 h and 4 h after the injection by perfusion of 4% formaldehyde (prepared from paraformol) buffered with Sorensen's solution (pH 7.3) and containing

0.1 mg/ml of tyrosine and 0.1% sucrose, through the lower abdominal aorta for 10 min (*Cantin et al.*, 1975; *Cantin et al.*, 1977). Fragments of the left renal cortex were kept in the same fixative for 4 h. They were then washed for 10 periods of 15 min each in the same buffer containing 0.1 mg/ml of tyrosine and 1% sucrose.

Radioautographic technique

The light and electron microscopic techniques as well as the light and electron microscopic radioautographic techniques used were as previously described (*Cantin et al.*, 1977; *Benchimol and Cantin* 1978a; 1978b; *Yunge et al.*, 1978).

Analysis of electron microscope radioautographs

Data were collected from 500 photographs and analyzed as already described (*Benchimol and Cantin*, 1978a; 1978b; *Yunge et al.*, 1978).

Determination of the relative specific radioactivity of organelles

The relative specific radioactivity of organelles was determined by expressing each grain count and circle count as a

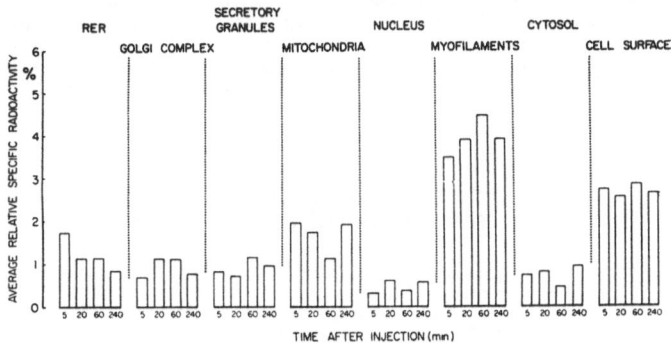

Fig. 1. Average relative specific radioactivity of juxtaglomerular cell organelles at various times after injection of L-Tyrosine 3,5 ³H

425

percentage and dividing grain percentage by the corresponding circle percentage (Fig. 1).

Results

Light microscope radioautography

The number of silver grains over the JGC increased slightly from 5 to 20 min and remained relatively stable thereafter.

Electron microscope radioautography

The distribution of silver grains on various JGC organelles was analyzed at 5 min, 20 min, 1 h and 4 h after the L-tyrosine-3,5^{3}H injection. At all time intervals, as can be judged from the chi-square values (p < 0.001), the grain distribution markedly differed from a random one. The data indicate that, at 5 min post-injection, the rough endoplasmic reticulum (RER) had a high relative specific radioactivity, while it was low in the Golgi complex and in secretory granules. The radioactivity regularly decreased with time in the RER while it rose at 20 min in the Golgi complex and

after 1 h in the secretory granules, where it became lower again after 4 h. There was a low level of radioactivity in the nucleus at all time intervals with small peaks at 20 min and 1 h. Radioactivity was already high in the mitochondria at 5 min. It decreased at 20 min and even more at 1 h to reach another high at 4 h. Radioactivity in the cytosol was low at all time intervals in contrast with peripherally located myofilaments, where it was high at all times. The radioactivity associated with the cell surface was already high at 5 min and remained so with minor variations at other time intervals

Discussion

The present results indicate that the protein moiety of renin, the main secretory protein of JGC is probably synthetized in the rough endoplasmic reticulum and, as judged from cytochemical studies (*Cantin et al.*, 1979), glycosylated in the Golgi complex, before reaching secretory granules.

REFERENCES

Benchimol, S. and Cantin, M., 1978a. Ultrastructural radioautography of the incorporation of tritiated leucine by the rat adrenal medulla in vivo. Cell Tiss. Res. 193: 179—199.

Benchimol, S. and Cantin, M., 1978b. Etude radioautographique de la synthèse et de la migration des glycoprotéines dans les cellules de la médullosurrénale du rat. Biol. Cell. (Paris) 33: 157—162.

Cantin, M., Araujo-Nascimento, M. de F., Benchimol, S. and Desormeaux, Y., 1977. Metaplasia of smooth muscle cells into juxtaglomerular cells in the juxtaglomerular apparatus, arteries and arterioles of the ischemic (endocrine) kidney. Am. J. Path. 87: 581—602.

Cantin, M., Desormeaux, Y., Chlebovicova, J., Benchimol, S. and Araujo-Nascimento, N. de F., 1975. Comparative ultrastructural cytochemistry of juxtaglomerular cell granules and renal tubular cell lysosomes. Lab. Invest. 33: 648—657.

Cantin, M., El-Khatib, E. and Yunge, L., 1979. Cytochimie ultrastructurale de l'appareil juxtaglomérulaire de la souris. Path. Biol. (in press).

Yunge, L., Benchimol, S. and Cantin, M., 1978. Ultrastructural cytochemistry of atrial muscle cells. VII.Radioautographic study of synthesis and migration of glycoproteins. J. Mol. Cell. Cardiol. (in press).

M. C., Département de Pathologie, Université de Montréal, 2900 boul. Edouard Montpetit Montréal, Quebec (Canada) H3T 1J4

RED CELL AGING AS A MODEL INFLUENCING PHARMACOLOGICALLY RED CELL DEFORMABILITY

H. G. GRIGOLEIT, H. LEONHARDT, R. SCHRÖER and F. LEHRACH

Hoechst Comp., Frankfurt/M., F.R.G., Steglitz Clinic of Free University of Berlin West and Hoechst Comp., Wiesbaden, F.R.G.

The geometries of erythrocytes and capillaries differ considerably, i.e. the mean diameter of these cells is higher than the mean width of most of the capillaries. Several states of disease are known (*Grigoleit* and *Leonhardt*, 1977) including peripheral arterial occlusive disease, (*Ehrly and Köhler*, 1976; *Reid et al.*, 1976) where red cell deformability is reduced. This led to the conclusion that reduced deformability might at least contribute partially to microcirculatory disturbances. Thus an increasing demand for methods to measure red cell deformability arose. In the past 15 years several methods were published (*Grigoleit er al.*, 1978) and we selected that by *Reid et al.* (1976) which allows estimation of the mean red cell deformability of erythrocyte populations from whole blood by filtration through filters with a pore diameter of 5 µm. To test drugs which may potentially have an influence on red cell deformability, it is essential to have a procedure which generates erythrocytes with reduced deformability in a reproducible manner. Red cells from freshly similar blood develop a continuous fall of this mechanical property (*Grigoleit et al.*, 1978) during short storage (up to 3 hours) and we used this model to evaluate the activity of pentoxifylline, theophylline and prednisolone. Several investigators have reported (*Grigoleit and Leonhardt*, 1977) that pentoxifylline increases red cell deformability. Theophylline was chosen as a comparative compound since its chemical structure is similar to that of pentoxifylline.

Materials and methods

In one experiment immediately after collecting the blood from 17 healthy volunteers, we measured blood viscosity with a capillary viscosimeter, red cell deformability and hematocrit. The purpose of this experiment was to find a possible interdependence between these parameters. In two further series of experiments we investigated the influence of pentoxifylline (10 and 20 µg/ml of blood) and theophylline (96,6 µg/ml of blood) and prednisolone (20 µg/ml of blood) versus a control. Blood was taken from 21 (pentoxifylline series) and 10 (theophylline and prednisolone series) healthy subjects, respectively. Isovolemic saline or the 3 compounds were added to 3 aliquots of blood from each subject and measurements at room temperature were carried out at times of 0, 45, 90 and 180 minutes after adding saline or the test compounds, respectively. For each series of experiments filters from one batch (pore diameter: 5 µm) were used to preclude all possibility of variation due to different filter batches. The mean red cell deformability derived from the method we used is given as the volume of whole blood passing through the filter per minute (ml/min). To preclude possible influences of pentoxifylline on the erythrocyte membrane, scanning electron microscopy of erythrocytes incubated in pentoxifylline solution (0.9—181 µg/ml plasma) for 3 hours was performed. The preparations were carried out according to *Dewar et al.* (1976) and *Hölke and Kemnitz* (1977) with magnifications of up to 20.000-fold. Statistical analysis of the data was made by Friedman's test and simultaneous comparison according to Nemenyi (*Miller, 1966*) or by linear regression analysis.

Results

No correlation was found between blood viscosity and red cell deformability using regression analysis, although this was found by other investigations. (*Leonhardt and Grigoleit*, 1977). The flow rate and hematocrit are plotted in Figure 1.

A correlation (p < 0.05) exists between the two parameters. Similar data were reported previously by *Leonhardt et al.* (1978).

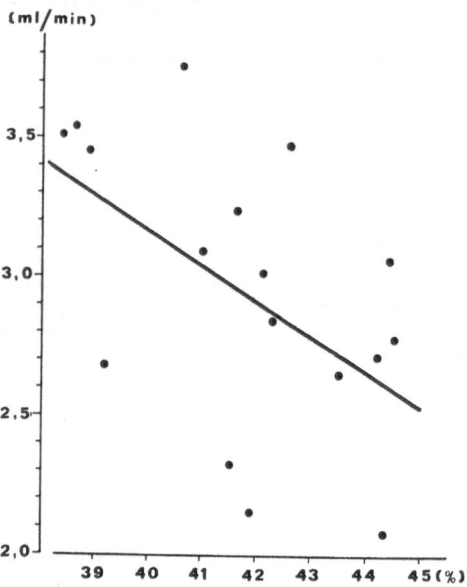

Fig. 1. Plot of hematocrit (%) versus flow rate. Linear regression analysis reveals a significant correlation (p < 0.05) between the parameters (n = 17; r = 0.520; y = 8.20 — 0.126x).

Figure 2 represents the results from the pentoxifylline series. The plot of the

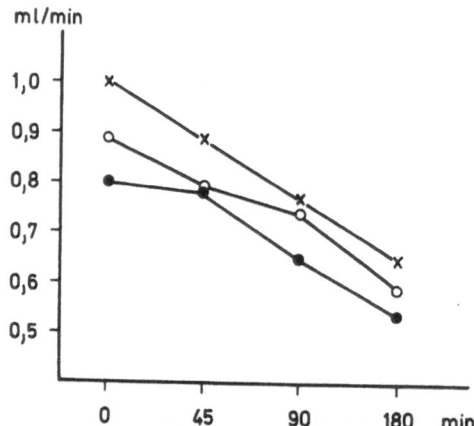

Fig. 2. Plot of flow rate (ml/min) versus time (● = control, ○ = 10 μg pentoxifylline/ml blood, x = 20 μg pentoxifylline/ml blood).

median values of flow rate against time shows a clear dose-response relationship. The compound has an immediate effect on the filtration rate as reflected in the results at time 0. The course of the control curve clearly indicates a time dependent

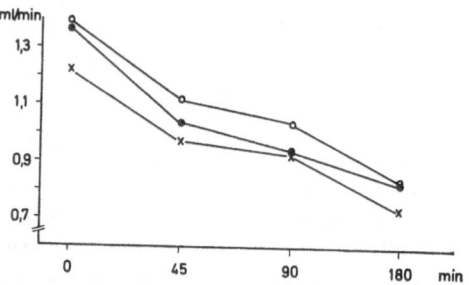

Fig. 3. Plot of flow rate versus time (● = control, ○ = 96,6 μg theophylline/ml blood, x = 20 μg prednisolone/ml blood).

decrease in the red cell deformability. Statistical analysis revealed a significant difference between the 20 μg group and the controls; the 10 μg group could be separated neither from the controls nor from the 20 μg group, i.e. there was a dose-dependent increase in the filtration rate. After 180 minutes a difference could no longer be established. In figure 3 are shown the data from the theophylline and prednisolone series. For both compounds statistically no difference from the control could be detected, though with theophylline over time a slight increase and with predni-solone a slight decrease in filtration rate was observed. The course of the control curve again proves that red cell deformability in our model considerably decreases in time.

Discussion

We assume that red cell aging is the most important physiological procedure in generating cells with impaired de-formability. The method described by *Reid et al.* (1976) is sufficiently precise for the quantification of the effect of different compounds. The handling of the filtration apparatus is simple and quick and, taking into account the methodological aspects previously reported by *Leonhardt et al.* (1978) provides data with good reproducibility. The results achieved with pentoxifylline confirm earlier data (*Grigoleit and Leonhardt*, 1977). The potency of pentoxifylline seems to be 10-fold higher in increasing red cell deformability than that of theophylline. It is not surprising that both compounds basically act in the same manner as their chemical structures are related. These investigations provide the first evidence to suggest that the differences in chemical structures of two methylxanthine derivatives affect their ability to influence red cell deformability in aging blood. A clear explanation of the effect of pentoxifylline cannot be given at the moment. It is assumed that the increase in red cell ATP content as reported by several investigators (*Grigoleit and Leonhardt*, 1977) might play an important role. A direct effect on the erythrocyte membrane can be excluded, based on scanning electron microscopy with magnifications up to 20,000.

REFERENCES

Dewar, C. L., Wolowyk, M. W., Hill, H. R. (1976): A simple method for processing erythrocytes for scanning electron microscopy. Amer. J. clin. Pathol. 6, 760—765.

Ehrly, A. M., Köhler, H.-J. (1976): Altered deformability of erythrocytes from patients with chronic occlusive arterial disease. VASA 5, 319—322.

Grigoleit, H.-G., Leonhardt, H. (1977): Rheology of blood and pentoxifylline. Pharmatherapeutica (Lond.) 1, 642—651.

Grigoleit, H.-G., Leonhardt, H., Schröer, R., Lehrach, F.: Die Erythrozytenalterung als Modell für die pharmakologische Beeinflussung der Erythrozytenverformbarkeit. Rheol. Acta (in press).

Hölke, D., Kemnitz, P. (1977): Formveränderungen von Erythrozyten unter dem Einfluss verschiedener Blutstabilisatoren im Rasterelektronenmikroskop. Dtsch. Gesund.-Wesen 32, 44—48.

Leonhardt, H., Grigoleit, H.-G. (1977): Effects of pentoxifylline on red blood cell deformability and blood viscosity under hyperosmolar conditions. Naunyn-Schmiedeberg's Arch. Pharmacol. 299, 197—200.

Leonhardt, H., Arntz, H.-R., Reinhardt, I. Methodische Untersuchungen zur Erythrozytenfiltration durch Polycarbonatfilter. Rheol. Acta (in press)

Miller, R. G. Jr. (1966): Simultaneous statistical inference. McGraw-Hill.

Reid, H. L., Dormandy, J. A., Barnes, A. J., Lock, P. J., Dormandy, T. L. (1976): Impaired red cell deformability in peripheral vascular disease. Lancet 1, 666—667.

Reid, H. L., Barnes, A. J., Lock, P. J., Dormandy, J. A., Dormandy, T. L. (1976): A simple method for measuring erythrocyte deformability. J. Clin. Path. 10, 855—858.

H. G. G., Medical Department Hoechst AG, P.O. Box 80 03 20, 6230 Frankfurt/M-80 F.R.G.

DIABETIC MICROANGIOPATHY

W. REDISCH

New York Medical College, New York City, U.S.A.

The details of mutual functional influences between micro-and macrocirculation have been more and more elucidated within the past decade. Understanding of the significance of this relationship for major clinical events, e.g. certain forms of circulatory failure, low flow syndromes, high viscosity syndromes, shock (8) has grown considerably.

It is by now accepted knowledge that hemodynamics alone can yield finally decisive parameters only as long as no structural abnormalities have developed within the arterial system (5), and that rheologic parameters gain significance for macroflow in direct proportion to the presence and degree of structural changes.

But deeper penetration into the clinician's mind is still needed. We must become more vividly aware of the enormous impact of microcirculatory changes upon the behaviour of the macrocirculation. Such awareness carries often immediate therapeutic awards such as the beneficial effects of vasodilators in a certain group of cases in congestive heart failure (12) or the prompt response to alert attention to rheologic parameters in a number of local flow disturbances (9) as well, as in the early phases of shock (4).

Recognition of inherent or acquired abnormalities in the microcirculatory system — so-called "microangiopathies" — have been recognized for some time to represent serious complications to the functioning of some physiological compensatory mechanisms in cardiovascular disease.

The specific example of microangiopathy which I have been asked to discuss with you is the probably best known inherent microangiopathy, namely the one which occurs specifically in diabetics (1).

The prevalence of diabetic microangiopathy has been assessed in various surveys: in early 1950, the literature recorded about half of all surveyed cases as involved (6); however, much higher prevalence (up to 85 and 90%) has been found in more recent surveys (13). Whether the "duration" of diabetes makes for the difference, remains a moot question; simply, because we are not capable of determining truly the onset of diabetes. Clinical manifestations are an unreliable and fallacious guide to the real "onset". There is little doubt that the sequelae of microangiopathy become more and more conspicuous as the diabetic patient ages. As our group has expressed it (1): "the longer the duration of diabetes, the longer has the patient lived with whatever factors are responsible for the microangiopathy".

Table I.

Macro- & Microangiopathy In Diabetes: Detailed Review Of 580 Patients.

PATHOLOGY	NUMBER	PERCENT
O A D	230	39.7
PROTEINURIA	126	21.7
RETINOPATHY	72	12.4
"MICROSCARS"	335	57.7

We have, as has been shown repeatedly, good reason to suspect that the "microangiopathy", seen as a structural and functional error within the vascular exchange system, is probably genetic and certainly inherent to the diabetic syndrome. Much detail work has been done to show the early evidence for diabetic microangiopathy (14) by investigations especially concerned with the comparison of microvessel parameters in prediabetics, chemical diabetics and overt diabetics.

Capillary basement membrane changes, morphologic and permeability changes in surface capillaries, conjuctival microaneurysms, changes in digital pulse morphology, plethysmographically ascertained perfusion changes are some of the better known published research findings which have accumulated over the years and by now are making up a fairly convincing mosaic to support the assumption of a genetic trait.

Table II.

DIABETIC MICROANGIOPATHY

MEASURABLE BASEMENT MEMBRANE THICKNESS

CHARACTERISTIC MORPHOLOGIC CHANGES IN SURFACE CAPILLARIES

OCCURRENCE OF CONJUNCTIVAL AND RETINAL MICROANEURYSMS

INCREASED CHANGES IN CAPILLARY PERMEABILITY

Clinical manifestation of diabetic microangiopathy may — for the sake of dogmatic teaching — be subdivided into two groups: 1) those representing direct results of malfunctioning of microcirculatory regulation and automatism; 2) those representing sequelae and repercussions in the macrocirculation (heart, arterial and venous systems) in connection with microflow disturbances.

The first group comprises in essence the manifestations of progressive "microcirculatory degeneration", as described

by Otfried Mueller 70 years ago, confusedly played with by several of his epigones (including myself) for decades and finally well summarized by *McMillan* in 1975 (7) as the "final deficit" in stages, as shown in Table III.

Table III.

STAGES OF "FINAL MICROCIRCULATORY DEFICIT"

(MC MILLAN)

1. ALTERED LOCAL BLOOD FLOW
2. PROGRESSIVE REVERSIBLE DILATION OF VENULES AND ARTERIOLES
3. ARTERIOLAR VASOCONSTRICTION
4. SCLEROSIS OF ARTERIOLES, CAPILLARIES AND VENULES
5. PROGRESSIVE MICROCIRCULATORY DECOMPENSATION

The organs most frequently and detectably affected are the eye, the kidneys, the skeletal muscle, the heart muscle.

The second group is characterized by presenting as a rather rapidly advancing form of occlusive atherosclerosis, most frequently affecting the coronary circulation, the brain and the extremities. While there is no essential difference in the atherosclerotic lesion per se, the deletary influence of microcirculatory decompensation calls for early therapeutic attention.

Diabetes has — after many years of effort on the side of a few investigators — finally been recognized as one of the major risk factors in the course of atherosclerosis (10). The consideration of its role in atherogenesis, however, must await clarification of the basic role of microvascular beds, specifically that of the vasa vasorum system in the arterial wall.

REFERENCES

1. *Camerini-Davalos, R. A., Opperman, W., Reddi, A. S., Velasco, C. A. & Redisch, W. (1977):* Diabetic Microangiopathy. In: Insulin and Metabolism (J. S. Bajaj, Ed.) Excerpta Medica, Amsterdam—London—New York.
2. *Chien, S., Usami, S., Taylor, H. M. et al. (1966):* Effects of hematocrit and plasma proteins on human rheology. J. Appl. Physiol. 21: 91.
3. *Chien, S. (1976):* Significance of macrorheology and microrheology in atherogenesis. In: Atherogenesis (R. A. Camerini-Davalos, E. L. Bierman, W. Redisch and D. B. Zilversmith Edts.) Annals of N. Y. Acad. of Sciences, Vol. 275.
4. *Dintenfass, L. (1976):* Rheology of blood in diagnostic and preventive medicine. Butterworth & Co., Sevenoaks, Kent.
5. *Kreulen, T. H., Kirk, E. S., Gorlin, R., Cohn, L. H. & Collins, J. J. (1975):* Coronary artery bypass surgery: assessment of revascularization by determination of bloodflow and myocardial mass. Am. J. Cardiol. 34: 129.
6. *Marble, A. (1966):* Controversy in Internal

Medicine (F. J. Ingelfinger, A. S. Rehman, & M. Finland, Edts.) W. B. Saunders Co, Philadelphia.

7. *McMillan, D. E. (1975):* Deterioration of microcirculation in diabetes. Diabetes 24: 944.

8. *Redisch, W. (1975):* Application of microcirculatory findings to the analysis of clinical disease. Vasa 4: 109.

9. *Redisch, W., Clauss, R. H., Messina, E. J., Terry, E. N. & Brodie, S. J. (1969):* Gangrene of microangiitis (9th Multidisc. Res. Forum), Am. Med. Ass. Chicago.

10. Report of the National Commission on Diabetes to the Congress of the United States. DHEW publication No. NIH 76-1018-1033, 1975.

11. *Rouen, L. R., Terry, E. N., Doft, B. H., Clauss, R. H., & Redisch, W.: (1972):* Classification and measurement of surface microvessels in man. Microvasc. Res. 4: 285.

12. *Schlant, R. C., Tragaris, T. S. & Robertson, R. J. Jr. (1962):* Studies on the acute cardiovascular effects of intravenous sodium nitroprusside. Am. J. Cardiol. 9: 51.

13. *Terry, E. N., Messina, E. J., Schwartz, S., Redisch, W. & Steele, J. M. (1967):* Manifestation of diabetic microangiopathy in nailfold capillaries. Diabetes 16: 595.

14. *Yodaiken, R. E., & Pardo, C. (1975):* Diabetic capillaropathy. Human Pathol. 6: 455.

PROBLEMS OF MICROANGIOPATHY, CAPILLARY FILTRATION AND NEUROCIRCULATORY CHANGES IN POTENTIAL AND MANIFESTED DIABETES MELLITUS

LUDMILA DVOŘÁKOVÁ, Š. FIGAR and J. VALNÍČKOVÁ

Charles University School of Pediatrics, Institute of Physiology
Czechoslovak Academy of Sciences, and Ophthalmology Department
of the Institute for Medical Postgraduate Education, Prague, Czechoslovakia

The relationship of microangiopathies in diabetes mellitus to capillary filtration values has been the subject of many studies, mostly resulting in finding of an increased capillary permeability. On the other hand, the relationship of these microangiopathies to neurocirculatory activities has not yet been studied as far as we know. Both of these relationships could be correlated. Therefore, we have studied the degree of microangiopathies, of capillary filtration and of vasomotor changes in potential and manifested diabetes mellitus.

Materials and methods

We have studied a group of 30 potential and 44 manifested diabetics, whom we have compared with another group of 25 healthy controls without any evidence of diabetes mellitus in their family. In all of them we have measured the values of the capillary filtration coefficient (CFC) by prolonged venous occlusion capacitance plethysmography. Ophthalmological examination was made in 53 cases (19 potential and 34 manifested diabetics) by ophthalmoscopy and by fluorescein angiography. We also registered the capacitance plethysmography vascular responses to a standard set of stimuli (sound, mental arithmetics, pain) in the fingers in 24 potential and in 30 manifested diabetics. The statistical evaluation was made by a t-test. Characteristics of the studied groups are shown in Table I.

Results

CFC values were significantly decreased in both potential and manifested diabetics as compared with healthy controls and represent about 55 per cent of the values found in the controls (Table II). When differentiating the manifested diabetics according to the duration of the disease and according to its treatment, we have not found any significant differences. Nevertheless, a certain tendency to increasing CFC values could be observed with prolonged disease. We have also not found any difference in the CFC values in potential diabetics differentiated according to the glucose tolerance test.

In potential diabetics all ophthalmological findings were physiological. In manifested diabetics, 12 cases exhibited 1st degree retinopathy, 11 cases retinopathy 2nd degree and 21 had normal finding.

Table I. The characteristics of the groups examined

	Number	Age ± SD	Duration of DM ± SD	Treatment Diet.	PAD	Insulin	Retinopathy —	I.	II. grad.
Control group	25 9 ♂ 16 ♀	40,3 ± 18.4	—	—	—	—	—	—	—
Potential diabetics	30 18 ♂ 12 ♀	37.8 ± 7.8	—	—	—	—	—	—	—
Manifest diabetics	44 27 ♂ 17 ♀	48.2 ± 15.9	11.5 ± 9.6	3	12	29	21	12	11

Table II. CFC values in groups examined

	CFC ml/100 ccm/ min/mm Hg $\varnothing \pm SE$	P difference from control group
Control	0.005759 ± 0.000751	
Potential diabetics	0.003180 ± 0.000446	0.01
Manifest diabetics	0.003155 ± 0.000368	0.01

When comparing CFC values obtained in cases with 2nd degree retinopathy with those obtained in diabetics with normal retina, no significant differences could be proved.

In the vascular reflexes, we have found a high percentage of abnormal responses (inversed vasodilator responses, transitory responses or no responses) in both potential and manifested diabetics (Fig. 1). Whereas abnormal responses in normal healthy controls occur only in 19.8 per cent of cases, in potential and manifested diabetics these responses are significantly increased to 64.1 and 67.9 per cent, respectively. Throughout the course of diabetes there was an increase in the frequency of no reactivity within the category of abnormal response. Comparison of all the values is given in Table III.

Discussion

Our finding of decreased CFC values in both potential and manifest diabetics is surprising considering the high capillary

permeability values recently found in diabetics by other methods of investigation based upon clearance of radioactive compounds (*Parwing* 1976). This discrepancy can be explained by the fact that CFC could be an expression of the total surface of the filtrating capillaries rather than of their permeability. The decrease in the total surface of the filtrating capillaries could be a result of a partial or complete constriction of a certain number of precapillary sphincters as a result of increased vasomotor tone (*Dvořáková and Figar*, 1977). Therefore, we feel that the decreased CFC values found by us are rather of a functional than of an organic nature and do not originate in thickening of the

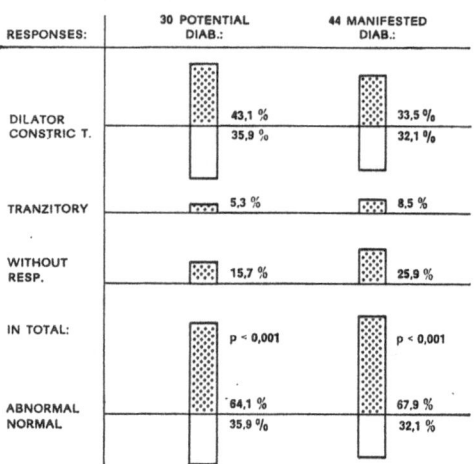

Fig. 1. Vascular responses in potential and manifest diabetics.

Table III. Comparison of the CFC values and abnormal vascular responses in potential and manifest diabetics and in healthy people

	CFC	abnorm. vascular responses
potential diabetics	0.003180 ± 0.000446	64.1%
manifest diabetics	0.003155 ± 0.000368	67.9%
healthy	0.005759 ± 0.000751	19.8%

basal membrane of the capillary wall. Our opinion is based on a completely negative finding on retinal capillaries in all our potential diabetics, whose CFC values decreased by the same amount as in manifest diabetics. Provided that diabetic microangiopathy develops as an universal process in all the capillaries of the body (*Syllaba*, 1973), we can take the state of the retinal capillaries as an indication of the state of the capillaries in all tissues. Futhermore, the decreased CFC values observed obviously do not correspond to the state of metabolism, because they were equal both in potential diabetics with normal and pathological glucose tolerance and in manifest diabetics with all degrees of control.

On the other hand, our findings of equally altered vasomotor responses in potential and manifest diabetics support our hypothesis of principally neural origin of the decreased CFC values in both types. All our present findings suggest that the neural tissue is attacked by the diabetic process earlier than capillaries. It seems that our results show a general process of changed neurocirculatory control independent of the state of metabolism, which is characteristic for all the stages of diabetes mellitus.

REFERENCES

Dvořáková, L., Figar, Š. (1977): Kapilární filtrace u cukrovky. Čas. lék. čes. 116, 814—817.

Parwing, H. H. (1976): Increased microvascular permeability to plasma proteins in short- and long-term juvenile diabetics. Diabetes 25, 884—889.

Syllaba, J. (1973): Diabetická mikroangiopatie. Diabetes mellitus, ed. Foit R., Syllaba J., Praha, Avicenum, 322—347.

L. D., Charles University School of Pediatrics, Vlašská 36, 118 33 Prague 1, Czechoslovakia

MUSCULAR BIOPSY IN DIABETIC MICROANGIOPATHY

E. PONTE, S. B. CURRI, R. VELARI and F. S. FERUGLIO

*Institute of Medical Clinic and Therapy, University of Trieste,
Centre of Molecular Biology, Milan, Italy*

The study of microcirculation in skeletal muscular tissue has always been of great interest in diabetes (*Bencosome et al.*, 1966, *Siperstein et al.*, 1968, *Vracko R.*, 1970, *Williamson et al.*, 1977). We have studied the histological morphology of muscular microcirculation in a large number of diabetic patients in various stages of the disease and also in non-diabetic controls.

Methods

Biopsies were taken from the left femoral quadriceps muscle, according to the "Bergström technique" (*Bergström J.*, 1962). These specimens were examined using an optic microscope.

There were 148 subjects (79 males and 69 females) with an average of 61 years for males, and 62.4 for females, with a range from 19 to 87 years. There were 49 non-diabetic, 10 prediabetic, 17 chemical and 78 clinical diabetic patients all together. The clinical diabetics were divided into different stages of the illness which are:

0—1 year	24 cases	17 male	7 female
1—5 years	9 cases	2 male	7 female
5—10 years	12 cases	6 male	6 female
10 years	33 cases	13 male	20 female

Results

Morphology in normal patients in the regulation of muscular microcirculation consists of:
a) capillary sphincters, in the conjunctiva or in the mesentery.
b) endo-arterial block-mechanisms, that are essentially of two types: 1) cushioned block-mechanisms with a large base, 2) polypoid peduncular block-mechanisms, that are round and long.

The third aspect of blood flow regulation is represented by an arrangement of muscular fibres in the arterial walls, with one external circulary layer and two or three longitudinal ones inside (as described by *Curri* 1972) in the arterioles of digital pulp.

Pathology in diabetes: It is possible to distinguish different stages of evolution:

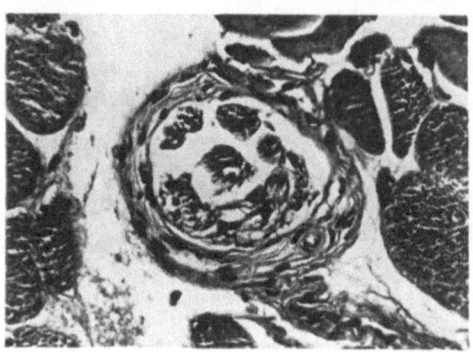

Fig. 1. e. e. ×180.

1) the oedema in the cushion (in the penis — *Rotter and Schuermann*, 1950) with disarrangement of muscular cells. The same phenomenon applies to the medial layer, but is not necessarily present.

2) the lysis of muscular cells that liquidify, as well as the destruction of smooth muscular cells of the cushion. (Fig. 1).

3) the replacement of the latter structures by connective tissue, presumably from the intima (and perhaps from fibrils produced from indifferentiated smooth muscular cells) (Fig. 2). This stage evolves in massive sclerosis with or without fixed reduction (Fig. 3).

Tortuosity and small enlargements with occasional aneurysm sacs can be found in the capillaries.

There are also wall enlargements in the venular efferential system.

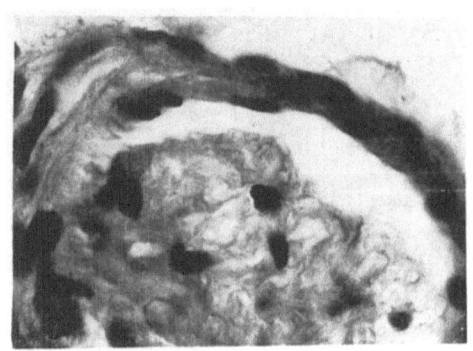

Fig. 2. P.A.S. × 1000.

Conclusions

We have found the presence of endo-arterial block-mechanisms in the muscle. We have observed normal findings and also abnormal ones in diabetic patients according to the evolution of the illness and of the patients' age (*Tischendorf and Curri*, 1974/75). As a result of the abnormalities found, there are profound changes of the microcirculatory blood flow of the muscle in movement or at rest. In red blood cells the blood pressure, stasis, and, presumably, sludging, have a negative effect on the morphological aspect of the endothelium and the basal membrane below. This can perhaps explain the presence of microaneurysms, capillary and venular enlargements. The whole blood circulation appears to have slowed down with stasis in the capillary and venular territories. It is important for us to find microvacuoles in the sarcoplasm during the lysis of muscular cells, when in liquidification. This aspect is similar to that found in the medial segment of the arterio-venous anastomosis of the digital pulp (typical sign of diabetes according to *Curri and Merlen*, 1975).

In conclusion, the problem of the diabetic microangiopathy in the muscular microcirculation appears to be more complex than so far realized. Block-mechanisms and basal membrane thickening are correlated with the profound alteration of the circulatory haemodynamics.

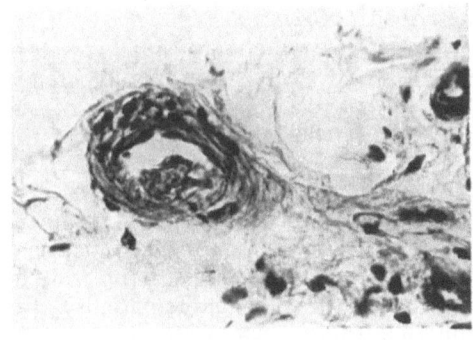

Fig. 3. P.A.S. × 250.

REFERENCES

Bencosme S. A., West R. O., Kerr J. W., Wilson D. L. (1966): Diabetic capillary angiopathy in human skeletal muscles. Am. J. Med. 40, 67.

Bergström J. (1962): Muscle electrolytes in man. Scand. J. Clin. Lab. Invest. 14 (Suppl. 68)

Curri S. B. (1972): The diagnostic significance of the fingertip biopsy in microangiopathies. Bibl. Anat. 11, 310.

Curri S. B., Merlen J. F. (1975): Histoangiopathies ou microangiopathies? Discussion nosologique. J. Scien. Méd. Lille 93, 255.

Gorgas K., Böck P., Tischendorf F., Curri S. B. (1977): The fine structure of human digital arterio-venous anastomoses (Hoyer-Grosser's Organs). Anat. Embryol. 150, 269.

Rotter W., Schuermann R. (1950): Die Blutgefaesse des menschliechen Penis. Virch. Arch. 318, 352.

Tischendorf F., Curri S. B. (1974/75(: The senile involution of arterio-venous anastomoses. Bioch. experimen. Biol. 11, 207.

Siperstein M. D., Unger R. H., Madison L. L. (1968): Studies of muscle capillary basement membranes in normal subjects, diabetic, and prediabetic patients. J. Clin. Invest. 47, 1973.

Vracko R. (1970): Skeletal muscle capillaries in diabetics. A quantitative analysis. Circulation 41, 271.

Williamson J. R.. Kilo C. (1977): Current status of capillary basement-membrane disease in diabetes mellitus. Diabetes 26, 65.

E. P., Via Monte Canino 3, 34149 Trieste, Italia

REACTIVE HYPEREMIA UNDER PLETHYSMOGRAPHIC CONTROL IN THE EARLY DIAGNOSIS OF DIABETES

J. MC COOK, A. ALDAMA, C. LÓPEZ, A. FERNÁNDEZ and S. MATEO.

Institute of Angiology; City of Havana, Cuba

It has been recognized (*Bloodworth*, 1963; *Berkman and Rifkin*, 1966) that microangiopathy may precede the clinical onset of diabetes and that the majority of early cases, and perhaps those of pre-diabetes, have a thickened basal membrane. The existence of a functional microangiopathy and its possibility to occur very early and sometimes before degenerative changes take place has been described (*Ditzel*, 1968; *Lundbaek*, 1971) and even that retraction of small vessels is abnormal after a postischemic hyperemia (*Christensen*, 1971). The objectives of our study are aimed at the appraisal of the efficacy of reactive hyperemia induced by temporary arterial occlusion and performed under plethysmographic control for the determination of the functional behaviour of microvessels of the foot in subjects with a high potentiality for suffering from diabetes mellitus.

Materials and methods

For the achievement of these objectives, 15 prediabetic cases (9 males and 6 females) descendant from diabetic parents were studied and also an equal number of normal subjects with similar ages and the condition of having no diabetic relatives. An oral glucose tolerance test sensitized with prednisone was performed in all the prediabetic cases. The reactive hyperemia test after 5 minutes of arterial flow arrest was used for the evaluation of vascular capacity and reactivity and the photoelectric plethysmography method for recording its results at the level of the first right toe during the following 7 minutes. In each one of the plethysmographic readings we measured: the time elapsed from decompression to the beginning of hyperemia or latency period (L. P.) and to the moment it reaches its maximum intensity (M. H.); the time elapsed from the beginning of hyperemia to the moment of maximum intensity or ascending hyperemia (A. H.) and to normalization or total duration (T. D.) and the time elapsed from the moment of maximum hyperemia to normalization or descending hyperemia (D. H.). The differences observed were appraised by means of the statistical t-Student test.

Results

A highly significant difference between the male and female control groups was observed (Graph I) specially concerning the ascending (p −0.01) and the maximum hyperemia periods (p −0.001) so we made

GRAPH I

DISTRIBUTION OF CASES (CONTROLS AND PREDIABETICS), MALES AND FEMALES, ACCORDING TO LATENCY AND ASCENDING PERIODS OF HYPEREMIA AND DIFFERENCES STATISTICALLY SIGNIFICANTS

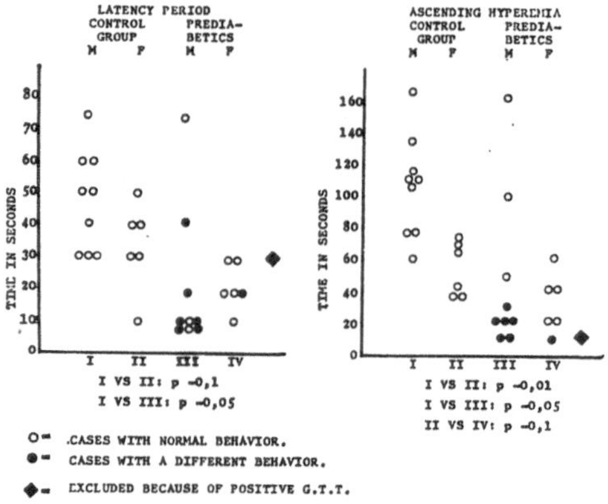

I VS II: p −0,1
I VS III: p −0,05

I VS II: p −0,01
I VS III: p −0,05
II VS IV: p −0,1

O= CASES WITH NORMAL BEHAVIOR.
●= CASES WITH A DIFFERENT BEHAVIOR.
◆= EXCLUDED BECAUSE OF POSITIVE G.T.T.

the comparison, taking into account the greater number of observations, between the male cases only. The differences between these two groups were found not only in the latency period and in the ascending and (Graph II) maximum hyperemia (p −0.05) but specially in the descending period and the total duration (p −0.01) as well (Graph III). The prediabetic cases that showed an abnormal behaviour and to which the

GRAPH II

DISTRIBUTION OF CASES (CONTROLS AND PREDIABETICS), MALES
AND FEMALES, ACCORDING TO MAXIMUM AND DESCENDING HYPEREMIA
PERIODS AND DIFFERENCES STATISTICALLY SIGNIFICANTS

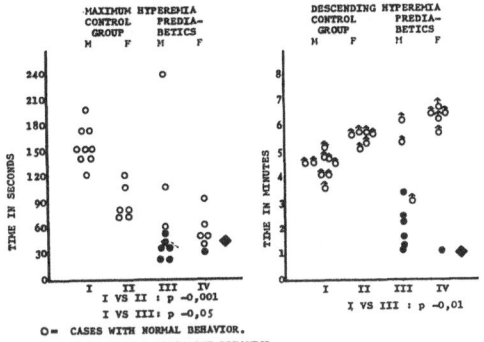

O= CASES WITH NORMAL BEHAVIOR.
●= CASES WITH A DIFFERENT BEHAVIOR.

◆= EXCLUDED BECAUSE OF A POSITIVE G.T.T.

Discussion

We suggest to be in possession of enough evidence to think that the pattern of abnormal behaviour identified consisting in a reduction of the ascending (less than 40 seconds) as well as of the maximum hyperemias (less than 60 seconds) and particularly of the descending period (less than $3^1/_2$ minutes) and the total duration of hyperemia (less than 4 minutes) is intimately related to the functional alterations found at the arteriolocapillary level consecutive or prior to hyalinization and thickening of the basal membrane. Since these phenomena may precede the disorder of carbohydrate metabolism, such pattern would become a tool of the greatest value for early diagnosis not only of diabetes in potential cases but also of microangiopathy itself in already known cases. Nevertheless, we consider that the follow-up study of our cases will dictate the final verdict on this matter. Though prediabetic cases selected for this study are at a greater risk of suffering the illness and perhaps the microangiopathy, they result relatively insignificantly within the great world of potential diabetes towards which the utilization of the method must be directed if we wish to be really useful from a social viewpoint. Finally, we should point out that clinical practice teaches us that the realization of a diagnosis generates, almost in all instances, a therapeutical responsibility. The reactive hyperemia test would permit an appraisal of the efficacy of the procedures used with the purpose of arresting, reverting or preventing diabetic microangiopathy at this localization.

differences encountered were imputable had as common features: a marked lowering of each of the mentioned parameters: A.H., M.H., D.H. and T.D. One case among the prediabetic females showed the same abnormal behaviour stated above and the whole group coincided with another case excluded from this study when a latent diabetes was detected by means of the G.T.T.

GRAPH III

DISTRIBUTION OF CASES (CONTROLS AND PREDIABETICS),
MALES AND FEMALES, ACCORDING TO THE TOTAL DURATION OF
HYPEREMIA. DIFFERENCES STATISTICALLY SIGNIFICANTS.

TOTAL DURATION

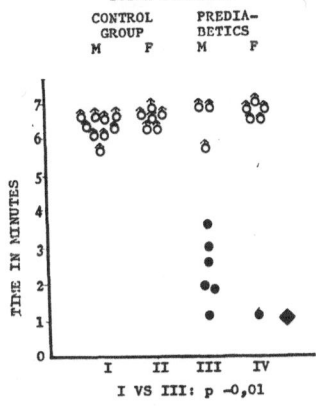

I VS III: p −0,01

O= CASES WITH A NORMAL BEHAVIOR.
●= CASES WITH DIFFERENT BEHAVIOR.

◆= EXCLUDED BECAUSE OF A POSITIVE G.T.T.

Conclusions

1. The reactive hyperemia test under plethysmographic control resulted an efficient mean for finding out the capacity and reactivity of microvessels of the foot and hence for offering information concerning their functional alterations. Highly significant differences between male cases of the control group and the prediabetics

439

were found in the following parameters: descending period and total duration of hyperemia (p −0.01) as well as in the ascending and maximum hyperemias (p−0.05).

2. Prediabetic cases that showed an abnormal behaviour had a characteristic pattern consisting in a marked reduction of the parameters previously described that presumably corresponds with diabetic microangiopathy, in which case an outstanding place should be awarded to the reactive hyperemia test in the early diagnosis of diabetes. The necessity is stated for future studies in larger groups of potentially diabetic populations.

REFERENCES

Berkman F. and Rifkin H. (1966): Newer aspects of diabetic microangiopathy. Ann. Rev. of Med. 17, 83—112.
Bloodworth, J.M.B. (1963): Diabetic microangiopathy. Diabetes 12, 2.
Christensen, J. (1971): Cit. by Lundbaek.

Ditzel, J. (1968): Functional microangiopathy in diabetes mellitus. Diabetes 17, 388—397.
Lundbaek, K. et al. (1971): The pathogenesis of diabetic angiopathy and growth hormone. Danish Med. Bull. 19. 1.

J. McC., Inst. of Angiology, Calz. del Cerro 1551, City of Havana, Cuba

CAPILLARY FUNCTIONS IN VASCULAR DISEASES

K. ROZTOČIL, I. PŘEROVSKÝ and I. OLIVA

Institute of Clinical and Experimental Medicine, Prague, Czechoslovakia

Clinical consideration in chronic arterial and venous diseases seems to be limited only to the large vessels. Nevertheless, the microcirculation is an integral component of the total cardiovascular system and can be involved either primarily or secondarily in a wide variety of clinical conditions. For these reasons, we tried to follow capillary functions in patients with occlusive arterial diseases and in those with chronic venous insufficiency.

The study was performed by measurement of the capillary diffusion capacity and capillary filtration rate. For measuring the capillary diffusion capacity we used the tissue clearance method of *Lassen* (1967), based on observations of the disappearance curves of two isotopes after injection into hyperaemic tissue. 133-xenon as a flow-limited and 131-I as a diffusion-limited tracer were used in our measurements.

The capillary filtration rate was assessed by the standard method of venous occlusion plethysmography using a mercury-in-rubber strain-gauge plethysmograph. The venous occlusion of 60 mm Hg was produced for 5 minutes and the filtration rate was calculated from the obtained volume changes (*Kitchin*, 1963).

These investigations were carried out in 18 patients with obliterating atherosclerosis and in 23 patients with chronic venous insufficiency. Investigations in 13 subjects without cardiovascular disease served as a control.

The mean capillary diffusion capacity in patients with arterial occlusions was significantly increased and the mean capillary filtration rate was not different compared with control findings (*Roztočil et al.*, 1975). The mean capillary diffusion capacity in patients with chronic venous insufficiency attained a value not differing significantly from that for the controls. The mean capillary filtration rate was significantly lower in these patients than in the control group.

The capillary diffusion capacity and capillary filtration rate represent different aspects of capillary permeability. Capillary diffusion capacity changes can reflect alterations either in available capillary surface area or in its permeability. As capillary filtration is determined almost exclusively by the surface area of the microvascular bed, simultaneous investigation of both these parameters can differentiate between the permeability and surface area changes. In patients with obliterating atherosclerosis we suggested that higher values of the capillary diffusion capacity could correspond to an increase in the capillary permeability. A decreased capillary filtration rate in patients with chronic venous insufficiency could be explained by reduced capillary surface area and then it must be determined if the normal capillary diffusion capacity reflects increased microvascular permeability.

It is more probable that both findings in patients with atherosclerosis as well as in venous insufficiency do not involve a primary affliction of the capillaries. It should be noted that adaptational changes oriented against the edema formation in one case and towards an increase in metabolism under conditions of inadequate blood flow in the second might be involved.

K. R., Institute of Clinical and Experimental Medicine, Vídeňská 800, Praha 4, Czechoslovakia

ABOUT THE DIABETIC MICROANGIOPATHY AND MACROANGIOPATHY

K. BUGÁR-MÉSZÁROS

István Hospital, Budapest, Hungary

The opinion that diabetic micro-angiopathy exists only in the retina and in the kidney is nowadays already untenable. Its occurrence in the extremities is also verified by own experience.

We have investigated the arteriolar system of the finger by registrating the reactive warming up of the skin according to the principle of *Herzog*, using the modificated method of *Burgár-Meszáros and Okos*. We got pathologic data in 42 percent of diabetic patients, which allows the conclusion that the arteriolae are in a narrowed state in many cases. In skin capillaries I found as an early change, dilatation of the connective part of the capillary loop by capillarmicroscope in 71 percent of adult diabetics as published already by *Weiss* and *Jürgensen*. We also found it in 66 percent of diabetic children aged between 3 and 16 (*Barta, Bugár-Meszáros, Okos, Rosta*). On examining the blood pressure of the skin vessels according to the method of *Herzog* we got pathologic low data in about half of the patients in harmony with the original examinations of *Herzog*. In 43 percent of our diabetic patients, suffering from occlusive arterial disease, we found the resistance of the capillaries low, which shows a close pathogenetic connection between the undoubtedly diabetogenic microangiopathy and the arteriopathy of diabetics. This connection seems to be manifested also by the fact that the diabetic retinopathy is more frequent among the arteriopathic diabetics, than among the diabetics without arteriopathy.

Apart from the angiochemical investigations of *Max Bürger, Hevelke, Randerath, Dietzel and other authors*, there are also clinical data demonstrating, that the occlusive arterial disease of the diabetic patients is not identical with arteriosclerosis obliterans and could maintain the denomination "angiopathia" or "macroangiopathia diabetica".

It is very important that the man-women ratio is greatly different between the patients suffering from arteriosclerosis obliterans and from macroangiopathia diabetica. Among 1565 arteriosclerotic patients we had only 279 women, which is only 17.8%, but among 222 patients suffering from diabetic macroangiopathy we had 101 women, to say 45.5 percent.

The diabetic macroangiopathy is not connected to age. We have observed it in a boy of 17 and in a woman, whose toe became gangrenous at the age of 21, after insulin-therapy of 5 years. It is interesting, that her retinopathy arose only at the age of 26, also her macroangiopathy preceeded her microangiopathy. Among our 222 macroangiopathic patients there were 11 below 40 years of age, that is 5 percent, but among 1565 patients with arteriosclerosis obliterans there was only one patient (0.06%).

We also observed a difference between the two diseases in the quality of the gangrene. Among 52 diabetic gangrene of the toes there were 50 humid ones in contrast with the arteriosclerotic gangrene which is in general dry.

Though between the arteriosclerosis obliterans and the macroangiopathia diabetica there are important differences, the atherosclerotic process probably may have also a role in the origin of the latter one. In this relation it is remarkable that the cholesterol and the total lipids of the blood serum are high also in macroangiopathia diabetica, moreover they are on the average higher, than in arteriosclerosis obliterans. The average difference between our group of 494 occlusive arterio-sclerotic patients and of 94 diabetic macro-angiopathic patients was 10 percent in relation of cholesterol and 25,8 percent in relation of total lipids.

REFERENCES

Barta, L., Bugár-Mészáros, K., Okos, G., Rosta, G. (1962): Über die Auswirkung der kindlichen Zuckerkrankheit auf das Gefässsystem. Acta Paediat. Hung. 3, 71.

Bugár-Mészáros, K., Okos, G. (1954): Untersuchung der Arteriolen mittels einer neuen Methodik der Messung der reaktiven Erwärmung. Acta Med. Acad. Scient. Hung. 5, 47—57.

Bürger, M. (1954): Angiopathia diabetica. Thieme. Stuttgart.

Herzog, F. (1941): Messung der reaktiven Erwärmung der Haut zur Funktionsprüfung der Arteriolen. Klin. Wschr. 20, 20.

Hevelke, A. (1958): Angiochemische Gefässver- änderungen beim Diabetes mellitus. III. Kongr. Internat. Diabetes Federation, Düsseldorf Thieme. Stuttgart.

Jürgensen, E. (1918): Mikrokapillarbeobacht-ungen und Puls der kleinsten Gefässe. Z. klin. Med. 86, 410.

Randerath, E., Dietzel, P. B. (1958): Morpho-logische Pathologie der extrarenalen Angio-pathie beim Diabetes mellitus. III. Kongr. Internat. Diabetes Federation, Düsseldorf 1958. Verh. Thieme, Stuttgart 1959.

Weiss E. (1916): Beobachtungen und mikro-photographische Darstellung der Hautkapil-laren am lebenden Menschen. Dtsch. Arch. klin. Med. 119. 1.

K. B.-M., István Hospital, IX. Nagyvárad tér 1., 1096 Budapest, Hungary

EXPERIMENTAL INVESTIGATIONS INTO THE 'RISK FACTOR'-SMOKING WITH SPECIAL EMPHASIS ON PLATELET FUNCTION AND BLOOD RHEOLOGY

M. MARSHALL, H. HESS, J. STAUBESAND and J. F. B. DE QUIROS

Med. Policlinic of the University, Munich and Anatom. Institute of the University, Freiburg, F.R.G.

In investigations into the initial effects of smoking, minipigs were exposed to cigarette smoke or CO-air mixtures or nicotine was administered intravenously. The studies were performed on 35 Hanford pigs with a weight of 42 ± 15.6 kg. In the inhalation experiments ($n = 26$) the non-anesthetized pigs were exposed in a smoke chamber to main-current cigarette smoke ($n = 8$) or synthetic air with 150, 200 or 500 ppm CO. In the CO studies the smoke chamber was first flushed with 30 l/min for 15 min and then constantly with 6 l/min of the CO-air mixture. The daily exposure time was 4 hours, the total duration of the experiment between 1 and 16 days. The arteries were removed in metomidate-azaperone anesthesia. For transmission electron microscopy the arteries were perfused in situ under arterial pressure with glutaric aldehyde for 30 min. In 17 experiments nicotine was administered intravenously to 9 non-anesthetized pigs in an average dose of 0.0521 mg/kg.

Results

In the experiments with cigarette smoke, maximum CO concentrations of 80 ppm were reached in the smoke chamber. With CO-air mixtures, concentrations about 80% of the supplied CO concentration were reached.

Humoral findings: The highest COHb values under cigarette smoke were 5%. Values around 10% were attained using CO-air mixtures up to 200 ppm CO; mixtures with 500 ppm CO led to values of about 35%.

The platelet aggregation (own modification of PAT I according to *Breddin*) (*Marshall et al.*, 1976)) increased by 1 step in tests with CO exposure up to 200 ppm CO ($n = 11$; $p < 0.0025$) and with 500 ppm ($n = 9$; $p < 0.05$). Measurements under cigarette smoke showed a rise by $0.5 - 1$ step. Recent investigations showed an increase in platelet adhesivity under cigarette smoke.

On exposure to cigarette smoke, a medium rise in the blood viscosity of 22% ($n = 3$) could be demonstrated. The hematocrit rose by 5.5% ($n = 4$). CO exposure up to 200 ppm caused no significant alteration of blood and plasma viscosity and hematocrit. In contrast, exposure to 500 ppm CO led to a distinct rise in blood viscosity from 3.71 to 4.32 cp ($n = 4$; $p < 0.0125$) and also a smaller rise in the plasma viscosity from 1.55 to 1.61. The hematocrit rose from 32.85 to 36.95 vol% ($n = 4$; $p < 0.0025$).

If compressed air was used instead of CO mixtures, no significant changes of all the humoral parameters could be observed.

After intravenous injections of nicotine there was a significant increase in platelet aggregation, blood and plasma viscosity and hematocrit (Tab. 1). The relative rise in blood viscosity was more pronounced the lower the shear rate.

Scanning electron microscopic findings: On the arterial endothelium no elements of the blood could be demonstrated unless there was irritation. After exposure to cigarette smoke or CO-air mixtures with COHb concentrations corresponding to those of a moderately heavy smoker, platelet adhesions in viscous metamorphosis on the superficially intact endothelium

Table I.

	value before nicotine injection	10	20	30	60 min after injection	(unit)	
PAT 1	1.4 ± 0.66	1.38 ± 0.6	1.57 ± 0.74[2]	1.86 ± 0.97[4]	2.09 ± 0.87[5]	(steps)	
blood viscosity (shear stress 78 sec^{-1})	3.6 ±0.43	3.85[3] ±0.5	3.81 ±0.43	3.92[2] ±0.59	3.85[2] ±0.53	(cp)	(n = 17)
(shear stress 39.6 sec^{-1})	4.12	4.49	4.54	4.76	4.58		
(shear stress 15.6 sec^{-1})	5.28	5.95	5.91	6.47	6.1		
(shear stress 7.8 sec^{-1})	6.63	7.65	7.76	8.38	8.04		
plasma viscosity	1.52 ±0.125	5.56[4] ±0.14	1.56 ±0.13	1.57[2] ±0.14	1.56 ±0.12	(cp)	
haematocrit	33.3 ±4.4	35.3[2] ±53.8	34.2 n.s. ±4.23	33.9 ±4.46	33.8 ±4.75	(vol.%)	
RBC	5.63	5.74	5.74	5.68		$10^6/mm^3$	(n = 3)
haemoglobin	10.93	11.03	11.2	11.0	11.1	g/100 ml	

n.s. = not significant; [1] = $p < 0.05$; [2] = $p < 0.025$; [3] = $p < 0.0125$; [4] = $p < 0.005$; [5] = $p < 0.0025$.

were frequently found. Especially at high CO concentrations there were advanced changes with dense, multilayered platelet incrustations and sometimes fibrin deposition, i.e. mixed microparietal thrombi.

Transmission electron microscopic findings: In preliminary studies adhesions of single platelets on the endothelium could also be observed after CO exposition. Prevailing, these adhesions could be determined by the proximity to an underlying focus of degeneration in the endothelial cell. Such foci could be seen after a single inhalation period.

Discussion

The behaviour of the pigs during the experiments, controls of hematocrit and pulse rate and the lack of changes in the experiments with compressed air indicate that the results cannot be related to stress effects. A striking finding is the different modification of blood viscosity: a marked rise with cigarette smoke and high CO concentrations and no changes at moderate CO concentrations. The rise in the blood viscosity can partly be explained by an increase in the hematocrit; this may well be catecholamine-induced, either as an effect of nicotine (Tab. I) or as a consequence of CO intoxication. An additional increase in viscosity could be explained by an increase in the free fatty acids, in fibrinogen and by changes in the flexibility and aggregation of the red blood cells. Such changes of erythrocyte rheology can be induced by hypoxia and obviously by nicotine (Tab. I).

An important result of these studies in the demonstration of platelet adhesions on a superficially intact appearing arterial endothelium under the influence of cigarette smoke and CO inhalation. Accordingly, CO may well have a decisive importance in inducing the changes described here, even on inhalation of tobacco smoke. Nicotine also influences platelet function (Tab. I).

Our findings lead us to consider a disturbed interaction between the flowing blood and the arterial wall as a crucial mechanism in the genesis of the obliterating arteriopathies induced by inhalation of cigarette smoke and also by other risk factors (*Marshall and Hess*, 1978). The sticking of platelets to the endothelium with the consequent effects initiated by the "release reaction" (*Mustard*, 1967; *Ross and Glomset*, 1973) appears to have a key role in the initial phase.

REFERENCES

Marshall M., De Quiros J. Fdez. B., Hess H. (1976): Wirkung von Nikotin auf Plättchen-aggregation und Blutviskosität beim Miniaturschwein in vivo. Vasa 5, 287.

Marshall M., Hess H. (1978): New findings concerning pathogenesis and nonsurgical treatment of peripheral arterial diseases. Vasa 7, 49.

Mustard J. F. (1967): Recent advances in molecular pathology: a review. Platelet aggregation, vascular injury and atherosclerosis. Exp. Mol. Pathol. 7, 366.

Ross R., Glomset J. A. (1973): Atherosclerosis and the arterial smooth muscle cell. Science 180, 1332.

M. M., Medical Policlinic of the University, Pettenhoferstr. 8a, D-8000 München 2, F.R.G.

VASCULAR DISORDER CAUSED BY VIBRATING TOOLS

F. SANO, A. NISHIMURA, Y. NAKANISHI, Y. MORITA,
Y. AKASAKA, N. UEDA and Y. KASAI

1st Department of Surgery, University of Hokkaido, Sapporo, Japan

In occupational Raynaud's phenomenon caused by vibrating tools, many studies have been made since the early report by *Loriga* in 1911. Since 1966, we have been studying the pathologic conditions in occupational Raynaud's syndrome caused by vibrating tools such as a chain saw. This paper proposes to elucidate the further etiologic mechanism and help to make a diagnosis, based on angiographic findings in the early stages of this disease.

The clinical material comprised 39 patients (76 extremities) with vibration disease including 11 without a previous history of Raynaud's phenomenon and the remaining 28 with a history of Raynaud's phenomenon. Seven patients (11 extremities) with nonoccupational Raynaud's syndrome were also studied. Forty five patients (66 extremities) were selected as a normal control group, which underwent angiography of the upper extremittes for the evaluation of trauma or tumor. In vibration disease, there was no significant difference between the group with a previous history of Raynaud's phenomenon and without a history of Raynaud's phenomenon with respect to age and to the duration of their employment using tolls.

Considering anatomical variations of the palmar arch, based on Coleman's classification, the complete superficial palmar arch was observed in 31 of 76 hands (41.5%) in vibration disease as compared with 50 of 66 hands (75.8%) in the control group. As for the incidence of the complete superficial palmar arch, there was no difference between vibration disease with Raynaud's phenomenon and without Raynaud's phenomenon, and also between the right and left hand. In non-occupational Raynaud's syndrome the complete superficial palmar arch was seen in 10 of 11 hands (90.9%). (Fig. 1). The

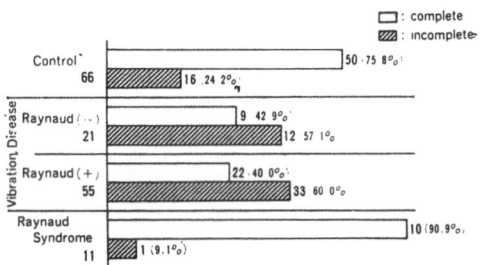

Anatomical Variations of the Superficial Palmar Arch

Fig. 1.

high incidence of complete deep palmar arch was observed in all the groups and this complete type account for more than 90% of all.

In vibration disease, three major changes in the ulnar artery and digital arteries are narrowing and irregularity of the arterial lumen and tortuosity called "kinking". Arterial occlusion or aneurysms were noted in a few cases. Irregularities of the arterial lumen can be divided into three groups: serrated, symmetric, and asymmetric types.

In evaluating the angiographic findings of the proximal ulnar artery, iregularities of the arterial lumen were seen in approximately 20% in all groups without significant difference compared with the control. But kinkings were observed in 52.4% of vibration diseases without Raynaud's phenomenon and 58.2% with Raynaud's phenomenon. The difference was statistically significant compared with 19.7%. of the control. And with the advancement of the disease, the more proximal portion of the artery is prone to be involved. Stenosis at the proximal ulnar artery was seen in few cases.

At the distal ulnar artery, irregularities were observed in 70.9% of vibration

447

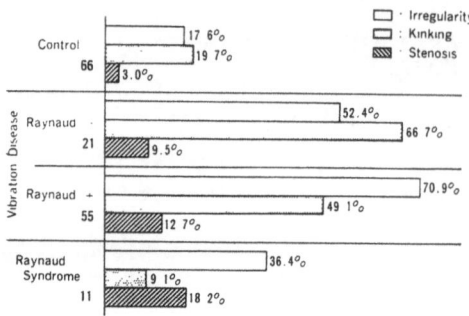

Fig. 2.

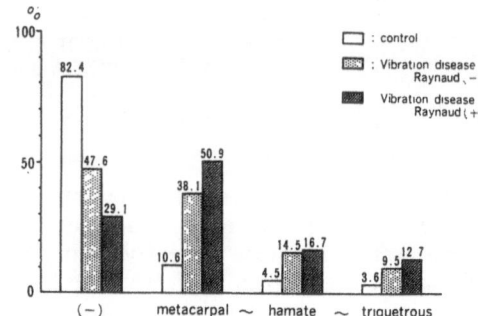

Fig. 3.

diseases with Raynaud's phenomenon and 52.4% without Raynaud's phenomenon and 17.6% of the controls. This figure is statis.ically significant compared with the controls. Kinkings were observed in 49.1% of vibration diseases with Raynaud's phenomenon and 66.7% without Raynaud's phenomenon. This figure is statistically significant compared with 19.7% of the controls. Incidence of stenosis was low in all groups. This was observed in 3.0% of the controls, 9.5% of vibration diseases without Raynaud's phenomenon and 12.7% with Raynaud's phenomenon. There were no significant differences among them. Stenosis seen in vibration diseases with Raynaud's phenomenon was located at the site of the metacrapal bone. In studying in detail the site of irregularities, these were observed most frequently at the site of the metacarpal bone. Irregularities at this site are present in 28 of the 55 hands (50.9%) for vibration disease with Raynaud's phenomenon and 38.1% whitout Raynaud's phenomenon. This figure is statistically high compared with

the control. In addition, at the hamate bone and triquetral bone, these irregularities were seen with a significantly high incidence compared with the control. This incidence correlated with the clinical stage of this disease.

Conclusions

1. In vibration disease with Raynaud's phenomenon caused by vibrating tools, incomplete superficial palmar arch was observed with high incidence. 2. In pathologic changes of the distal ulnar artery, irregularities were most frequently observed at the site from the hamate bone to the fourth metacarpal bone, which occurred in 42.1% of cases. This region is more distal to the area afflicted with Conn's Hypothenar Hammer Syndrome. 3. In cases of third and fourth degree based on Galanina's classification, tortuosities were often observed in the proximal ulnar artery and with the advance of the disease, a more proximal portion of the artery appears to be involved.

REFERENCES

Benedict, K. T. Jr., Chang, W., McCready, F. J. (1974): The hypothenar hammer syndrome. Radiology 111, 57—60.
Nishimura, A., Sano, F., Nakanishi, Y., Koshino, I., Kasai, Y. (1974): Occupational Raynaud's syndrome: Hemodynamic and angiographic characteristics of the upper extremity. Angiologia-VII, 231—240.
Porter, J. M., Snider, R. L., Bardana, E. J., Rösch, J., Eidemiller, L. R. (1975): The diagnosis and treatment of Raynaud's phenomenon. Surgery 77, 11—23.

F. S., Ist Department of Surgery, University of Hokkaido N-15, W-7, Sapporo, Japan

DIGITAL CIRCULATION IN CASES WITH RAYNAUD'S PHENOMENON, AND TREATMENT WITH HYDERGIN

O. THULESIUS and S. L. NIELSEN

Departments of Clinical Physiology, Central Hospital, Växjö, Sweden and Herlev Hospital, Herlev, Denmark

Objective evaluation of vasospastic disorders of the digital circulation is a difficult problem due to labile circulatory changes, which are not readily reproduced in a laboratory situation. Estimation of digital systolic pressure after local cooling of the middle phalanx seems to be a dependable procedure which can be applied quantitatively.

Material and methods

The present investigation applies this method and compares the results with a semi-quantitative evaluation of the severity of the clinical disturbance.

A total of 123 patients was investigated. The characteristics of the population are evident from table I. One hundred patients were screened with pulse plethysmography before and after local cooling of the fingers in a water bath of 15 °C for 10 minutes. Digital pulse curves were recorded from one finger of each hand (one which presented maximal symptoms) using plastic cups applied to the terminal phalanx with a pressure sensing system using air transmission.

Digital systolic arterial pressure was determined using a mercury in-rubber strain gauge, applied to the terminal phalanx in order to sense changes in finger volume and pulsations. The occluding cuff at the middle phalanx was water-filled and could be utilized for local cooling by perfusion with cooled water. To ensure thorough local cooling, the finger circulation was arrested for 5 minutes with another, more proximally applied, tourniquet. Cooling was performed stepwise from 35° to 5° with steps of 5 °C. Control blood pressure was also frequently checked with another cuff and strain gauge applied to an uncooled finger. In addition, the brachial artery pressure was measured using the auscultatory method.

Table II. Effect of chronic treatment with Hydergin on digital artery pressure upon cooling. Improvement was considered if pressure fall was reduced by at least 35 mm Hg.

	improvement	no effect	number of cases
Raynaud (total)	9	8	17
Raynaud with critical closing	4	4	8

Treatment with Hydergin was performed in 6 patients with intramuscular administration and in 17 patients after 5 and thereafter 10 mg orally per day over 3 weeks. The patients were evaluated with digital artery pressure measurement before and after the treatment periods, in the acute study 30 minutes after injection.

Results

The correlations between the objective parameters of pulse curves and finger systolic pressure versus the subjective grading of Raynaud symptoms are given

Table I. Total patient material and subgroups (secondary Raynaud phenomena = = vibration induced)

	n	men/women	mean age	Primary/secondary
Hydergin (0.5 mg) acute	6	6/1	27	0/6
Hydergin (5—10 mg) 3 weeks + 2 weeks	17	11/6	40	6/11
Raynaud screening	100	75/25	44.5	19/81

in Figures 1 and 2. From these diagrams it can be seen that parameter ΔP max is a better and more quantitative discriminator of the severity of the vasospastic circulatory disturbance.

The effect of treatment with Hydergin was therefore exclusively evaluated with the digital pressure technique and this is shown in Figure 3. Figure 3 shows the results of acute administration of 0.5 mg Hydergin given by intramuscular injection. It can be seen that there was no measurable improvement in finger circulation. Chronic administration, however, resulted in marked improvement in about 50% of the cases. Most patients (7 out of 9) responded favourably after 3 weeks treatment with 5 mg Hydergin per day. Increasing the dosage to 10 mg only resulted in further minor changes.

Discussion

Local cooling of the finger in cases with Raynaud's-phenomenon leads to a reproducible reduction in the digital artery pressure, the extent of which seems to be roughly parallel to the severity of the distrubance. In about half of the cases the finger blood pressure was not measurable after cooling to $15-5\ ^\circ C$. This seems to be an example of a critical closing phenomenon, which occurs as a result of enhanced smooth muscle tone.

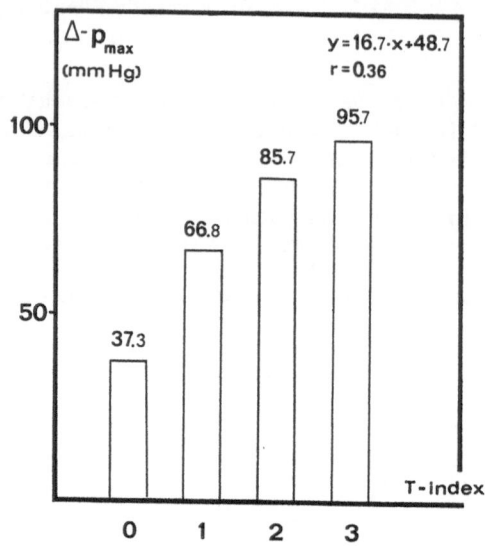

Fig. 2. Grading of severity of vasospastic finger systolic pressure drop ($\Delta - P$ max) versus Taylor index.

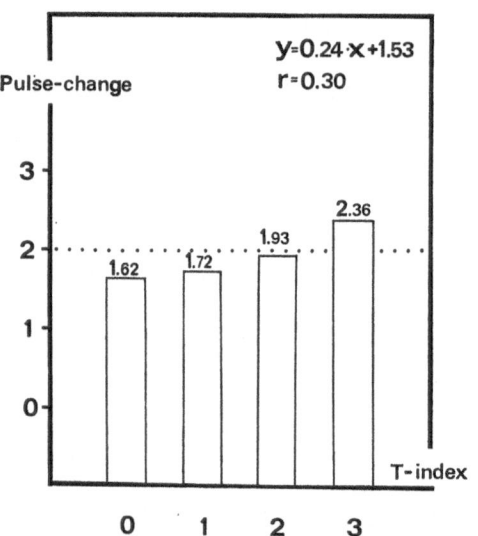

Fig. 1. Grading of severity of vasospastic pulse wave changes versus Taylor index.

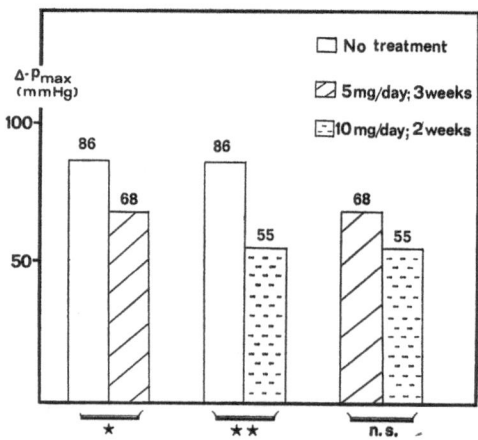

Fig. 3. Result of acute administration of Hydergin, evaluated by finger systolic pressure.

O. T., Dept. Clin. Physiol., Central Hospital, Växsiö, Sweden

GENETIC FACTORS IN TAKAYASU'S DISEASE

I. ISOHISA, F. NUMANO, N. MASHIMO,
M. YAJIMA and H. MAEZAWA

Dept. of Internal Med., Tokyo Medical and Dental University, Tokyo, Japan

Takayasu's disease[1,2] is well known for its characteristic clinical feature of "pulselessness" due to obstructive changes in the vessel wall, mainly the aortic arch and its main branches. Almost all patients suffering from this pathological condition are young females. Epidemiological studies performed in Japan in 1975 confirmed that 2.148 patients had Takayasu's disease and 89% of all patients were female[3]. This disease may be related to racial differences as cases of this pathlogical condition usually occur in Asian or South American contries, with very few incidences in Western countries. The etiology of the disease remains obscure.

Recently we encountered monozygotic twin sisters with Takayasu's diseases.[4] A causative factor which would induce this pathological condition could not be found in either twin. One brother and two sisters of the twins were quite healthy. All these five children were born and raised in the same contryside in Japan. The parents are first cousins.

This case led us to search for genetic factors in the pathogenesis of Takayasu's disease. HLA typing of all familly members was performed using the lymphocyte microcyte toxicity test devised by Terasaki and McClelland(S), using 396 types of anti-HLA sera to determine the haplotype of HLA A11-BW40 in the factor which had been passed to the twins and not to the other three children.

Ten cases, including the above mentioned twin sisters have been reported in Japan as family cases of Takayasu's disease.

Table I.   **HLA Phenotypes in TAKAYASU disease**

A locus		A - 2	A - 9	A -10	A- 11	AW 33
TAKAYASU disease (65)	No. of patients	23/	46/	23/	8/	6 /
	frequency	35.4%	70.7%	35 %	12.3%	9.2 %
JAPANESE (128)		38.3%	64.8%	11.7%	16.4%	0.8 %
χ^2		0.2	0.7	15.3	0.6	8.8
p value				$<10^{-4}$		$10^{-3}<p<10^{-2}$

B locus		B - 5	B - 7	B -12	B -13	BW-15	BW-16	BW-17	BW-22	BW-35	BW-40
TAKAYASU disease (65)	No. of patients	41/	2/	11/	1/	10/	7/	1/	8/	1/	26/
	frequency	63.1%	3.1%	16.9%	1.5%	15.4%	10.7%	1.5%	12.3%	1.5 %	40.0%
JAPANESE (128)		32.0%	16.4%	12.5%	2.3%	11.7%	6.3%	0.8%	14.0%	18.8%	35.9%
χ^2		17.0	7.3	0.7	0.1	0.5	1.2	0.2	0.1	11.3	0.3
p value		$<10^{-4}$	$10^{-3}<p<10^{-2}$							$<10^{-3}$	

451

Parents in 3 families were first cousins. HLA typing of all family members in 6 families was analyzed and we found that an associated haplotype with Takayasu's disease could be predicted at the level of 7.8 in χ^2 test.

Furthermore a population study on HLA analyses of HLA typing for 52 patients with Takayasu's disease was performed and compared with findings in 128 healthy Japanese[6]. Table I shows the phenotypes in a patient with Takaysu's disease. HLA A9, A10, B5 and BW40 were seen with a high frequency in patients with the disease and statistical analysis certified a significantly high frequency of HLA A10 ($P < 10^{-4}$) and B5 ($P < 10^{-4}$) in Takayasu patients as compared with these values in healthy Japanese.

The close association of B5 with Takayasu's disease should be given close attention as the frequency of B5 antigen is high in Japanese, American Indians and South Americans.

To confirm the close association of HLA B5 with Takayasu's disease, the association with BW51 and BW52, subgroups of B5 was studied in 82 patients with Takaysu's disease. There was a significantly high frequency of BW52 as compared with that in 128 healthy Japanese[7] (Table II). These data suggest that a genetic or disease-sensitive factor may play an important role in the pathogenesis of Takaysu's disease.

Table II.

Association between HLA-BW52 and Takayasu disease

	Takayasu Disease (N=82)	Healthy Japanese (N=128)	x^2	cP-value	RR
BW51	12.2% (10)	19.5% (25)	1.94	NS	0.6
BW52	43.9% (36)	12.5% (16)	26.46	cP < 3x10^4	5.5

NS = not significant
cP = corrected P

REFERENCES

1. *Takayasu, M. (1908):* A case with peculiar changes of the central retinal vessels. Acta Soc. Ophthalmol. Jap. (in Japanese) 112: 554.
2. *Ueda, H., Ito, I., Okuda, R., Inoue, G., Yamada, H., Matsuyama, K., Saito, S. and Gondaira, T. (1963):* Jap. Heart. J. 4: 224.
3. Committee report: Clinical and pathological studies of Takayasu's disease. Ministry of Health & Welfare, Japan.
4. *Numano, F., Isohisa, I., Kishi, Y., Arita, M. and Maezawa, H. (1978):* Circulation 58: 173.
5. *Terasaki, P. I. and McClelland, J. D. (1964):* Nature 204: 998.
6. *Numano, F., Kochi, K., Arita, M., Tamaki, H., Numano, F., Maezawa, H. (1976):* J. Jap. Soc. Int. Med. 65: 34.
7. *Isohisa, I., Numano, F., Maezawa, H., and Sasazuki, T. (1978):* Tissue Antigens: in press.

F. N., Dept. of Int. Med., Tokyo Med. and Dental Univ., Yushima-1, Bunkyo-ku, Tokyo 113, Japan

INCREASED VASCULAR PERMEABILITY IN DEVELOPING COLLATERAL PATHWAYS OF RABBITS AFTER FEMORAL ARTERY LIGATION

A. SEKI, T. TANAKA, S. TOMONO and J. FUJII

Institute for adult diseases. Asahi life foundation. Tokyo, Japan.

Introduction

An increase in the vascular permeability of arterioles plays an important role for developing hypertensive vascular disease. During our recent study on vascular lesions in rabbits with two − kidney Goldblatt hypertension, we by chance found an increase in the vascular permeability of the peri-ureteric collateral arteries. These observations have led us to the hypothesis that vascular permeability increases in developing collateral arteries. Little is known about vascular permeability of the collateral vessels. The present study was carried out to verify our hypothesis.

Methods

Male rabbits weighing 2.0 to 2.5 kg were used. The right femoral artery was occluded by ligation at a proximal site just after bifurcation of the cranial femoral artery in 141 animals and a sham-ligation was performed in 12 animals. Colloidal carbon (Pelican C11/1431a) was injected intravenously at various intervals after ligation. The intervals were 3 hours in 16, 6 hours in 17, one day in 36, 2 to 3 days in 20, 6 to 8 days in 21 and 14 to 180 days in 31 animals. Colloidal carbon was also injected in 6 animals 6 hours and in 6 animals one day after sham-ligation. All animals were killed from 2 hours to 7 days after injection of colloidal carbon. Collateral vessels, corresponding arterial trees of contra-lateral legs and those of legs with sham-ligation were dissected, and were examined grossanatomically and microscopically. An increase in the vascular pemeability was identified by the presence of visible carbon deposits on the vascular walls. Postmortem angiography was carried out in 25 animals using barium sulphate.

Results

Prominent collateral arteries extended from the internal iliac, the deep femoral and the cranial femoral artery.

Carbon deposits were frequently found on developing collateral arteries when colloidal carbon had been injected within a few days after ligation. Collateral arteries on the sciatic nerve were the most favourable site for detecting carbon deposits. (Fig. 1). Carbon deposits were occasionally found on the intramuscular small arteries of the thigh, which were components of the collateral system. (Fig. 2). Carbon deposits were found on limited segments of the collateral pathways. Observation through a magnifying glass revealed that they were situated in small arteries of 0.1 to 0.3 mm in diameter which were intermediate segments of the collateral system and they appeared as a ring-like arrangement. (Fig. 2). Larger arteries which were the stem or the re-entrant segments of the collateral system were free of carbon deposits.

Microscopic observation demonstrated that the carbon particles were situated on the arterial wall. (Fig. 3). The arteries

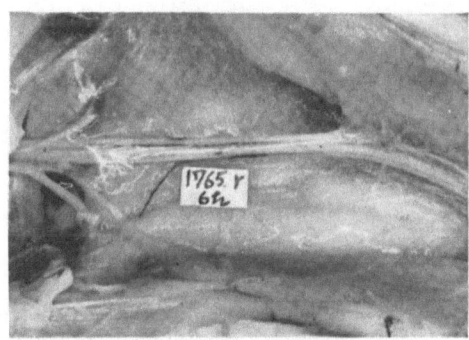

Fig. 1. Visible deposits of carbon on small arteries of collateral pathways along the sciatic nerve. This animal was treated with colloidal carbon 6 hours after ligation of the femoral artery and was killed the next day.

with carbon deposits also showed various structural changes, such as fragmentation of the internal elastic layer, degeneration of the medial muscle and deposition of fibrinoid material. (Fig. 3).

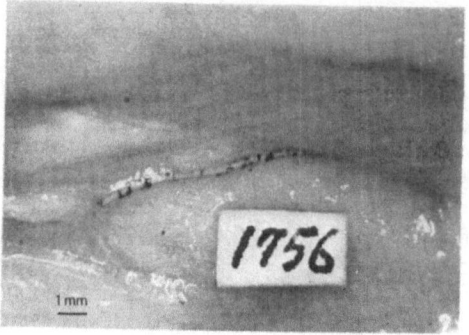

Fig. 2. Ring-like arrangements of carbon deposits on an intramuscular artery. This animal was treated with colloidal carbon one day after ligation of the femoral artery and was killed 2 hours later.

The presence of visible carbon deposits indicated that the arterial endothelia were permeable to colloidal carbon at the time of colloidal carbon injection. As mentioned above, carbon deposits were frequently found on developing collateral arteries.

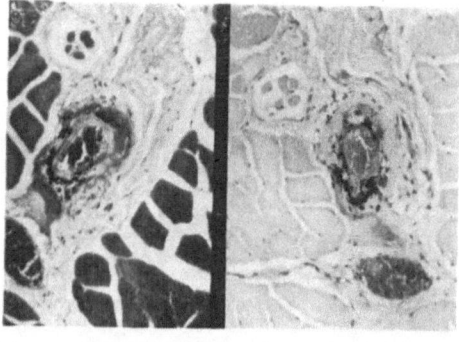

Fig. 3. Carbon deposits, fragmentation of the internal elastic layer, degeneration of the medial muscle cells and deposition of fibrinoid material in a small intramuscular artery of an animal which was treated with colloidal carbon one day after ligation of the femoral artery and was killed 2 hours later.
right: H. E. stain. left: Masson-Weigert's stain.

On the other hand, there were no carbon deposits on any of established collateral arteries when colloidal carbon had been injected more than 14 days after ligation of the femoral artery. These established collateral arteries showed marked thickening of the vascular walls as a result of fibrocellular hyperplasia.

The incidence of animals with increased vascular permeability of the collateral arteries at various times after ligation of the femoral artery is as follows: the increase in vascular permeability observed in 3 of 16 animals after 3 hours, in 15 of 17 animals after 6 hours, in 32 of 36 animals after one day, in 16 of 20 animals after 2 to 3 days, but only in 5 of 21 animals after 6 to 8 days and in none of 31 animals more than 14 days after ligation.

Discussion

The present study demonstrated that vascular permeability of developing collateral arteries started to increase almost immediately after ligation of the femoral artery, reached a peak within one day, remained increased for several days and returned to normal later.

Recently, much attention has been focused on the role of vasodilatation in the pathogenesis of hypertensive vascular disease. (*Giese*, 1964., *Wiener*, 1969., *Jellinek*, 1969). Several investigators have reported that dilated segments of arteries were permeable to colloidal carbon in experimental hypertensive animals. (*Giese*, 1964., *Goldby*, 1972).

The increase in vascular permeability of developing collateral arteries can be more simply accounted for by the vasodilatation theory than with hypertensive vascular disease. The increase in the vascular permeability was limited to the intermediate segments of the collateral pathway which have been described as the segments with the most striking vasodilatation. (*Longland*, 1953).

Morphological observations of the collateral arteries have been reported (*Eriksson*, 1970., *Borgers*, 1970), but the

early changes have not been fully elucidated. The present study pointed out that
increased vascular permeability and the
structural changes of developing collateral arteries took place a few days after
ligation of the femoral artery.

REFERENCES

Borgers, M., Schaper, J. and Schaper, W. (1970):
Acute vascular lesions in developing coronary
collaterals. Virchows Arch. A. Pathol. Anat.
351: 1.

Eriksson, I. (1970): Histology of collateral arteries. Scand. J. Thor. Cardiovasc. Surg. 4: 231.

Giese, J. (1964): Acute hypertensive vascular
disease. 2. Studies on vascular reaction patterns and permeability changes by means of
vital microscopy and colloidal tracer technique. Acta Pathol. Microbiol. Scand. 62: 497.

Goldby, F. S. and Leilin, L. J. (1972): Relationship between arterial pressure and the permeability of arterioles to carbon particles in acute
hypertension in the rat. Cardiovasc. Res. 6:
384.

*Jellinek, H., Nagy, Z., Huttner, I., Balint, A. and
Kerenyi, T. (1969):* Investigation of the permeability changes of the vascular wall in
malignant hypertension by means of colloidal
iron preparation. Brit. J. exp. Pathol. 50: 13.

Longland, C. J. (1953): The collateral circulation
of the limb. Ann. Roy. Coll. Surg. Engl. 13: 161.

*Wiener, J., Lattes, R. G., Meltzer, B. G. and
Spiro, D. (1969):* The cellular pathology of
experimental hypertension. 4. Evidence for
increased vascular permeability. Amer. J.
Pathol. 54: 187.

*A. S., Institute for Adult Diseases. Asahi Life Foundation,
Shinjuku-ku Nishishinjuku 1-9-14, Tokyo 160, Japan*

VASCULAR REACTIVITY IN SKIN AND MUSCLE AFTER MYOCARDIAL INFARCTION

EVA KELLEROVÁ, MARGITA KITTOVÁ and S. CAGÁŇ

Institute of Normal and Pathological Physiology, Slovak Academy of Sciences and Department of Medicine, Municipal Hospital, Bratislava, Czechoslovakia

Introduction

Several studies have differentiated subjects with coronary heart disease from healthy people by an increased humoral response to adrenergic stimuli. The peripheral circulation which is of clinical relevance and in man represents a sensitive indicator of sympathetic discharge, was investigated only in acute cardiac emergencies. These studies revealed constriction of resistance and capacitance vessels in the calf and hand in the acute phase of myocardial infarction. There is no information on the peripheral vasomotor reactivity of subjects who had suffered from myocardial infarction. The present study was undertaken to examine the response of resistance and capacitance vessels of skin and muscle and of blood pressure to procedures which stimulate the sympathetic system.

Materials and methods

Studies were performed in 45 patients — men, ranging in age from 24 to 53 years (mean 41.6 ± 7.5 years) who had sustained a myocardial infarction 1—36 months previously. None of them manifested clinical evidence of overt congestive heart failure. Vasoactive drugs, if used, were discontinued several days prior to the study. 20 healthy subjects similar in age represented the control group.

All subjects were investigated in a supine position at rest and during vasomotor reactions to deep breathing and to mental arithmetic. The blood flow in skin (hand) and muscle (forearm) measured by venous occlusion plethysmography and local vascular resistance calculated by means of simultaneously registered blood pressure values, were used as indicators of the resistance vessel reactivity. The reactivity of the capacitance vessels in the skin was assessed as an absolute value of voluminal change of the investigated segment, which corresponds to the active change in venous tone.

Results

The resting blood pressure values and their variability in patients with MI and in the control group were not significantly different. Nonetheless, during the test of mental arithmetic the lability of systolic blood pressure significantly increased and the customary elevated systolic as well as diastolic blood pressure values (longer than 1 min after MA) was significantly more frequent (P < 0.02) in the group of patients as compared to the controls.

The vasoconstrictor reactions in skin to both stimuli were significantly prolonged

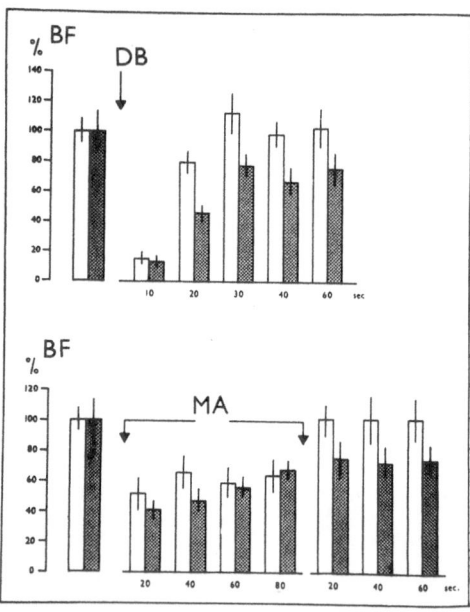

Fig. 1. Changes in skin blood flow following deep breathing (DB) and a test in mental arithmetic (MA) in subjects with coronary heart disease (dotted bars) and in controls (white bars).

456

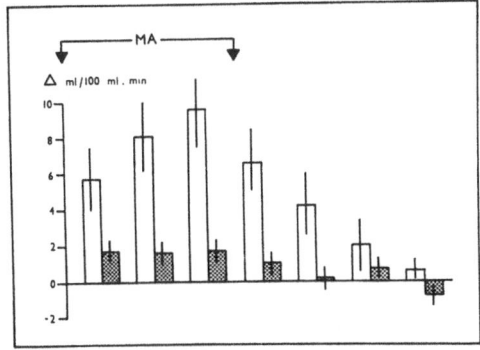

Fig. 2. Changes in muscle blood flow during and after the test of mental arithmetic, measured at 20 sec. intervals. Subjects with coronary heart disease (dotted bars), control subjects (white bars).

after cessation of stimuli in resistance vessels (after DB longer than 50 s; after MA longer than 60 s), as well as in capacitance vessels (after DB longer than 100 s; after MA longer than 110 s) in patients, as compared to the course of the reactions in control subjects: in resistance vessles (30 s after DB; 20 s after MA) (Fig. 1) and in capacitance vessels (60 s DB and 50 s MA) (Fig. 3). The amplitude of the vasoconstrictory reactions in the skin, expressed as the blood flow change (Fig. 1) and or as an absolute volume change (Fig. 3) was significantly greater in subjects after myocardial infarction.

The resting blood flow in the muscle 2.7 ml/100 ml min was significantly ($P < 0.01$) lower in patients than in controls (6.4 ml/100 ml min). The vasodilatatory reaction to the mental arithmetic test was less pronounced and shorter (Fig. 2).

Discussion

Our findings of the preponderance and prolongation of the vasoconstrictory type of reactions in patients after myocardial infarction indicate a general increase in sympathetic discharge to the stimuli of everyday life, perhaps associated with a predominant increase in norepinephrine secretion.

Spontaneous anginal attacks occur frequently with sympathetic nervous discharge. In all these circumstances the prolonged peripheral vasoconstriction to the above-mentioned and other stimuli, by increasing the peripheral resistance, may increase the energy requirements of the heart and aggravate the myocardial ischemia.

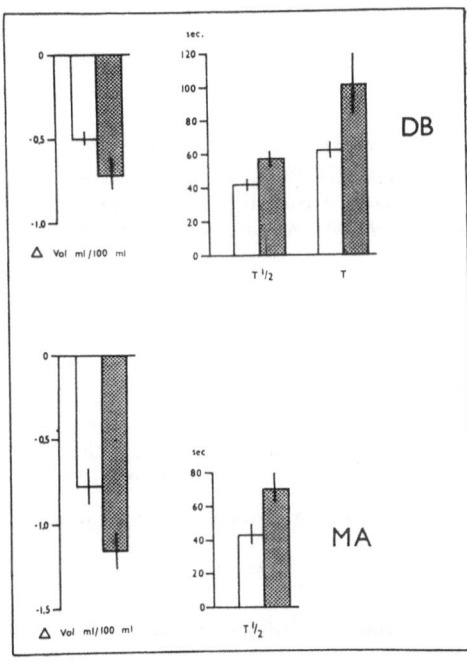

Fig. 3. Response of the capacitance vessels in the skin to deep breathing (DB) and to mental arithmetic (MA), indicated as voluminal changes of the segment (ml/100 ml of tissue). $T_{1/2}$ indicates the time after the reaction, in which 50% of the resting volume of the segment is regained.

E. K., Institute of Normal and Pathological Physiology, Slovak Academy of Sciences, Sienkiewiczova 1, 884 23 Bratislava, Czechoslovakia

ACTION OF PIRACETAM ON SERUM-INDUCED SPASMS IN PIAL ARTERIOLES OF RABBITS

SUZANNE REUSE-BLOM,

Free University of Bruxelles, Belgium

Subarachnoid haemorrhages are often accompanied by longlasting cerebral arterial spasms leading to further neurological pathology.

Although numerous and excellent methods are now available for the study of total or regional cerebral blood flow, this particular problem needs investigation at a local level, and the quite old method of looking directly at vessels at the inframillimetric level still has its uses, as it allows recording of long duration without too much interference with the physiological conditions (*Edvinsson and Mackenzie* 1977).

Methods

Rabbits of ± 4 kg are anesthetized with pentobarbital. The animals breath spontaneously through a tracheal canula throughout the experiment.

The skull is then opened by trepanation and the dura mater carefully resected allowing for a "window" of about 2.5 cm^2 where the leptomeningeal vasculature can be observed through a microscope.

The preparation is illuminated by a powerful (450 W) cold light brought by fiber glass to an angle of 45° to avoid glare and is kept moist by a continuous drip of mock cerebrospinal fluid of stable pH.

Continuous recordings are made with a TV camera and magnetoscope and measurements of diameters made on play back of the videotapes. This allows for continuous measurements for 35 minutes.

Spasms of the arterioles are induced by topical application of fresh serum. These spasms last as long as there is serum present on the territory.

As soon as the spasm has been observed on the monitoring screen, I. V. injection of the drug is made and the recording goes on until the end of the tape.

In experiments testing the eventual "protection" to the spasm, the drug is administered either "per os" before anaesthesia, or by I. V. injection after anaesthesia.

In the experiments reported here, we used papaverine as a reference drug (1 mg/kg) and tested various concentrations of piracetam. Chemically, piracetam is 2-oxo-1-pyrrolidine acetamide and shows a kinship with GABA (gamma-amino-butyric acid, the ring in its formula can be obtained by simply removing a molecule of water followed by cyclization).

Results

1) I. V. injection of various doses of piracetam provokes mild vasodilatation (Fig. 1).

2) I. V. injection of piracetam made 1 minute after the visual observation of a spasm induced by topical application of 0.5 ml of fresh serum of same species alleviates the spasm within a few seconds

Fig. 1.

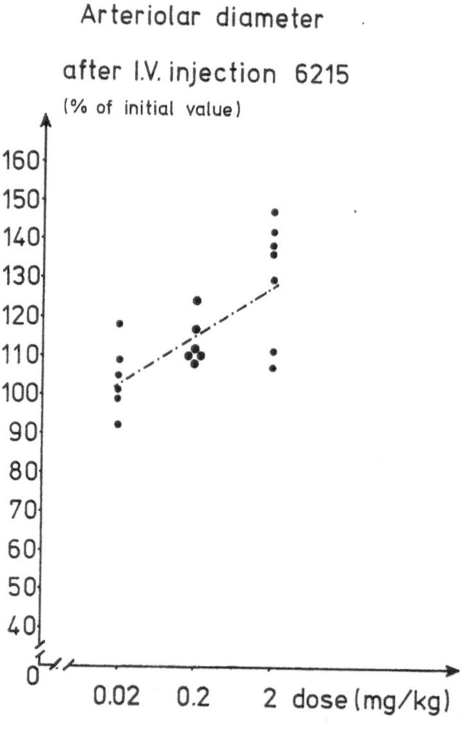

Arteriolar diameter

after I.V. injection 6215

(% of initial value)

(the spasm persists if serum is present for more than 300 minutes in the absence of the drug). (Fig. 2).

3) Pretreatment by piracetam either per os (one hour before, I. V. 20' before topical application of serum) does not prevent the onset of spasm but the spasm is often incomplete and in all cases very brief. (Fig. 3).

Conclusions

Other workers have shown that piracetam is not a vasodilator. Our results suggest only mild vasodilaion (the limits of spontaneous changes of diameters are about 15% either way). Therefore one cannot suspect piracetam of inducing the dangerous steal phenomenon. On the other hand, piracetam acts very rapidly on the spasm induced by serum-well within on the spasm induced by serum — well within the dangerous 3 minutes — and dilates those very vessels which were spasmed and this effect lasts, while the antispasmodic effect of papaverine is short lived.

REFERENCE

Edvinsson and MacKenzie (1977): Amine mechanisms in the cerebral circulation. Pharm. Rev. 20, 275.

Increase (in %) of diameter

after spasm plus I.V. injection of 6215

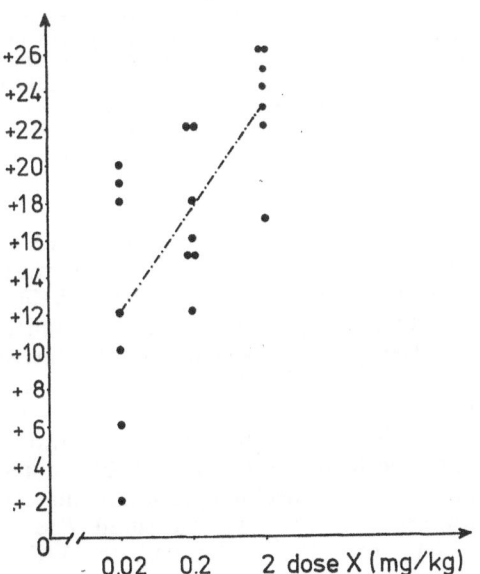

Fig. 2.

Pretreated orally length of spasm.

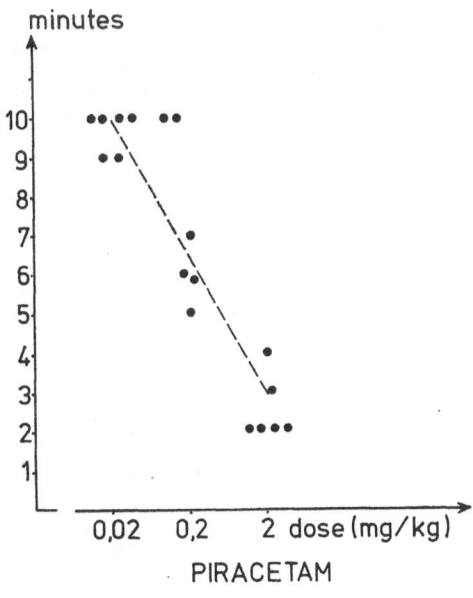

Fig. 3.

S. R-B., Laboratoire de Physiologie, 2, rue Evers, 1000 — Bruxelles, Belgium

DO THE DIFFERENCES IN ANGIOARCHITECTURE BETWEEN NORMOTENSIVE (NR) AND SPONTANEOUSLY HYPERTENSIVE RATS (SHR) INFLUENCE THE ARTERIO-VENOUS PO₂ BALANCE?

R. HERTEL, H. HENRICH and R. ASSMANN

Institute of Physiology, Würzburg, F.R.G.

Introduction

Compared to NR, the precapillary microvasculature of SHR is characterized by an elevated intravascular pressure (*Hertel et al.*, 1978) and by fewer arterioles of different branching order ('rarification', *Henrich et al.*, 1978). These peculiarities in SHR contribute to the over-all increased blood flow resistance, though the individual precapillary microvessel of SHR is shorter and has a wider inner diameter (*Henrich and Hertel*, 1977). A considerable elevation of tangential wall stress of precapillary arterioles (+120 to 140%, *Hertel et al.*, 1978), on the one hand, and a thickened arteriolar vessel wall of SHR on the other hand (*Folkow et al.*, 1970) favour the idea of influencing the exchange of substances between blood and tissue. As a sensitive indicator of the metabolic process, the analysis of arterio-venous PO₂ balances can be valuable.

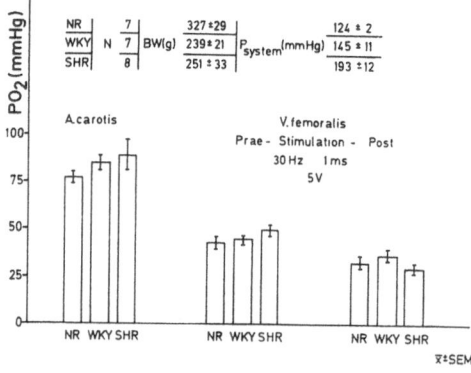

Fig. 1. Comparative analysis of blood PO₂, measured in the carotid artery and in the femoral vein before and after stimulation of the femoral nerve in the left hind limb. Abbreviations: see legend of table.

Methods

Experiments were performed on the mesentery preparation and hind limb of sex-matched pairs of NR and SHR (Okamoto-Aoki, strain of Wistar-Kyoto rats, established hypertension; body weight (BW), hematocrit (Hkt) and systemic blood pressure, measured in the carotid artery under chloralose-urethane anaesthesia (10 and 50 mg/100 g BW i. m., see the table). The preparation of animals is described elsewhere (*Henrich et al.*, 1978). For the experiments with stimulation of the left femoral nerve, we took blood from the right hind limb for the 'before-stimulation' analysis and from the left hind limb for measuring the 'after-stimulation' value. For gaining lymph, we canulated the main intestinal lymph duct and the mesenteric artery. For measurements of PO₂, PCO₂ and pH we used the blood-gas analyser.

Results and discussion

The table shows averaged data ±SEM of PO₂ measurements in the carotid artery and in the femoral and mesenteric veins. The arterio-venous differences are added (*Δ*). Using another group of normotensive controls (Wistar-Kyoto-rats), a significant difference of blood PO₂ cannot be established in spite of the elevated hamatocrit of SHR (and WKY) compared to NR. Checking pH as a parameter for shock control, we measured 7.38 ± ± 0.02 for NR, 7.37 ± 0.02 for WKY and 7.36 ± 0.03 for SHR; the averaged PCO₂ (NR, WKY and SHR) did not differ significantly and reached 46.6 ± 2.2 mm Hg. Furthermore, there is no significant difference in the PO₂ of the venous blood of mesentery of muscle nor in the pH under these experimental i.e. resting conditions. The analyzed the oxygen balance in the hind limb before and after stimulation of the femoral nerve (30 Hz, 1 ms, 5 V) exceeded the significance level

Table I. Analysis of PO$_2$ in the arterial and venous blood of Wistar-Kyoto rats (WKY) and rats of the Okamoto-Aoki-strain with normotensive (NR) and spontaneously hypertensive (SHR) nlood pressure.
N = number of animals, BW = body weight, P$_{system}$ = blood pressure, measured in the carotid artery, HKT = hematocrit. Further explanations in the text.

	N	BW (g)	P$_{system}$ (mmHg)	HKT (%)	PO$_2$ (mmHg) A.carotis	V femoralis	Δ	V mesenterica	Δ
NR	29	300 ±15	119 ±4	46.9 ±0.7	88.9 ±2.2	41.3 ±1.7	47.6	44.1 ±2.9	44.8
WKY	20	254 ±13	121 ±7	56.6 ±0.7	89.9 ±3.6	40.4 ±1.7	49.5	43.4 ±1.7	46.5
SHR	36	211 ±9	191 ±5	55.7 ±0.7	87.4 ±2.4	42.1 ±2.9	45.3	40 6 ±2.1	46.8

x̄±SEM

for NR, a difference of 8 mm Hg was measured at a PO$_2$ value of 35 mm Hg after stimulation, for WKY the difference was also 8 mm Hg (post-stimulatory value: 37 mm Hg). In SHR, the before/after stimulation difference was 20 mm Hg with the post-stimulatory value of 30 mm Hg (Fig. 1). The data suggest a difference in the oxygen extraction during muscle work between NR or WKY versus SHR. The higher extraction in SHR could be a consequence of augmented blood flow in connection with the elevation of tangential wall stress in precapillary vessels. This would be consistent with our findings of augmented permeability ($+55\%$) of pre-capillary arterioles for a water soluble low-molecular fluorescent tracer in SHR even under resting conditions (Hertel and Henrich, 1978). The relatively low post-stimulatory value of SHR compared to NR and WKY could point to effective compensation of rarification in the microvasculature. For NR, the analysis of PO$_2$ in the intestinal lymph (46 ± 6 mm Hg) as well as in the mesentery vein (45 ± ± 5 mm Hg) shows values which do not significantly differ (Fig. 2): the same is reported for experiments with other animals, unfortunately without listing of the over-all blood pressure (Yoffey and Courtice, 1970). Thus, we measured a PO$_2$ of 46 ± 1 mm Hg in the mesenteric vein of SHR but a PO$_2$ of 62 ± 3 mm Hg in the intestinal lymph, which represents a difference of 35% compared to NR. The statistics, shown in Fig. 2, as well as our findings of a higher lymph flow rate ($+63\%$) of SHR (Hertel et al., 1978) emphasize the significance of our data. Consequently, we feel induced to postulate either an active tracer for O$_2$ in the lymph a higher tissue pressure (osmotic and/or oncotic) in SHR or a different solubility coefficient α, which would allow a higher PO$_2$ in the intestinal lymph of SHR.

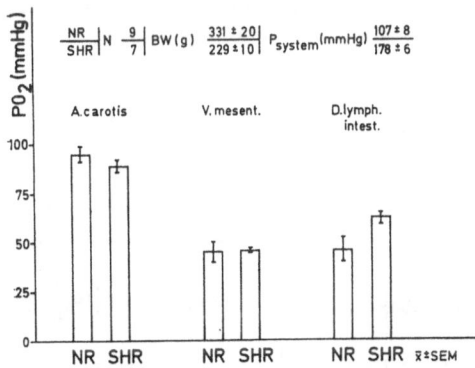

Fig. 2. Comparative analysis of blood PO$_2$, measured in the carotid artery, in the mesenteric vein and in the lymph of the main intestinal lymph duct. Abbreviations: see legend of table.

REFERENCES

Folkow, B., Hallbäck, M., Lundgren, Y., Weiss, L., (1970): Background of increased flow resistance and vascular reactivity in SHR. Acta Physiol. Scand. 80, 93—106.

Henrich, H. and Hertel, R. (1977): Comparative network analysis of the ileocecal mesentery vasculature in SHR and NR. Microvasc. Res. 13, 268.

Hertel, R. and Henrich, H. (1978): Comparative analysis of fluorescent tracer leakage in microvessels of SHR and NR. Pflügers Arch. 373, R 64.

R. H., Physiologisches Institut der Universität, Röntgenring 9, D-8700 Würzburg, F.R.G.

CRITICAL LESIONS OF CERVICAL ARTERIES INDUCE RETINAL A—V ANASTOMOSES IN CASES OF OCCLUSIVE THROMBOAORTOPATHY (TAKAYASU'S DISEASE)

K. ISHIKAWA, K. ASAYAMA, M. UYAMA and C. KAWAI

*Department of Internal Medicine, Department of Ophthalmology,
Kyoto University, Kyoto, Japan, Department of Ophthalmology,
Kansai Medical University, Osaka, Japan*

Occlusive thromboaortopathy (OTAP), Takayasu's arteritis, pulseless disease and Takayasu's disease are all the same entity. Patients were classified into four groups according to evidence of Takayasu's retinopathy, secondary hypertension, aortic regurgitation and aortic or arterial aneurysm, attributed to OTAP.

In the 20 year period from 1957 to 77 we encountered 69 Japanese patients with OTAP. Twenty-four (34.8%) of the 69 had Takayasu's retinopathy. We report here the relation of the main cervical arterial lesions to retinal vascular impairment and to cerebral circulation time in these 24 patients and in 5 patients with normal ocular fundi in OTAP. All of the 29 but one were females. The average age at the time of established diagnosis was 31 years. Most patients were under 40.

Estimation of the severity of Takayasu's retinopathy was made according to *Uyama and Asayama's* classification (1976): stage 1 — 13 cases; vascular dilatations, stage 2 — 4 cases; microaenurysm formation, stage 3 — 6 cases; arteriovenous anastomoses and stage 4 — 1 case; ocular complications. Granding of lesions of the four cervical arterial systems consisting of the bilateral common carotid and vertebral arterial systems was carried out by supravalvular aortography. The grading was expressed in terms of the sum of each percentage reduction of the original luminal diameter assessed on the basis of the immediate proximal or distal uninvolved segment. For example, if each of these four arterial systems shows a 50% narrowing in one patient, the sum totals

a 200% narrowing. Cerebral circulation time was simultaneously estimated at the time of serial aortography with mainly 80% angio-conray. This was defined as the time interval between the beginning of filling of the aortic arch and either of the bilateral internal jugular veins.

The relationship of narrowing of the cervical arteries to retinal severity in 28 cases is shown in Figure 1. Mean percent narrowing in patients in normal, stage 1, stage 2 and stages 3 and 4 groups was 116 (SE = 43), 146 (SE = 30), 303 (SE = 23)

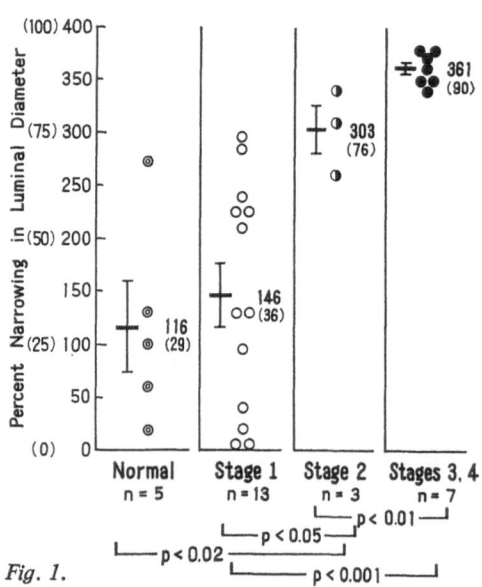

Relation of Narrowing of Cervical Arteries to Retinal Severity in 28 Cases of Occlusive Thromboaortopathy (Takayasu's Disease)

Fig. 1.

and 361% (SE = 5), respectively. Retinopathy of patients in two groups in stage 2 and stages 3 and 4 was dependent on the degree of narrowing.

The relationship between cerebral circulation time and retinal severity in 20 cases is shown in Figure 2. The mean cerebral circulation time of patients in normal, stage 1, stage 2 and stages 3 and 4

"normal" cerebral circulation time reported by *Gilroy*, 1963.

It is suggested that the critical lesions of the cervical arteries which lead to retinal arteriovenous anastomoses in this disease represent over a 320% narrowing in the luminal diameter and that the cerebral circulation time is over 7 seconds.

The correlation between log percent patency of the cervical arteries and cerebral circulation time in 20 cases is shown in Figure 3. The vertical scale gives the cerebral circulation time and the horizontal scale, the logarithm of percent patency in the luminal diameter. There was a good inverse correlation ($r = -0.80$) between these two parameters. The linear least squares regression line was shown with equation, $y = -2.4 \log x + 10.2$.

Thus, we emphasize that further lsight

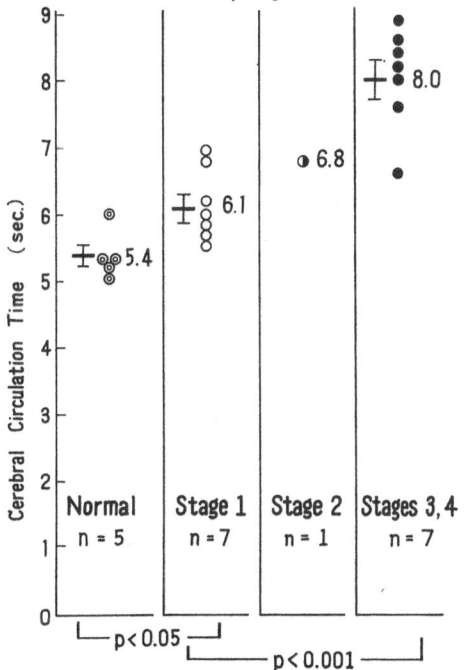

Relation between Cerebral Circulation Time and Retinal Severity in 20 Cases of Occlusive Thromboaortopathy (Takayasu's Disease)

Fig. 2.

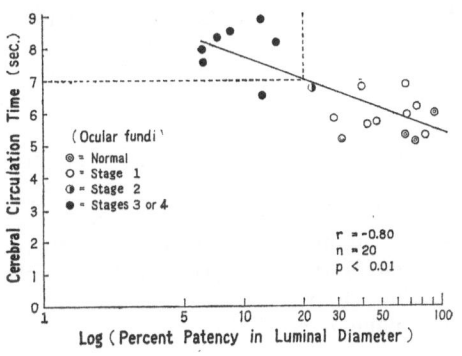

Correlation between Patency of Cervical Arteries and Cerebral Circulation Time in Occlusive Thromboaortopathy (Takayasu's Disease)

Fig. 3.

groups was 5.4 (SE = 0.16), 6.1 (SE = = 0.20), 6.8 and 8.0 seconds (SE = = 0.29), respectively. Prolongation of cerebral circulation time was seen with an increase in severity of the retinopathy. The value of the cerebral circulation time in patients in the normal ocular fundi group is compatible with that of the

reduction in the lumen of the cervical arteries with pre-critical lesions, which give rise to retinal microaneurysms, may rapidly lead to "critical" lesions of these vessels and may induce practically irreversible retinal arteriovenous anastomoses.

K. I., 3rd Div., Dept. of Internal Med., Faculty of Medicine, Kyoto University, Kyoto 606, Japan

MICROCIRCULATION AND OXYGEN UTILIZATION IN SKELETAL MUSCLES OF SPONTANEOUSLY HYPERTENSIVE RATS (SHR)

H. HENRICH, AGNES HECKE, R. HERTEL and R. ASSMANN

Institute of Physiology, Würzburg, F.R.G.

Introduction

Spontaneous hypertension is character-ized by an increased blood flow resistance in series as well as in parallel coupled sections of the vasculature (*Henrich et al.*, 1977). 'Rarification' of the small resistance vessels and capillaries is found in the cremaster muscle of pre-hypertensive rats (*Hutchins and Darnell*, 1974), in the mesentery vascular bed of SHR suffering from established hypertension (*Henrich et al.*, 1978) and also in the gracilis muscle, as will be shown. Vascular smooth muscle hypertrophy narrowing the vessel lumen is seldom seen under intravital conditions; rather an increased diameter is found very often. The experiments presented are aimed at answering the question of whether a stepwise pressure reduction would eliminate the differences in the arteriolar size between SHR and normo-tensive control rats (NR). Of further interest is the nutritive situation in the 'rarified' hypertensive system during he-morrhagic hypotension.

Materials and Methods

Experiments were carried out on the gracilis muscle preparation of SHR of the Okamoto-Aoki strain, and on NR with an age of 14—16 weeks. The animals were anesthetized with chloralose-urethane (10 or 50 mg/100 g body weight) i. m. The systemic blood pressure was measured continuously in the carotid artery. Pressures given are mean systemic arterial pres-sures. The diameters of the arterioles were continuously measured by a Video-Angiometer (*Assmann and Henrich*, 1977). This technique evaluates differences in light intensity between the vessel wall and tissue as differences of the video voltage. Red cell velocity as an estimate of the blood flow velocity in capillaries was mea-sured by use of a Video-Photometric Analyzer (IPM, San Diego, U.S.A.) in combination with a Tracking Correlator. The method is actually base on dual-slit velocimetry (*Wayland and Johnson*, 1967).

Blood gas pressures and metabolic parameters were measured by use of a Blood Gas Analyzer (Mod. 213 IL, Boskamp). Venous blood of the rats' hind limb was sampled from the femoral vein; arterial blood was taken from the carotid artery.

Results and Discussion

Perfusion pressure in the gracilis muscle vascular bed was indirectly lowered by

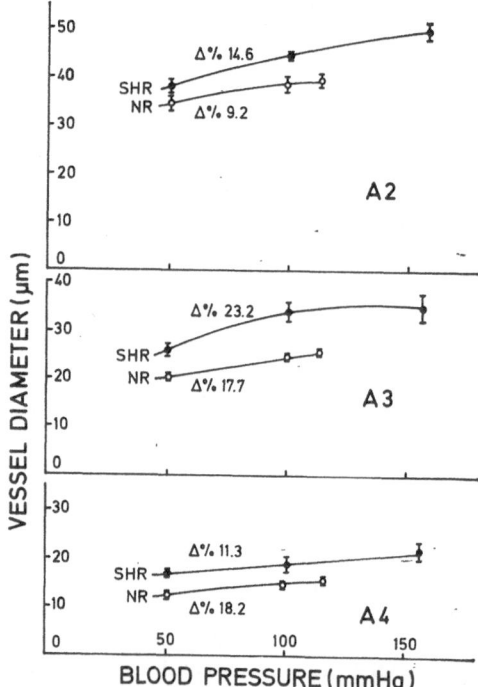

Fig. 1. Changes in vessel diameter after pressure reduction by hemorrhage. Control diameters are significantly greater in SHR vs NR. A2 = large arterioles, A3 = terminal arterioles A4 = pre-capillary arterioles

Table 1. Blood parameters of relevancy before and after hemorrhage

	P_system (mmHg)	Age (weeks)	Body weight (g)	CONTROL (art.)				HEMORRHAGIC HYPOTENSION (ven.)									
								P_{system} → 100 mmHg					→ 50mmHg				
				HCT %	pH (art.)	S.B. mval/l	PO$_2$ mmHg	HCT %	pH (ven.)	S.B. mval/l	PCO$_2$ mmHg	ΔPO$_2$ mmHg	HCT %	pH (ven.)	S.B. mval/l	PCO$_2$ mmHg	ΔPO$_2$ mmHg
NR	126 ±7	15 ±1	246 ±15	47 ±1	7.36 ±0.01	24.4 ±0.6	95.7 ±4.0	45 ±1	7.35 ±0.01	25.3 ±0.7	53.1 ±2.0	52.3	44 ±1	7.34 ±0.01	24.9 ±0.8	53.7 ±1.4	68.1
SHR	209 ±5	14 ±0	184 ±3	57 ±1	7.35 ±0.02	24.7 ±0.6	97.1 ±6.3	54 ±1	7.34 ±0.01	25.5 ±0.7	56.3 ±2.4	59.0	51 ±1	7.34 ±0.02	24.7 ±0.6	54.1 ±2.9	71.8

reducing the systemic arterial pressure by hemorrhage. As fig. 1 shows, arteriolar diameters differed significantly (p at least <0.001) under control conditions, i.e. the small resistance vessels of SHR had a wider lumen compared with NR. These unexpected peculiarities are not simply caused by differences in the distending intravascular pressure because a reduction of the systemic pressure to 100 mm Hg in both groups of animals did not adjust the diameters of the arterioles of different branching order to the same size. The same was also true at a pressure level of 50 mm Hg. Differences in vessel size are evidently caused by structural properties in hypertensive animals.

The reduction in the vessel number was found to be extended even to the capillary bed, where the capillaries are reduced in number to 61% in SHR as compared to NR (*Henrich et al.*, 1977). As a consequence, red cell velocity in the capillaries of skeletal muscle of SHR exceeded that in NR by 58% (0.41 mm/s in SHR vs 0.26 in NR). As Fig. 2. shows, the effect of pressure reduction on the erythrocyte

flow velocity was more distinct in SHR than in NR. At 100 mm Hg, flow was still higher in capillaries of SHR, but further pressure reduction to 50 mm Hg induced an overproportional flow reduction to 0.10 mm/s in SHR vs 0.16 mm/s in NR partially caused by an increase in the number of plasma capillaries by 23% of the control value.

The hypertensive microvascular system apparently needs an elevated perfusion pressure. The extremely augmented wall stress in the microvessels of SHR (*Hertel et al.*, 1978) at control pressures may be substituted by an overproportional narrowing of the lumen and thickening of the arteriolar wall after pressure reduction followed by a corresponding decrease in capillary blood velocity or flow. Control of the hematocrit, standard bicarbonate and pH (Table I) in the femoral vein excluded any shock situation possibly caused by the hemorrhage. Under control conditions the arterio-venous pO$_2$ difference did not differ significantly indicating that oxygen supply to the skeletal muscle tissue was sufficient, at least under

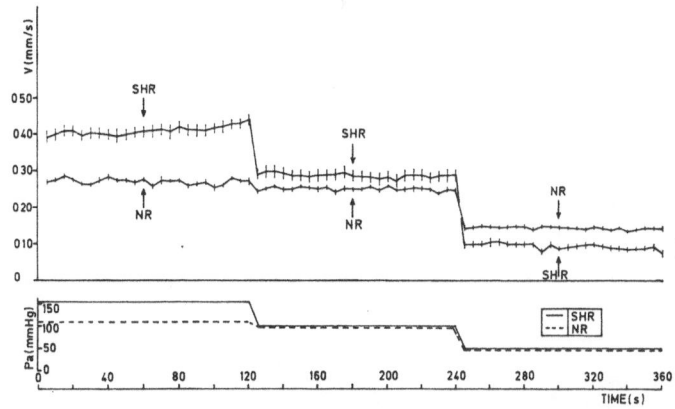

Fig. 2. Effect of hemorrhagic hypotension on blood flow velocity profiles in SHR and NR ($\bar{x} \pm s\bar{x}$)

resting conditions. A similar conclusion may be drawn with respect to the av-pO_2 difference after reduction of the systemic arterial pressure: ΔpO_2 52.3 vs 59.0 mm Hg at 100 mm Hg, 68.1 vs 71.8 mm Hg at 50 mm Hg perfusion pressure. From this data the authors concluded that rarification of the microvasculature in SHR does not affect the oxygen supply to the tissue and with it the metabolism of the skeletal muscle. Overperfusion of the single microvessel might contribute as an additional compensatory effect.

REFERENCES

Assmann, R. and Henrich, H. (1977): A new video-angiometer device for on-line measurement of diameters in microvessels. Bibl. Anat. 16, 354—357.

Henrich, H., Assmann, R., Hertel, R., and Hecke, A. (1977): Die Stromstärke als geregelte Größe der essentiellen Hypertonie — Quantitative Untersuchungen der Mikrozirkulation in SHR und NR — In: Hoher Blutdruck, Steinkopff, Darmstadt.

Henrich, H., Hertel, R., and Assmann, R. (1978): Structural differences in the mesentery microcirculation between NR and SHR. Pflügers Arch. 375, in press.

Hertel, R., Henrich, H. and Assmann, R. (1978): Intravital measurement of arteriolar pressure and tangential wall stress in NR and SHR (established hypertension) Experientia (Basel) 34, in press.

Hutchins, P. M. and Darnell, A. E. (1974): Observation of a decreased number of small arterioles in spontaneously hypertensive rats. Circulat. Res. 34/35, 161—165.

Wayland, H. and Johnson, P. C. (1967): Erythrocyte velocity measurement in microvessels by a two-slit photometric method. J. appl. Physiol 22, 333—337.

H. H., Physiologisches Institut der Universität, Röntgenring 9, D-8700 Würzburg, F.R.G.

HISTOMORPHOMETRIC STUDIES AT THE MICROCIRCULATORY BED IN SPONTANEOUSLY HYPERTENSIVE RATS (SHR).

H. J. HERRMANN, R. BAUMANN, V. MORITZ and P. MÜHLIG

Inst. for Res. of Heart and Circul. Regul., Berlin, and
Inst. for Microbiol. and Exp. Ther., Jena, Acad. of Sciences of G.D.R.

Introduction

The pathophysiological investigations of *Folkow et al.* (1970), *Finch and Haeusler* (1974) and others strongly suggest structural reactions of blood vessels (b.v.) in SHR. But there are apparently no investigations for this hypertension model indicating histomorphometric increases in the thickness of the wall of anatomically undefined arterial blood vessels of the microcirculatory bed including the smallest precapillary vessels. The histomorphological behaviour of the various parts of the microvascular system in different stages of spontaneous hypertension and in different organs is only partially known. A newly developed histomorphometric method has made it possible to answer some of these questions.

Materials and methods

32 SHR aged 2, 4, and 12 months were compared with 20 control animals. 14 of the latter were inbred in our institute (contr. animals A) and 6 were wistar rats "Schönwalde" (contr. animals B). For details see Figure 1. Specimens of musculus rectus femoris, pancreas, and heart were analyzed. Blood pressure ante mortem: 2-months old SHR, group 1: 166 ± 19 mm Hg (systol.), group 2: 138 ± 19 mm Hg (systol.), 83 ± 12 mm Hg (diastol.); 12 months old SHR: 248 ± 17 mm Hg (systol.), 155 ± 6 mm Hg (diastol.). In 15-week old SHR we measured 211.5 ± 28.5 mm Hg, systolic (*Baumann et al.*, 1976). For a selective visualization of all the b.v. $< 10.5 \mu m$ and the polyphosphatase-positive b.v. $< 10.5 \mu m$ specimens were prepared by a special variation of the Wachstein-Meisel-Mg-ATPase reaction. Measurements were made by means of the automated image analyser Quantimet 720 and the Hewlett-Packard computer 9100 B after fulfilling certain requirements of specimen preparation and test principles. The number ($N_{b.v.}$) and projected whole wall area of b.v. ($A_{b.v.}$) were measured. Statistical testing of the differences between the experimental and control animals was carried out by comparing these results with the normal variation in more than 20 control animals by 2-factorial variance-analysis. Ascertainment of the thickening of the walls of b.v. based on the measurement of a significantly increased number of b.v. with an external diameter (e.d.) in formalin-fixed cryostat specimens $< 10.5 \mu m$ and a significantly increased projected vessel wall area ($A_{\Sigma b.v.}$) of all b.v./unit measuring area of the organ specimen. A significantly increased number of b.v. $< 10.5 < 21 \mu m$ and/or of b.v. $< 21 \mu m$ indicates a thickening of the wall of b.v. with an e.d. prior to the pathogenetic influence below the lower limit of the respective class. The mean b.v. area ($A_{b.v.}$) was calculated from the projected whole b.v. area and the number of all b.v. with a maximal chord $< 10.5 \mu m$. A significant increase indicates a thickening of the walls if the number of b.v. $< 21 \mu m$ did not decrease.

Results and conclusions

1. The significantly increased number of b.v. $< 10.5 \mu m$ as well as the significant increase in the projected whole vessel wall area and in the mean b.v. area (Fig. 1) indicate a thickening of the wall of arterial b.v. of the microcirculatory bed. Thus, the fundamental conception of *Folkow et al.* (1973) concerning the development of structural b.v. reactions in SHR is histomorphometrically corroborated for the microvascular system. — 2. The skeletal muscle (group 1 and 2) and pancreas (group 2) exhibit an increase of the mentioned parameters in the stage of borderline hypertension. The differences between groups 1 and 2 of the 2-months old SHR mainly result from higher values of the measured parameters in control rats inbred in our institute compared with wistar control rats (unpublished results). This emphasizes the necessity of comparison of SHR-results with different control

animals. – 3. The pathogenetic influence is mainly restricted to the b.v. of the microcirculatory system with an e.d. > 10.5 μm in skeletal muscle and pancreas. – 4. The behaviour of the microvascular system of the heart is very different from that of both the other organs. Structural reactions could only be found in the late stage of hypertension, which is moreover characterized by signs of increased performance of the smallest precapillary vessels.

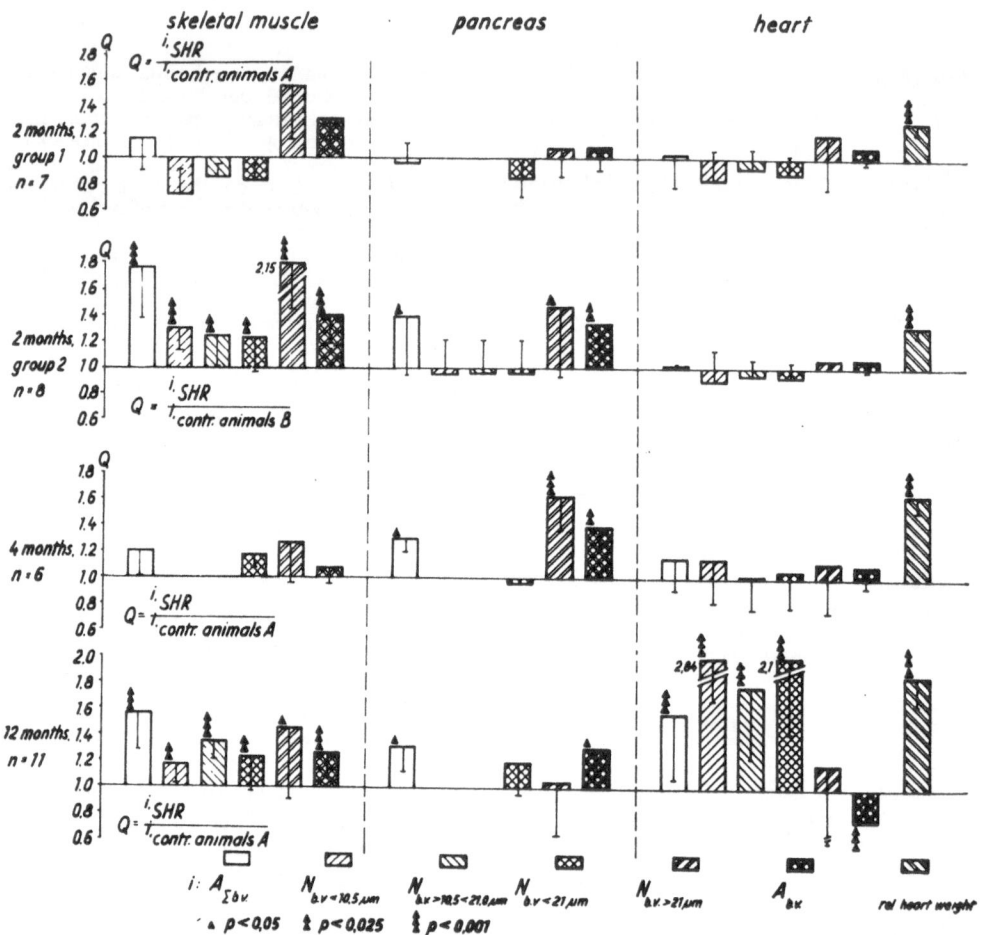

Fig. 1. Behaviour of the projected whole vessel wall area (A$_{\Sigma b.v.}$), the mean b.v. area (A$_{b.v.}$), the number of b.v. (N$_{b.v.}$) of various external diameters, and of the relative heart weight (mg heart/g body weight) in 2-, 4-, and 12-months old SHR. Control animals A: inbred of the institute; control animals B: wistar rats.

H. J. H., Central Institute for Res. of Heart AS, Wiltbergstr. 50, 1115 Berlin, G.D.R.

INDUCTION MECHANISMS OF METASTATIC HEPATIC CANCERS VIEWED FROM BLOOD VESSEL CONSTRUCTIONS AND THEIR HISTOMORPHOLOGICAL FORMS

K. OHMURA, K. MATSUO, K. MIZUOCHI and S. OHTSUKA

1st Dept. of Internal Medicine, School of Medicine, Toho University, Omori, Tokyo, Japan

Much clinical information on the occurrence and proliferation of metastatic hepatic cancer remains unknown. Metastatic hepatic cancer was induced experimentally via the portal vein in rabbits weighing 3 kg. We studied the process of occurrence and proliferation of hepatic cancer with intrahepatic vascular changes from the morphological point of view. Cell suspensions were prepared by mixing $5 \times 10^4/0.1$ ml of VX_2 carcinomatous cells under sterilization. Experimental subjects consisted of two groups. In one group isolated transplantation was performed in the subcapsular area of the liver. In the other group transplantation was performed via the portal vein. In both

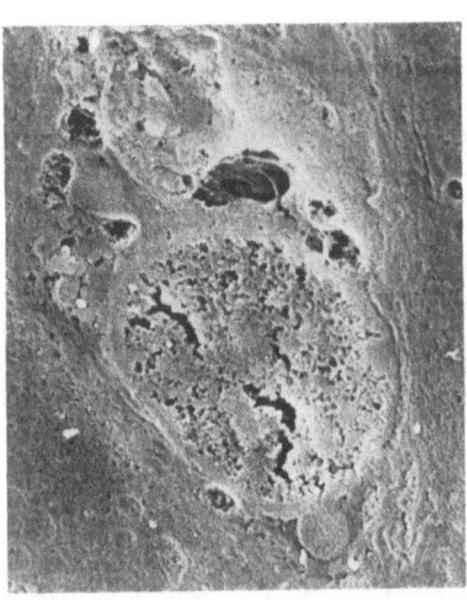

Fig. 2. Electronmicroscopic (scanning). Observation of emboli of portal carcinomatous cells.
(X 10000)

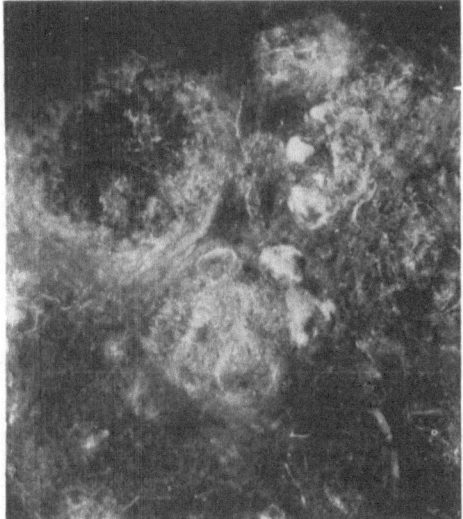

Fig. 1. Microangiogram of the group with transplantation of VX_2 carcinomatous cells via the portal vein.

groups, the vascular architecture was observed on the microangiogram. Histological findings were compared using a light electron microscope and electron-microscopic (translucent and scanning) observation. In the group with isolated transplantation, the arterial branches showed hypervascularity in the carcinomatous area and in the surrounding areas and the portal branches showed a sawtooth-like interruption around the carcionomatous area. The porto-hepatic shunt was not observed in the carcinomatous area. The histological findings revealed the remaining hepatic arterial branches and

469

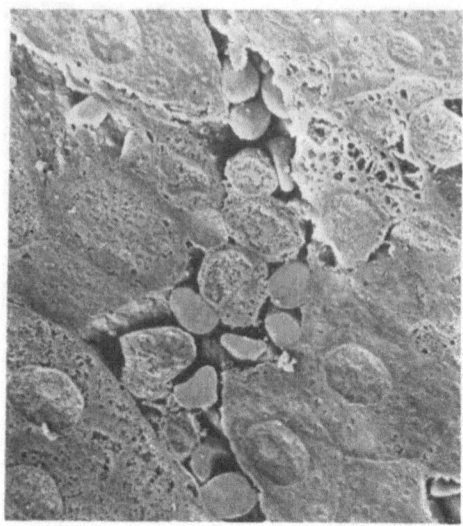

Fig. 3. VX$_2$ carcinomatous cells extending to the sinus.   (X 2000)

proliferation of neoplastic blood vessels. The portal branches had a tendency to disappear. The fine structure of the neoplastic blood vessels was characterized by the presence of endothelial cells which grew irregularly and peculiarly, adjusting to the vascular cavity, and by the presence of a basal mebrane consisting of connective tissues, including collagen. As shown in photo 1, the group with transplantation via the portal vein displayed hepatic metastasis with multiple nodes in the border of the liver. Hepatic angiography showed hypervascularity in a 2 × 3 mm minute nodular carcinoma and also necrotic centre with vascular findings in the border of the carcinoma was larger than 3 × 5 mm. In a large carcinomatous node, the blood vessels were filled only in the border of the carcinomatous area and non-carcinomatous area. The core of the lesion was necrotic. The portal vasography showed a sawtooth-like interruption around the carcinoma and dead branch-like structure in some parts of the carcinoma. Histological examination revealed portal embolism due to carcinoma, degeneration of the branches of the hepatic artery due to the carcinoma and dilation

of the carcinomatous sinus. Furthermore, with enlargement of the carcinoma, branches of the hepatic artery became decreased and dilation of the carcinomatous sinus and necrotic center became marked. The manner of development of hepatic metastasis is shown in photo II. Embolization due to carcinoma was induced in the portal vein and the arterial branches surrounding the portal vein were intact. As shown in photo III, the portal branches with the emboli of the carcinoma showed dilation of the sinus, in which carcinomatous cells separated from the erythrocytes were present. In addition, photo IV shows the changes with time. Emboli of the carcinoma were partly reopened: The carcinomatous cells destroyed the portal wall and proliferated the surroundings of the portal vein. The hepatic arterial branches degenerated due to the carcinomatous cells. In the group with transplantation via the portal vein, the type of metastasis of the carcinoma in the liver consisted of two groups. In one group the carcinomatous cells moved from the carcinomatous emboli in the portal

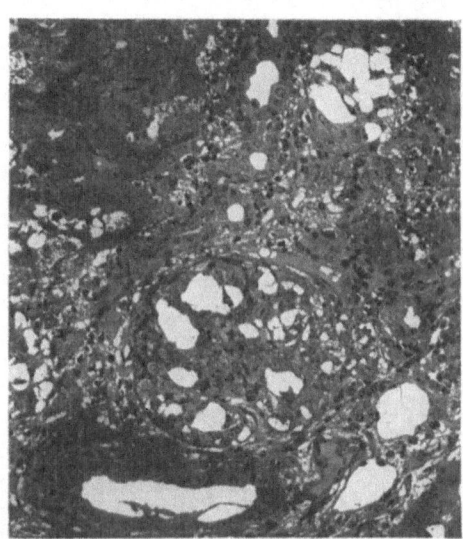

Fig. 4. The carcinomatous cells extending from the emboli of the portal carcinoma have destroyed the portal vein and have swollen and proliferated in the surrounding areas.   (X 40)

470

vein into the sinus of Glisson's sheath. In the other group, the carcinomatous cells destroyed the portal wall and proliferated and expanded into the surroundings of the carcinomatous area. The hepatic arterial branches were degenerated and destroyed with proliferation of the carcinomatous cells. These findings correspond to the fact that a minute carcinomatous nodule shows hypervascularity and an enlarged carcinoma became central lucent. These results also suggest that metastatic hepatic cancer causes the necrosis of the core from the beginning. Neoplastic blood vessels observed in the minute carcionomatous nodules of the metastatic carcinoma were the same as the fine structure of the neoplastic blood vessels of the isolated transplantation. Intrahepatic development processes of the VX_2 carcinomatous cells could be studied from the fine structure.

K. O., Ist. Dept. Int. Med., Sch. Med., Toho Univ., Omori, Tokyo, Japan

VENOUS AND LYMPHATIC CIRCULATION

THE INFLUENCE OF DRUGS ON HUMAN VENOUS TONE

R. LAVEN, H. P. BRUCH, E. SCHMIDT and G. WINTER

Department of Surgery, University of Würzburg, Würzburg, F.R.G.

The influence of the volume and pressure of the venous part has been recognized to be important for heart action and efficiency. The quality and quantity of circulation, especially that of the extremities, highly depends on the tone of venous smooth muscle. It was tried to find drugs capable of changing the venous tone either by contraction or by dilatation. Many substances were tested experimentally and therapeutically, but definite evidence of the desired effect was difficult to obtain. There were many confusing results depending on the mode of application, the place of activation — for example extremities or brain, respectively — and the kind of species.

Immediately after resection during operation, the human saphenous veins were cut into spiral strips. These muscle strips were suspended in a chamber perfused with Tyrode's solution and aerated with O_2 and CO_2 constant pH and temperature. They were stretched to about 30%, which is the approximate in situ length. All tensions were related to the muscle cross-sectional area. In total we used 60 vein strips.

In Figure 1 the difference of reaction depending on the degree of varicosis is shown. The left column is the normal control, and the next three columns are classes of light, medium, and severe heavy varicosis. This classification is more or less arbitrary, so we will give the results for normal veins. All effects are related to the tension development after depolarization with a potassium-rich solution. The maximum contraction capacity is set to 100%.

Effect of noradrenaline: Concentrations below 10^{-2} g/ml prove to be ineffectual. The maximum effective dose is seen at

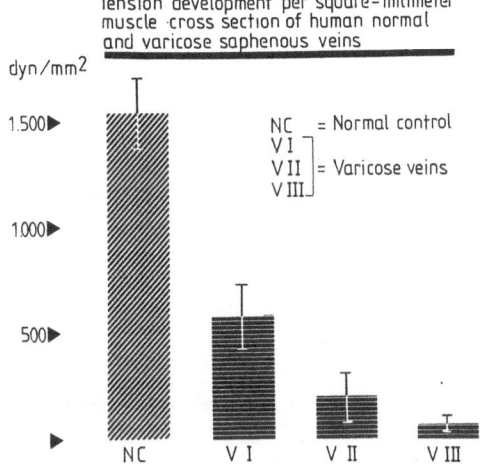

Tension development per square-milimeter muscle cross section of human normal and varicose saphenous veins

NC = Normal control
V I
V II = Varicose veins
V III

Fig. 1.

1−2 g/ml. This value is in the range of concentration found nearly in all types of smooth muscle for maximum activation. In relation to potassium we got 60 ± 12%.

Effect of papaverine after activation: At 10 g/ml papaverine we found a complete elimination of the contractions, and even a reduction of the venous muscle basic tone. This neutralization amounted to −64 ± 9% for potassium activation.

Effect of naftidrofuryl: The relaxation caused by naftidrofuryl amounts to −58 ± ± 5%. Even higher concentrations cannot increase the dilatation.

Effect of bencyclane: At 10 g/ml bencyclane we have a relaxation down to −44 ± 15%. At concentrations more than 10 g/ml the delating effect of bencyclane increases up to about −200%.

The drug Rutin, the horse-chestnut extract, and Dihydroergotamine used for venous tone never showed an effect on isolated human saphenous veins.

475

In Figure 2 the effect of the drugs papaverine, naftidrofuryl, and bencyclane after potassium-induced contractions of human saphenous veins is summarized. In general, there is no significant difference between these drugs when given at the same dosage of 10 g/ml each. These result derived from normal veins, that means there were no varicose changes. On varicose veins we found the same quality and relative quantity of the shown effects, but the reactivity of varicose veins is extremely diminished (Fig. 1). As a consequence, it is not possible to contract or relax these vessels. The diameter and therefore the volume of the venous system will more or less remain unchanged under the drugs we reported on. It is obvious that in therapy only nonpathologically chenged vessels can be influenced, but on varicose veins the success of therapy is questionable with regular drugs.

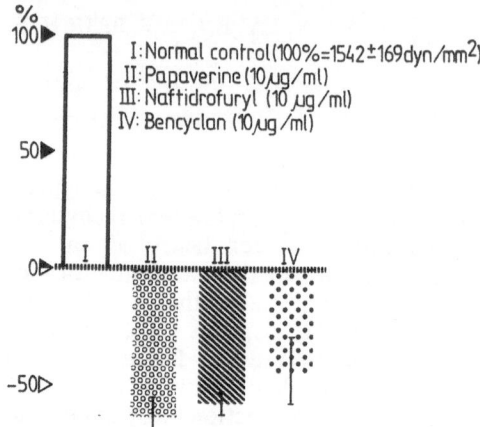

I: Normal control (100% = 1542 ± 169 dyn/mm^2)
II: Papaverine (10 μg/ml)
III: Naftidrofuryl (10 μg/ml)
IV: Bencyclan (10 μg/ml)

Tension changes after potassium-induced contractions of human saphenous veins   *Fig. 2.*

R. L., *Department of Surgery, University of Würzburg, Josef-Schneider-Str. 2, D-8700 Würzburg, F.R.G.*

DEVELOPMENT AND STRUCTURE OF THE VENOUS WALL

JITKA KOČOVÁ

*Institute of Histology and Embryology, Medical Faculty,
Charles University, Plzeň, Czechoslovakia*

Introduction

Extensive as the phlebological biblio-graphy is, works studying the structure of veins by methods of comparative morphology (*Hochstetter*, 1891, *v. Kügelgen*, 1955, *Kočová*, 1974, *Vankov*, 1974) are but rare exceptions. The present report aims to complement data missing in literature, and hence we have investigated both prenatal and postnatal development of the venous wall in the limbs of man and selected mammals, adopting different ways of locomotion, i.e. quadrupeds and the flying.

Materials and methods

Out of specimens of the embryonic collections assembled by our Institute we arranged develop-mental rows in man, in the domestic sheep, white rat, and bat. Postnatally we studied the veins in man (in 2 newborns, 3 sucklings, and 4 children, aged 4, 5, 7 and 10 years) further in sheep, rats, cats, dogs, and bats of various ages. Altogether we evaluated 150 series: 90, of them were embryologic, demonstrating the limbs of embryos and fetuses, and 60 were histologic series of the blood vessels, obtained from exci-sions in the postnatal period. Paraffin sections were stained both by the usual methods for distinguishing connective tissue and muscle ele-ments, and especially by our combination of Verhoeff's hematoxylin and green trichrome that

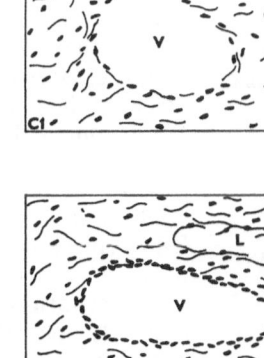
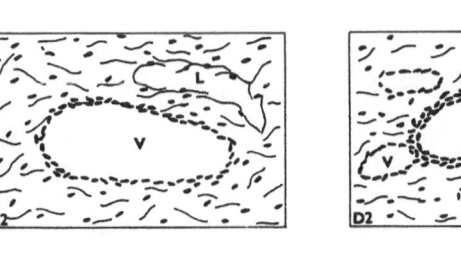
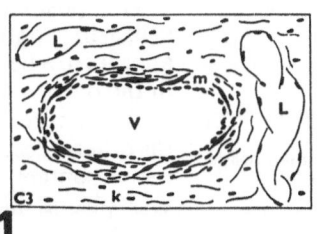
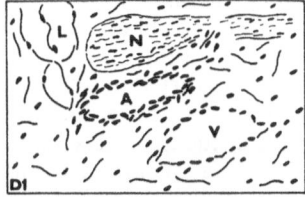
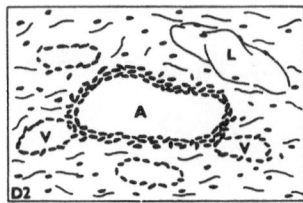
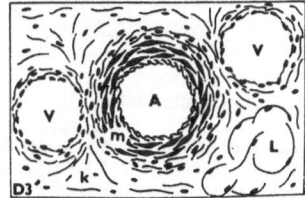

Fig. 1. Scheme illustrating the development of super-ficial (C_{1-3}) and deep limb veins (D_{1-3}) during the terms as follows:
terms as follows: 1) 6th week — the main veins are only in the central region; 2) beginning of the 3rd month — in the region of the forearm and shin; 3) beginning of the 4th month — in the same region as under 2) A — artery, V — vein, L — primordium of lymphatic vessels, N — nerve, e — elastic fibres, k — collagen fibres, m — muscle cells.

allows to demonstrate elastic and collagen fibres as well musculature in the same preparation. (In figures marked by+) Reticular fibres were made prominent according to Gomori, muco-polysaccharides by the PAS reaction and Alcian Blue.

Results and Discussion

In the limbs of mammals, both the superficial and deep system of veins occurs as considerably variable. In the vena saphena magna and parva we have found most striking differences as to the course, largeness and structure. The mightiest vein draining off most blood from the pelvic extremity in the dog and sheep is the vena saphena parva. Within the thicker wall of this vein there are more muscular and elastic elements than in the vena saphena magna, that ac-companies in these animals the persisting arteria saphena inside the common con-nective-tissue sheath. In rats, the system of superficial and deep veins cannot be distinctly separated. Both the vena femoralis and vena saphena magna, ac-compannying the artery, posses the pro-minent membrana elas.ica interna char-acteristic of its kind. At variance with older literary data (*Benninghoff*, 1930 and others), we have found smooth muscle cells inside the wall of the pulsing veins in the flying membrane of the bat.

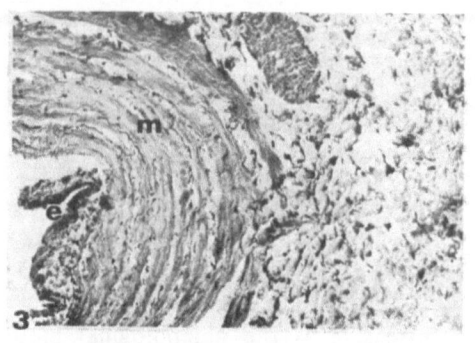

Fig. 2. Human fetus, 24 weeks, cross-section, (+), 3.2 × 25. Vena saphena magna in the region of the shin, with a developing membrana elastica interna (e). The tiny muscular bundles of the media run circularly (m).

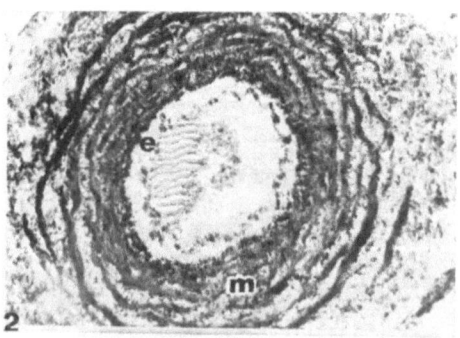

Fig. 3. Girl, 10 years old, cross-section, (+), 3.2 × 25. Vena saphena magna-the region of the shin. The well-formed membrana elastica interna (e) and numerous elastic fibres of the adventitia are stained black. The strong muscle bundles (m) in the media run circularly. Both in the intima and adventitia the muscular cells run longitudinally.

In the prenatal development we have established-according to Hochstetter, 1891 – that both in phylogeny and ontogeny the superficial marginal veins are laid down earlier than the deep veins (Fig. 1). In the superficial, independently running veins, which are functionally more loaded than the veins accompanying the arteries, the fibrous, and muscular elements appear earlier than those in the deep veins and in the v. saphena magna in mamals where the a. saphena has been preserved. During the second half of intrauterine life there occur even elastic fibrils and muscular bundles in the superficial veins (Fig. 2), while muscle cells appear in deep veins. The typical structure of superficial and deep veins forms early before birth.

In newborns and sucklings we observed-similarly as Riechenbacher, 1966 – a surprisingly thick muscular media and internal elastic membrane in the v. saphena magna.

The postnatal growth 3 – of muscle cells, in contrast to the prenatal one appears to be relatively more rapid just in the deep veins (*Vankov*, 1974). The vein wall structure is considerably variable, and the differences as to muscle and connective tissue contents may be noted even in the v. saphena magna in the region of the shin and thigh (*v. Kügelgen*, 1955, *Švejcar et al.*, 1962, *Kočová*, 1974). (Fig. 3).

Conclusion

We studied the development and structure of veins in the limbs of mammals using different ways of locomotion. In the superficial veins which are developmental older and are exposed to greater functional stress than the deep veins, collagen, elastic, and muscle elements appear sooner than in the deep veins. During the process of adaptation of man to bipedalism the deep veins acquire gradually a decisive role in draining off the blood from the pelvic limbs.

REFERENCES

Benninghoff, A. (1930): Venen. Handbuch der mikroskopischen Anatomie des Menschen. VI/1, 1—161, Springer, Berlin.

Hochstetter, F. (1891): Über die Entwickelung der Extremitätsvenen bei der Amnioten. Morph. Jb. 91, 368—393.

Kočová, J. (1974): Study of the development and structure of the veins in mammalian limbs (in Czech). Thesis, Plzeň.

Kügelgen, A. von (1955): Über das Verhältniss von Ringmusculatur und Innendruck in menschlichen grossen Venen, Z. Zellforsch. 43, 168—183.

Riechenbacher, J. (1966): Zur Entwickelung der Venen der unteren Extremitäten. Zbl. Phlebol. 5, 6—14.

Švejcar, J., Přerovský, I., Linhart, J., Kruml, J. (1962): Content of Collagen, Elastin, and Water in Walls of the Saphenous Vein in Man. Circulat. Res. 11, 296—300.

Vankov, V. N. (1974): Strojenije ven. Medicina, Moskva.

J. K., Inst. of Histology, Charles University, Lidická 1, 301 67 Plzeň, Czechoslovakia

THE "RISK FACTORS" OF PHLEBOTHROMBOSIS AND THROMBOPHLEBITIS

U. SIBUL, J. MÄNNISTE, E. SEPP, T. TAMM and A. JAKONSON

Central Hospital, Dept. of Surgery, Tallin, U.S.S.R.

Phlebothrombosis and thrombophlebitis are always complications of miscellaneous diseases or occur in the post-traumatic or post-natal period. In all these cases numerous factors favouring thrombosis are presest — they are the "risk factors". In order to avoid the vein diseases and even the frequently lethal embolism of pulmonary arteries, these risk factors should be known and taken into consideration.

We figured out the frequency of occurrence of the risk factors of thrombosis in cases of phlebothrombosis, thrombophlebitis and embolism of pulmonary arteries in groups consisting of 115 patients each. We also found the most characteristic combinations of factors leading to thrombosis. Every patient gave evidence of several risk factors, whereas in more serious cases the number of them was greater.

The groups under observation were chosen only from among those cases of phlepothrombosis and thrombophlebitis that were operated on (thrombectomy, by-passes). In this way it was possible to determine histologically whether it was a case of primary phlebothrombosis or thrombophlebitis — i.e. if there was a clot or an inflammation in the wall of the vein. In the later stages of the disease the inflammation was always present.

We also examined the mast cell count (heparinocytes) in the vein-wall and the regional lymphatic nodes as well as their functional state (degranulation step). This enabled us to observe the protective reactions of the organism in case of thrombosis. In connection with the above-mentioned we recorded also the blood coagulation and fibrinolytic activity in venous blood and in the basin of regionally venous stasis.

The frequency of the risk factors in case of phlebothrombosis, thrombophlebitis

Table I.

Clinical risk factor	Thrombosis $\% \pm m$	Thrombophl. $\% \pm m$	Embolism $\% \pm m$
Over-7-days bed regime	53.9 ± 4.2	5.1 ± 1.3	93.0 ± 2.3
Heart-trouble	45.3 ± 4.2	7.1 ± 1.2	$74.7 \pm 4\,0$
Age over 50	41.7 ± 4.1	28.7 ± 4.1	86.9 ± 3.1
Clinically expressed atherosclerosis	$39\,5 \pm 4\,1$	39.5 ± 4.1	85.2 ± 3.3
Surgical infection	32.3 ± 3.9	64.7 ± 4.0	53.9 ± 4.6
Infusion of hypertonic and vein-irritating solutions	30.9 ± 3.9	54.7 ± 4.0	63.4 ± 4.4
Varicose veins in low extremities	26.6 ± 3.7	93.3 ± 1.3	15.6 ± 3.3
Trauma	25.9 ± 3.7	24.4 ± 3.6	20.8 ± 3.7
Anaemia	25.9 ± 3.7	5.7 ± 1.9	28.7 ± 4.2
Post-operative period	24.4 ± 3.6	17.9 ± 3.2	51.3 ± 4.6
Pulmonary diseases	19.2 ± 3.3	19.9 ± 3.3	39.1 ± 4.5
Pregnancy, post-natal period gynaecological diseases	17.9 ± 3.2	6.3 ± 1.2	22.6 ± 3.9
Application of procoagulants	15.9 ± 3.1	5.7 ± 1.9	22.6 ± 3.9
Malignant tumor	7.9 ± 2.2	7.9 ± 2.2	34.7 ± 4.4
Adiposity	5.7 ± 1.9	5.7 ± 1.9	13.9 ± 3.2

and embolism was as follows: (Table I).

In cases of phlebothrombosis and pulmonary embolism the most frequent combinations consisted of 3 to 4 risk factors (bed regime, anaemia, infusion of hypertonic and vein-irritating solutions) occurring in 20 to 26 per cent of patients, i.e. in every 4th or 5th patient. In cases of thrombophlebitis the combination — varicose disease, trauma, infection — predominated, thus giving rise to an inflammation of the superficial veins.

In cases of thrombophlebitis, factors in connection with changes in vein-walls and regional haemodynamics predominated, whereas in cases of phlebothrombosis and embolism disturbances in central haemodynamics dominated.

In cases of recent phlebothrombosis and some of pulmonary embolism the mast cells in the vein-wall and regional lymphatic node were degranulated due to their activity (index of degranulation 2.5 − 2.8 on 3-mark system). The count of mast cells had risen in the wall of the vein as vein as well as in the regional lymphatic node at thrombophlebitis. The mast cells were found in all the three stages, the index of degranulation was within 1.7 − 2.3.

In cases of phlebothrombosis and pulmonary embolism we observed a rise in venous blood coagulation without any increase, but even a considerable restraint, in fibrinolytic activity. At thrombophlebitis the rise in blood coagulation did not occur, but fibrinolytic activity increased especially in the venous blood punctured from the inflammated area.

The exhaustion of the mastocytic system together with the rise in coagulation and decrease in fibrinolysis is a sufficient factor to cause phlebothrombosis and pulmonary embolism. If any of the above-mentioned clinical risk factors is added to them, the probability of thrombosis or embolism is even greater.

Our clinical experience proved that the patient having 5 to 6 risk factors in in need of intensive prevention of phlebothrombosis, that is at the same time prophylaxis again embolism of pulmonary arteries.

U. S., Central Hospital, Dept. of Surgery, Karl Marx Street 16. Tallin, U.S.S.R.

CHRONIC VENOUS INSUFFICIENCY FOLLOWING SURGERY ON THE INFERIOR VENA CAVA AND THE LARGE VEINS

A. PODZIMEK and M. ANDĚL

Surgical department, Faculty of Medicine, Charles University, Plzeň, Czechoslovakia

Ligature or plication of the inferior vena cava (IVC) used in prophylaxis of pulmonary embolism (PE), division of the IVC in order to perform the meso-caval shunt causes obstruction to the returning venous blood flow. In the periphery of the lower limbs different signs and symptoms of chronic venous insufficiency (CVI) can occur.

In this paper we are presenting an evaluation of CVI in 20 patients operated upon IVC in the past 12 years.

Patients and methods

The patients are divided in two groups: Group A consists of 14 patients following IVC interruption at the age of 25—70 years in whom 3 different procedures were performed (ligation and plication 9×, plication and phlebectomy of the comm. iliac vein 2×, ligation of the superficial femoral vein 3×). Group A included 8 men and 6 women. In 12 patients the indication was recurrent pulmonary embolism and the last two patients were operated prophylactically following pelvic surgery. Out of them 7 patients had 3 attacks of PE. The source of the emboli was found to be thrombosis of the venous system of the lower limbs or of pelvic veins. These patients were operated on in the years 1967—1976.

Group B. In this group there are 6 patients following meso-caval shunt and one 4 year — old child after resection of IVC for tumor. These patients were operated on in the years 1967—1976.

Long-term clinical results — Group A

Only one woman out of 14 patients died 2 months after ligation of IVC of causes not related to the operation.

In no patient gross edema of the lower limbs comparable to that seen in ileofemoral thrombosis was observed. Only one woman aged 70 years, in whom the lower segment of IVC following plication thrombosed, had progressive signs of CVI

and venous ulcer developed four years following surgery. In this case the thrombosis of IVC occurred in connection with discontinuation of anticoagulant therapy. Symptomatic varicosities confirmed by thermography developed in two cases. The decrease in blood flow at rest and after exercise tested by means of occlusive plethysmography and the prolongation in clearance of intramuscularly injected isotopes helped us to discover a serious

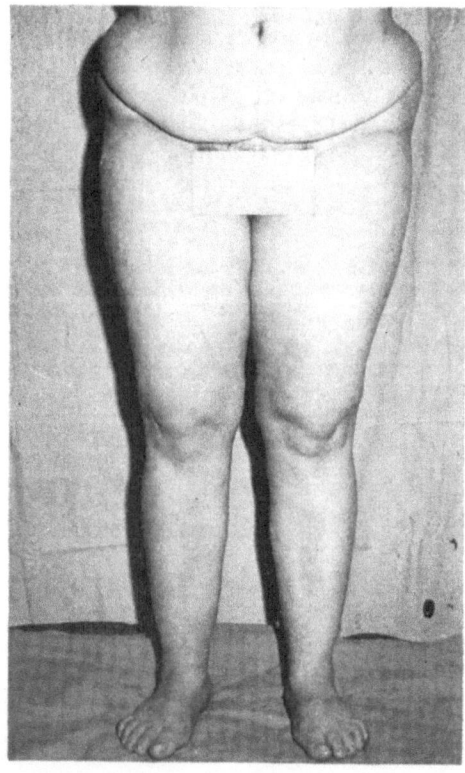

Fig. 1. 31 years-old woman -- 11 years following meso-caval shunt.

degree of CVI in 3 patients, who underwent ligation of, the superficial femoral vein. These 3 patients had markedly more pronounced painful sensation in the operated limb than those following surgery on IVC/clearance activity: 43.5%, 55.5%, 45.3%-normal rate 20 $\pm$ 2.77 — var. coef. 13.9% to 20 min. Venous manometry: 85, 70, 80 torr, plethysmography: BF 0.5 to 1 ml/100 ml/1 min, FF 4.3 ml — norm: BF 2.6, FF 11.9) (occlusive — Fluvoscript).

Group B — patients with division of IVC due to meso-caval shunt. This group includes 3 women, 3 children and 1 man. In these patients we have not observed any serious haemodynamic disturbances unless there was residual coexisting thrombosis of the peripheral or pelvic veins. The longest follow-up has been in a 31 year-old woman in whom a meso-caval anastomosis was performed in 1968 and who delivered a normal child by Caesarian section 11 years following operation. At present she has CVI with following findings: (Fig. 1). Higher BF in plethysmography (11.7 ml/100 ml/1 min.), venous pressure 45 torr and no remarkable varicosity is present. The collateral veins which developed at the thoracoepigastrical region cannot be seen well due to obesity, but were well recorded by thermography. She has only a moderate dependent edema without stasis changes in the malleolar region.

In the two children, operated for prehepatic thrombotic obstruction of the portal vein in 1973 and 1974 we observed subcutaneous venous collateral pathways on the abdominal wall and on the chest. Neither varices, nor swelling on the lower limbs have been observed, both boys are lively and without any difficulties when taking physical exercises or training. The third child, aged 4 years, was operated upon for ganglioneuroma growing around the subrenal segment of IVC; a follow — up in June this year showed that the child was in good health and no varicosity was observed.

The next two women who underwent the meso-caval shunt in 1975, 1976 have visible subcutaneous venous network with mildly dilated veins on their limbs. The younger one, 24 years old, is pregnant and should deliver this August. The dependent edema is very moderate and there are no trophical changes.

The postoperative course was unfavorable in a single case of a 63 year — old man who died on the 4th day after reintervention for recurrent bleeding from esophageal varices. The cause of his death was PE due to massive thrombosis of the pelvic and peripheral veins.

Discussion

Venous drainage following IVC ligation or plication is established through 3 channels: 1. the saphenous vein to thoracoepigastric veins, 2. the deep femoral vein to hypogastr. vv., 3. the pelvic

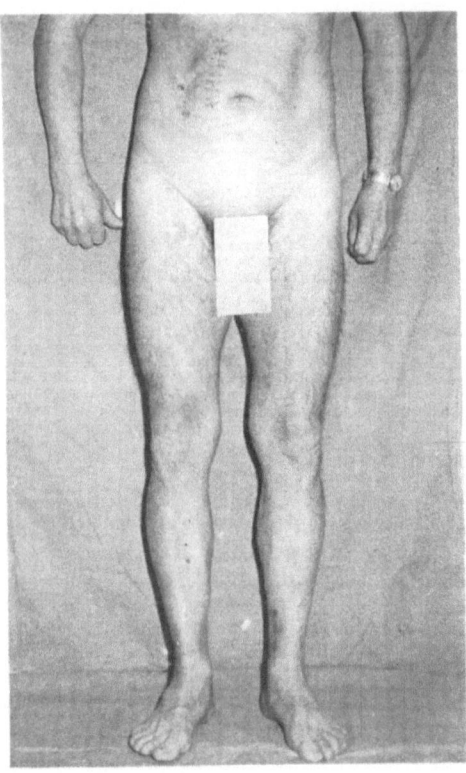

Fig. 2. 61 years-old man — 4 years following plication of the IVC — 10 days following cholecystectomy.

crossover from the fem. vein in the affected limb to the contralateral side (*Haller*, 1967). Signs of collateral circulation usually appear within the 1st year (*Anděl*, 1975). Venous hypertension does not appear in the absence of extensive thrombosis (*Anděl*, 1975). The typical postthrombotic disease with severe pain associated with brawny dependent edema and cellulitic stasis ulcers can be effectively prevented by strict avoidance of chronic edema. We have applied the usual postoperative care with anticoagulants (*Klioner et al.*, 1973)

We kept the patient in a slight Trendelenburg position for at least 3 weeks. Ambulation is begun at the end of the 1st postoperative week and elastic stockings with high compression are recommended.

All our younger patients returned to their work. The elder ones were capable to take care of themselves without assistance at home, one man underwent un uneventful cholecystectomy four years after ligation of IVC, and two younger women became pregnant. (Fig. 2).

REFERENCES

Anděl, M. (1975): Chronic venous insufficiency. Thesis II., Plzeň.
Haller, J. A. (1967): Deep thrombophlebitis. W. B. Saunders Co., Philadelphia a. London.

Klioner, L. I. (1973): Problems of vascular surgery (Voprosy sosudistoj chirurgii), Moscow, T XXIV.

M. A., Dept. of Surgery, Faculty of Medicine Charles University, Marxova 13, 3016 Plzeň, Czechoslovakia

INCIDENCE OF CALF VEIN THROMBOSIS
AFTER EXTRACORPOREAL CIRCULATION

M. E. MONTEIRO, P. LAUWERS, G. STALPAERT, R. SUY
and R. VERHAEG

Departments of Internal Medicine, Anesthesiology and Cardiovascular Surgery, University of Leuven, Leuven, Belgium

Introduction

The incidence of deep vein thrombosis is high in patients undergoing elective abdominal surgery when sensitive and accurate techniques are used for its detection (1, 6, 9). Fewer studies have been performed in thoracic surgery (10) and a literature search did not reveal any data on the incidence after surgery requiring extra-corporeal circulation. Therefore, in the present study radiolabeled fibrinogen tests were carried out in a series of patients undergoing coronary surgery and heart valve replacement.

Patients and methods

Relevant clinical data on the 45 patients studied are summarized in Table I. For extra-corporeal circulation partial haemodilution was used; the priming solution consisted of sorbitol

Table 1. Patient data.

Patient	Coronary surgery	Heart valve replacement
number	35	10
mean age	49	47
(years)	(30—60)	(27—72)
sex (m/f)	31/4	8/2

(16—20 ml per kg body weight). Heparin (3 mg per kg body weight) was injected before the perfusion was started and neutralized with protamine sulphate after the pump was stopped. Patients undergoing coronary surgery received an intravenous infusion of Dextran 40 for the first three postoperative days (30 ml per hour); in those with heart valve replacement oral anticoagulants were started on the third postoperative day. Active mobilization of the legs under

supervision of a physiotherapist was started on the second postoperative day in all patients.

For analysis of the results, the increase in the ratio between the highest and lowest counts on the same calf on any two occasions was calculated (2). Five patients undergoing coronary surgery were excluded from the analysis: three because of technical failure of the radiolabeled fibrinogen test and two because of excessive bleeding on the first postoperative day requiring reintervention leading to too low counts over the legs.

Results

None of the examined patients developed symptoms or clinical signs of deep vein thrombosis in the legs. The results of the radiolabeled fibrinogen tests are summarized in Table II. In none of the patients

Table II. Results of radiolabeled fibrinogen tests.

	Number of legs	Change in ratio of calf counts*
valve replacement	20	−0.01 ± 0.02
coronary surgery		
— all legs	60	0.13 ± 0.05
— legs with vein taken out	33	0.28 ± 0.09
— legs without vein taken out	27	−0.05 ± 0.03

* data expressed as mean ±SE.

with heart valve replacement did the change in the ratio over the calf reach 0.56, a value which is indicative of the presence of developing thrombus (2, 7). Ten legs of nine patients undergoing coronary surgery had at some time a ratio higher than the critical value; the saphenous vein had been taken from the calf in nine of these legs and from the thigh in the tenth. Phlebography was carried out in five of the nine latter patients; none of them showed evidence of an occlusion of the calf veins.

Discussion

The fibrinogen uptake test is well established as a valuable sensitive and specific screening method for early detection of calf vein thrombosis. The labeled protein behaves in the same manner as endogenous fibrinogen and thus is concentrated preferentially in a forming thrombus. Normally, an increase of 20 percent in radioactivity over the leg compared to the heart on any day is indicative of deep vein thrombosis [7]. However, in patients who undergo cardiac or coronary surgery requiring extracorporeal circulation, several problems hamper the application of this test. If labeled fibrinogen were injected before surgery was started, the blood loss and the expansion of the circulating volume that accompanies extracorporeal circulation would result in a considerable decrease in radioactivity over the legs in the postoperative period. For this reason, in the present study, the ^{127}I-fibrinogen was injected only at the end of the surgical procedure. Furthermore, the counts over the sternal region cannot be used as a reference to evaluate the radioactivity because of the thoracic surgery. Therefore radioactivity was measured as absolute counts and the change in the ratio of the highest to the lowest counts on the same calf on any two occasions was calculated [2, 7].

Finally, when veins are taken out of the calf or thigh for bypass surgery, minor local bleeding may cause false positive results. This is suggested by the significantly higher change of the ratio in legs with veins taken out compared to those without veins taken out and is demonstrated by the absence of calf vein thrombosis in all patients with a change in ratio indicative of thrombus formation who were subjected to phlebography.

The absence of any definite evidence for calf vein thrombosis in the present series of patients is rather surprising and even more so since exposure of circulating blood to artificial surfaces as during extracorporeal circulation is known to induce a hypercoagulable state [4, 8] and may therefore be expected to predispose to intravascular thrombosis. Several reasons may help explain this unexpected findings. First, all patients received systemic heparinization throughout the duration of the extracorporeal circulation; this probably prevents effectively early thrombus formation in the deep venous system since it is increasingly evident that postoperative venous thrombosis actually develops during the surgical procedure [5]. In addition, mobilization of the legs in the immediate postoperative period was carried out as a routine measure for prevention of deep vein thrombosis [3].

Finally, patients with coronary surgery were infused dextran daily while those with artificial heart valves were placed on oral anticoagulants; both treatment regimens are valuable in lowering the incidence of postoperative calf vein thrombosis [11]. The combination of these measures in the present series of patients was highly effective in preventing calf vein thrombosis.

REFERENCES

1. *Becker, J. and Schampi, B. (1973):* The incidence of postoperative venous thrombosis of the legs. A comparative study on the prophylactic effect of dextran 70 and electrical calf muscle stimulation Acta Chir. Scand., 139, 357.
2. *Flanc, C., Kakkar, V. V. and Clarke, M. B. (1968):* The detection of venous thrombosis of the legs using ^{125}I-labelled fibrinogen. Brit. J. Surg. 55, 742.
3. *Flanc, C., Kakkar, V. V. and Clarke, M. B. (1969):* Postoperative deep-vein thrombosis. Effect of intensive prophylaxis. Lancet, 1, 477.

4. *Harker, L. A. and Slichter, S. J. (1972):* Platelet and fibrinogen consumption in man. N. Engl. J. Med. 287, 999.
5. *Heimbecker, R. O. (1977):* Systemic heparin in major vascular operations. Surg. Gynec. Obstet. 144, 753.
6. *Kakkar, V. V. (1972):* The diagnosis of deep vein thrombosis using the I^{125}-fibrinogen test. Arch. Surg. 104, 152.
7. *Kakkar, V. V. (1977):* Fibrinogen Uptake Test for Detection of Deep Vein Thrombosis. A Review of Current Practice. Sem. Nucl. Med. 7, 229.
8. *Kendall, A. G. and Lowenstein, L. (1962):* Alterations in blood coagulation and hemostasis during extracorporeal circulation. Can. Med. Assoc. J. 87, 786.
9. *Lambie, J. M., Mahaffy, R. G., Barber, D. C., Karmody, A. M., Scott, M. M. and Matheson, N. A. (1970):* Diagnostic accuracy in venous thrombosis. Brit. Med. J. 11, 142.
10. *Nicolaides, A. N., Dupont, P. A., Desai, S., Lewis, J. D., Douglas, J. N., Dodsworth, H., Fourides, G., Luck, R. J. and Jamieson, C. W. (1972):* Small doses of subcutaneous sodium heparin in preventing deep venous thrombosis after major surgery. Lancet, II, 890.
11. *Verstraete, M, (1976):* The prevention of postoperative deep vein thrombosis and pulmonary embolism. Surg. Gyn. Obstet., 143, 981.

M. M., Kapucijnenvoer 35, Leuven, Belgium

THROMBOSIS OF FEMORAL AND ILIAC ARTERY AFTER CATHETERISATION

MILADA KRČÍLKOVÁ and A. KRČÍLEK

Medical faculty, Charles University, Prague, Czechoslovakia

Thrombosis of the femoral and iliac arteries can occur as a complication after catheterization of the artery, particularly using the Seldinger technique and after extracorporal circulation. Acute thrombosis of the femoral artery is frequently overlooked, as it has only mild symptoms and signs: The patient has only paresthesias in the lower limb, numbness and tingling or mild pain in the foot. Trophic changes of the skin or gangrene usually do not develop. The foot is a litle paler and colder in comparison with the other healthy foot. Peripheral arterial pulsation of the leg is absent, oscilations are diminished and the skin temperature is lower. After several weeks a light atrophy of the leg develops and the patient has intermittent claudication after walking a long distance.

Our observation: S. L., a 24 year-old woman. One year ago, an operation for heart disease (atrial septal defect) was performed with extracorporal circulation. No thrombosis was diagnosed at that time. The women complained of cramps in the left calf after a longer walk, mainly when walking uphill.

On the thorax can be seen the scar after the operation of the heart, in the groin two scars after extracorporal circulation. The left calf is 1 cm thinner in circumference. In the left groin there is systolic murmur. Peripheral arterial pulsation of the extremity is absent and oscillations diminished. The foot is pale on elevation. Arteriography shows obliteration of the cranial segment of the left iliac artery with sufficient collateral circulation, the femoral artery is well filled. Phlebography + femoral and iliac veins are quite free. Function test: on flat ground the woman can walk as far as 3 km without any discomfort, but walking uphill produces cramps in the left calf.

Our vascular surgeons suggested a by-pass operation of the obliterated segment with a graft, but as it caused the woman little discomfort the operation was postponed.

On the other hand, thrombosis of the femoral artery in a child has more serious results: The growing of the child's extremity is slowed down and shortening of the limb develops. Prevention of thrombosis, early diagnosis and intensive therapy in children with thrombosed femoral arteries are therefore very important.

Our experience with thrombolytic therapy: We treated 7 patients with acute thrombosis of the femoral and iliac artery with Streptase. The age of the children treated was $9-11$ years. The reason for catheterisation of the femoral artery was that 3 children had aortic stenosis and the catheterisation was made for levography of the heart. 1 child had agenesis of one kidney-nephrography was performed, 1 child had epilepsy (brain angiography), 1 adult had obliteration of the femoral artery (peripheral arteriography), one had hematuria.

The doses for children were $1/3-1/2$ that for adults. The initial dose was 100 000 U, the maintenance dose 50 000 U per hour. The therapy was discontinued as soon as peripheral arterial pulsation of the limb appeared, usually after 10 hours of treatment.

Results:

In 6 of 7 our patients recanalization of the thrombosed artery was achieved, on an average after 10 hours of thrombolytic tratment. In one child, where the thrombolytic therapy was started 8 days after catheterization, during which the artery was lacerated and sutured, we failed to recanalize the thrombus. The therapy was stopped because of epistaxis in the child.

The dosage of Streptase for adults was: 250 000 U as an initial dose and 100 000 U per hour as a maintenance dose.

Complications

There were 4 cases of bleeding from the puncture in the groin. Light compression of the artery was able to control the bleeding in all cases. Suture of the artery was never performed. It was necessary to watch the children during the thrombolytic therapy because the bleeding from the puncture was sometimes very intensive. *Prevention* of thrombosis after catheterisation of the artery:

1. The size of the catheter must correspond to the size of the child's artery.
2. After the catheterisation it is necessary to examine every 2 hours for a period of 24 hours: The color and the temperature of the foot and the peripheral arterial pulsation of the limb should be noted.
3. Diminished arterial pulsation of the limb is a indication for immediate application of papaverin and procaine and, if this is not effective.
4. Thrombolytic therapy must be applied.

Conclusion

Acute thrombosis of the femoral and iliac artery after Seldinger catheterisation is discussed. Early treatment with streptokinase and heparin in 7 cases established recanalisation of the thrombosed artery. The importance of prevention, early diagnosis and thrombolytic therapy of the thrombosed artery are emphasized.

REFERENCES

Bergentz, S. E., Hanson, L.O ., Norbäck, B. (1966): Surgical management of complication to arterial puncture. Ann. Surg., 164, s. 1021.

Donner, L., Krčílek A.: Thrombolytische Therapie mit Stretase. Behringwerke Mitteilungen 1964. Frankfurt, Hoechst, 1967.

Krčílek, A., Krčílková, M.: Thrombose der Femoralarterie bei Kindern nach der extracorporalen Zirkulation. Angiolog. Kongres in Essen 1966.

Lang, E. K. (1963): A survay of the complication of percutaneous retrograde arteriography, Seldinger technic. Radiology, 81, s. 275.

A. K., IVth Internal Clinic, Faculty of Charles Univ.
U nemocnice 2, 128 08 Prague 2 Czechoslovakia

ABOUT REACTIVITY CHANGES IN ORGANISM IN CASE OF THROMBOTIC DISEASES IN THE VEINS OF LOWER EXTREMITIES

J. MÄNNISTE, U. SIBUL, V. VALDES, R. LEVINA and T. TAMM

Central Hospital, Tallin, U.S.S.R.

The change in organism's reactivity is a general conception for the concrete estimation of which there are numerous possibilities.

In the present study we have tried to determine the reactivity changes in the organism in case of thrombotic diseases in the veins of low extremities:

a) by means of the estimation of mast cell activity in the wall of the damaged vein and the regional lymphatic node;

b) through some immunological tests: determination of rosette-forming cells, determination of the deep autoflora of the skin and the study on the skin bactericide activity (methods recommended by N. Klemparskaya).

The number of mast cells was estimated in 40 fields of vision with $300 \times$ magnifying. The functional condition of the mast cells was determined according to the degranulation index:

$$x = \frac{(1 \times a)(2 \times b)(3 \times c)}{100}$$

whereas:

a — the number of mast cells in the 1st stage of activity (homogeneously granulated protoplasm, intensive coloration)

b — the number of mast cells in the 2nd stage of activity (the cells are bigger, swollen, well-definded, brightly granulated)

c — the number of mast cells in the 3rd stage of activity (the cells have exploded, their contures perished, granules have emerged from the cells — shows the phase of degranulation at the time of active functioning.

In case of recent phlebothrombosis degranulated forms were in the majority in the vein-wall ($x = 2.5 - 2.8$). In the regional lymphatic node the number of mast cells exceeded the number of the mast cells in the vein-wall, whereas the degranulation index was high ($x = 2.25$ to 2.8).

In case of acute superficial thrombophlebitis the number of mast cells in the vein-wall as well as in the regional lymphatic node had increased, but the degranulation index approached the normal ($x = 1.7 - 2.3$), i.e. the degranulation index of the mast cells in the inflammation-free vein-wall and lymphatic node.

In case of an arrested inflammation in postthrombotic vein-wall the degranulation index was also low ($x = 1.2 - 2.2$), but the number of mast cells was considerably reduced. The mast cells retain their activity longer in the lymphatic node than in the vein-wall (x 2.3 in over 50 per cent of cases), whereas in case of the trophic ulcer in the leg lots of plasma-cells could be detected in the fields of vision as well.

Assuming that the mast cells secrete heparin, serotonin is characteristic of the rise in fermentactivity of tissues in case of thrombotic processes.

In case of ileofemoral thrombosis the deep microflora of the skin increased (AF — $6.8 - 28.4$ colonies, in the control group $2.8 - 0.8$), basically on the account of patogenic mannitepositive microbes.

In case of thrombophlebitis and especially in postthrombotic syndrome of the patient having a chronic ulcer in the leg, the number of rosette-forming lymphocytes increased ($10.9 - 12.2$, normally $1.3 - 0.2$). In all cases of the thrombotic diseases in veins the bactericide activity of the skin diminished (48.7 — 58.8, normally 92.1 — 1.2).

The changes in the activity of mast cells in regional lymphatic nodes and vein-walls in various cases of thrombosis, the enrichment of the skin autoflora with mannitepositive patogenic colonies, the decrease in bactericide ability, the increase of the number of rosette-forming lymphocytes and the multitude of plasma cells in the cell content of a lymphatic node evidence the essential changes in the reactivity of organisms in case of thrombotic diseases of veins.

In addition to the need of replenishing the heparin reserve of the tissues in the early stages of thrombosis the desensibilitating treatment as well as avoiding septic complications play an important role.

J. M., Central Hospital Tallin, Karl Marx Street 16, Tallin, U.S.S.R.

NEW ASPECTS OF POST-THROMBOPHLEBITIC SYNDROME

S. CARONNI, A. BAGLIANI and R. MOIA

Institute of Vascular Surgery, University of Pavia, Italy

This paper deals with new aspects of the post-thrombophlebitic syndrome.

After a more accurate study of the different sites of the deep veins of the lower limbs and of the possible collateral compensatory blood circulation using the Doppler flowmeter in addition to the standard diagnostic procedures, the authors wist to propose a new classification for the post-thrombophlebitic syndrome.

171 phlebographies were performed on a group of 140 patients; the classification we suggest is as follows:

Post-Tibio-Thrombophlebitic Syndrome (in cases of obstruction of the anterior and/or posterior tibial veins): 94 phlebographies.

a) Obliteration of the anterior tibial veins (12 phlebographies): collateral blood circulation takes place:
   1) through the surface venous system with a greater overload on the long saphenous vein, only in the leg;
   2) through the deep venous system of the posterior tibial veins;
   3) through Vernuil's emergency blood circulations;
b) Obliteration of the posterior tibial veins (14 phlebographies): the compensatory blood circulation channels are through the short saphenous veins, the anterior tibial veins and Vernuil's emergency blood circulation;
c) Obliteration of the anterior and posterior tibial veins (most frequently observed) (59 phlebographies).

In these cases the collateral blood circulation channels are the following:
1) through the surface circulation of both saphenous veins;
2) through Vernuil's pathways;
3) through the secondary deep venous system.

Post-Femoro-Thrombophlebitic Syndrome (in cases of obliteration of the femoro-popliteal axis) (39 phlebographies).

The following collateral blood circulations can be distinguished:

a) through the surface venous system of both saphenous veins with reversion of the circulation at the level of the high communicating veins of the leg and return of the circulation into the deep venous system, according to the site and the importance of the obstruction, through the communicating veins of the thigh and the sapheno-femoral junction;
b) through the secondary and collateral deep blood circulation. The latter is especially involved when the deep femoral vein is patent.

Post-Iliaco-Thrombophlebitic Syndrome: (9 phlebographies).

Different kinds of compensatory blood circulation are observed:

a) the first has been widely described by Martorell and is represented by the abdominal collateral veins and the heterolateral iliac vein;
b) the second type of compensatory blood circulation is through the hypogastric vein;
c) the third can be found in the parietal veins which drain the blood towards the upper part of the inferior vena cava and towards the superior vena cava.

Post-Thrombophlebitic Syndrome (29 phlebographies) only in cases with obliterations in tibial veins together with the femoro-popliteal axis and iliac vein.

It is quite understandable that symptomatology in these cases will affect the abdominal wall.

Remarks

The seriousness of the post-thrombo-phlebitic syndrome will largely depend on the efficiency and rapidity of the flow-rate in this blood circulatin.

Although we feel that this paper represents a further step in this research field, it is also aimed at further investigation into the trends and application fields of surgical therapy.

We think that study of the post-thrombophlebitic syndrome on the basis of this new classification which reflects different post-thrombophlebitic syndromes, will lead to different trends in surgical therapy: long total saphenectomy; short total saphenectomy; long saphenectomy peculiar to the leg or to the thigh; ligament or interruption of the incontinent perforating veins; creation of new venous by-passes; operations directly involving the deep venous circulation etc...

At presently we cannot give a more detailed analysis of surgical therapy, as this paper is more an experimental clinical hypothesis for a new classification of the post-thrombophlebitic syndrome and for a better understanding of the surgical procedures pertaining to it, rather than an analysis of our experience.

S. C., Istituto di Chirurgia Vascol., Università di Pavia, Pavia, Italia

LITTLE TRICKS OF THE TRADE IN THE SURGERY OF VARICOSE VEINS

R. MOIA, S. CARONNI and A. BAGLIANI

Institute of Vascular Surgery, University of Pavia, Italy

The aim of this paper is to give some advice on the surgical therapy of varicose veins that may lead to discussion.

In particular, it should be remembered that this therapy must be atraumatic, radical and aesthetic as well.

The authors consequently think that the surgeon should:

1) never operate on areas overlying phlogosis in cases of surface thrombophlebities or of varico-thrombophlebities, to prevent lymphorrhagias and avoid necrotic cutaneous areas;

2) perform long total saphenectomy by introducing the stripper upwards and by stripping downwards to prevent injury to the saphenous nerve;

3) incise in the groin in a parallel direction to it, 2—3 cm above the inguinal told and at the level of the inner malleolus, above and crosswise;

4) fasten and section all the adjacent collateral veins to the sapheno-femoral junction to avoid further operations;

5) identify the whole femoral vein and fasten the long saphenous at the level of the cross;

6) limit the number of cutaneous incisions of the leg and on the thigh in order to remove all the collateral veins with a sub-cutaneous extractor (avoid ligaments); possibly perform small and medial incisions and always follow the cutaneous lines;

7) section and fasten the communicating veins in the underfascial area (they are fastened under the aponeurosis that is closed only in cases of severe hypertension) by using, whenever possible, former incisions;

8) perform short total saphenectomy only when varicose veins are present on the back of the leg;

9) tampon and empty the sub-cutaneous hematomas with manual pressure;

10) suture the skin without tension in order to prevent superficial necroses;

11) apply a double elastic bandage during the post-operative period and raise the legs;

12) remove nonabsorbable sutures as soon as possible.

The time the surgeon needs to perform these surgical steps is short and the advantages are many.

The complications and inactivity period following the operation are thus considerably reduced and the aesthetic results achieved are excellent.

R. M., Istituto Chirurgia Vascol., Università di Pavia, Pavia, Italia

A TIME-SAVING AND SUCCESSFULL TECHNIQUE OF VARICOSE VEIN OPERATION

G. W. HAGMÜLLER and H. DENCK

1st Surgical Department, Hospital Vienna—Lainz, Austria

Since the introduction of intraluminal stripping of the saphenous vein at the beginning of our century, the central status of this step in varicose vein operations is fixed in every operation plan (*Babcock* 1907, *Hagmüller et al.* 1976). The next important advance, introduced in surgical therapy, was the crossectomy, the high ligation of the internal saphenous vein with entire removal of all branches in the fossa ovalis (*Haeger* 1966). Even complete saphenectomy from the internal malleolus to the groin is no longer a matter of discussion. The greatest variations still exist in the surgical treatment of varicose branches and insufficient perforating veins. They range from stitchligations (*Romich* 1935) up to, the recently published "surgical sclerotherapy" (*Lerma* 1974).

Methods of operation (Hagmüller et al. 1976)

We differentiate 5 steps in our varicose vein operation plan:

1. Crossectomy with a transversal suprainguinal skin incision. Thus the saphenous orifice is exactly to be reached, and on the other hand the inguinal entering lymphatic vessels cannot be hurt.

2. Premalleolar finding of the internal saphenous vein and introduction of the stripper from distal towards proximal part. The curled head of newly developed one-way strippers renders it nearly every time possible to pass the entire saphenous vein. When extracting the stripper from the groin, simultaneously a thin vaccuum drainage is pulled into the subcutaneous bed of the withdrawn vena saphena. Leaving this drain 2—3 hours after operation diminishes saphenous bed haematomas.

3. Immediate sterile compression bandage following the stepwise extraction of the stripper is performed.

4. The preoperatively exactly marked varicose branches and perforating veins are percutaneously dissected with the Klapp-scalpel (*Klapp*, 1923) (Figs. 1 and 2).

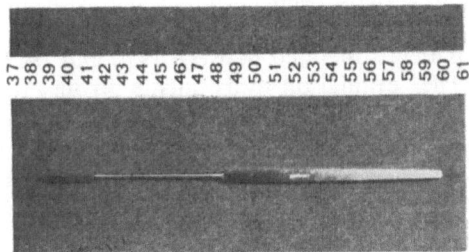

Fig. 1. Klapp scalpel with one-side sharpened blade.

5. Separate extraction of great varicose convolutes and subfascial ligature of larger perforating veins recognized by phlebographic examination and clinically by the blow-out phenomenon.

Klapp scalpel

Since 1970 we have been using the Klapp scalpel for percutaneous dissection. We took this method over in 1970 from Hejhal (Prague) and operated since then on more than 1000 patients successfully. In western Europe this instrument, introduced in 1923 by R. Klapp for varicose vein operations, has obviously fallen into oblivion.

Advantages: a) Quick and exact destruction of marked varicose branches
b) Good cosmetic results because of few skin incisions

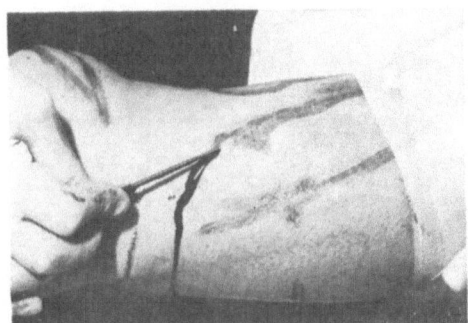

Fig. 2. Operation situs with percutaneous dissection of a marked varicose branch.

c) No scars after percutaneous dissection.

Disadvantages: Extensive haematomas after insufficient blood expression and insufficient compression bandage.

Results

To evaluate this technique for operation on varicose vein insufficiency with the Klapp scalpel we checked up all our patients operated between 1970 and 1975. The evaluation was made from the clinical and cosmetical point of view as well. The results were termed after Haeger standards published in 1966. The appraisal was classified as -very good-, -satisfactory- and -unsatisfactory-.

983 patients operated upon in this period were examined 2 to 5 years after operation. 40.9% were termed very good, 54.4% satisfactory and 4.7% unsatisfactory.

Postoperative phlebographic control examinations showed also satisfactory results after percutaneous dissection (Fig. 3).

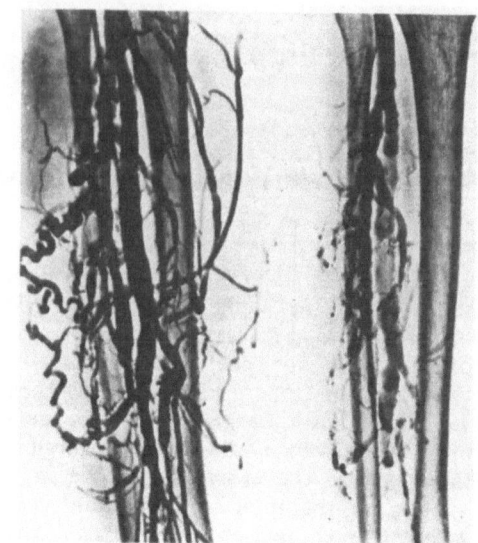

Fig. 3. Preoperative (left) and postoperative (right) phlebogramm of a patient with internal saphenous insufficiency, insufficient perforating veins and significant varicose branches. Operation was performed by stripping and Klapp discission.

REFERENCES

Babcock, W. W. (1907): A new operation for extirpation of varicose veins of leg. New York Med. J. 86, 153.

Haeger, K. (1966): Five Year Results of Radical Surgery for Superficial Varices with or without Coexistant Perforator Insufficiency. Acta Chir. Scand. 131, 38.

Hagmüller, G. W., Denck, H. (1976): Die Verwendung des Klappschen Messers in der Varicen-Chirurgie. Aktuelle chir. 11, 219.

Hagmüller, G. W., Denck, H. (1976): Die Varizenoperation unter besonderer Berücksichtigung der "Gamaschenzone". Wiener klin. Wschr. 88 (12), 388.

Klapp, R. (1923): Experimentelle und klinische Studie über Varizen. Arch. f. klin. Chir. 127, 817.

Lerma, M. (1974): Sclerose Chirurgicale des Varices. 5th Intern. Congress Phlebol., Mailand.

Romich, S. (1935): Vier Hauptforderungen bei der Varizenoperation. Med. Klinik 14, 445.

G. W. H., I. Chirurgische Abteilung, Krankenhaus der Stadt Wien—Lainz, Wolkersbergerstr. 1, A 1130 Wien, Austria

COMPLETE RECONSTRUCTION OF THE SUBCLAVIAN VEIN OCCLUDED AT THE COSTOCLAVICULAR LEVEL

M. A. BEAUJEAN

Institute of Surgery, University of Liege, Belgium

The chronic, repetitive or accidental compression of the subclavian vein in the scapulo-thoracic passage is more frequently produced at the level of the costo-clavicular space. It results in two main types of alterations:

Type 1: Extrinsic compression without significant lesion of the vein wall. The narrowing of the lumen of the vessel varies widely according to the position of the arm and shoulder with regard to the thorax.

Type 2: Segmental stenosis or occlusion by a localized intraluminar thrombosis, usually occurring at the point where repeated crushing of the vein wall in a narrowed costo-clavicular slit produces a fibrous reaction. In addition, in such cases, the last valve of the subclavian vein is frequently found to be implanted precisely in this progressively atrophied segment, thus completing obstruction of the vessel. This valve itself may constitute the only stenotic element present (case n°4), but usually, this combination of factors may finally lead to the formation of a connective tissue plug in the proximal part of the subclavian vein (cases 1, 2, 3); consistent collateral compensation is usually developed; the clinical symptoms, at this stage, may be absent or more or less disabling in relation to its efficiency. There is no relation between the more or less functional impairment of mucsular activity and the phlebographic aspect of the lesion surrounded by its often impressive collateral network. Either the two types of lesions mentioned above may be complicated by an acute, rapidly extending, venous thrombosis (cases 1,3) if the previously "stabilized situation" is disrupted by an accidental circumstance. Intense muscular work of the arm (effort thrombosis), which produces a contusion of the vein wall clearly visualized in case n°3;

From the site of compression, the thrombosis always progresses peripherally, occluding the ostia of collateral veins and therefore producing a sudden distal swelling, of the limb. (Paget-von Schrötter Syndromcases n°1,3). In rare cases, the clot also progresses proximally, involving a slight risk of pulmonary embolism. The degree and duration of the venous congestion depends on the capacity of the collateral vessels still patent to compensate for the obstructed vessel during the early and late period, in all conditions of physical activity. It is "classicaly" assumed that lysis and recanalization of the clot, assisted by anticoagulant therapy, in connection with developement of a collateral venous network, very often lead to an almost complete recovery. However, it has been more recently demonstrated that 70% of the patients who where treated conservatively after extensive acute thrcmbosis sustain moderate to serious "postthrombotic" sequelae. Venous thrcmbectomy (preferably through the axillary approach) or fibrinolysis performed scon after initiation of the acute thrcmbosis can completely unclog the vessel, which is restored to normal, if its structure has no been previously modified by traumatic injuries (Type 1). The organic cause of the extrinsic compression must be removed at the same time: excision of the first rib — also through the axillary route — is usually preferred to claviculectomy. If a previous segmental intraluminar thrombosis is present (Type 2), classical thrombectomy or fibrinolysis can only evacuate the recent clot from the main deep vein and the orifices of the collateral vessels, but will have no effect on the former lesion which is permanent and may lead to recurrence of the thrombosis. In such cases, at first, removal of the costo-clavicular "bottle-neck" by costectomy or claviculectomy is always mandatory: It can improve the circulation in the "first rib collateral veins" only, and if the phlebography has demonstrated that venous return is further impaired by the compression of these veins in certain positions of the arm (hyperabduction...). The "by-pass" of the venous stenosis by a venous graft involves problems of diameter discrepancy, difficulties of maintaining the anastomosis widely open under low pressure blood flow and the need for a temporary A. V. shunt which is an additional somewhat handicapping operation. In addition, the origin of recurrent centrifugal thrombosis – the "fibrous plug" persists. For similar reasons, segmental replacement of the lesion, also using a venous graft, has not proved satisfactory. The direct reconstruction of the altered segment of the subclavian vein associated with resection of the first rib appears to be the only logical solution in still active patients remaining severely disabled. Simple removal of the obstacle followed by direct suture of the phlebotomy are impossible in almost all cases, due to the atrophy of vein walls in the fibrotic portion. In 4 cases with segmental organized lesions of the subclavian vein at the costoclavicular level, (– Two with an acutely recurring Paget – Von Schrötter Syndrom after anticoagulant

therapy and fibrinolysis; – One with a very crippling clinical condition; – One in whom the only stenotic element is only the valve itself;) corrections have been successfully performed by a combination of:
– First rib resection;
– Endophlebectomy with excision of the

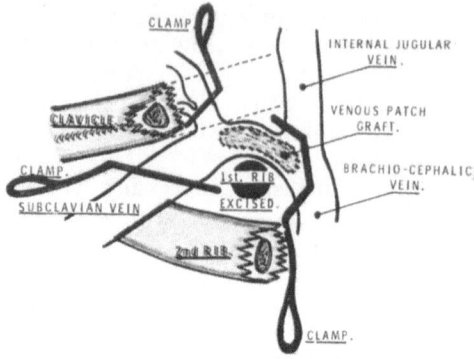

Fig. 2. Diagram of the reconstruction performed.

terminal valve of the subclavian vein, which, in case was included in the intraluminar fibrotic tissue;
– Plastic enlargement of the junction of

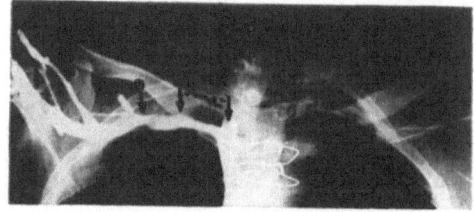

Fig. 3. Case N° 1. Post-operative phlebography the arrow indicates the location of the venous patch graft.

the subclavian and the brachiocephalic veins;
– Closure of the subclavian phlebotomy with a large and rectangular autologous saphenous vein patch graft. (Figrs 1., 2., 3.)
These procedures have been performed using a combined subclavian and partial unilateral sternotomy approach permitting

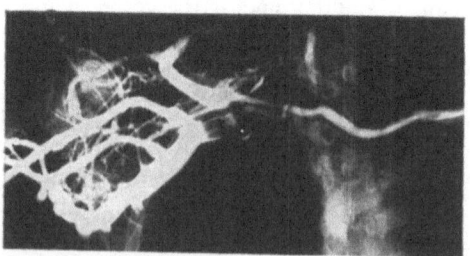

Fig. 1. Case N° 1. Pre-operative phlebography.

lateral retraction of the clavicle and the 2 first ribs. The final cosmetic aspect is more satisfactory than after claviculectomy. All clinical symptoms immediately disappeared in all cases and phlebograms demonstrated a restoration of the venous return. These results still persist since 4 to 20 months and the patients soon resumed complete physical and professional activity. Temporary A. V. shunt fistulae or post-operative anticoagulant therapy is not needed. The sternal split is remarkably easily tolerated. Such complete corrections of lesions of the subclavian veins have not yet been reported.

REFERENCES

Beaujean, M. A.: Proceedings of the Symposium "Pain in shoulder and hand" ed. University of Limburg. The Netherlands, in press.

Beaujean M. A. and Honore D.: Proceedings of the "Journées d'Angéiologie" Paris 1978; in press.

M. A. B., Inst. de Chirurgie, Univ. de Liège, 80/101 Ave Blonden, 4000 Bruxelles, Belgique.

SURGICAL MANAGEMENT OF VARICES OF SHORT SAPHENOUS VEIN AS INDICATED BY TWO-DIRECTIONAL PHLEBOGRAPHY

H. GOTO, H. MATSUMURA, M. KOHNO,
and A. MATSUMOTO

*First Department of Surgery, Yokohama City University Hospital
and School of Medicine, Yokohama, Japan*

Introduction

Although the stripping operation of varicose veins of the leg is now widely performed, it has been recently reported that a relatively large number of patients suffer from their recurrence during a long follow-up period (*Aremander*, 1960, *Lofgren*, 1971, *Keith*, 1974).

Several reasons responsible for the recurrence include an inadequate groin dissection, residual varicose tributaries, persistence of perforating veins and the short saphenous vein (*Agrifoglio*, 1961, *Carter*, 1964). It is important that adequate operative procedures should be performed in the first place, but more emphasis is placed on careful preoperative assessment as well as accurate identification of diseased veins if one attempts to obtain good results. The purpose of this paper is to stress the importance of evaluating the pathophysiologic changes of superficial veins phlebographically and operatively, with special reference to the short saphenous vein, in the hope that good results could be achieved by the operation once and for all.

Methods and materials

Many methods of phlebography have been studied by many authors (*De Weese*, 1959, *Massell*, 1957). The phlebography of our method presented previously (*Goto*, 1975) is as follows: the patient is placed in supine position and a rubber-hand tourniquet is tightly placed just above the ankle to obtain an obstruction of the superficial venous system. Forty ml of 76% Urografin is then injected into a vein running in the dorsum of the foot over a period of two minutes. Immediately after the injection the patient is forced to walk to and stand close to the long X-ray cassette which is set up in erect position. One minute after the injection, a postero-anterior exposure is made followed by a lateral exposure to another set of cassettes.

By our method of two-directional phlebography which is a combination of active move-

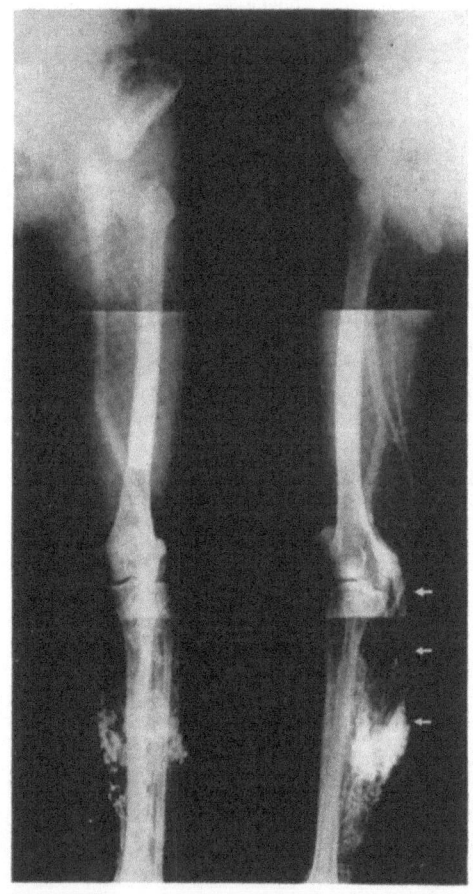

Fig. 1. Two-directional phlebography Arrow shows dilatation and regurgitation of the short saphenous vein.

500

ment of walking and standing in erect position, we can observe simultaneously the filling phase as well as the regurgitation phase of the deep and superficial veins. Comparing the two films, it is possible to obtain a three-dimensional projection and estimate with reasonable accuracy the location of many abnormal veins. Generally speaking, the postero-anterior projection is most useful for identification of the long saphenous vein trunk and the lateral projection is useful for identifying the short saphenous vein trunk (Fig. 1).

During the period from January 1965 to March 1978, 553 phlebograms using our method were performed on 402 patients who were subjected to the stripping operation. One hundred and forty-eight were male and 254 female. The side of the diseased leg was the right leg in 254, the left leg in 299 patients, totalling 553. The phlebograms in the present subjects are divided into three groups. Although there were more or less abnormal perforating or communicating veins a in all cases, a highly abnormal finding was observed in the long saphenous trunk in 426 legs (77%), whereas the abnormality extended to the long and short saphenous trunks was seen in 109 legs (20%) and the abnormality confined only to the short saphenous trunk was seen in 18 legs (3%). We determined the surgical indication these patients on the basis of our findings on their phlebograms.

Results

One hundred and twenty-seven legs of these patients (23%) had abnormalities of the short saphenous trunk that were identified by their phlebograms and findinds during operation. The surgical procedures are presented in Table I. Ninety patients had undergone the stripping operation of long and short saphenous

Table I. Surgical Procedures (402 Patients)

Stripping or Ligation of Main Trunk	No. of Legs	
1. St. of Long Saphenous Main Trunk	426	(77%)
2. St. of Long and Short Saphenous Main Trunk	90	(16%)
3. St. of Long Saphenous Main Trunk plus Lig. of Short Saphenous Main Trunk	19	(4%)
4. St. of Short Saphenous Main Trunk	18	(3%)
Total	553	(100%)

St. : Stripping
Lig. : Ligation

Jan. 1965 — May 1978
Yokohama City University Hospital and School of Medicine

main trunk, 19 patients were subjected to stripping of long saphenous main trunk and ligation of short saphenous main trunk, and 18 patients stripping of only short saphenous main trunk or stripping of long saphenous vein trunk below the knee. As a result, varices in short saphenous vein occurred in 23% of all cases. In addition to these operative procedures, pathologic perforators or communicating veins were ligated or excised according to the phlebographic findings. Excluding minor recurrences, six of 402 patients (1.5%) had a recurrence of sufficient severity to require another operation (Table II). Two of these patients had severe venous ulcer and complete stripping

Table II. Résumé of 6 Recurrent Cases after Vein Stripping

No. of Cases	Sex	Age	Ulcer	Finding at Reoperation
1. S.H.	M	47	(+)	residual distal long
2. Y.S.	M	52	(+)	and short saphenous vein
3. T.I.	M	32	(+)	perforating vein
4. T.I.	F	43	(−)	
5. R.N.	F	35	(−)	intact long saphenous vein
6. A.O.	F	39	(−)	accesory saphenous vein stripping

Jan. 1965 — May 1978

was not feasible because of severe subcutaneous fibrosis. At the reoperation, residual distal long and short saphenous veins under the ulcer were confirmed. In two patients, the reason of the recurrence was inadequate excision and dissection of the perforating vein. In the last two patients, accessory long saphenous vein stripping had been performed and the long saphenous vein was intact.

REFERENCES

Agrifoglio, G., Edwards, E. A. (1961): Results of surgical treatment of varicose veino. J.A.M.A. 178, 138.

Aremander, E. (1960): Hemodynamic effects of varicose veins and results of radical surgery. Acta chir. scandinav. 260, 7.

Carter, B. N., Johns, T. N. (1964): Recurrent varicose veins: anatomical and physiological observations. Ann. Surg. 159, 1017.

De Weese, J. A., Rogoff, S. M. (1959): Functional ascending phlebography of the lower extremity by serial long film technique. Am. J. Roentg. 81, 841.

Goto, H., Matsumura, H., Yamamoto, H., Yo-shida, S., Matsumoto, A., Wada, T. (1975): Surgical management of severe venous leg ulcer of the leg indicated by two directional phlebography. Atti di Angiologia 1, 365.

Keith, L. M., Turnipseed, W. D. (1974): Systematic approach to saphenous system stripping. Am. J. Surg. 128, 612.

Lofgren, E. P., Lofgren, K. A. (1971): Recurrence of varicose veins after the stripping operation. Arch. Surg. 102, 111.

Massell, T. B., Heringman, E. C., Greenstone, S. (1957): The problem of perforator localization in varicose veins. Arch. Surg. 74, 112.

G. H., Yokohama City Univ. Hosp. and School of Med., 3-46 Urafunecho, Minamiku, Yokohama, Japan

CURRENT ASPECTS ON THE MANAGEMENT OF SECONDARY SAPHENO-FEMORAL VALVULAR INCOMPETENCE

D. CHAVATZAS and G. JANTET

Department of Surgery, Hammersmith & King Edward Memorial Hospital, London, U.K. and Athens General Hospital, Greece

Introduction

From the time of Hippocrates to the first half of our century, the applied anatomy, physiology, pathophysiology and phlebodynamics of chronic venous insufficiency have not been given proper attention in the various methods of the treatment of varicose veins. This work as an exercise of application of the above knowledge aims at emphasizing what is necessary and what is unnecessary in the treatment of cases with secondary valvular incompetence.

Materials-methods-results

We have studied 320 legs in 216 patients with secondary sapheno-femoral valvular incompetence (Fig. 1). The diagnosis was based on data from the patients' history of the disease and from clinical examination. The usual complaint was the appearance of varicose veins in the lower legs, which had gradually spread upwards, without any evidence of iliac or deep vein thrombosis. On examination it was confirmed that the venous filling was mainly from below, although in 123 legs cough impulse at the sapheno-femoral opening and thrill was also detectable. In the majority of cases the causative factor was not found. In the rest of cases the secondary valvular incompetence was attributed to minor traumatic thrombotic episodes in the leg perforators involving the valve cusps, to alterations in the

thrombotic and lytic properties of blood and vessels, to arteriovenous shunts, possibly to the administration of hormones and to heredity and congenital factors. Prolonged standing was not considered as a causative, but as an aggravating and accelerating factor. Out of the 320 legs, 287 were treated by compression sclerotherapy (*Fegan* 1967). A 3% sodium tetradecyl sulphate solution was injected into the incompetent perforator, as shown in Fig. 2. In the remaining 33 legs injection-compression was avoided. Incompetent perforators in large legs, in patients unable to walk or with a history of multifactorial allergy, perforators at difficult sites for compressions and large-sized perforators were treated surgically by ligation as is diagrammatically shown in Fig. 2. Following injection-compression or ligation of the incompetent perforators the long saphenous vein, reassessed three months later, gave no signs of incompetence. It was interesting to note that the cough impulse at the sapheno-femoral opening and thrill which was felt in 123 legs on the first examination, disappeared in 106 legs three months after therapy. Other symptoms and signs such as night cramps, tireness in legs, pain in the veins, ulceration, eczema, phlebitis and oedema were reduced or had disappeared. Only in 17 legs the long saphenous veins remained after injection-compression failing and dilated and had to be excised at a second stage.

Discussion

It is known that a leak from a perforating vein which is not adequately compensated will ultimately result in the

Fig. 1. In primary valvular incompetence the venous valve has been irreparably damaged, while in secondary valvular incompetence the cusps of the valve are normal, but fail to meet due to an increase in the diameter of the vein.

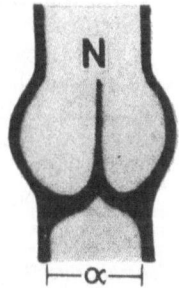
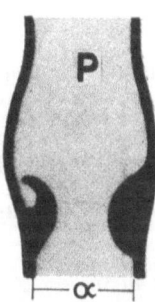
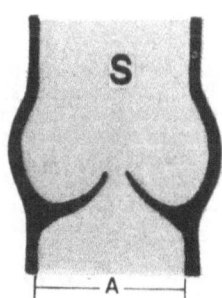

appearance of symptoms and signs of secondary sapheno-femoral valvular incompetence. Amongst the commonest known described causes of this leakage was post-traumatic leg thrombosis of a perforating vein, followed by recanalization, dilatation of superficial veins, incompetence of the valves of the superficial veins, regurgitation into the superficial veins from the deep veins and from the termination of the long saphenous vein (Fig. 2). In the latter stage of incompetence at the sapheno-femoral opening the valve cusps are normal, but fail to meet due to an increase in the diameter of the vein (Fig. 1). The leakage of blood into a segment of the vein below the valve often leads to turbulent retrograde flow, which further enhances the vascular trophic

changes and the venous dilatation (*Švejcar* 1964). Venous dilatation leads to the reduction of blood flow velocity and favours stagnation and thrombosis according to the principle $V = F/A$, which says that the velocity (V) in a tube with a constant volume flow (F) is inversely proportional to the total cross-sectional area A of the tube (*Chavatzas* 1977).

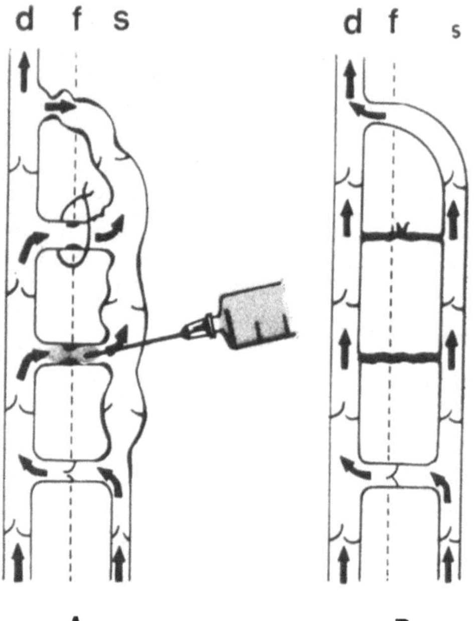

Our study showed that secondary valvular incompetence did not cause irreparable damage to the cusps in the majority of legs studied. Out of 320 legs, 303 showed that the damage was reversible since the vein wall regained normal function. The latter was achieved after the abnormal pressures from below, responsible for the initial venous dilatation, were relieved following obliteration at the point where the trouble began (Fig. 2). This was manifested by the disappearance of the dilated veins, saphena varices and thrill three months after treatment. As has been mentioned earlier, only in 17 legs the long saphenous vein remained dilated and failing. This was attributed in 11 legs to permanent damage in the venous wall which, after severe trophic changes and stretching, was not any longer reversible, in 4 legs to technical error during injection-compression and in 2 legs to factors of underlying primary valvular incompetence following proximal obstruction and deep vein damage.

In conclusion, obliteration of the responsible failing perforator by injection-compression or ligation is the only treatment required in the large majority of cases with secondary valvular incompetence. It is essentially based on the principle of restoring the pumping capacity of the multiple pumps in the foot, calf and thigh, rather than on the habit of unnecessary eradication of the superficial varices. It is worth bearing in mind that the proximal half of the long saphenous vein in one of the best "spare parts" that the human being carries, and should not be light-heartedly stripped out.

Fig. 2. a) Diagramatic presentation of secondary valvular incompetence showing the regurgitation into the superficial vein from the termination of the long saphenous veins.
b) Note the restoration of normal venous flow after the obliteration of the responsible failing incompetent perforators by injection or ligation.

D. Ch., Dept. of Surgery, Athens General State Hospital, Cholargos, Athens, Greece

NEW OPERATING METHODS OF SURGICAL HEALING OF VARICES IN LOWER EXTREMITIES, ACCORDING TO LUŽA

E. LUŽA

*1st Surgical Clinic, Faculty of Medicine of the Charles University,
Prague, Czechoslovakia*

Since 1970, we have developed many efforts to introduce new progressive elements into surgical treatment of varices in lower extremities. We have determined the following aims: 1. full radicality of action, 2. removal of cumbersomeness, 3. simplification and acceleration of the operation, 4. elimination of numerous incissions and punctures, 5. perfect cosmetic effect. During the years from 1971 to 1973, we have gradually elaborated new surgical procedures for all types of varices and designed original instruments for them.

Our instrumentary to operations of varices contains the following items: 1) Coniform Striptor, 2) One-, Two-, and Three-crowned Venedeletor, 3) Communicotome, 4) Spiny needle. As far as it is known to us from the available world literature, this is the first complete and complex surgical instrumentary of its kind at all.

An operation of varix is commenced by a carefully executed crossectomy. A 4 to 5 cm long cut is led (performed) directly in the inguinal fold. Thereat, care is to be taken that all the venous inflows are interrupted, and as far as possible far off distantly from the great saphena, that its ligature is made directly on the junction with the thigh vein without leaving any blind arm or a narrowing swaging of the vena femoralis.

The stripping of the great saphena is principally carried out from periphery to central direction. Our coniform striptor is introduced into the magna from a small longitudinal incission before medial knucle after having been interrupted and its peripheral end ligatured. In an absolute majority of patients, a penetration of the striptor is succeeded up to the inguinal region from which the great saphena is extracted "in toto".

Our coniform striptor consists of a soft-steel litz wire to the one end of which a small leading olivary body is welded on, while an extractive piece is fastened to the other having a form of a flat pyramide. While extracting, the vein is deposited into the piece in accordion shape, the role of the piece consists in just extending the tissues. Veal branches are torn off far from the trunk; therefore, a bleeding and traumatization of tissues are restricted.

With an insufficience of the small saphena, we also carry out a crossectomy within the region of orifice above all and, thereafter, the stripping of the trunk.

Ectatic and varicose branches of the great and small saphena are removed from punctural 4 to 5 mm longitudinal incissions with the aid of the venedeletor. As little as possible incissions are made, namely in the way enabling to reach and remove in all directions varices from one point. Also incissions from which saphenas had been removed are utilized thereat. Often three or four cuts along the whole extremity enough thereto.

The deletor consists of an about 25 cm long steel wire. On its one end, an S-bent blade knife is welded, transitting into a hollow funnel-shaped crown fitted with several teeth. The wire is fixed into a handle by means of a screw. It is penetrated from the subcutaneous incission in a rectilinear way up to the point where the vein is getting lost. The penetration needs not proceed intraluminaly, the varices are sufficient to be pricked in several points.

505

Under systematical rotation of the instrument, the varicose vein is extirped. To remove great varicose convolutions, a multiple-crown deletor is used. For a hemostasis, an elevation and compression of the extremity for one minute by hand is enough.

In order to interrupt insufficient connecting veins, our communicotome is applied. A flat hook is welded into an about 25 cm long steel wire. The leading edge of the hook is of a cigarshaped curvature, while the internal one is semilunar and sharp. The other wire end is fixed into a handle.

It is penetrated with the instrument from an about 1 cm long incission made in the point, where no secondary skin alterations are found, up to the muscle fascia, and thereafter, using a reasonable pressure, along the fascia close by beside and behind the insufficient joint. With a reverse traction, the interruptor is pressed so that the connecting vein gets under the cutting hook edge by which it is disrupted. An elevation and compression of the extremity for 2 minutes is sufficient for hemostasis.

In order to remove goal-form, cobwebby or reticular microvarices, a spiny needle is used. This is designed with tiny spines arranged in a helical line in about 3 – 5 cm extent; the other wire end is screw-fixed in a handle.

It is penetrated from a pointed scalpel puncture either through all the microvarices or they are destroyed by transversal leading the instrument. The main collecting vein must be interrupter thereat, too.

In order to close all the incissions, one or two stitches are sufficient for each.

A compression by hand for about 1 minute suffices for hemostasis.

After the operation, the compressions is healed completely for about two to three weeks by an elastic bandage IDEAL and six weeks by zinc-glue dressings. After discharge from hospital, compressive rubber stockings are recommended to be worn by loading the extremities, and to women, in addition, in premenstruation periods.

E. L., 1st Surgical Clinic, Faculty of Medicine, Charles University, U nemocnice 2, 12 808 Prague 2, Czechoslovakia

PRACTICAL ASPECTS IN THE DIFFERENTIAL DIAGNOSIS OF LYMPHEDEMA OF THE EXTREMITIES

A. SCHIRGER and J. A. SPITTELL, Jr.

Mayo Clinic and Mayo Foundation, Rochester, Minnesota, U.S.A.

Whether affecting one leg or both, lymphedema may be idiopathic or secondary. Of the two forms of idiopathic lymphedema, congenital lymphedema appears at birth or shortly thereafter. Lymphedema praecox has onset in the teens or early twenties, and the late form of idiopathic lymphedema — which is rare — appears at the beginning of the fifth decade of life.

Lymphatic obstruction causing lymphedema usually is due to malignant growth (primary or metastatic) or to treatment for such disease — the vessels having been interrupted by resection of suspect nodes or closed by fibrosis resulting from radiation therapy.

Of inflammatory lymphedema, the nontropical type is due most often to non-hemolytic streptococci. Trichophyton infection, by causing excoriation and maceration of the skin, may provide ready portals for repeated entry of the streptococci and recurrent episodes of lymphedema. Filariasis is the most common cause of tropical inflammatory lymphedema.

Precise diagnostic distinction between idiopathic and secondary lymphedema is of paramount importance to the patient because of its prognostic significance. The introduction of lymphography into clinical medicine by *Kinmonth et al.* (1955) the use of contrast and radioisotope venography, and the recent revolutionary impact of computer-assisted tomography have provided the clinician and surgeon with powerful means of diagnostic investigation, whose accuracy and precision would have escaped the imagination of even farsighted clinicians 30 years ago. However, these new techniques impose a responsibility to use them wisely and to keep these resources easily available to physicians and patients in need of them. Consequently, clinicians must sharpen their clinical observation and bedside deduction rather than fall into undue reliance on costly laboratory tests.

It is the purpose of our communication to reiterate basic clinical tenets of the bedside diagnosis of lymphedema, based originally on our observation of 211 patients seen at the Mayo Clinic over a 5-year period and confirmed in ensuing years by repeated clinical observations in many other cases. (*Schirger et al.*, 1962, *Smith et al.*, 1963).

Idiopathic lymphedema usually begins with onset of swelling in the first four decades of life (Table I). More men than women are affected, and the course is punctuated by single or recurrent episodes of lymphangitis or cellulitis in 13% to 20% of cases.

In contrast, secondary lymphedema of the obstructive type usually begins in the fifth decade or later. Comparison of our two series indicates a clear separation,

Table I. Age at Onset of Lymphedema, by Type

Age at onset, yr	Primary		Secondary	
	Congen- ital	Idio- pathic	Malig- nancy	Infec- tion
0—9	8	5	0	0
10—19	...	47	0	2
20—29	...	48	0	1
30—39	...	20	1	7
40—49	...	3	5	10
50—59	...	0	5	13
60—69	...	0	18	6
70—79	...	0	5	4
80—89	...	0	1	0

allowing – in our opinion – for secure distinction between idiopathic lymphedema and secondary lymphedema of the obstructive type on clinical grounds alone in the majority of instances. Further, in secondary lymphedema the cause of obstruction can be predicted with a moderate degree of confidence from the sex of the patient: in men, carcinoma of the prostate dominates other forms of malignancy affecting the lymphatic system, whereas in women lymphoma is the most common cause of lymphatic obstruction.

In the early phases of secondary obstructive lymphedema, the differentiation from thrombophlebitis related to the underlying malignancy may be difficult. Under these circumstances we have found radiopaque contrast venography to be of aid. In our institution, lymphangiography is reserved for the staging of lymphomatous disease, whether with lymphedema or not, and it is rarely employed to determine the cause of an apparently lymphedematous swelling of the leg. We have been reluctant to employ lymphangiography in such cases for fear of making a new portal of entry for bacterial infection.

In contrast, during the past 18 months we have come to rely increasingly on computer-assisted tomography for detection of intrapelvic and intra-abdominal masses causing lymphedema. This advanced diagnostic method has revolutionized the noninvasive approach to occult malignancy by demonstrating tumors and lymph-node enlargements too small to be detected otherwise. Tissue biopsy may be helpful in determining the type of neoplastic process, but it usually is the last diagnostic resort (Table II).

Table II. Usefulness of Means for Distinguishing between Idiopathic and Secondary Lymphedema of Extremities

| | Idiopathic | | | | Secondary | | |
| | Congenital | | Praecox | Late form | Obstructive | | Inflammatory |
	Simple	Familial			Carcinoma	Lymphoma	
History	+++	+++	+++	++	++	++	+++
Physical examination	...	...			++	++	++
Laboratory							
General					++	++	++
Venography	...	...	...	+	++	++	+
Lymphangiography	...	...	...	+	++	++	...
Computer tomography	...	...	...	...	+++	+++	...
Tissue biopsy	...	...	...	...	+++	+++	...

+++ maximal, ++ moderate, + minimal usefulness.

REFERENCES

Kinmonth J. B., Taylor G. W., Harper R. W. (1955): Lymphangiography: a technique for its clinical use in the lower limb. Br. Med. J. 1: 940–942.

Schirger A., Harrison E. G., Jr., Janes J. M. (1962): Idiopathic lymphedema: review of 131 cases. JAMA 182: 14–22.

Smith R. D., Spittell J. A. Jr., Schirger A. (1963): Secondary lymphedema of the leg: its cha characteristics and diagnostic implications. JAMA 185: 80–82.

A. S., Section of Publications, Mayo Clinic, 200 First St. S. W., Rochester, MN 55901, U.S.A.

ISOTOPE LYMPHOGRAPHIC EXAMINATIONS FOR THE CRITICAL APPRAISAL OF FUNCTIONAL CONDITION OF LYMPHATIC FLOW

N. KLÜKEN and K. U. TIEDJEN

Dept. of Angiology, University Essen, F.R.G.

The magnitude of aetiopathogenetic possibilities causing a swelling of the lower extremities require examination methods facilitating a sufficient differentiation of oedema concerning the different causes. The colour test with patent blue eight or eleven p. c. dilution injected intra- or subcutaneously gives via the lymphflow only a broad orientation value. It should be considered merely a search test.

The adrenalin urtica method only informs about the condition of the lymphflow in the lymphatic ducts of the skin.

With the help of the contrast medium lymphography only definite lymphatic ducts can be shown. The initial and prelymphatic ducts cannot be demonstrated by this method. It should also be considered that the mechanical injection under pressure may lead to a change of the morphology of the lymphatics as well as of the functional condition. With the usual technique of x-ray lymphograms only the prefascial lymphatics of the lower extremities can be shown. Furthermore there are contraindications (Table I) as well as complications (Table II).

Considerable lipoedem, organized lymphoedema, pachydermosis and papillomatosis may complicate the execution of contrast medium lymphography or even make it impossible.

Table I.

contraindications of the contrast medium lymphography

a) allergy to iodine or patent blue
b) deminishing of pulmonary sufficiency
c) heart failure with right-left shunt
d) gravidity
e) iodine loading with hyperthyreosis

Table II.

complications of the contrast medium lymphography

a) rhexis of lymphatics depend on high pressure and rapid injection
b) pulmonary embolism (cerebral e.)
c) additional irreversible damage of predamaged lymphatics by the oily contrast medium

Contrary to the above mentioned the isotope lymphogram has certain advantages. It requires simply a needle injection into the subcutaneous tissue and not into the lymphatics directly.

This method presents the following statements:

1. the demonstration of the lymphatic nodes (systemic diseases or metastases)
2. measuring the lymphoutflow of the tracer from the point of injection or the inflow into the regional lymphnodes in relation to time.

Whereby the latter method shows under certain conditions the function or better said capability of the lymphatic system.

Such examinations of lymphatic drainage were already carried out since 1955 by *Hultborn* a.o. with colloidal aureum. In a standardised particle size of five or 30 nanometers is in our opinion even today the aureum 198 colloid the substance of choice contrary to 125 or 131 iodine albumen. Because the albumen is not completely transported by the lymphatics as it will also be resorbed by venoles. The storage of this substances in the lymphnodes is not constant and its fate in metabolism is not known.

Technetium-99 m-colloid is not considered as optimal as its particle size is not given as constant. However it is well suited for the lymphscintigraphy.

Therefore we have selected for our measuring sequence 198 Au-colloid, whereby we injected depending on the clinical status for the determination of the function of the prefascial lympha ic system into the first interdigital fold of the forefoot in the soft subcutaneous tissue.

For the determination of the subfascial system the injection is made into the muscles of the calf (Fig. 1).

After the injection the outflow rate is measured from the activity depot exclusively. The inflow into the inguinal region is considered as important criterion. Due to the multiple variations of the inguinal lymphnodes it is not precise enough to measure the inguinal nodes with a two or five inch detector. Also the percentage storage of the colloidal tracer in the lymphatic nodes is different. It can be demonstrated that a part of the substance passes through the lymphnodes and reaches the liver.

These facts require large area detectors as the scintillation camera by Anger. This covers the total pelvic region including the inguinal nodes.

It should be observed critically that even

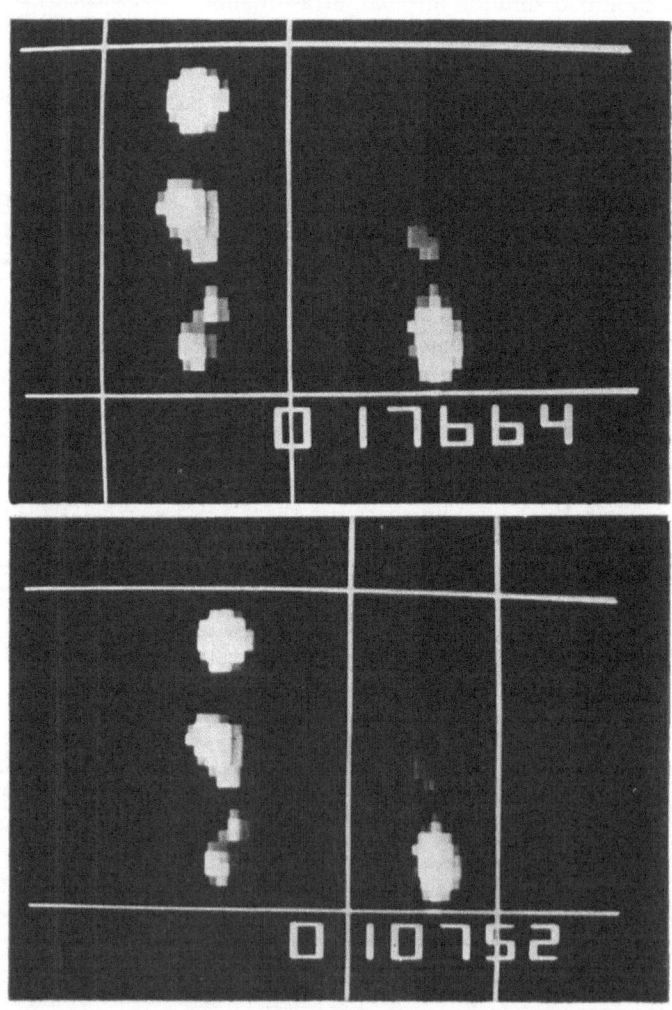

Fig. 1. Asymmetry of the inguinal and pelvic lymphnodes of a healthy proband.

here exact measuring data cannot be obtained due to the anatomical variations of the storing lymphnodes as already slight differences in depth of the lymphnodes lead to considerable variations of the impulse rates.

Fig. 1 shows a lymph-scintigram of the inguinal region of a healthy proband. The considerable asymmetry of the lymphnodes with side difference of impulse rate is evident.

Based on the above we selected for our examinations the customary 198 Au-colloidale of Behring comp. in the particle size of five nanometers. (Table III).

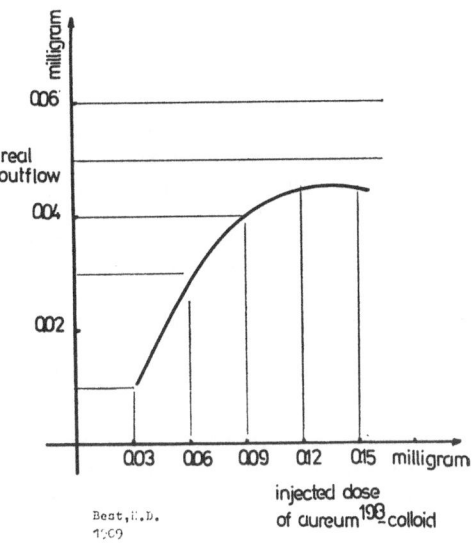

Fig. 2. The saturation effect with increasing dose of the injected Au-colloid.

Table III. Aureum[198]-colloid

components:

goldcolloid	3.5	milligram
glucosis	200	milligram
sodiumchloride	5	milligram
gelatine	30	milligram
aqua destillata	1	milliliter

pH 5—7   (Douis, M., 1963)

dose: 0,5 milliliter = 1,75 milligram aureum colloidale 10 microCurie per injection

particle size: 5 nanometer = 50 Ångstroem

In order to keep the dose of activity and the volume of injection as constant as possible a mixture of active and inactive colloid in a volumen of 0.5 ml gold solution or 1.75 gold-colloid respectively was injected.

We have kept the activity between 1.5 and 10.0 mikro-Curie as low as possible, since only the outflow at the point of injection is measured in percentages of relativity. We have disregarded the addition of hyaluronidase as the effect of the hyaluronidasis is variable. As proven by *Földi* and *Casley-Smith* hyaluronidase in addition causes an immediate damage of the lymphatics.

After the injection of 0.5 ml Au colloidale only a part of the substance participates in lymphatic outflow. With doses more than 0.12 mg Au colloidale a saturation effect is noted, which increases with increasing doses of colloid, which means

that the local transport capacity of the lymphatic system exhausts. The saturation effect is probably a fixation of gold-colloid particles by reaction of the connective tissue. The impulse rates were measured at a rate of sixty and 120 minutes, if required also 2, 4, 6 and 24 hours after injection. For orientation the inflow rate into the region of inguinal nodes and into the liver is noted.

Research by *Lofferer and Mostbeck* as well as animal experiments by *Földi* have shown that there is no sizable lymphatic outflow under rest condition. Only under motion a considerable increase of filtration and of the lymphatic flow takes place, whereby the movement of the muscles play an important role. For this reason a number of authors have put movement phases inbetween. For example *Thewes* with bicycle ergometer, *Sage* with temporary walking phases, *Földi* with foot seesawing. These movement variations however have the disadvantage that they lack the exact control over the cooperation of the patient.

Therefore one of us (*Tiedjen*) has developed with *Földi* an instrument. Seating and with horizontal positioning of the legs a passive movement is carried out by an electric motor with 50 revolutions per minute and with a maximal bending of the legs with 160 degrees.

A further advantage of this arrangement is the avoidance of orthostatic pressure components on the lymphflow, which is present while walking and with the usual bycicle ergometers. The measures are carried out with a scintillation counter and the impulses per minute were shown. There is no measuring on a definite point but the values of the whole forefoot are measured. Therefore a dermal-epidermal reflow of the tracer, which could occur, can be traced, which otherwise would be regarded incorrectly as lymphoutflow.

With an injection in the muscles of the calf an exact measuring of the point of injection in an angle of 90 degrees is of advantage. A tide collimator 7 centimeter lower diameter is used.

The activity in the inguinal lymphnodes is measured by a wide collimator through centering of the probe onto the middle of the white band under skin contact.

The radiation load is not relevant. Table IV substantiates the details by the manufacturers and by *Wolf and Haas*.

Table IV.

radiation loading	rad/μCi	rad/150 μCi
	Behring comp.	Wolf and Haas
lymphonodi/side	1 — 5 rd	30 rd
wholebody	0.02 mrd	few mrd
ovarians	— —	700 mrd
testes	— —	100 mrd
injection point	— —	1000 rd

Obviously the radiation load is highest at the point of injection. It should be noted, that *Wolf and Haas* have used an injection volume of 1.0 ml.

The low activity used by us have shown no side effects and no local irritations by the tracer.

There is only a slightly blueblack dot, which is comparable to a pigmentation of the rest depot of the colloidal gold. This pigment dot will become pale during the following months.

The methodology of examination used by us for the measuring of the lymphatic outflow has been proven successfull in numerous examinations. It is essential, this should be emphasized again, that an exactly dosed passive movement is applied.

N. K., Dept. of Angiology, Hufelandstr. 45, Essen, F. R. G.

LYMPHOSCINTIGRAPHY IN THE STUDY OF LYMPHATIC CIRCULATION

D. SALVO, A. MORATTI, M. PAOLICELLI and D. SERAFINI

*1st Radiology Department, Angiology Department, Hospital
Santa Maria Nuova, Reggio Emilia, Italy*

The use of radioisotopes in the exploration of the lymphatic apparatus is not a recent method; originally, radioactive drug were used primarily for therapeutic purposes. Later was employed a very original method using I^{135} to make Lipiodol radioactive, thus associating the preparation diagnostic use with the therapeutic action of the radionuclide on the lymphonode. On the other hand, all these methods presupposed the direct injection of the radiocompound, by surgical insulation of a collecting duct. Therefore, they started research for into a radioactive drug that, after being introduced into tissues, could be carried by the lymphatic system and reach the lymphonodes in the affected area (indirect technique): this purpose, they used the colloidal Au^{198}.

Methods

All detections were made using a linear scanner and only later, when Tc^{99m} was introduced,

was a gammacamera used. This method has undeniable advantages in comparison with traditional lymphography, as it avoids traumatic operations and can be repeated and applied even in areas that cannot be examined by radiologic lymphoadenography; however, it yields inferior morphostructural findings compared to the latter.

This radioisotopic method provides very interesting functional data and we have paid attention to this aspect, applying it in the study of the lower limb lymphatic circulation. We used a gammacamera, equipped with Microdot apparatus, for transferring the scintigraphic image to radiographic film and a Scintiscan system for automatic scanning, thus following the progress of the radioactive drug in the lymphatic collecting ducts. We injected colloidal antimonium sulfide bound with Tc^{99m} (total average dose 6 mCi) into the interdigital spaces under skin.

In order to study changes in the lymphatic circulation of the lower limbs, we have considered:

1 — detection of the radioactive drug progress in lymphonodal collecting ducts, carrying out series scanning.

2 — examination of the radioactive drug flow

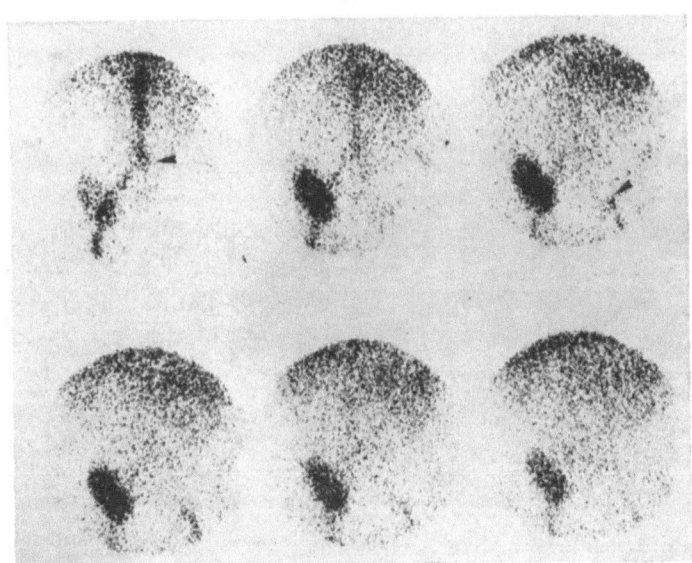

Fig. 1. Precocious congenital lymphedema with hypoplasia of collecting ducts and lymphonodes.

curves detected at the level of the thigh third middle area.

3 — time of appearance of the radioactive drug in the inguinal lymphocentres (normally 10 min—15 min)

4 — the time of appearance of hepatic uptake (normally 15 min—20 min)

Results

Our 150 lymphoadenoscintigraphies of lower limbs in different pathological situations, has provided us with various morphological and dynamic data, summarized as follows:

1. *Lymphonodal metastases*

Lymphatic ducts and lymphonodes of areas affected by metastatic dissemination present an unhomogeneous aspect, with total exclusion of the lymphonode or lymphonodal groups. The slow flow of the radioactive compound in the prelymphonodal ducts on one side, as well as the visualization of derm lymphatic system and the reduced, late or no-fixation in the inguinal lymphocentres or liver, show metastatic presence in the areas under examination.

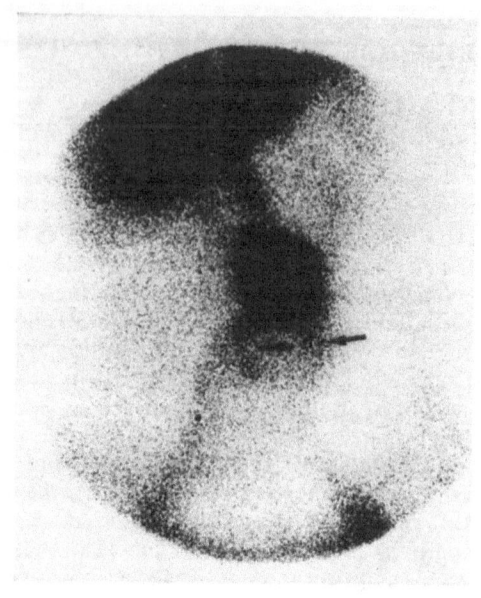

Fig. 2. Right post-lymphangitis lymphedema.

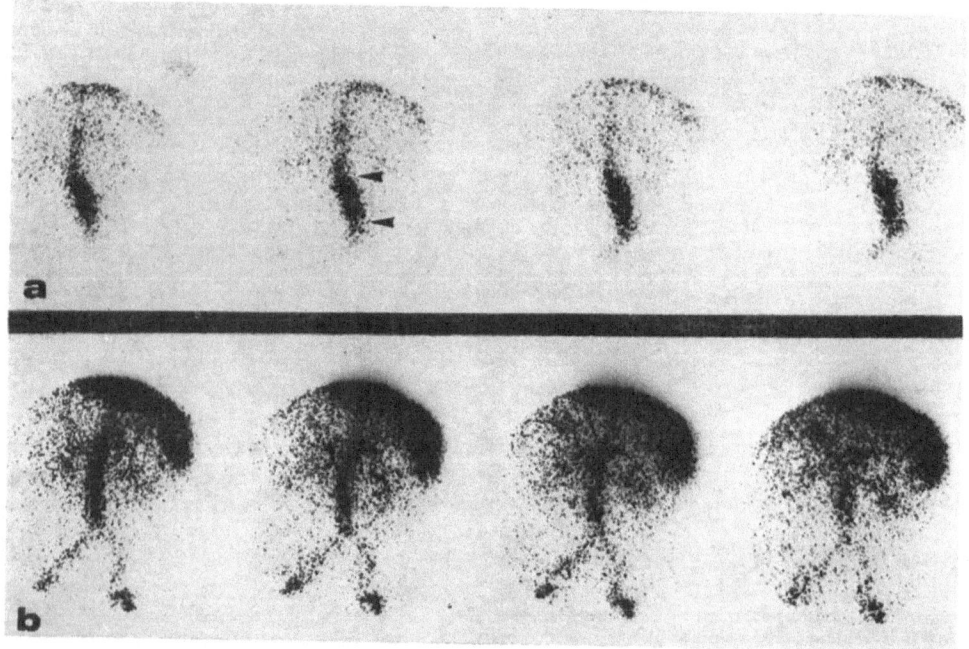

Fig. 3. Left lower limb thrombophlebitis.

514

2. Lymphomas and lymphogranulomas

Even though our cases are limited, we have observed an increase in the lymphonode volume of lymphomas, with almost regular fixation of the radioactive drug and normal or extended lymphatic circulation time.

On the contrary, lymphonodal fixation in lymphogranulomas is poor and the lymphatic flow is sometimes accelerated.

3. Edemas

a) We noted a remarkable slowing down of the lymphatic flow in lymphatic edemas, with nearly flat curves or late increment (Figrs 1 and 2).

b) In our post-phlebitis cases, we noted a remarkable increase in the lymphatic flow in venous edemas, with a sharp increment in the flow curve and a fixation of the radioactive drug at level of inguinal lymphocentres and hepatic parenchyma. (Fig. 3).

4. Post-therapy checks

We noted a remarkable acceleration of the lymphatic flow after radiation therapy or chemotherapy, with intense fixation of radioactive drugs in the liver, while it is late and poor in lymphonodes with reduced volume.

On this basis, we can state that radiologic lymphoadenography is unquestionably the best method in the morphostructural study of lymphonodes and in the detection of collateral circulation, while lympho-adenoscintigraphy has undeniable advantages, thanks to its repeatability and to the accurate study of the lymphatic flow.

D. S., Via Gorizia, 65/1, 42100 Reggio Emilia, Italia

CARDIAC LYMPH IN VENTRICULAR FIBRILLATION: AN EXPERIMENTAL STUDY

A. TAIRA, M. YAMASHITA, K. ARIKAWA, Y. HAMADA,
H. TOYOHIRA and H. AKITA

*Department of Surgery, Kagoshima University School of Medicine,
Kagoshima, Japan*

This experiment was attempted to clarify the relationship between cardiac function and cardiac lymph. On the basis of our knowledge, obtained from previous experiments (2, 3) on cardiac lymph, further study was contemplated on the heart with electrical ventricular fibrillation (EVF) under cardiopulmonary bypass (C−P bypass). EVF was induced by continuous direct current stimulation of the heart. Normothermic perfusion with diluted homologous blood (30% in hematocrit) was used. Experimental animals were divided into two groups of flow velocity and flow volume measurements. Thirty mongrel dogs were subjected to the former and 30 to the latter.

Flow velocity of cardiac lymph was indicated by measurement of the time needed for the cardiac lymph node to become stained after injection of the dye into the apex myocardium of the left ventricle. The time measurement was performed in two ways. One was the measurement immediately after the commencement of EVF and the other was two hours following continuous EVF. The

data of the two groups were compared with each other and also with our previous experimental results of flow study on cardiac lymph on the heart with hypoxia, hyperoxygenation, exsanguination, coronary sinus ligature (congested myocardium) and control (Table I). Twenty dogs whose flow velocity was measured immediately after the commencement of EVF revealed 417 ± 25 seconds SE, while the 10 measured after two hours revealed 115 ± ± 14 seconds SE. Markedly retarded flow velocity at the commencement of EVF became fast after two hours. The difference between the two values was statistically significant (p < 0.01).

Flow volume was collected from an afferent lymphatic duct by means of a small tube insertion. Other afferent lymphatic ducts were all ligated. Ten dogs were subjected to the collection of cardiac lymph under beating condition without C−P bypass (control). Further 10 dogs were studied in beating non-working hearts with C−P bypass. The remaining 10 were placed under continuous EVF with C−P bypass. The

Table I.

Groups	Cases	Time (sec)	LV dp/dt (mmHg/sec)	LV press. (mmHg)
1 Control	16	137 ± 13 (SE)	2428 ± 258 (SE)	152 ± 10 (SE)
2 Mypoxia	9	151 ± 15	3233 ± 418	171 ± 13
3 Hyperoxygenation	14	227 ± 30	2373 ± 271	102 ± 7
4 Exsanguination	9	241 ± 32	1357 ± 263	59 ± 4
5 Congestion	10	77 ± 13	2590 ± 384	117 ± 14
6 Fibrillation				
at the commencement	20	417 ± 25		
after 2 hours	10	115 ± 14		

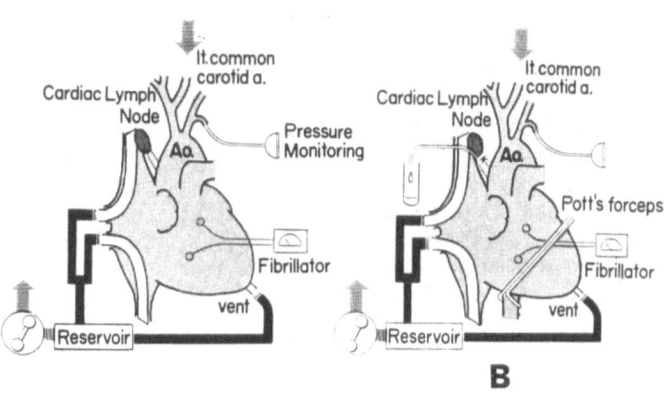

Fig. 1. A: Experimental model of flow velocity study is presented. The time needed for the cardiac lymph node to become stained after injection of, the dye into the apex myocardium was measured on the fibrillating heart under C—P bypass.
B: Experimental model in flow volume study is presented. Cardiac lymph was collected from an afferent lymphatic duct by inserting a small cannula. Perfusion pressure was kept at 100 mmHg by means of manipulation of a clamp placed on the descending thoracic aorta.

experimental model was depicted in Figure 1. Perfusion pressure was kept at 100 mm Hg by means of manipulation of a clamp placed on the descending aorta. Lymph collection was carried out for two hours in three groups. A linear increase of lymph volume was seen in the control group. Gradual increments of lymph volume with the passage of time were observed in the remaining two groups. The influence of diluted extracorporeal circulation might be cause of gradual increment of flow volume in both situations with C—P bypass. The initial depression of flow volume was dominant in the EVF group. This depression of flow volume is considered to be a result of retarded cardiac lymph flow due to lack of transport-mechanism of contractile movement of the heart. Depression of cardiac lymph production under EVF is not probable.

Our previous study on cardiac lymph clarified the interrelationship between flow velocity of cardiac lymph and congestion of the myocardium and augmentation of cardiac contractility. Both congested myocardium and increment of the contractile force of the heart apparently influenced the cardiac lymph flow as accelerating factors. Therefore, lack of contractility of the heart with EVF closely relates to initial depression of lymphatic

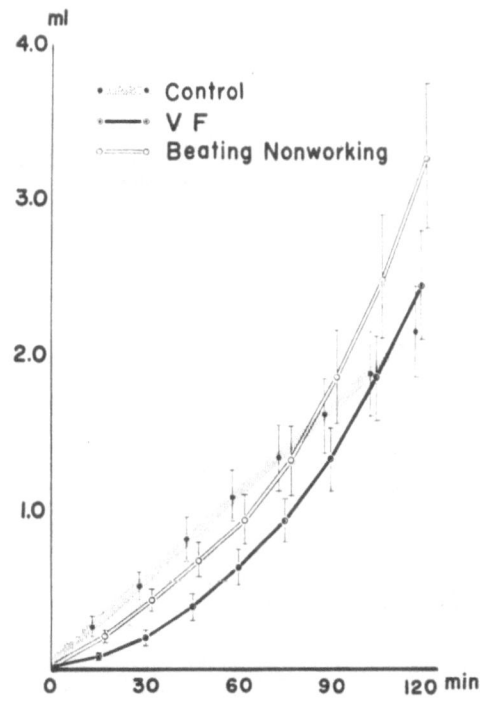

Fig. 2. Patterns of flow volume in three groups of control, beating nonworking heart under C—P bypass and fibrillating under C—P bypass are presented in the same graph. Initial depression was significant in the fibrillating heart. The total amount of flow volume was the greatest in the group with beating nonworking heart under C—P bypass. The flow of cardiac lymph in fibrillated heart was probably influenced by increased interstitial pressure, which had been produced by retarded transportation and augmented production of cardiac lymph.

517

transportation of the heart. Subsequent accumulation of cardiac lymph in the tissue might result in a later augmentation of the flow volume due to elevation of interstitial pressure. Augmentation of lymph production after continuous EVF was probably connected with an unphysiological condition of the myocardium derived from absent contractibility. The component of cardiac lymph with collected samples, such as protein, electrolytes and enzymes in both situations in fibrillating and in beating hearts under C−P bypass revealed an insignificant difference. The present result, from the point of view of cardiac lymph dynamics, accorded with the concept of recent studies of pathophysiology of EVF clarified by Hottenrott and others. (1) The results obtained from our experiment offer a possible explanation of the problem with respect to the continuous use of EVF in cardiac surgery.

REFERENCES

1. *Hottenrott, C., et al., (1974):* Studies of the effects of ventricular fibrillation on the adequacy of regional myocardial flow. III. Mechanism of ischemia. J. Thorac Cardiovasc Surg, 68 634−645.
2. *Taira, A., et al., (1976):* Cardiac lymph and contractility of the heart. Jap. Circul. J., 40, 665−670.
3. *Taira, A., et al., (1977):* Flow velocity of cardiac lymph and contractility of the heart: An experimental study. Ann. Thorac. Surg., 23, 230−234.

A. T., Dept. of Surgery Kagoshima University School of Medicine, Usuki-cho 1208-1, Kagoshima City 890, Japan

LYMPHOVENOUS ANASTOMOSES OF THE HEART

O. ELIŠKA and M. ELIŠKOVÁ

Department of Anatomy, Charles University, Prague, Czechoslovakia

In 35 dogs patent blue was injected after thoracotomy carried out under general anaesthesia in order to demonstrate the course of the lymphatic vessels of the heart. Then the main lymphatic trunks in the cardiac atria, the aorta and the truncus pulmonalis were ligated and severed. The dogs were divided into two groups: acute and chronic experiment. In the chronic experiment (dogs 13–35) the animals were left to survive ligation of the lymphatic trunks for 2 to 132 days. The animals of the acute group (dogs 1 to 12) were sacrificed 30 min. after ligation of the lymphatic vessels. Immediately after death, a mixture of India ink and 4% gelatine was injected into the lymphatic vessels demonstrated by patent blue. The lymphatic vessels were filled with a pressure of 30–100 mm H_2O; when pressure rose to more than 200 mm H_2O, damage to lymph vessels and extravasation occurred. Approximately in one half of the heart specimens, this injection was supplemented by an intravenous injection of 6% gelatine containing a pigment dye.

Observations and results

In a normal heart no lymphovenous anastomoses (LVA) are present. After direct injection into the lymphatic vessels, the injected substance spreads from the apex towards the base of the heart; after retrograde injection, the lymphatic vessels are not filled at all because of the well functioning valves, and if the pressure increases, the wall bursts and extravasation takes place.

In the second group of 23 dogs surviving ligature of the cardiac lymphatic trunks for 2–132 days, the following changes were observed: The subepicardial lym-

phatic vessels were dilated, varicose and tortuous. By the second or third day even some of the side branches of the main trunks were partly filled after retrograde injection. This collateral filling of the

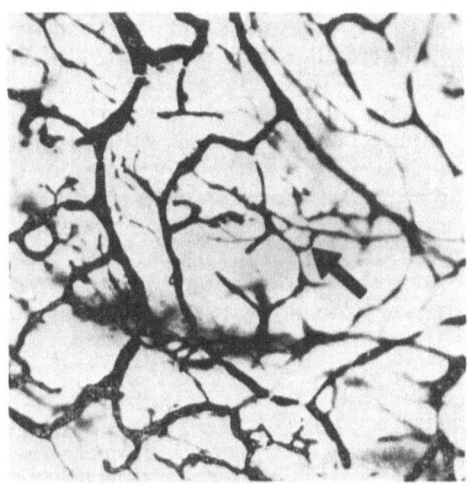

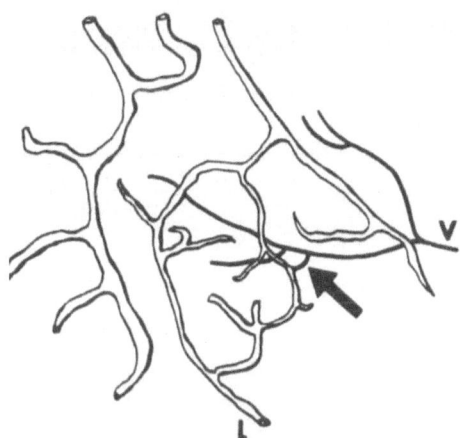

Fig. 1. Lymphovenous anastomosis, 50 μm. in calibre, in a clarified specimen on seventh day after ligature of lymphatic trunks. (L — lymph, V — vein).

519

lymphatic network was the rule in all cases observed. The shunts between lymphatic trunks and their branches were made visible (between the anterior and posterior left and those of the right truncus). The collateral between the right and left truncus lymphaticus, running across the origin of the truncus pulmonalis was obviously thickened. Between the seventh and 14th day, lympho-lymphatic anastomoses started to develop between the regions below and above the ligation, first as a network of thin, later of thick vessels (between the aorta and the truncus pulmonalis). In five heart specimen (7 – 28 days after ligation) shunts between lymphatic vessels and a vein were observed (Fig. 1). Their presence was already indicated after direct injection of the lymphatic vessels by the penetration of the injected mass into the vein. Some of the arched anastomoses split up into smaller branches, approximately 20 μm. in calibre, most of them running straight for a distance of 40 to 60 μm. LVA were most frequently found on the anterior aspects

of the ventricles. Lymphovenous anastomoses appeared in the heart specimens seven to 14 days after ligation of the lymphatic trunks, in one case they persisted up to 28 days. In cases, lasting more than one month, lymphovenous anastomoses were no longer found. At the same time, in three out of the five specimens referred to above, lympho-lymphatic anastomoses were found on the seventh, 14th and 28th day after ligation of the lymphatic trunks.

It should be assumed that the development of LVA is indirectly dependent on the development of lympho-lymphatic anastomoses. If lympho-lymphatic anastomoses have developed by the seventh day, a substituting drainage of lymph and the interstitial fluid via the LVA is not required and LVA do not develop. If, howewer, the drainage of lymph via the lympho-lymphatic anastomoses is insufficient, both forms of lymph drainage may exist simultaneously. This is borne out by the cases of the three out of five heart specimens with LVA referred to above.

REFERENCES

Eliška O., Elišková M. (1975): Contribution to the solution of the question of lymphovenous anastomoses in heart of dog Lymphology, 8, 11.

Patek P. R. (1939): The morphology of the lymphatics of the mammalian heart. Amer. J. Anat. 64, 203.

Vajda J. M., Tomcsik W. J. van Dooremaalen (1972): Connections between the venous system of the heart and the epicardiac lymphatic network. Acta Anat. 83, 262.

Zerbino D. D., Gavrish A. S. (1970): Lymphovenous shunts in lymph outflow from obstruction the heart (Experimentalmorphological research). (Russ). Bjulleten Experimentalnoj Biologii i Med. 8, 106.

O. E., Department of Anatomy, U nemocnice 3, 120 00 Prague 2, Czechoslovakia

VASCULAR TUMORS OF THE EXTREMITIES

F. H. SIM, R. B. IRWIN and A. SCHIRGER

Mayo Clinic and Mayo Foundation, Rochester, U.S.A.

Vascular tumors of the extremities are, on a whole, relatively rare phenomena. Aside from the more common and usually inocuous soft tissue entities of various forms of benign hemangiomata, these can be challenging orthopedic problems. The Mayo Clinic experience with hemangioma and hemangioendothelioma of bone and hemangiopericytoma of bone and soft tissue is indicative of the serious nature of these lesions and their treatment.

On recent review of the Mayo Clinic files, 69 bone tumors of vascular origin were found, 56 of them being hemangiomas. Of these, two were found to be multicentric only four of them occurred in patients less than 20 years of age, and 36 of the 56 occurred in females. Only ten, or less than 20 percent were asymptomatic, while he remainder presented with local pain, swelling, or both. Most of these lesions presented the usual roentgenographic picture of zones of rarification with scattered trabeculae, but several showed more destructive appearing areas requiring definitive biopsy for diagnosis, Histologic study by and large revealed either cavernous or capillary spaces lined by small endothelial cells and were readily differentiated from its malignant counterpart, hemangioendothelioma or angiosarcoma.

Treatment of these hemangiomas included curettage, total excision, or resection-debulking in areas where complete surgical removal was impossible. This was the case in 7 of the 13 vertebral lesions, surgical decompression then being followed by radiation therapy. Follow-up of 47 of the 56 cases revealed the above treatment plan to give excellent results in all but two cases, one with persistent disease in the leg, and the other requiring reoperation for spinal cord decompression five years after initial treatment.

Added to the 9 hemangioendotheliomas in our files were 13 hemangioendothelioma in our consultation files. This entity was found to be twice as frequently occurring in males, 19 of the 22 occurred in patients over the age of 30 years, and 6 were found to have multifocal disease. Although there was found slight predilection for the vertebral column, any bone can be involved, and most patients presented with local pain with or without swelling. Roentgenographically the lesions were lytic without reactive new bone formation and the roentgenographic "aggressiveness" was found to correlate well with the histologic grading of the tumor.

The essential microscopic feature was that of blood vessel formation lined by neoplastic, usually cuboidal cells with large nuclei, plus stromal neoplastic cells between blood vessels. Histologically the hemangioendothelioma tumors of bone were readily divided into three grades. Grade I lesions were characterized by good vasoformation, little mitotic activity and little nuclear atypia, while Grade III lesions showed little vasoformation, much atypia, and much mitotic activity, while Grade II lesions were intermediary in histologic appearance. This histologic grading was found to be prognostically significant in that only 4 of the 13 Grade I lesions were dead at follow-up, while all 5 of the Grade III lesions were dead with metastatic disease at 1 month to 2 years, and 2 of the 4 Grade II lesions had succombed at 5 and 20 months. Treatment in terms of prognosis is difficult to assess, but its our feeling the complete surgical removal, preferably en bloc, is the treatment of choice, with radiation being employed only in those cases that are surgically inaccessible.

Table 1. Hemangioendothelioma of Bone.

No. of patients	22
15 male, 7 female	
Age range	7 to 74 years
Average follow-up	3.4 years
Mortality	
Grade I	4 of 13 dead
Grade II	2 of 4 dead
Grade III	5 of 5 dead

Hemangiopericytoma of bone is really quite rare and was found in only 4 of the 69 vascular tumors in our files. These occurred equally in men and women at an average of 44 years and did not exhibit any significant physical findings. Roentgenographically there was various forms of destructiveness seen and microscopically these demonstrated small spindle cell (pericyte) tumors surrounding blood vessels lined by a single layer of endothelial cells. Reticulin staining can be used to differentiate between hemangioendothelioma and hemangiopericytoma as, in the latter, the reticulin is seen to surround each pericyte and separate them from the inner, non-reticulin-lined single layer of endothelial cells, while in hemangioendothelioma the reticulin stain accentuates the intravascular location of the aniplastic cells. Histology was found not to be of help prognostically as increased cellularity

Table II. Hemangiopericytoma of Soft Tissue

No. of patients	60
28 male, 32 female	
Age range	4 to 72 years
Prognosis	
% metastasis	
Grade I (Benign)	0
Grade II (Borderline)	37.5
Grade III (Malignant)	78

and greater mitotic activity did not correlate with decreased survival and we, in fact, feel that hemangiopericytoma of bone is an unpredictable lesion.

Hemangiopericytoma of solft tissue, however, is more predictable. Although this lesion is uncommon, we have followed 60 patients, the 24 survivors being followed from 11 months to 22 years. These lesions were found to occur equally as often in males as females, from the ages of 4 to 72 years, but most often in the fifth and sixth decades, and were widely distributed over the body in location, although 25 percent of these lesions occurred in the anterior thigh or groin. Approximately three-fourths of the patients complained of soft tissue mass, and one-half of these also complained of pain. Roentgenographically a soft tissue density was noted in one-half of the patients, while approximately one--third had negative x-ray examinations. Histologically these lesions, as in those of bone, demonstrated a spindle cell stroma with occult vascular spaces lined by endothelial cells, but classification was possible in benign (12 lesions) borderline malignant (16 lesions) and malignant (32 lesions). The borderline lesions were characterized either by 1 mf/10 hpf with slight cellular anaplasia or 1 mf/20 hpf with moderate cellular anaplasia. These borderline malignant lesions were found to follow a malignant course with 37.5 percent metastasizing, and six exhibiting local recurrence after excision. Seventy-eight percent of the frankly malignant histologic variety were found to metastasize while none of the histologically benign tumors did so. More alarmingly, metastasis was found to be possible at late follow-up as 11 percent of the malignant and 7 percent of the borderline lesions were found to metastasize after five years of disease-free existence after excision. Complete surgical oblation then is the recommended treatment, amputation being necessary if en bloc removal from normal tissue is not possible.

F. H. S., Mayo Clinic, 200 First St. S. W., Rochester, MN, U.S.A.

LYMPHANGIOGRAPHY IN MODERATE DISTURBANCES OF LYMPHODYNAMICS IN THE LOWER LIMBS

H. BUJAR

Department of Radiology, "N. Gh. Lupu" Institute of Internal Medicine, Bucureşti, Romania

This study was carried out to analyze the causes, frequency and persistence of moderate lymphodynamic disturbances of the lower limbs secondary to certain local pathological states. It is well known that such troubles are not considered as an indication for lymphangiography, their diagnostic and therapeutic implications being overlooked by both clinicians and radiologists.

Materials and methods

The study was based on 87 complementary lymphangiographies of the lower limbs selected from 211 such examinations performed in patients with various diseases requiring investigation of the sub-diaphragmatic lymph nodes. None of these patients showed lymphodynamic troubles due to lymph node involvement. The classical technique described by Kinmonth was used, Ultrafluid Lipiodol being injected at a slow rate of 1 ml/10 min. At the end of the injection and 24 hrs later, frontal and profile X-ray pictures of the legs and thighs were taken.

The lymphangiographies obtained were divided into three categories according to the presence or absence of clinical symptoms (S+, S—) and of pathologic history in patients (H+, H—): I group: 53 patients S+ H+; II group: 23 patients S— H+ and III group: 11 patients S+ H—. All the cases reported had pathological local antecedents dating over more than two years. The lymphangiographic aspects taken into consideration were: dermal — back-flow, opacification of deep lymphatic vessels, extravasation, changes of vascular caliber and/or tract. The explored territory was the satellite of the internal saphenous vein.

Results

As shown in Table I, 53 patients of the first group reported 67 pathologic antecedent symptoms. Eighty three lymphangiographic aspects were observed — the most frequent of them were extravasations (in 54% of cases). Strictly localized dermal back-flow occured in 34% of cases (in phlebitis, skin diseases, contu-

Table I. Distribution of lymphangiographic aspects in 53 patients with a past history and clinical symptoms in the lower limbs

History	Nr. of symptoms	Lymphangiographic aspects				
		dermal back-flow	deep vessels	extra-vasation	changes of caliber	tract
phlebitis	19	6	3	15	2	3
arthrosis	13	—	—	2	4	7
skin diseases	10	8	—	2	—	3
hurts	8	1	—	6	—	2
fractures	7	—	—	6	1	1
burns	4	2	—	—	1	1
arteritis	3	—	1	2	1	—
penetrating wounds	2	2	1	2	—	2
irradiation	1	1	1	1	—	—
Total	67	18	5	34	9	17

Table II. Clinical symptoms in 53 patients*

History	Nr. of symptoms	Clinical symptoms			
		slight evening oedemas	skin lesions	venous ectasias	pain
phlebitis	19	13	4	6	7
arthrosis	13	3	—	—	10
skin diseases	10	4	6	—	—
hurts	8	3	—	2	3
fractures	7	3	1	1	2
burns	4	2	2	—	—
arteritis	3	—	1	—	3
penetrating wounds	2	—	2	—	—
irradiation	1	—	1	—	—
Total	67	28	17	9	25

* Same as in table I.

sions, burns, penetrating wounds and after high-dose irradiation). Only 5 cases (9%) showed opacification of deep vessels. The most frequent clinical symptoms encountered, as shown in Table II, were small vesperal oedemas (53% of cases) and pains (47%). The most varied clinical symptomatology was phlebitis.

In 23 patients of the second group, with pathologic antecedents but without symptoms, we also noted the frequency of phlebites (52% of cases) and among lymphangiographic aspects of extravasations (52% of cases). Dermal back-flow occured only once (4% of cases); only one case of deep vessel opacification was recorded in this group (4% of cases). (Table III).

In the last group of 11 patients young women aged up to 25 years (who couldn't recall any past history except recurrent attacks of influenza) we observed a unique symptom, small vesperal oedemas, mostly distal. The predominant lymphangiographic pattern was diffuse extravasation.

Discussion

As follows from the mentioned data, many sufferings of the lower limbs are accompanied and/or followed by moderate lymphodynamic disturbances. Their radiologic pattern is non-specific, depending on the intensity of the primary disease, on the anatomophysiologic state of the regional lymphatic network and on the preco-

Table III. Distribution of lymphangiographic symptoms in 23 patients with a past history but without clinical symptoms

History	Nr. of cases	Lymphangiographic aspects				
		dermal back-flow	deep vessels	extra-vasation	changes of caliber	changes of tract
phlebitis	12	—	—	7	5	—
arthrosis	5	—	—	—	—	5
skin diseases	3	1	—	3	—	—
fractures	2	—	—	2	—	—
hurts	1	—	1	1	—	—
Total	23	1	1	13	5	5

ciusness and effectiveness of treatment, very often neglected or insufficient.

It has been shown that persist moderate lymphodynamic disturbances for a long time after the primary disease. Most of these troubles are accompanied by a very annoying symptomatology, which becomes chronic. In the cases investigated, the frequency of lymphangiographic aspects was in an evident relationship with that of clinical symptoms (53 patients showing 83 radiologic aspects, 43 of them with collateral circulation, mentioned 79 clinical symptoms, while 23 patients with 25 lymphangiographic aspects, 6% of which had collateral circulation, were free of symptoms).

The presence of collateral localized circulation and its relationship to clinical symptoms raise the question of the compensation degree of this network. We feel that the 11 cases with diffuse extravasations but without a past local history are lymphoedemas by vascular hyperpermeability (primary or secondary).

We should like to emphasize the necessity of paying more attention to the various pathologic events affecting the lower limbs and to their early and correct treatment which might prevent many moderate lymphodynamic disturbance, often accompanied by chronic clinical symptoms.

H. B., Dept. of Radiology, "N. Gh. Lupu" Institute of Internal Medicine, Bucureşti, Romania

LONG TERM RESULTS OF MEDICAL AND SURGICAL TREATMENT OF LYMPHEDEMAS OF LEGS

R. C. MAYALL, J. FREITAS, J. C. MAYALL and A. C. D. G. MAYALL

Hospital da Gamboa, Rio de Janeiro, Brasil.

The treatment of lymphedemas of the lower limbs is based always on etiology, physical and laboratory findings, radiological examinations and if possible on the histopathologic studies.

The radiological examinations include: a) The superficial lymphography by the *Kinmonth's* technique; b) The deep lymphography of the posterior tibial lymphatics; c) The arteriography by the femoral artery injection or by direct punction of the popliteal artery, or by retrograde method using the punction of the dissected posterior tibial artery; d) ascending phlebography on standing position under fluoroscopic control or a selective phlebography by injection of the posterior tibial vein that is dissected together with the artery and the deep lymphatic in the retromalleolar region.

The conservative medical treatment is always considered when there are infections, inflammation, hyperkeratosis or acanthosis and a big lymphedema or fibredema, without a complete block of the lymphatic and venous flow. The conservative medical treatment in most of patients is the first stage of the surgical treatment to prepare correctly the skin for a more radical surgical treatment. For this treatment the following conditions must be met: a) the absolute bed rest with an elevation of 30 cm of the foot side of the bed; b) broad spectrum antibiotic therapy by intra-arterial proximal injections, or oral and intravenous routes; c) antiallergic and antiinflammatory drugs, like corticosteroids and glucomethacin compounds orally; d) anticoagulant drugs and fibrinolytics; e) hyaluronidase injections of 2000 T. U. every six hour by intraarterial proximal injection or intravenously; f) poor

salt and low caloric diet; g) correction of anemia and dysproteinemia, hormonal defects and salt retention; h) intensive intravenous, intraarterial or oral use of benzopyrones (coumarin-rutin) as lymphokinetic drugs and to increase the phagocytosing activity of the reticulo-endothelial system; i) when there is no more infection of inflammation, the intermittent use of pneumatic compression instruments as Jobst, Hadomer or Alpha-Bed followed by local massage of the extremity according to the principles of Vodder method. To speed up the absorption of the edema the *Van der Molen's* method of latex tubes is very good, when followed by the continuous use of the high pressure elastic stockings.

When there is a failure or incomplete reduction of the edema, or when there is persistence of the fibredema, the surgical treatment is considered basing on the following principles: a) when there are arteriolo-venular communications producing hyperostomy findings on arteriography, they must be ligated on the thigh, on the mid-leg, around the ankle and foot to prevent the venous and lympho-stasis. b) The Charles operation modified by Josias technique is recommended only when there is a good deep lymphatic and venous circulation. c) With a complete block of lymph flow in the inguinal region, the skin pedicled lymphangioplasty by Rodriguez-Azpurua's-method is very useful, if performed together with a complete liberation of the fibrosis that commonly produces a partial block of the venous flow, and associated with a direct lymphatic-vein anastomosis by the techniques of *Degni* and *Cordeiro*. d) When the lymphedema is secondary to a superficial lymphostasis and there is a good superficial venous circulation we recommend only the direct lymphovenous anastomosis by the techniques of *Degni* and *Cordeiro* at different levels of the leg followed by the use of intermittent pneumatic compression, high pressure elastic stockings and benzopyrones compounds for a long post-operative period.

When rules are held to the follow-up results are very satisfactory both from esthetic and functional point of view. The breeches appearance below the knee is uncommon. The patients are able to wear normal clothes and shoes. The incidence of inflammatory attacks has been completely eliminated in the majority of the operated cases. The weight of the bulky part is reduced.

The best results were observed on secondary inflammatory lymphedema due to post-phlebitic syndrome and iatrogenic lymphedemas following operations on the groin and leg.

REFERENCES

Cordeiro, A. K., Baracat, F. F., Moreira Jr., F., F., Mayall, R. C.: (1977): New techniques of lymphovenous anastomosis for surgical treatment of lymphedemas of the lower limbs and postmastectomy lymphedema of upper limbs. In: Progress in Lymphology. Plenum Press, New York, 347—359.

Degni, M.: (1977), New technique of lymphatic-venous anastomosis for the treatment of lymphedema. In: Progress in Lymphology. Plenum Press, New York, 319—328.

Földi, M.: (1977), New Aspects in the Therapy of Lymphedemas. In: Progress in Lymphology. Plenum Press, New York, 299—302.

Kinmonth, J. B.: (1972), The Lymphatics. Edward Arnold, London.

Mayall, R. C.: (1976), Sindrome de Hiperostomia — Contribuição au seu Estudo Clinico e Radiológico. Ed. Graf. Villani Filhos Ltda., Rio de Janeiro.

Mayall, R. C., Freitas, J., Barbosa, C., Azevedo, M. A. F.: (1970), Medical and Surgical Treatment of Lymphedemas. In: Progrès Cliniques et Thérapeutiques dans la Domaine de la Phlébologie. Stenvert & Zoon, Apeldoorn.

Van der Molen, H. R.: (1977), Medical Treatment of Lymphedema. In: Progress in Lymphology. Plenum Press, New Yrok, 303—318.

R. C. M., Caixa Postal 1822 ZC-00, 20.010 Rio de Janeiro (RJ) — Brasil

PHARMACOLOGY AND THERAPY
OF VASCULAR DISEASES

EFFECTS OF VARIOUS DRUGS ON EXPERIMENTAL AND CLINICAL ATHEROSCLEROSIS

Introduction to the Symposium of Pharmacology

DANA HORÁKOVÁ and J. POKORNÝ

Research Laboratory of Angiology, Charles University, Prague, Czechoslovakia

When Harvey described the circulation almost 400 years ago, the main causes of death were infection, starvation and violent death. Now the pattern of mortality has changed so that diseases of the circulatory system have become the main cause of death in most industrialized countries. Since atherosclerosis underlies most cardiovascular disease — a major cause of death and disability in modern society—, it has been subject of a great deal of research. Studies in man and in experimental animal models reveal that the atherosclerotic process can be defined as a variable combination of changes of the intima of arteries characterized by the focal accumulation of lipids, complex carbohydrates, blood and blood products, fibrous tissue and calcium — deposits and associated with medial changes. In the discussion concerning the etiology of atherosclerosis, it is becoming apparent that, rather than being a disease entity, this complex condition is composed of a number of different clinical patterns, relating respectively to the location of the disease (peripheral, coronary, cerebrovascular etc.), the type of lesion (obliterative etc.) and to the rate of development of the disease. A distinction has to be made between atherogenesis and progression of the disease, particularly in view of the extensive development that has taken place in the field of reconstructive surgery.

Certain markers (factors) have been identified in subjects long before symptoms or clinical signs of atherosclerotic process and its complications appear. Consistently high blood pressure, high serum concentrations of certain lipids and cigarette smoking, singly or in combination, frequently characterizes these who develop atherosclerotic circulation lesions. Many other habits, enviromental factors and altered biochemical variables, have been put forward as so called risk factors. And this can represent a great field for the treatment possibilities.

There have been many studies employing various agents including antiproliferative and antiinflammatory drugs in animal models to learn if the course of experimental atherosclerosis can be modified by these therapeutic agents. In the study of *W. M. Lee and K. T. Lee* (see above, p. 25), the effects of hydroxyurea and pyridinol carbamate were investigated in in 33 yound Yorkshire pigs weighing average 11 kg. The intimal cells of the abdominal aorta of all animals were partially denuded using a balloon catheter. Where this procedure was combined with an atherogenic diet, the two processes appeared to act synergistically to produce lesions, the extent and thickness of which were far greater than those expected by summing up the effect when these two procedures were used separately. The lesions produced by this combined method have many of the characteristics of advanced human lesions. Each pig received the atherogenic — hypercholesterolemic diet plus either hydroxyurea (50 mg/kg/ /day) or pyridinol carbamate (50 mg/kg/ /day) for six months. The control group received the hypercholesterolemic diet only (without drug treatment). At the end of six months, all pigs were secrificed. The extent of intimal surface and medial wall involved by atherosclerotic lesions were significantly less in drug treated animals than in untreated control group (see above, p. 26). The cholesterol contents in the serum, aorta and liver among the followed groups were not significantly different. On the basis of this study it is possible to conclude that hydroxyurea and pyridinol carbamate retarded progression of experimental atherosclerotic lesions in animals produced by combination of the balloon injury and the hypercholesterolemic-atherogenic diet.

These mentioned Lee's observations and similar studies of other authors (*Shimamoto, Adams, Kritchevsky, Reiniš, Terry* et al.) can indicate that endothelial integrity and modification in permeability appear to be at the core of progression of atherosclerosis. The concept of endothelial changes is common to all theories, current or past. *Shimamoto and Numano* demonstrated that protection of the integrity of the endothelial layer may be possible. Many authors attempted to apply their experimental findings in laboratory animals to patients using the treatment with pyridinolcarbamate, vasodilators and other drugs. Many authors then believe that it may become feasible to other methods already customarily taken, protection of the endothelial integrity and permeability in an attempt to reduce or even arrest progression of atherosclerosis (*Terry*).

It was not possible in this introductory part to discuss all the problems of pharmacotherapy — nevertheless we believe in the usefullness of demonstrating and determining the effectiveness of various vasoactive drugs in the following studies. Though we must accept the fact that we are still in ignorance of the etiology and the causal treatment possibilities of atherosclerosis, it is certainly possible to influence some risk factors (blood pressure, smoking habits and blood lipids) in the population.

D. H., IV. Medical Clinic, Charles University, U nemocnice 2, 12000 Prague 1, Czechoslovakia

PHARMACOLOGICAL CONTROL OF AORTIC ENZYMES INVOLVED IN ATHEROGENESIS

OLGA MRHOVÁ, D. URBANOVÁ and L. KAZDOVÁ

Institute of Clinical and Experimental Medicine, Prague, Czechoslovakia

Studies of enzymes of the vascular wall in experimental animals and man indicate that changes in the activity of some enzymes of basic metabolic cycles accompany, or even precede the pathologic changes in the vessel that lead to atherosclerosis (*Kirk*, 1963; *Zemplényi*, 1968). Decreased activity of the enzymes of Krebs and glycolytic cycles and increased activity of some phosphomonoesterases marked the processes resulting in lipid deposition, alteration of connective tissue, and atherosclerotic lesions in the vessel wall.

We assume that one of the defence mechanisms of a healthy arterial wall against the consequences of injury is its intact respiration and oxydative phosphorylation with unimpaired capacity to synthetize ATP and proteins, including enzymes. We propose therefore that a favourable effect on the metabolism of the vascular wall, such as activation of its respiratory enzymes might increase vascular resistance against lipid accumulation and other pathologic changes. Therefore the need and rationale of studies of the effect of drugs on vascular wall metabolism and its possibilities are self-evident.

We studied above all the effect of drugs on those vascular enzymes, whose activity changes sensitively as early as during the preatherosclerotic period. The enzymes involved are of the Krebs cycle, namely MDH, SDH, glycolyses — LDH and its fractions, phosphomonoesterases, mainly acid and alkaline phosphatases, adenylpyrophosphatase and 5 mononucleotidase.

Our preliminary screening experiments with some "lipid affecting" drugs as Vasolastin, Neopeviton, Heparin, Atromid and some other drugs as Venalot and Pyridinolcarbamate indicate that arterial enzyme activities can be artificially changed. Some changes, in particular those of Krebs cycle enzymes, could be desirable on the basis of our previous findigs (*Mrhová*, 1971; *Zemplényi*, 1967; *Mrhová*, 1972).

Metabolism was affected most by oral PDC. Therefore we present here the result of our studies of the effect on vascular wall metabolism by this drug. It has been established that PDC is neither a hypocholesterolemic agent nor a vasodilatator. However, it reduced triglycerides in serum and liver mitochondria, inhibits a sub-

Table I.   IN VIVO EFFECT OF PDC ON ARTERIAL WALL ENZYMES AT NORMAL AND PATHOLOGICAL CONDITIONS

EFFECT	TCA cycle enzymes	glycolytic enzymes	phosphomono-esterases	anaerobic fract. of LDH
OF PDC IN RATS	↗ p < 0.001	↗ p < 0.005	→	↘ p < 0.05
OF PDC IN RATS FED THE HIGH-FAT DIET	↗ p < 0.01	↗	→	↘ p < 0.01
OF EXCESS OF CALCIFEROL IN RATS	↘ p < 0.005	↘	↗ p < 0.001	↗ p < 0.05
OF PDC IN CALCIFEROL INTOXICATED RATS	↗ p < 0.005	↗ p < 0.005	→	↘ p < 0.05
OF ALLYLAMINE IN RATS	↘ p < 0.001	↘ p < 0.001	↗ p < 0.005	↗ p < 0.001
OF PDC IN ALLYLAMINE INTOXICATED RATS	↗ p < 0.025	↗ p < 0.05	→	↘ p < 0.05
OF EXPERIMENTAL RABBIT ATHEROMATOSIS	↘ p < 0.05	↘	↗ p < 0.001	↗ p < 0.05
OF PDC IN EXPERIMENTAL RABBIT ATHEROMATOSIS	↗ p < 0.025	↗	→	↘ p < 0.01

endothelial entry of plasma substances including LDL by reducing the contractive and phagocyte activity of arterial endothelial cells. Finally, it significantly reduces platelet aggregability which results in antithrombotic activity (*Shimamoto*, 1976; *Kritchevsky*, 1971). In our experiments we studied the effect of PDC on the activity of the above enzymes in the vascular wall of rats and rabbits in response to injuries eliciting pathologic changes more or less resembling atherosclerosis.

The specific and favourable effect of PDC on the activity of enzymes mentioned above is reviewed in Table I.

Line 1 shows that after eight weeks of 30 mg/kg/daily PDC, the activity of TCA cycle enzymes in the aortic wall of rats increased, including rats on high fat and cholesterol diets. (Line 2.)

In contrast to PDC, for example Atromid-S combined with the standard diet, enhanced the activity of TCA and glycolytic enzymes, but added to a high-fat and cholesterol diet, Atromid-S either did not affect the enzymes studied, or had an opposite effect than after Atromid plus standard diet. Therefore the diet used in Atromid treatment may change the effect of this drug (*Mrhová*, 1971).

Line 4 shows that given to Calciferol intoxicated rats for 9 weeks, PDC prevented decreased activity of TCA cycle enzymes, normally seen in later stages of hypervitaminosis D (*Mrhová*, 1963).

In contrast to calciferol injury which according to Duguid causes mediocalcinosis in rat arteries, allylamine injected parenterally induced arterial necrosis in rats. Histological control showed the aortic medial edema and cellular reaction of the adventitia in the aorta of allylamine-treated rats.

The middle part of the aortic media with negative activity of MDH showed areas of medial necrosis. Its negative activity was much smaller after allylamine plus PDC. (Fig. 1, 2).

PDC treatment elevated aortic activity of TCA and glycolytic enzymes to the levels seen in control animals both during allylamine and calciferol intoxication. (Line 6.)

Similarly, rabbits fed with cholesterol

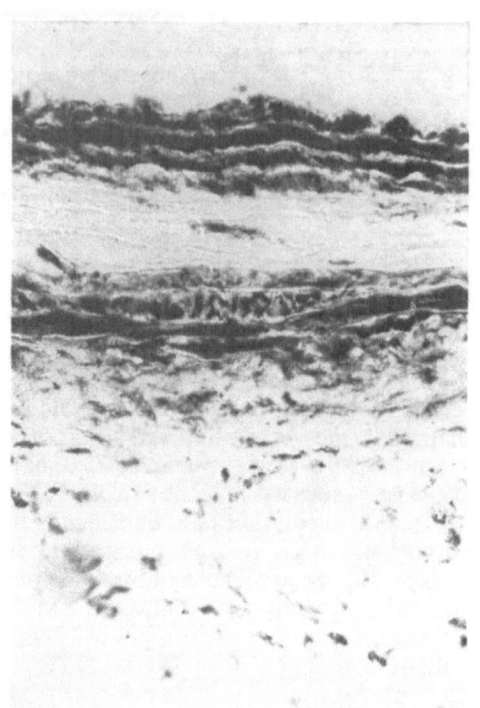

Fig. 1. The middle part of the aortic media with negative activity of MDH after the allylamine treatment without PDC. MDH, 270×.

showed a decrease of TCA cycle enzymes and an increase of phosphomonoesterases activity, which was accompanied by the formation of arterial plaques. As in all models of experimental injury of arterial wall studied so far, PDC prevented a decrease of TCA cycle enzymes. (Last line.)

In preliminary experiments we attempted

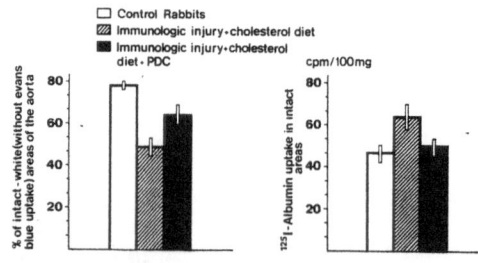

Fig. 2. The negative activity od MDH is smaller after the allylamine treatment with PDC. MDH, 270×.

also to determine the effect of PDC on vascular wall permeability in rabbits with atherosclerosis induced by a cholesterol diet and immunological vascular wall injury by i.v. bovine albumin. (Fig. 3). Endothelial integrity observed by means of Evans blue and permeability determined by labelled albumin showed that the number of sites of intact endothelium, that is the sites at which Evans blue did not accumulate, was higher after simultaneous administration of PDC with cholesterol than after cholesterol without PDC. Similarly, albumin uptake after PDC was lower at the intact sites than in the cholesterol-fed group without PDC added. In addition, the results showed that PDC has not a very conspicuous effect at sites with disturbed endothelial integrity. On the other hand, at still intact sites, PDC obviously decreased permeability, as compared with intact segments of the vascular wall of rabbits fed PDC-free cholesterol.

Let me now draw your attention to the effect of PDC on the anaerobic muscle fraction of LDH. (Last column.) Decrease of this fraction shows an improved situation in the vessel, as far as energy production is concerned (*Dawson*, 1964).

On the other hand, in pathological conditions increased phosphomonoesterases activity was not influenced by PDC. (Column 3.) Since the increase in acid phosphatase is related to intensified connective tissue metabolism, we speculate that PDC does not influence the metabolism of ground substance in the aorta.

The effect of PDC manifests itself mainly in the TCA and glycocity clycle enzymes. This entrancing effect of PDC is believed to contribute to the production of ATP, which is not only the key substrate in protein synthesis and repair process, but also the precursor of cyclic AMP, which is known to correlate with the tone of vascular actomyosin and platelet aggregability (*Shimamoto*, 1975).

At this stage we cannot interpret our results in relation to the mode of action. Moreover, the role of the metabolism of the vascular wall in the contractibility of endothelial cells — a major causal factor of vascular permeability — is still obscure. Nevertheless, if intact metabolism is one of the mechanisms protecting the artery against pathologic changes, there may be a relation between the antiatherosclerotic effect of the drugs tested, and its effect on TCA and glycolysis cycle enzymes. We believe that investigation of the means of preventing or at least reducing metabolic impairments of the vascular wall bring a new aspect to the research of atherosclerosis.

REFERENCES

Kritchevsky, D. and Tepper, S. A. (1971): Influence of Pyridinolcarbamate on oxidation of cholesterol by rat liner mitochondria. Arzneim Forsch. (Drug Res.) 21, Nr. 1, 146—147.

Mrhová, O., Grafnetter, D., Janda, J., Linhart, J. (1971): The effect of Atromid-S on the activity of vascular enzymes in rats. Biochem. Pharmacol. 20, 3069—3076.

Mrhová, O., Shimamoto, T., Numano, F. (1972): The metabolic effect of PDC on rats. Acta Path. Jap. 22, 353—361.

Mrhová, O., Zemplényi, T., Lojda, Z. (1963): The effect of cholesterol fat feeding on the activity of rabbit aorta dehydrogenase systems. Quart. J. Exp. Physiol. 48, 61—66.

Shimamoto, T., Numano, F., Yamazaki, H. and Murase, H. (1975): Cyclic AMP phosphodiesterase inhibitors in the treatment of senile mental deterioration cerebellar afaxia and thrombotic and atherosclerotic disorders. Front. intern. Med. 110—114, (Karger, Basel 1975).

Shimamoto, T., Takashima, Y., Kobayashi, M., Moriya, K. and Takahashi, T. (1976): A Thromboxane A_2 — antagonistic effect of Pyridinolcarbamate and Phtalazinol. Proc. Japan. Acad. 52, 591—594.

Zemplényi, T. and Mrhová, O. (1967): The effect of some drugs and hormones on the activity of vacular enzymes. Progr. Biochem. Pharmacol. 2, Karger, Basel, 141—146. (Eds. D. Kritchevsky, R. Paoletti, D. Steinberg).

Zemplényi, T., Mrhová, O., Urbanová, D. and Kohout, M. (1968): Vascular enzyme activities and susceptibility of arteries to atherosclerosis. Am. N. Y. Acad. Sci. 149, 682—698.

O. M. IKEM, Vídeňská 800, 14622 Prague 4, Czechoslovakia

PHYSIOLOGICAL AND ELECTRONMICROSCOPICAL OBSERVATIONS IN EXPERIMENTAL ISCHEMIC HEART DISEASE

A. NEMES, S. JUHÁSZ-NAGY, L. SOLTÉSZ, E. SOMOGYI
and P. SÓTONYI

*Institute of Vascular Surgery and Institute of Forensic Medicine,
Semmelweis University Medical School, Budapest, Hungary*

To study the pathophysiology of the heart muscle, a hypoxic model was worked out in 100 dogs imitating the situation of human angina pectoris. A left thoracotomy was performed under anaesthesia and a carotico-coronary or mammary-coronary bypass was prepared. Hypoxic pulses were elicited during 30 min by repeated 30 sec clampings of the graft with 30 sec unclamped periods. Cessation of the reactive hyperaemic response indicated the exhaustion of the adaptive

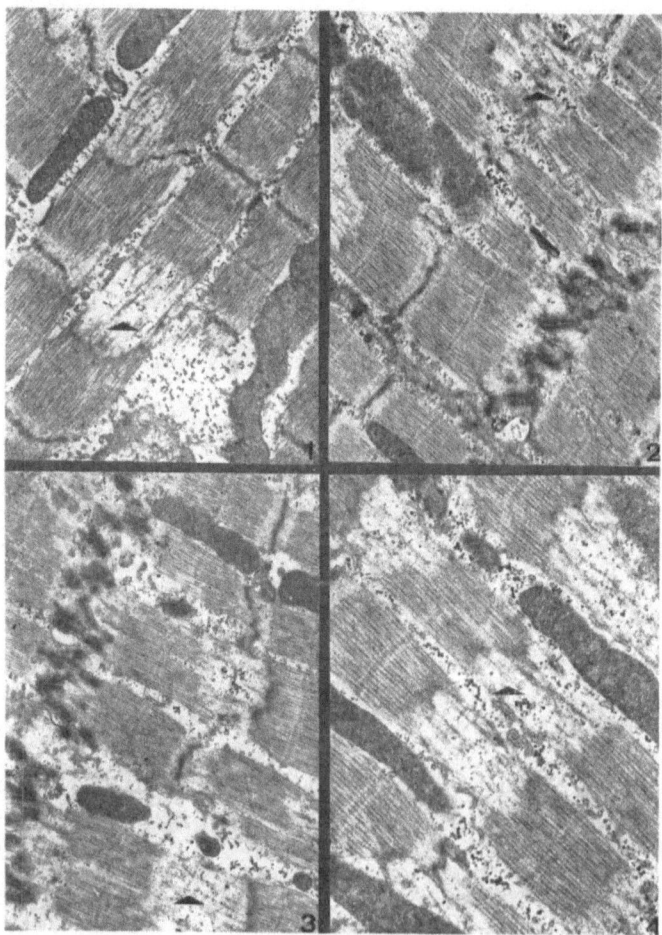

Fig. 1—4. The reactive hyperemia was ceased almost completely. There were places of focal (mosaic-like) destruction of the I-band, loss of actin filament, irregular Z-band and giant mitochondria.
18.000×, 18.000×,
24.000×, 18.000×.

capacity of the coronary. Blood streaming was monitored by an electromagnetic flow-meter or by a rotameter. Ventricular contractility was measured by a strain gauge. Electron-microscopic studies were performed partly after immersion, partly after perfusion glutaraldehyde fixation. Small blocks were excised from the papillary muscle and the subendocardial ventricular wall. As hypoxia was induced on the anterior left ventricular wall, the posterior one, namely the supply territory of the arteria circumflexa, served as control. The early signs of intermittent hypoxic loading were the appearance of giant mitochondria, dilatation of the sarcotubular system and a moderate decrease of the creatine phosphate level. Prolongation of the duration of hypoxic loading brought about a cessation of reactive hyperaemic response and concomitant structural and functional alterations. With the tracer method disturbances in membrane permeability, pericapillary, interstitial and interfibrillary edema were detected. The damages of the Z-membrane, actin and myosin filaments developed in a mosaic-like pattern. (Fig. 1—4.) Cytochemical and Ca^{45}-uptake studies revealed an increase in Ca^{2+} content. Tissue ATP and creatine phosphate levels decreased markedly. The morphological pattern corresponded to diffuse necrosis. The model system shows well reproducible

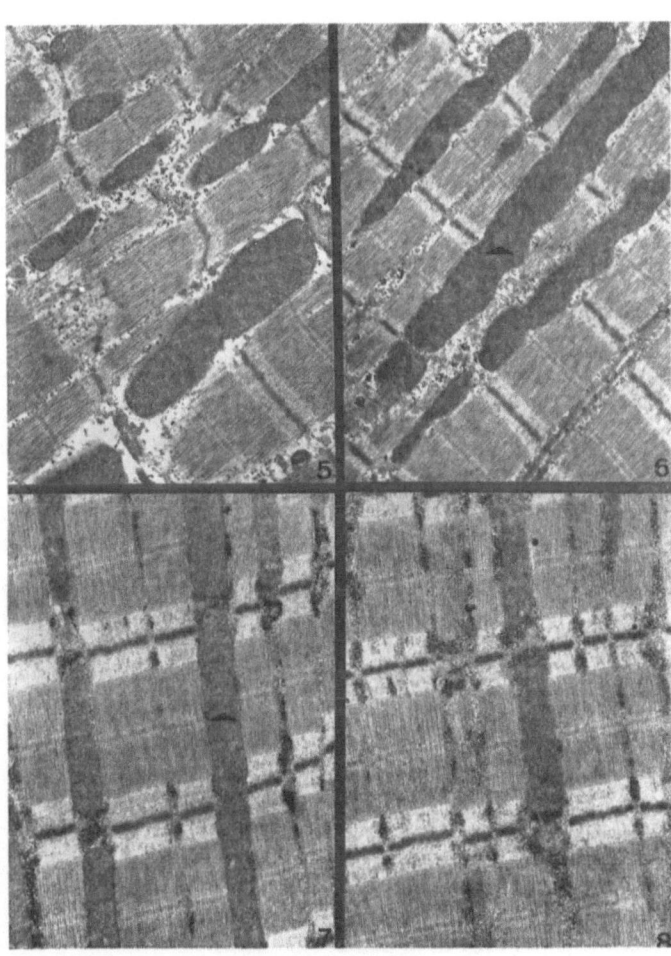

Fig. 5—8. After applying Solcoseryl (blood dialysate) only some mitochondria were present, with partial disruption of the I-band. 18.000×, 18.000×, 18.000×, 18.000×.

alterations; therefore it is thought to be suitable to test various protective agents. For that end, an intermittent ligature of the left anterior descendent coronary was performed. The intravenous or intra-coronary administration (1 ml/kg) of Sol-coseryl (Solco. Basel) increased tolerance against hypoxia. Mitochondrial destruction diminished and less macroerg phosphate compounds were lost indicating an activation of energy production and conservation. (Fig. 5—8.) Isoptin (Knoll. Ludwigshafen) administered intravenously in 1 mg/kg doses countered the disturbances of Ca^{2+}-transport of the sarcolemma and mitochondrial membranes. This was unequivocally demonstrated by cyto-chemical and liquid isotope studies. (Fig. 9—12.) Inosine (desaminated adenosine. Chinoin. Budapest) in 50 mg/kg had a favourable effect on microcirculatory restitution and acted against formation of diffuse necrosis. In countering the effects of hypoxia, the correction of the disturbance of energy supply, increase of membrane resistance and the restoration of impaired Ca^{2+}-transport proved to be essential. Using the intermittent hypoxic experimental model, early changes of coronary diseases can be studied electron-microscopically. The exhaustibility of coronary adaptation suggests that no single parameter can characterize myocardial blood supply from the clinical

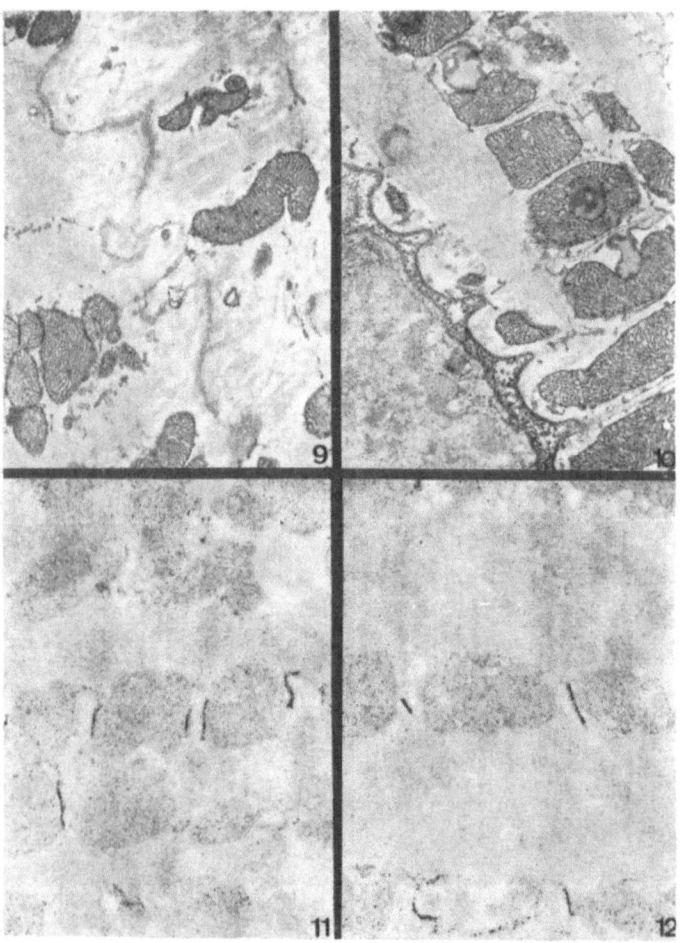

Fig. 9—12. After intermittent hypoxia mitochondria showed massive Ca^{2+} accumulation. (9—10). By Isoptin administration the mitochondrial Ca^{2+} accumulation could be delayed or prevented (11—12). 18.000×, 18.000×, 18.000×, 18.000×.

point of view. Structural and functional alterations can be elicited without coronary occlusion. Our model system seems to be particularly suitable for testing protective agents. This type of protection is now an important aim of research with special regard to the clamping of the aorta during extracorporeal operations. The model can also be applied in research into compounds for transcoronary cooling or infusion cardioplegia. Our results provide data for the formation of the so called "stone heart" which seems to be the joint result of energetic insufficiency and disturbance of Ca^{2+}-transport. According to our experience in the arrest of heart function Ca^{2+}-antagonists, Isoptin, whereas in starting it Solcoseryl and Inosine are useful.

REFERENCES

For any references please contact authors.

A. N., Institute of Vascular Surgery, Semmelweis University Medical School, Városmajor. u. 68, 1122 Budapest, Hungary

PROTECTIVE ACTION AGAINST CEREBRAL ISCHEMIA BY A NEW IMIDAZOLE DERIVATIVE (Y-9179) AND PENTOBARBITAL: A COMPARATIVE STUDY OF CHRONIC MIDDLE CEREBRAL ARTERY OCCLUSION IN CATS

A. TAMURA, T. ASANO, K. SANO, T. TSUMAGARI* and A. NAKAJIMA*

Department of Neurosurgery, University of Tokyo, Tokyo, Japan
* Research Institute of Yoshitomi Pharmaceutical Industries LTD, Fukuoka, Japan

The protective action of barbiturates against cerebral ischemia has been repeatedly demonstrated in animal experiments as well as in clinical trials (*Yatsu et al.*, 1972; *Michenfelder et al.*, 1976; *Marshall et al.*, 1977). The very high dose of barbiturates, however, precluded their clinical administration to severely ill or preoperative patients in whom a strict regimen of respiratory and circulatory cares could be afforded. Hence, the effort to search for alternate drugs with less adverse effects than barbiturates enabling their use for the whole spectrum of stroke seems justified. It was recently reported that a new imidazole derivative (Y-9179) posesses a remarkable cerebral protective effect against cerebral ischemia and/or anoxia in animal experiments using mice or rats (*Yasuda et al.*, 1978). The anti-anoxia or anti-ischemia effect of this agent was observed even with a very small dose which induced neither sedation nor motor depression. For the purpose of investigating the possibility of clinical application a comparative study with Y-9179 and pentobarbital was carried out using the chronic middle cerebral artery (MCA) occlusion model in cats.

Materials and methods

A total of 33 adult cats of both sexes were anesthetized by inhalation of halothane. The horizontal portion of the MCA was exposed by the transorbital approach under an operating microscope. The MCA was occluded at the lateral margin of the optic nerve by a clip with a short and straight blade.

Thirty minutes after the clip application, administration of drugs was started and continued for three days according to the schedule (Table I).

The animals were then transferred to a cage and observed with regard to the posture, vital signs, body weight, blood exams and the neurological status at regular time intervals for six days. For the purpose of maintaining the fixed experimental condition, no such cares as artificial ventilation, forced feeding or parenteral fluid supply were performed. On the seventh postoperative day, all the surviving cats were again anesthetized with halothane and the brains were fixated in situ by perfusion with Karnovsky's solution via the bilateral carotid arteries. The brains were sliced at four fixed coronary planes and examined microscopically for the extent of the infarction. The focal and the perifocal areas were differentiated according to the severity of tissue destruction. The infarction ratios of these areas were separately calculated as percentages of the total areas of both hemispheres. In several cats of each group EEG was recorded pre- and postoperatively with implanted epidural electrodes. The stored EEG recordings were later analyzed by a computer.

Table I.

Time (Hr)		Observation Items
-25.5	Observation(A-K) / Fasting	A. Posture
-1.5	Atropine 0.75mg/kg i.m.	B. Respiratory Rate
-1.0	Halothane Anesthesia	C. Heart Rate
-0.5	MCA Clip / 5% Dextrose 20ml s.c. / Kanamycin 200mg i.m.	D. Rectal Temperature / E. Body Weight / F. Pinna Reflex / G. Pupillary Light Reflex
	Halothane Turn Off	H. Pain Response / I. Neurological Evaluation / J. EEG / K. Appetite

Time (Hr)		Drug Administration (3 Days)			
		Cont.	Y-9179 6.25	12.5	PBT* 25
0 3 6	Observation(A-J)	--- i.p.-	2.5	5.0	10
9	(A-J)	--- s.c.-	1.25	2.5	5
16		--- s.c.-	1.25	2.5	5
24	(A-J)	--- s.c.-	1.25	2.5	5
		(* mg/kg/day, -:Vehicle)			
96	Observation(A-K)				
120	(A-K)				
144	(A-K*)	Evans Blue 2.5ml/kg i.v.			
	Brain Perfusion				

Results

There were no significant differences between each group as to mortality and vital signs (Fig. 1). The neurological scores showed a transient increase during the period of drug administration in both Y-9179 and pentobarbital groups, which later recovered. The infarction ratios are shown in the figure (Fig. 2). A pronounced

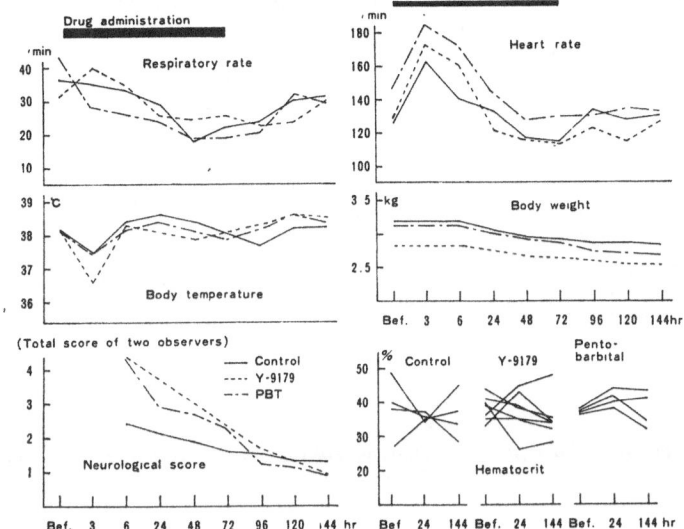

Fig. 1.

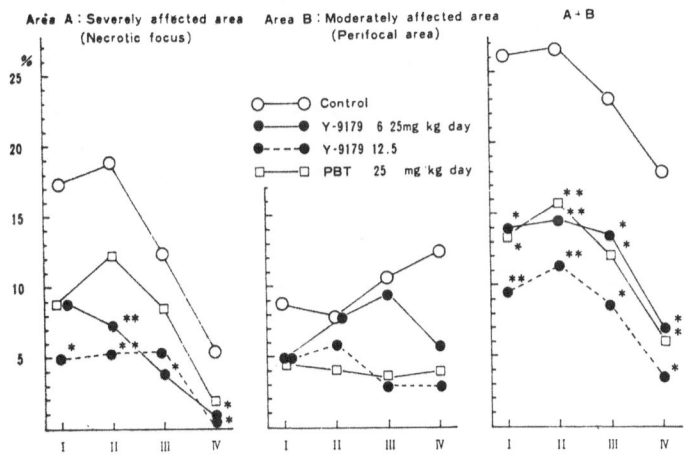

	mg kg	Area A	Area B	A - B
Control	–	12 62 ± 2 59 ·8	10.17 ± 4.19 ·8	22 79 ± 2 82 ·8
Y-9179	6 25	4 90 ± 1.76 8· ** *	7.30 ± 1.88 ·8·	12.20 ± 2 41 ·8· **
	12.5	4.00 ± 0.87 ·4· *	4.04 ± 2.45 ·4	8 04 ± 2 43 ·4· **
PBT	25	7.63 ± 1.30 ·8·	3.86 ± 1.52 ·8	11.49 ± 2.52 ·8· **

Fig. 2.

Statistical analysis was performed using variance analysis method. Mean ± SE(N)
**P<0.01, *P<0.05

cerebral protection from ischemia was revealed with both Y-9179 and pento-barbital. The protection by Y-9179 covered both the focal and perifocal areas and dose dependency is also seen. A pronounced cerebral protection against ischemia was confirmed with Y-9179 which was apparently superior to that of pento-barbital. This unique property of Y-9179 seems to be far more advantageous in clinical application than barbiturates.

All through the postoperative period, there was a tendency that the slowing of the basal rhythm in the irfarcted side was less severe in the Y-9179 and pentobarbital groups as compared with the control group.

REFERENCES

Marshall, L. F., Shapiro, H. M. (1977): Barbiturate control of intracranial hypertension in head injury and other conditions: Iatrogenic coma. Acta. Neurol. Scand. 56 (Suppl. 64): 156—157.

Michenfelder, J. D., Milde, J. H., Sund, T. M. Jr. (1976): Cerebral protection by barbiturate anesthesia: Use after middle cerebral artery occlusion in Java monkeys. Arch. Neurol. 33: 345—350.

Yasuda, H., Shuto, S., Tsumagari, H., Nakajima, A. (1978): Protective effect of a novel imidazole derivative against cerebral anoxia. Arch. Int. Pharmacodyn. 33: (in press).

Yatsu, F. M., Diamond, I., Graziano, C., Lindqist, P. (1972): Experimental brain ischemia: Protection from irreversible damage with a rapid-acting barbiturate (Methohexital). Stroke 3: 726—732.

A. T., Department of Neurosurgery, University of Tokyo, Hospital Hongo, Bunkyo-ku, Tokyo, Japan

THE EFFECT OF Ca^{++} ANTAGONISTS ON THE LIMB BLOOD FLOW

F. SOLTI, E. TURBÓK, J. FRANK, Z. SZABÓ, M. ISKUM and G. BEKE

Institute of Vascular Surgery, Budapest, Hungary

It is well-known that some types of Ca^{++} antagonistic agents have antiarrhythmic and coronary vasodilating properties. Some years ago we could observe in a patient suffering from both angina pectoris and peripheral obliterative arterial disease an unexpected remarkable increase of the claudication distance during Adalat administration. Therefore it seemed worth to study the effect of some Ca^{++} antagonists on the limbs circulation.

Materials and methods

The investigations were carried out in 36 patients suffering from peripheral obliterative arterial disease. Among them 12 had already rest pain, while 24 suffered from intermittent claudication; mean age: 62.3 years (32—75), sex: male = 31, female = 5. Two types of Ca^{++} antagonists were used for this investigations: 1. Verapamil (Isoptin) 2. Nifedipin (Adalat). Isoptin was administered in slow i. v. drop infusion, dosis: 5 mg, while Adalat orally — in capsules, dosis: 5 mg.

The extremital — limb — blood flow was determined by using the venous isotope-dilution method with double punctures of the collecting femoral vein (*Solti et al.* 1966).

The perfusion pressure of the limb was measured by the Doppler ultrasonic method.

After prolonged Adalat therapy (3 × 5 mg

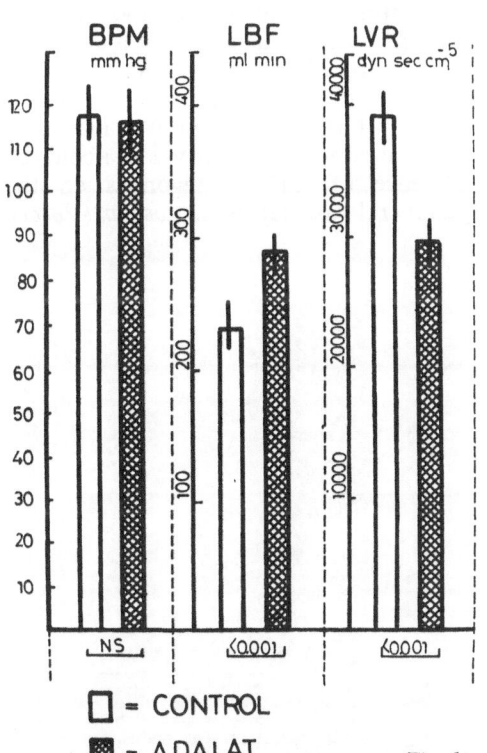

= CONTROL
= ADALAT

Fig. 1a

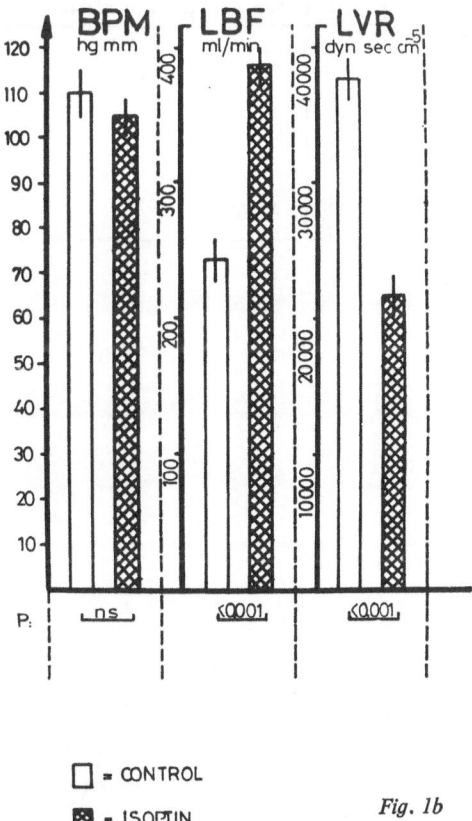

= CONTROL
= ISOPTIN

Fig. 1b

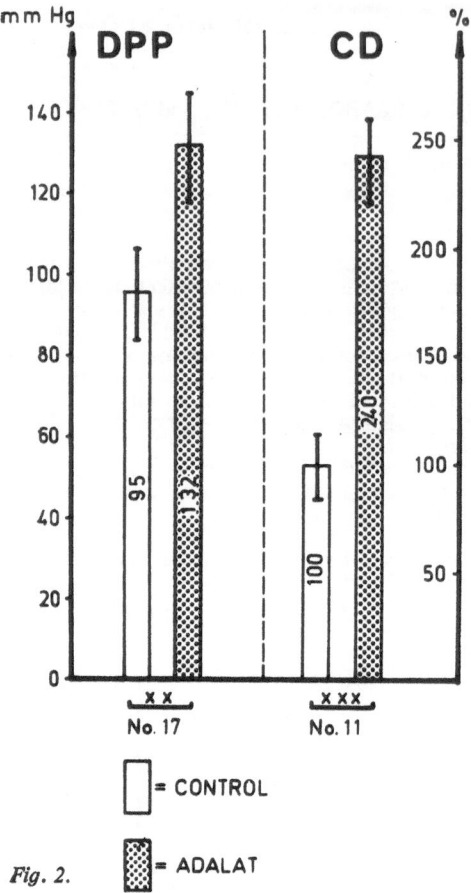

Fig. 2.

□ = CONTROL

▨ = ADALAT

per os for 4—12 weeks) the changes in the claudication distance and the distal perfusion pressure of the limb were controlled in 18 patients. For the statistical analyses of the experimental data the Student's one-sample "t-test" was used.

Results

The acute effect of Ca^{++} antagonistic agents showed a significant increase in the limb blood flow and a pronounced diminution of the extremital vascular resistance. The influence of Isoptin and Adalat on the extremital circulation was quite similar. (Fig. 1a and 1b).

After prolonged administration of Adalat there was a significant increase in the distal limb perfusion pressure and a very marked increase of the claudication distance. A characteristic improvement can be noticed in the Figure 2 on the effect of Adalat administration.

Discussion

According to our present investigations the Ca^{++} antagonists Isoptin and Adalat have a very favourable effect on the extremital circulation in pathological conditions of the peripheral vascular area. There are only few literary data about the influence of Ca^{++} antagonists on the peripheral vascular area. *Ross and Jorgen*

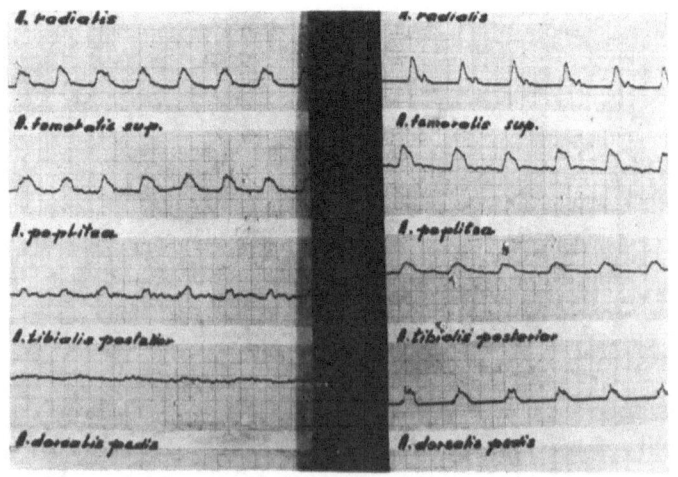

Fig. 3.

(1967), as well as *Greenberg and Wilson* (1974) observed a decrease in the total — peripheral — vascular resistance after the administration of iproveratril. In animal experiments *Angus et al.* (1976) detected a diminution of vascular resistance in the femoral artery after verapamil administration. We could now establish a pronounced increase of the limb blood flow and a very marked decrease of the extremital vascular resistance in obliterative peripheral vascular disease after the acute effect of Isoptin and Adalat. After administration of Adalat for a longer period, a significant increase of the perfusion pressure of the limb and of the claudication-distance could be observed, too. On the Figure 3 a characteristic improvement of the pathologic ultrasonic pressure curves of the lower limb can be noticed after the acute effect of Adalat administration.

Conclusions

1. Ca^{++} antagonists (Adalat, Isoptin) have a favourable effect on extremital circulation in pathological conditions.

2. The limb blood flow increases and the limb vascular resistance decreases the acute effect of Isoptin or Adalat.

3. The pathomechanism and therapeutic effect of Ca^{++} antagonists on peripheral circulation deserve further detailed studies.

REFERENCES

Angus, J. A., Richmond, D. R., Dhuma-Upakoru, P., Cobbin, L. B., Goodham, A. H. (1976): Cardiovascular action of verapamil in the dog with particular referenc to myocardial contractility and atrioventricular conduction. Cardiov. Res., 10, 623. t

Greenberg, S., Wilson. W. R. (1974): Iproveratril: A nonspecific antagonist of peripheral vascular reactivity. Canad. J. Physiol. Pharmacol. 52, 266.

Ross, G., Jorgensen, C. R. (1967): Cardiovascular action of iproveratril. J. Pharmacol. Exper. Therap. 158, 504.

Solti, F., Krasznai, I., Iskum, M., Rév, J., Nagy, J. (1966): Measurement of blood flow in the brain and lower extermities in man by venous dilution. Cor Vasa 8, 178.

F. S., Institute of Vascular Surgery, Városmajor Str. 68., 1122 Budapest, Hungary

CA-ANTAGONIST DRUGS FOR THE STUDY AND TREATMENT OF ANGIOSPASTIC SYNDROMES

L. SAVI, P. POLA, A. DAL LAGO and A. PINELLI

Department of Internal Medicine, Catholic University of Sacred Heart,
Faculty of Medicine and Surgery, Rome, Italy

Recent studies tend to admit an identity between the mechanisms that regulate the contraction of vascular smooth muscle and those that regulate muscle from other areas because the same proteins are involved.

Among physiological factors regulating vasomotility an important role is due to calcium-ions. Contraction results from an interaction between proteins and free intracellular calcium-ions with energy liberated by the enzyme ATPase, which is activated in turn by calcium. The kinetics of the interaction are regulated by the cytoplasmic concentration of free calcium-ions. Only when this concentration reaches a certain level are the calcium-ions able to bind with specific receptors on troponin. This binding causes modifications on which the interaction between actin and myosin depends, and the process of muscular contraction is thereby realized. On the other hand an insufficient intracellular level of calcium-ions results in relaxation of the vascular musculature.

Because of its particular effect of the mechanism of contraction of vascular smooth muscle, we used Nifedipine as antagonist of calcium-ions.

The quantity of endocellular ionic calcium depends exclusively on the equilibrium between association and dissociation of the ions with the structures controlling this process, such as the mitochondria, the superficial vesicles, the extracullular space, the plasmatic membrane and the sarcoplasmic reticulum.

Therefore, by interfering with these processes, Nifedipine lowers the endocellular level of free calcium-ions and causes relaxation of vascular smooth muscle.

Materials and methods

Our research was carried out on 10 subjects with angiospastic syndrome of the superior limbs. Their ages ranged from 18 and 39 years and averaged 32 years.

In every subject rheography of a forearm and photoplethysmography of a finger of the same hand were carried out.

After the basic tracings each subject was administered one placebo capsule, making recordings every ten minutes up to fifty minutes to evaluate possible modifications of the sphygmic wave. To verify whether the substance has a protective capacity on angiospastic crisis, a cold test was them carried out keeping the hand of the patient for one minute in water at a temperature of 4 °C, and after five minutes were examined sphygmic variations.

After 3 days the same tests were executed on the same subjects, administering a 10 mg capsule of Nifedipine instead of placebo.

Rheography was performed by a Duorheograph from the ATE Company, connected to a three channel Cardioline poligraph.

Photoplethysmography was done with a Cardioline unit connected to the aforementioned poligraph; the photoelectric recorder was placed in correspondence to the distal phalange of the second finger of the hand.

All the tracings were recorded at a paper speed of 25 and 50 mm/sec. For each tracing a careful study was made of the form ang amplitude of the pressure pulse contours and of the rheographic quotient (PR) in order to chart both modifications in the caliber of the arterial tree and variations in its vascular tone.

The rheographic quotient (PR) allows us to establish, in units per thousand, the haematic volume relative to the pulse in the area being studied utilizing the formula A/RT, where A is the amplitude of the wave, R is the resistance, in ohms, of the tissues to the passage of current, and T is the total time of the wave.

To evaluate the eventual protective efficacy of the substance from angiospastic crises, each subject was told to record every angiospastic crisis for three months. No treatment was given in the first and third month, while 3 capsules of Nifedipine were given in the second month.

Table I. Average values of PR and amplitude in 10 subjects with angiospastic syndrome before and after placebo and nifedipine

Number of subjects : 10	PR in $^o/_{oo}$		Amplitude	
Average base values	29.78	27.28	13.67	10.53
	Placebo	Nifedipine	Placebo	Nifedipine
Average maximum values	33.38	43.43	16.22	21.32
Average variations	+3.6	+16.15	+2.55	+10.79
Percent variations	+12.08%	+59.2%	+18.56%	+102.46%
t	±1.5868	±2.9278	±0.8301	±2.1961
p	<0.10	<0.005	<0.2	<0.01

Results

The PR and amplitude values observed before and after administration of placebo and Nifedipine are summarized in Table I. The percentage variations following placebo are negligible and not statistically significant either for PR or for amplitude, while after Nifedipine there is a 59.2% increase in PR and 102.46% increase in amplitude. The two latter values are both statistically significant.

Table II carries the values of PR and amplitude observed after cold testing carried out following the maximum vascular response provoked by placebo and Nifedipine. Placebo administration does not prevent angiospasm produced by cold testing with the consequence of a reduction in PR and amplitude. On the other hand, Nifedipine exerts a protective action even after cold testing.

Table III shows the angiospastic crises reported by each patient a month before Nifedipine therapy, during the month of treatment and the month following suspension of the drug. In the period of therapy, 7 out of 10 subjects had no angiospastic crisis and the remaining 3 had a noticeable reduction in the frequency of crises. The month after therapy only 5 patients had angiospastic crises.

It is important to point out that 2 months following suspension of Nifedipine,

Table II. Average values of PR and amplitude in 10 subjects with ang ospastic syndrome following cold testing performed immediately after maximum vascular response provoked by placebo and nifedipine

Number of subjects : 10	PR in $^o/_{oo}$		Amplitude	
Average base values	29.78	27.28	13.67	10.53
	Placebo	Nifedipine	Placebo	Nifedipine
Average values after cold testing	23.48	38.77	7.72	16.78
Average variations	−6.3	+11.49	−5.95	+6.25
Percent variations	−21.15%	+42.11%	−43.52%	+59.35%
t	±1.2818	±3.0435	±1.028	±2.4566
p	<0.15	<0.005	<0.15	<0.01

Table III. Number of angiospastic crises in 10 subjects with angiospastic syndrome one month before, during and one month after treatment with nifedipine

| Case | Number of angiospastic crises | | |
	Before treatment	During treatment	After treatment
1	6	0	2
2	4	0	1
3	8	1	4
4	3	0	0
5	7	2	4
6	4	0	0
7	6	0	0
8	6	0	0
9	8	2	3
10	7	0	0
Average	5.9	0.5	1.4

8 of the subjects studied had a relapse of the clinical process observed before starting the treatment.

Discussion

The study of the vasomotility by using calcium-ions antagonist drugs is clinically interesting for both diagnostic and thera- peutic reasons. In fact the possibility of pharmacologically provoking relaxation of vascular smooth muscle facilitates a dif- ferentiation between functional and organic clinical forms. Its use has until now been limited to the therapy of ischemic car- diopathy. We have considered these agents useful in the study and therapy of peripheral angiopathies. Nifedipine can reduce the passage of calcium-ions from the extracellular space to the intracellular space, and inhibit its release by cellular structures such as the sarcoplasmic reti- culum, the site of myofibrillar ATPase. Because this enzyme is activated by calcium, a reduction of its endocellular availability results in a decreased splitting of ATP and therefore insufficient energy for contraction.

The result is a vasodilation that involves many areas, including the peripheral. The improvement in haematic flow manifests itself 10 min after the administration of the drug and is long lasting.

The intense and persistent action of Nifedipine permits to use it in an active therapeutic program for angiospastic syndromes.

L. S., Cent. of Angiopathies, Dept. Int. Med., Cathol. Univ., Via Pia di SCO 26, 00139 Roma, Italy

CLINICAL EXPERIENCE WITH PROSTAGLANDIN E_1 IN SEVERE PERIPHERAL ARTERY DISEASE

A. G. OLSSON

King Gustaf V Research Institute and Department of Medicine, Karolinska Hospital, Stockholm, Sweden

Prostaglandin E_1 (PGE_1) increases blood flow to the extremities in healthy subjects when injected locally intra-arterially (*Bevegård and Orö*, 1969). It inhibits platelet aggregation (*Bergström et al.* 1968). These findings have prompted us to study the effect of PGE_1 in subjects with severe peripheral artery disease. We have earlier reported often striking beneficial effects on ischemic pain and ulcer healing both when PGE_1 has been given locally with intraarterial infusions (*Carlson and Eriksson*, 1973) and with intravenous infusions (*Carlson and Olsson*, 1976). The intravenous infusion technique required the administration of 1000 ml of saline every 24 hours. As the saline infusion itself could theoretically have beneficial effect on blood flow properties and as this method under certain circumstances could precipitate congestive heart failure, we have used intermittent intravenous injections of PGE_1 thereby giving the same 24 hour dose of the substance in a minimum of vehicle.

Materials and methods

Thirteen subjects (one woman) (mean age 68 years) with advanced peripheral atherosclerotic disease and ischemic ulcer(s) of the foot (feet) were studied. Four subjects had diabetes. All subjects were treated by specialists before PGE_1 and ulcers had been present and stable for at least three months.

Twenty μg PGE_1 diluted in 5 ml of saline was given in 7 daily slow intravenous injections every second hour for three days. Thereby the patients received the same 24 hour dose as in the constant infusion method. In most cases treatment was repeated with monthly intervals one or more times. During treatment the patients stayed in hospital for four days.

The effect of PGE_1 on ulcer healing was studied by colour photos.

Results

The effects of treatment with PGE_1 were with this technique as striking as with the other methods (Table). During the treatment the ulcer oedema diminished and the ulcer surface dried up. The colour of the edges got a pink instead of grey tone. Epithelialisation started and con-

Case nr	Nr. of treatments	Follow up time, months	Healing effect	Complete healing	Notes
1	2	3	+	No	Diabetes
2	5	15	+++	Yes	
3	2	3	++	No	
4	2	10	+	No	Diabetes
5	4	6	++	No	
6	2	5	++	No	
7	5	12	+++	Yes	
8	2	3	−	No	Diabetes, distal gangrena
9	2	8	+++	Yes	
10	2	6	++	No	Diabetes
11	1	3	+++	Yes	
12	1	1	+++	Yes	
13	2	3	−	No	

tinued after treatment had stopped. Ulcer pain disappeared.

During the varying follow up time until now the ulcers of five of the thirteen subjects have healed completely. Two subjects did not respond, the ulcers of the remainder showed varying degree of healing.

Discussion

The present study confirms that ischemic ulcers of the lower limbs heal after treatment with PGE$_1$ in a majority of cases.

This effect is thus maintained if PGE$_1$ is given as intermittent injections with negligible amounts of saline. The mechanisms behind the healing effect have so far not been studied. Possible mechanisms are vasodilatation (less likely), inhibition of platelet aggregation (more likely) or metabolic effect of the tissues including stimulation of epithelial growth (*Bentley-Phillips*, 1977).

The findings are striking enough to prompt us to perform controlled studies on the effect of PGE$_1$ on ischemic ulcer healing.

REFERENCES

Bentley-Phillips, C. B. (1977): The effects of Prostaglandins E$_1$ and F$_{2\alpha}$ on epidermal growth. Arch. Derm. Res. 257, 233. .

Bergström, S., Carlson, L. A., Weeks, J. R. (1968): The prostaglandins: A family of biologically active lipids. Pharmacological Reviews 20, 1.

Bevegård, S., Orö, L. (1969): Effect of Prosta-glandin E$_1$ on forearm blood flow. Scand. J. clin. Lab. Invest. 23. 347.

Carlson, L. A., Erikssson, I. (1973): Femoral-artery infusions of Prostaglandin E$_1$ in severe peripheral vascular disease. Lancet i, 155.

Carlson, L. A., Olsson, A. G. (1976): Intravenous Prostaglandin E$_1$ in severe peripheral vascular disease. Lancet ii, 810.

A. G. O., Department of Medicine, Karolinska Hospital, Stockholm, Sweden

THE PRESENT STATUS OF VASODILATOR THERAPY. AN ANALYSIS OF UNDERLYING MECHANISMS

J. LINHART, J. SPÁČIL and A. BROULÍKOVÁ

Research Centre of Cardiovascular Diseases of the Institute for Clinical and Experimental Medicine, Prague, Czechoslovakia

We have demonstrated that vasodilator drugs increase blood flow through the ischemic foot provided loss of heat from the vasodilated skin is prevented. On the contrary, no increase in flow is observed in the same patients, if dissipation of heat is not prevented (*Linhart, Frič and Spáčil*, 1974). The aim of the present paper was to compare the hemodynamic mechanisms of the "effective" (i.e. properly performed) with the "ineffective" (i.e. not properly performed) vasodilatation.

Methods

Foot blood flow was measured by venous occlusion plethysmography using a mechanical air transmission system. Plethysmography was also employed to measure systolic ankle blood pressure. Peripheral resistance in the foot was calculated from ankle blood pressure and foot blood flow, and collateral resistance from the arm-to-ankle pressure gradient and foot blood flow. Oral temperature was measured sublingually before and after each vasodilator infusion. The duration of vasodilator effect was also measured. Reactive hyperemia in the foot was studied after five-minutes arterial occlusion.

Results

Oral temperature was measured before and after vasodilator infusion (*Linhart,*

Table I.

Vasodilator infusion: oral temperature (N = 18)

uncovered:	control	36.9	
	infusion....	36.5	
	diff........	−0.4	$P < 0.001$
covered:	control	36.9	
	infusion....	36.8	
	diff........	−0.1	n.

Frič and Spáčil, 1974) on two consecutive days (Table I). With the subjects uncovered, there is a significant decrease in the temperature while in the subjects covered with blankets there is no change in oral temperature.

The hemodynamic mechanism of an "effective" (i.e. properly performed) vasodilatation in the covered subjects is shown in a typical example in Figure 1. With no change in systemic blood pressure and a slight increase in distal ankle pressure, the calculated collateral resistance as well as the resistance in the foot decrease. Consequently, there is a definite increase in foot blood flow.

The hemodynamic mechanism of an "ineffective" (i.e. not properly performed) vasodilatation in the uncovered subjects is shown in Figure 2. A striking increase in collateral resistance along with a drop of distal ankle pressure are observed. Thus

EFFECTIVE VASODILATATION

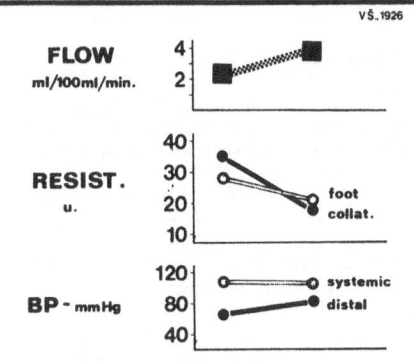

Fig. 1. Hemodynamic mechanism of "effective" vasodilatation. The patient is covered to prevent loss of heat. Note the decrease in collateral resistance. See text for the details.

INEFFECTIVE VASODILATATION

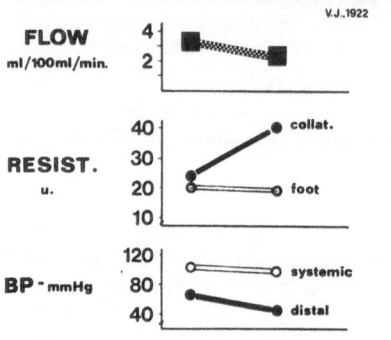

Fig. 2. Hemodynamic mechanism of "ineffective" vasodilatation. The patients is not covered. Note the increase in collateral resistance. See text for the details.

the flow of blood through the foot decreases.

The duration of vasodilator effect: after the infusion, the increase in flow persists for a least two hours (*Spáčil and Linhart, in press*).

Reactive hyperemia almost doubled foot blood flow before the infusion as well as after its termination (*Spáčil and Linhart, in press*).

Discussion

Our data indicate that with proper technique of vasodilator administration, it is the decrease in collateral resistance

that enables the elevated inflow of blood to the ischemic foot. However, if loss of heat is not prevented by covering the patients, the resulting decrease in core temperature brings about a compensatory vasoconstriction with an increase in collateral resistance and paradoxical decrease in foot blood flow. Thus the collaterals are not permanently dilated as some authors have believed.

The increase in foot flow even after termination of the vasodilator infusion is of obvious clinical value. It is also of interest that the pharmacological vasodilatation is not maximal. It may well be that the additional increase in flow caused by the reactive hyperemia is due to enhanced accumulation of vasodilator substances in ischemic foot muscle.

It is well known that venous occlusion plethysmography does not provide information on distribution of blood. Ideally, the increase in total flow should be accompanied by increase in capillary flow and clinical improvement. These aspects have been investigated in a separate study (*Linhart et al., in preparation*).

In conclusion, it has been shown that the circulatory drugs is primarily due to the reaction of collateral vessels, which in turn depends upon the conditions of drug administration. In patients covered with blankets to prevent heat loss, the collaterals dilate and secure an increased blood flow through the ischemic foot.

REFERENCES

Spáčil, J. and Linhart, J.: The increase in foot blood flow in ischemic extremities following pharmacological vasodilatation. The duration of the effect. Angiology, in press.

Spáčil, J. and Linhart, J.: Foot blood flow during reactive hyperemia in patients with ischemic disease of lower extremities. VASA, in press.

Linhart, J., Frič, M. and Spáčil, J. (1974): Vasodilator therapy: the effect of external conditions on blood flow through ischemic feet. Angiologia III, Proceedings of the IX. International Congress of Angiology, Florence, pp. 65—68.

Linhart, J., Spáčil, J. and Dejdar, R.: The effect of treatment with a series of vasodilator infusions on foot blood flow and clinical condition of patients with ischemic extremities. (In preparation).

J. L., IKEM, Vídeňská 800, 14622, Prague 4, Czechoslovakia

CLINICAL EXPERIENCE WITH PYRIDINOL CARBAMATE

E. N. TERRY, L. R. ROUEN, R. H. CLAUSS and W. REDISCH

Departments of Surgery, Medicine and Physiology
New York Medical College, New York, U.S.A.

Introduction

Atherosclerosis has been defined as:
"... a variable combination of changes of the intima of arteries (as distinguished from arterioles) consisting of the focal accumulation of lipids, complex carbohydrates, blood and blood products, fibrous tissue and calcium deposits, and associated with medial changes."
(Study Group: Classification of atherosclerotic lesions. WHO Tech. Rep. Ser. 143: 1–20, 1958).

Since atherosclerosis underlies most cardiovascular disease – a major cause of death and disability in modern society, it has been the subject of a great deal of research. Though the two major and still accepted hypotheses concerning the pathogenesis of atherosclerosis date back to the 1850's (*Rokitansky K.*, A Manual of Pathological Anatomy, Vol. 4 translated by G. E. Day) London Sydenham Society, 1852, p. 261–272) (*Virchow R. L. K.*, Cellular Pathology as based upon physiological and pathological histology (translated from the second German edition by *F. Chance*) New York, Dover Publications, 1971, p. 230–254) we are still in total ingorance of the etiology of atherosclerosis. Common however to all theories, current or past, is the concept of endothelial changes (*Shimamoto T.*, J. Atheroscleros. Res. 3: 87–102, 1963). *Shimamoto* demonstrated that protection of the integrity of the endothelial layer may be possible (*Shimamoto T., Numano F.* in Atherosclerosis III, *Schettler K., Weizel A.*, Eds.: 89–92 Springer Verlag, N. Y., Heidelberg, Berlin, 1974). We attempted to apply his experimental findings in laboratory animals to patients.

Methods and materials

Our study, dealing with the effects of Pyridinol Carbamate (PDC) on the progression of atherosclerosis in patients with advanced disease in the lower extremities, consisted of 2 parts.

A total of 94 patients were entered into the study and were attributed randomly to either of 2 groups, receiving either PDC 200 mg or an identical looking placebo 4 times a day.

In part I of the study, patients were followed for 2 years under tightly controlled double-blind conditions.

Subsequently, following evaluation of the effects of the treatment regimen and breaking of the code, a number of patients continued to undergo treatment with either PDC or placebo, under single-blind conditions. This period lasting for 18–24 months is referred to as part II.

Detailed descriptions of methods used in this study have been published (*Redisch W., Terry E. N., Rouen L., Clauss R. H.*, In Atherogenesis II, Eds: *Shimamoto T., Numano F.*, 287–294, Excerpta Medica Amsterdam, 1973).

A small number of these patients have been followed for an additional 2 years. To assess their condition a questionnaire was designed.

Results

In part I 38 patients, 22 on PDC, 16 on placebo, completed the planned course of treatment: progression of atherosclerosis as defined for the purposes of this study (*Redisch W. et al.*, 1973) seemed to be arrested in 19 of 22 patients on PDC 200 mg q.i.d. and 1 of 16 patients on placebo.

In part II 28 patients were followed. Atherosclerosis did not progress, according to the criteria used in this study in 16 of 18 patients on PDC and 1 of 10 patients on placebo.

It is thought to be of particular significance that among the patients on PDC who did not present with progression of atherosclerosis were 3 patients who in part I of the study had been in the placebo group and during that period had shown evidence of progression of atherosclerosis.

Adverse effects, primarily gastrointestinal problems such as diarrhea and nausea required discontinuation of treatment in 21 patients, of whom 19 were found to have been on PDC and 2 on placebo.

Details on the fate of all those taking part in the study have been published (*Terry E. N., Rouen L. R., Clauss R. H., Katz M. C., Redisch W., Zilversmit D. B.,* Aun., N. Y., Acad. Sci. 275: 379 – 385).

Sixteen patients filled out the questionnaire given to them. Six had been on PDC in the preceeding parts of the study, 10 had received placebo during this period. Progression or non-progression of their atherosclerosis during the after-study period is being assessed in part based on the subjective statements made by the patients, in part on their interim medical history.

Of the 6 ex-PDC patients, 3 showed no further progress since discontinuation of PDC administration. The others progressed, one (=88) requiring amputation, one (=5) requiring a by-pass operation. The third (=66) evidenced a considerable decrease in walking ability. These 3 patients had not responded to PDC during the preceeding treatment periods, their condition having progressed relentlessly since first seen by us in 1971 (=5), 1972 (=66) and 1973 (=88) respectively.

Of the 10 ex-placebo patients, 2 had not progressed, one of whom had not shown any signs of progression since first seen in 1971 (=2). The others continued to present with signs of progression of atherosclerosis, not necessarily limited to the periphery: one patient had suffered a stroke (=63),one a myocardial infarction (=40). One patient had to undergo amputation of an extremity (=23).

Discussion

In the ongoing discussion concerning the etiology of atherosclerosis, it is becoming apparent that, rather than being a disease entity, this complex condition is composed of a number of different clinical patterns, relating respectively to the location of the disease (coronary artery, cerebrovascular, aortic, peripheral etc.), the type of lesion (obliterative, aneurysmal, predominantly lipid-filled or largely occupied by fibrous connective tissue and dense mucopolysaccharides) and to the rate of development of the disease. Type of lesion and rate of development may be related (*Smith E. B., Smith R. H.* in Atherosclerosis Reviews, i, Eds. *Raoletti E., Kotto A. M.* in Raven Press N. Y. 1976, p. 119 – 136). A distinction has to be made between atherogenesis and progression of the disease, particularly in view of the extensive development that has taken place in the field of reconstructive vascular surgery. Reconstructive, as all other surgical procedures still carry a certain risk and thus can only be justified if upon re-establishment of blood flow, continued deterioration in the vascular system can be brought to a halt, or at least slowed down.

Endothelial integrity and modification in permeability appear to be at the core of progression of atherosclerosis. Since in our study (*Terry* 1976) we were able to show that other factors, such as platelets and lipid levels, had not been measurably affected, one has to assume that the inhibition of progression observed related to effects on the endothelium, perhaps similar to those occurring in laboratory animals and described by *Shimamoto* (*Shimamoto T.* 1974). It may thus become feasible to add to other measures already customarily taken, protection of the endothelial integrity and permeability in an attempt to reduce or even arrest progression of atherosclerosis.

E. N. T., New York Medical College, Departments of Surgery, 10 East End Ave, New York, N. Y. 10021 U.S.A.

THE EFFECT OF NITROGLYCERIN IN ACRAL PULSE CURVE AND ACRAL CIRCULATION IN THE UPPER LIMB

S. GOLDBERG

„Heinrich Braun" County Hospital, Zwickau, G.D.R.

It is of clinical importance to differentiate between functional and organic vascular disturbances in acral circulation. This differentiation should distinguish vasospastic (functional) from truely occlusive (organic) symptoms. In medical terminology functional vascular disturbances comprise a complex of symptoms consisting of circulatory disturbances in the hand with different clearly distinguishable etiologies. On closer scrutiny it becomes evident that the symptoms can be differentiated from each other. They are different in their natural time course, manifestation and etiology. Ischaemia of fingers is also often seen in consequence of arterial occlusion. But occlusions in the upper extremities are often without symptoms and are overlooked because the incidence of arterial occlusions is higher in the lower than in the upper limb. Also the branching of these arteries shows many variations which were investigated and based on our own experience. Further diagnostic and therapeutic measurements hinge on an acurate assessment of acral vascular disturbances. In consequence of this, they should be defined separately in order to institute causal therapy after careful investigation.

The so-called "nitroglycerin test" is of help in this differentiation. Acral volume pulse is registered every three minutes after oral application of 0.8 mg nitroglycerine. It could be demonstrated that rheography is a very useful and evident method of investigation which gives the possibility to establish quantitative data on the circulation-time-volume of a certain measuring region. After application of nitroglycerine the change of the pulse curve, its shape and the form and timing of the dicrotic notch are all taken into consideration. This test is easily administered, repeated and evaluated. In 38 patients with Raynaud's phenomenon the arteriography of the upper limbs was performed. In 10 patients, all older than forty, who showed progression of ischemic symptoms on the fingers, arterial obstructions were seen.

The oral effectiveness of nitroglycerin was tested in 100 patients with Raynaud's phenomenon. The patients consisted of 22 men mean age 38 years (range 20−56) and 78 women, mean age 32 years (range 18−58). All patients were without cardiac disease. The subjects were recumbent for 15 minutes in a room with an air temperature between 22−24 °C before measurement was started. Except for bare legs they were normal clothing. All patient received a single dosis of 0.8 mg nitroglycerine. 78 patients had a good response to nitroglycerin which is rapidly absorbed. The pulse curve and the relative pulse volume showed a significant difference between the two groups. Along with the reduction of the peripheral resistance following the application of nitroglycerin the final part of the catocrotic limb rapidly drops to the baseline where such pulse waves adopt the shape of symmetric peaks.

No effect was seen in 10 patients with occlusive arterial disease. We found a more gradual and often pulseless baseline shift. Also no significant difference was seen in patients with and without stenoses of arteries of the fingers. Smaller arteries of the muscle type react to nitroglycerin more strongly than the large elastic arteries.

Nevertheless, judgment of the acral volume pulse according to formation criteria and according to the quotient from the time of the increase of pulse to the time of decrease of pulse before and after administration of nitroglycerin allows a diagnostic estimation of the microcirculation as well as recognition of functional prodromal stages of Raynaud's phenomenon.

REFERENCES

Böhme, H. (1975): Der "Nitroglyzerin-Test" zur Beurteilung funktioneller peripherer Gefäßstörungen. Herz/Kreisl. 7, 666—671.
Delius, L. (1961): Die funktionellen peripheren Gefäßstörungen. Internist 2, 676—684.
Koziak, P. (1966): Oszillographische Funktionsprüfung der Extremitätenarterien bei Anwendung von Nitroglyzerin. Dtsch. Gesundh.-Wes. 21, 207.
Lemmens, H. A. J. (1977): Raynaud-Phänomen-Asphyxia manus et digitorum; Digitus mortuus sive Digitus moriens. Vasa, Band 6, Heft 3, 295—299.

S. G., 95 Zwickau, Bundschuhweg 11 B, G.D.R.

VEINOUS-OCCLUSION-PLETHYSMOGRAPHIC EXAMINATIONS ON THE BEHAVIOUR OF RESTING-BLOOD-FLOW AND REACTIVE HYPEREMIA DURING INTRA-VEINOUS LONG-TERM-THERAPY WITH VASOACTIVE DRUGS

D. WITT, E. WITT and H. HEIDRICH

Free University Berlin, Berlin West

The behaviour of resting-blood-flow and reactive hyperemia after intra-venous long-term-therapy of peripheral arterial occlusive disease with vasodilative drugs is — due to diverging opinions on the therapeutical value of such substances — of general clinical interest. However examinations on this topic are rare — often concerning only acute-trials and usually concerning only one substance. There are no independent controlled comparative studies with several substances on intra-venous long-term-therapy with measurement of the quantitative blood-flow. That is why we examined whether:

1. 14-day intra-venous infusion-therapy with different vasoactive substances causes a change of quantitative extremity-perfusion in peripheral arterial occlusive disease whether

2. different vasoactive substances change the perfusion-rate similarly or differently, and whether

Table I. Means of resting-blood-flow (RBF), peak-flow (PF), peak-flow-time (PFT), and painfree walking distance (PWD) before and after 14-day-therapy or observation

	RBF (ml/100 ml/min)	PF	PFT (sec)	PWD (m)
CONTROL				
before	3.2846	15.1437	8.0208	187
after	3.9365	14.9771	7.0000	248
difference	+0.6519	−0.1666	−1.0208	+61
difference %	+20	−1	−13	+32
BENCYCLANE				
before	3.8172	13.2321	9.5000	111
after	3.5483	12.5750	12.0000	214
difference	−0.2689	−0.6571	+2.5000	+103
difference %	−7	−5	+26	+93
NAFTIDROFURYLE				
before	4.1711	9.3861	23.5277	88
after	4.1731	11.3028	17.6944	221
difference	+0.0020	+1.9167	−5.8333	+133
difference %	+0	+20	−25	+151
PENTOXIFYLLINE				
before	3.6647	12.0000	12.6451	186
after	3.6559	13.9935	10.3870	332
difference	−0.0088	+1.9935	−2.2581	+146
difference %	−0	+17	−18	+78
RAUBASIN				
before	3.9700	12.8036	10.7500	99
after	4.6900	13.6786	9.0000	186
difference	+0.7200	+0.8750	−1.7500	+87
difference %	+18	+7	−16	+88

3. there is a dependence of possible changes upon seriousness or type of occlusion.

The examinations were carried out on in total of 100 patients with an arterial occlusive disease (Fontaine-stage II—IV) by means of a mercury-strain-gauge-plethysmograph (Gutman/Eurasburg). Just before and one day after a 14-day intra-venous infusion-therapy with ben-cyclane, naftidrofuryle, pentoxifylline or raubasin resting-blood-flow, peak-flow and peak-flow-time were measured. Like in earlier studies of our team we chose substances which were monosubstances, of different chemical structure, ranked with newer groups of vasoactive pharmaca, are indicated in peripheral arterial occlusive disease, and are used most frequently according to market-analyses. The at-tachment of the patients to the different substances occurred by chance, and i.v. infusions were given twice daily for two hours at a time. The single dose per infusion was 200 mg of bencyclane, nafti-drofuryle, or pentoxifylline and 50 mg

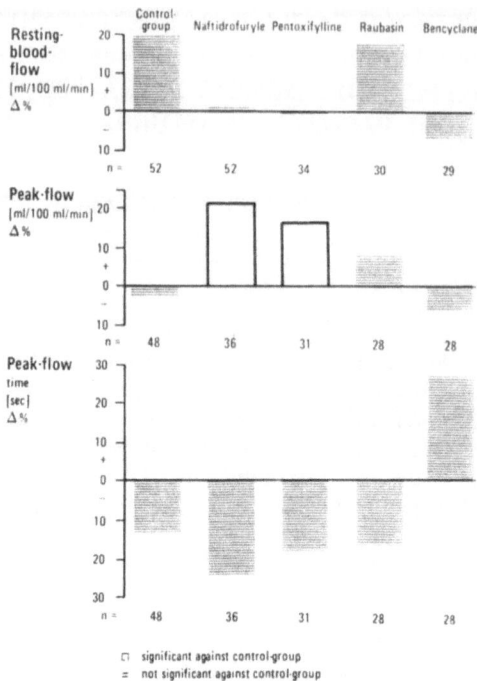

Fig. 2. Change in % of resting-blood-flow, peak-flow, and peak-flow-time after therapy in comparison to before therapy.

of raubasin respectively. Hence the total daily dose was 400 mg of bencyclane, naftidrofuryle or pentoxifylline and 100 mg of raubasin respectively.

In parallel with these treated groups, resting-blood-flow and reactive hyperemia were measured in comparable patients before and after a 14-day interval but no therapy was carried out. The behaviour of blood-flow in the substance-groups was compared with that of the untreated control-group.

The significance of changes in particular perfusion values was computed by the t-test at $p = 0.05$, the dependence of blood-flow-change upon seriousness or type of occlusion within each group by analysis of variance and f-test, the comparison of the different groups by Wilcoxon-test.

The results were (Table I, Fig. 1 and 2):

1. resting-blood-flow was not improved significantly by any of the tested substances

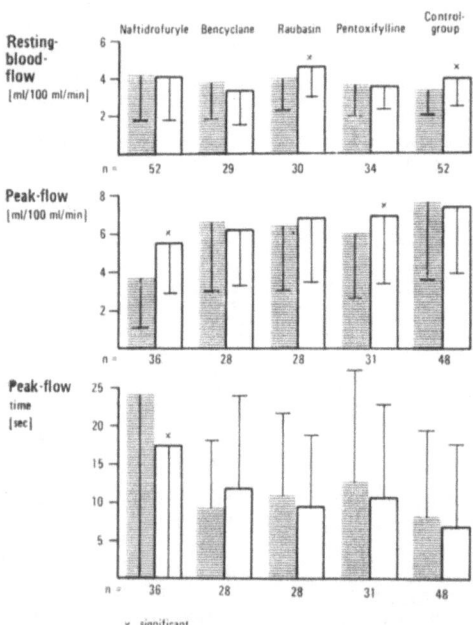

Fig. 1. Resting-blood-flow, and peak-flow-time before (left column) and after (right column) therapy or observation.

558

in comparison with the control-group after 14-day infusion-therapy. Merely the control-group showed a significant improvement of resting-blood-flow in comparison with the bencyclane-, naftidrofuryle- and pentoxifylline-group. The increase of resting-blood-flow in the raubasin-group by $+18\%$ corresponded to the increase by $+20\%$ of the untreated control-group.

2. On the contrary peak-flow as a measure of reactive hyperemia improved by $+20\%$ in the naftidrofuryle-group and by $+16\%$ in the pentoxifylline-group. These changes in the naftidrofuryle- and pentoxifylline-group were statistically significant in comparison to the control-group. On the contrary peak-flow was changed neither in the bencyclane- and raubasin-, nor in the untreated control-group.

3. In comparison with the untreated control-group none of the substance-groups showed a significant reduction of peak-flow-time. A reduction of peak-flow-time by 25% under naftidrofuryle and by 18% under pentoxifylline was significant merely in comparison with the bencyclane-group.

4. There was no statistically significant correlation between a change of blood-flow in the different groups and the seriousness or the type of occlusion of the disease.

These results demonstrate that naftidrofuryle and pentoxifylline, when given intra-venously, led to a significant increase of reactive hyperemia, measured with the peak-flow, in comparison with the untreated control-group while bencyclane and raubasin merely showed a similar behaviour as the untreated control-group. Thus some of the tested vasoactive substances are able — despite numerous reservations — to improve the blood-flow-reserve when given intravenously as long-term-infusion.

Under the here chosen therapy- and test-conditions there is a correlation between the increase of the blood-flow-reserve under naftidrofuryle and pentoxifylline and a simultaneously observed increase of the painfree walking distance. Thus, those substances meet the theoretical suppositions for their clinical use by intravenous application and objectify clinic-empirical observations of an improvement of peripheral arterial occlusive disease.

D. W., Free University of Berlin, Klinikum Westend, Grunewaldstr. 27
1000 Berlin 41 — West

ERGOTISM — A SEVERE COMPLICATION DURING TREATMENT OF HEADACHE

U. ST. MÜLLER, R. KOCH, J. VAN DE LOO, F. BENDER,
K. LANGENBRUCH and J. SCHÜTZ

*Medical Clinic and Policlinic of Radiology of the University Münster,
Department of Roentgenology and Nuclear Medicine Knappschafts
Hospital, Dortmund, F.R.G.*

Since rye has been cleaned of the fungus claviceps purpura, chronic intoxications by ergot have become rare. Today, these intoxications, so called ergotism, may be observed after suicidal intake of drugs containing ergot and during treatment of headache and hypotension. The present paper describes a case of ergotism, which was angiographically investigated during and after intoxication.

A 34 year old woman, suffering from migraine and hypotension since 1970, was treated with Cafergot(R)-PB. The patient took 2 to 5 capsules daily containing 2 to 5 mg ergotamintartrate. Since November 1976 she suffered from intermittent claudication of the legs. Therefore, an arteriography was performed in February 1977. Obliteration of the femoral artery in the adductor canal on both sides (Fig. 1), which was more pronounced on the left side, and a very narrowed lumen of the popliteal artery on the same side were noted. The alterations of these arteries were not suited for operative therapy.

In May 1977, the woman was referred to our University Hospital with occlusions of the femoral arteries of degree IIb on the right side and degree III to IV on the left side. The femoral arteries were palpable, but not the pulses of the popliteal, posterior tibial or dorsalis pedis arteries.

The ergotamine drug was discontinued and treatment with heparin, papaverine and pentoxifyllin was initiated. Two days after the beginning of this treatment the pulses of the right lower limb were normally palpable, on the left leg the pulses

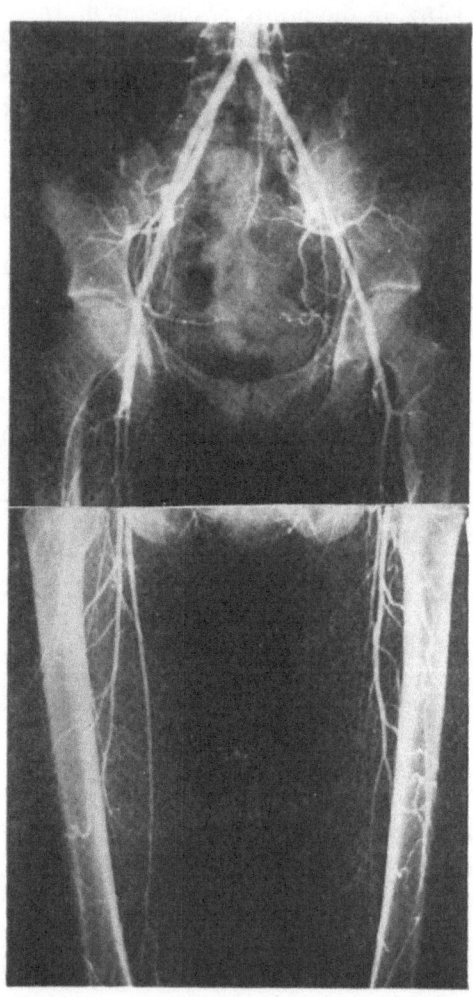

Fig. 1a. Arteriography after injection of contrast medium into the distal part of the abdominal aorta (February 1977)

appeared somewhat reduced and there was a vascular murmur in the middle of the adductor canal of the left side. The patient could walk about half a kilometer at 120 steps/min. three weeks after discontinuing the ergotamine treatment.

In July 1977 a second arteriography was performed, which showed a narrowed lumen and limited stenosis in the middle of the adductor canal on the left side and signs of arteriospasm in the adductor canal of the right side (Fig. 2). The systolic arterial blood pressure was 30 mm Hg lower in the left foot than central systemic blood pressure, as measured by the ultra-sonic Doppler-method.

It is supposed that the rate of severe complications during treatment with drugs containing ergotamine is about 0.01% (5). The beginning of the symptoms of ergotism can be acutely serious (3) as well as mildly chronic (1, 6). Usually, the occlusions of the arteries caused by ergotism are completely reversible, but cases have been described, in which the peripheral obliterative arteriopathy progressed after

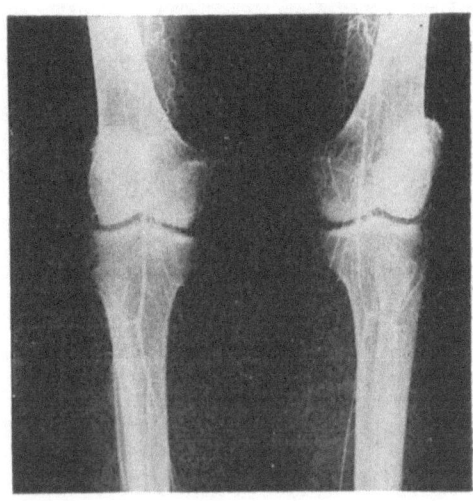

Fig. 1b. Arteriography after injection of contrast medium into the distal part of the abdominal aorta (February 1977).

discontinuing ergotamine treatment (4, 2). It is supposed that the chronic spasm of the arteries caused an alteration of the vessel wall and subsequent thrombosis.

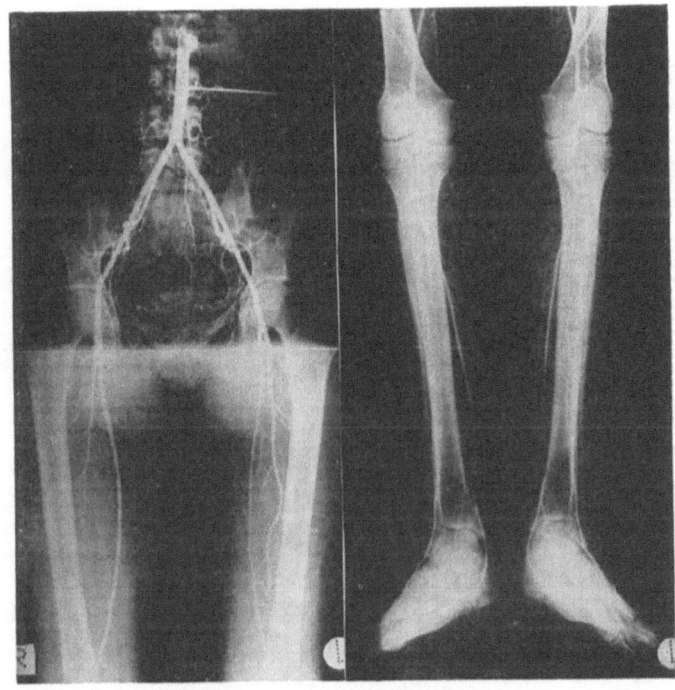

Fig. 2. Arteriography of the same case, repeated in July 1977.

561

REFERENCES

Bollinger, A., Preter, B.: (1973): Spasmen der muskulären Stammarterien nach Einnahme von ergotamintartrathaltigen Medikamenten. Dtsch. med. Wschr. 98, 925.

Heberer, G., Rau, G., Schoop, W., (1974): Angiologie, G. Thieme, Stuttgart.

Johnson, K. A. (1962): Angiography in two cases of ergotism. Acta radiol. (Stockh.) 57, 280.

Korth, Kl., Ploner, J. (1977): Ergotismus als Ursache peripherer arterieller Durchbluttungsstörungen. Fortschr. Röntgenstr. 127, 448.

Von Storch, T. J. C. (1938): Complications following the use of ergotamine tartrate, their relation to the treatment of migraine headache. J. Amer. med. Ass. 111, 293.

Tüttenberg, K. et al. (1976): Periphere Durchblutungsstörungen bei der Migränebehandlung mit Ergotamin. Med. Welt 27, 1938.

U. St. M., Med. Klinik und Poliklinik der WWU Münster, Westring 3, 440 Münster, F.R.G.

CONTINUOUS INTRAARTERIAL INFUSION-THERAPY OF PROSTAGLANDIN E 1 FOR ISCHEMIC ULCERATION OF THE EXTREMITY

S. SHIONOYA

Department of Surgery, Nagoya University Branch Hospital, Nagoya, Japan

Thirty-two patients with intractable ischemic ulcers of the extremity were submitted to continuous intraarterial infusion-therapy of prostaglandin E 1 (PGE 1): Buerger's disease in 29, arteriosclerosis obliterans in 1, scleroderma in 1 and lupus erythematosus in 1. They were no candidates for arterial reconstruction, and all but 3 cases had undergone sympathetic denervation in the affected limb formerly.

PGE 1 was continuously infused through a catheter, 1 mm in diameter, into the artery by means of a portable infusion-pump: A. femoralis in 30, A. peronea in 1 and A. brachialis in 1. When a percutaneous insertion of the catheter like Seldinger's method was not feasible, cut-down was performed. Correct insertion of the catheter was always certified by arteriography. The catheter was detained mostly above the knee in the femoral artery.

The solution in the infusion-bag consisted of 1) 0.1 ng/kg/min of PGE 1, 2) 1.000 units/day of heparin and 3) 500 mg/day of AB-penicillin. The capacity of the bag was 25 ml and 5 ml of the solution was infused each day.

Clinical evaluation of the infusion-results was as follows:

1. Excellent (14 cases): Ulcers healed with 9 to 135 days' infusion (average: 33 days). In this group, intractable pain promptly disappeared within a few days after initiation of the infusion.
2. Good (11 cases): Ulcers improved remarkably but did not completely heal with 5 to 140 days' infusion (average: 44 days).
3. Unchanged (7 cases): No improvement of ulceration was seen with 3 to 31 days' infusion (average: 16 days). Four of the 7 cases were Buerger's disease and development of the disease was very progressive. Other two were collagen disease. In another one, thrombotic occlusion due to insertion of the catheter occurred on the 3rd day, and thrombectomy salvaged the affected limb. Six of the 7 patients underwent amputation of the extremity afterwards: of the thigh in 1, of the leg in 3, of the foot in 1 and of a toe in 1.

In all the cases, PGE 1 was at first infused at a dose of 0.1 ng/kg/min.

In 11 of the 32 cases, swelling or pain was noticed around the knee or ankle joint, and the troubles promptly disappeared when the dose of PGE 1 was reduced to 0.05 ng/kg/min. When the initial dosage of PGE 1 was not effective, the dosage was twofold increased in 4 cases with good result in two: the dosage was fourfold increased in another case with good effect. During the continuous intraarterial infusion of PGE 1, the blood pressure value did not change not only on the level of the arm or the ankle. There was no abnormal as well variation in laboratory studies. However, C-reactive protein test was intensified in 12 cases only during the infusion-therapy.

Recently, an attempt to use PGE 1 for treatment of peripheral vascular disease was reported (*Carlson and Eriksson*, 1973). They infused PGE 1 into the femoral artery at a dose of 10 ng/kg/min for 10 min. every hour for 24—72 hrs.

When 100 ng/kg of PGE were infused into the femoral artery of the dog over a period of one minute, the blood flow in the anterior tibial muscle at rest, measured by the Xe-133 clearance method, increased in 6 of 7 dogs (average: 3.5 → 9.2 ml/100 g/min.) (*Shionoya et al.*, 1976). This effect continued one min. after completion of the infusion, and lumbar sympathetic denervation had no influence on the effect of PGE 1. However, the maximum muscle blood flow after ischemic exercise did not increase with PGE-infusion.

The general pathophysiological basis in occlusive arterial disease is the reduced flow rate of blood in the microvascular circulation, and the microvascular blood flow at ischemic condition is considerably influenced by the blood flow properties.

By the tracer technique with a diffusable substance, 99 mTc pertechnetate, measurement of both arterial and capillary blood activity as well as the diffusion interface for the injected tracer is possible (*Gerritsen et al.*, 1974). Therefore, a radioactive tracer technique with 99 mTc pertechnetate under reactive hyperemia seems to be a reliable and atraumatic method to evaluate microcirculation in the peripheral region of the extremity.

In the time activity curves in the toes and foot, by intravenous injection with 10 mci of 99 mTc pertechnetate, shortening of the arrival time and increasing of the counts were seen after this intraarterial infusion of PGE 1 in some cases (Fig. 1).

A possible pharmacological mechanism of therapeutical usefulness of PGE 1 on ischemic ulceration might be an improvement of microvascular circulation in the distal area of the extremity. An intraarterial insertion of the catheter itself seemed to be very harmful for the patients with collagen disease.

Continuous intraarterial infusion-therapy of PGE 1 was useful for intractable ischemic ulceration in the patients for whom no surgical procedure was feasible, because of rapid disappearance of the pain and of complete healing of ulceration within a short-term period of the infusion.

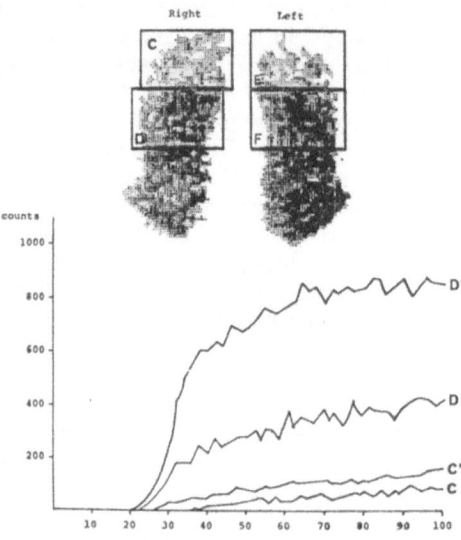

Fig. 1. Time activity curves of two regions of interest in the right foot. The insert demonstrates the regions of interest.

C and E: region including whole toes
D and F: region neighbouring to C and E
C′ and D′: before treatment
C and D: after two months' infusion of PGE_1
Shortening of the arrival time and increase of the counts are seen.

REFERENCES

Carlson, L. A., Eriksson, I. (1973): Femoral-artery infusion of prostaglandin E_1 in severe peripheral vascular disease. Lancet January 20, 155—156.

Gerritsen, H. A., Kazem, I., Hasman, A., Kuypers, P. J. (1974): A new approach to the evaluation of peripheral vascular disease using the gamma camera. Radiology 112, 115—121.

Shionoya, S., Ban, I., Nakata, Y., Matsubara, J., Shinjo, K., Hirai, M., Miyazaki, H., Kawai, S. (1976): Continuous intraarterial infusion-therapy of prostaglandin E_1 for peripheral arterial occlusive disease. Gekachiryo 34, 213 to 218.

S. S., Dept. of Surgery, Nagoya University Branch Hospital, 2-12-1 Higashisakura, Higashi-ku, Nagoya, Japan

ADAPTATION OF ARTERIAL WALL TO PHYSICAL STRESS BEFORE AND AFTER PENTOXIFYLLINE ADMINISTRATION

G. BREVETTI, S. ABATE*, G. LAVECCHIA,
G. P. FERULANO*, G. PAUDICE, S. FASANO*

*Institute of Special Medical Pathology, *Institute of Surgical Anatomy,
University of Naples, Italy*

In most patients with peripheral arterial insufficiency, the exercise induces in the affected limb a reduction in blood flow, at least partially responsible for the claudication (*Zetterquist*, 1968). Since this hemodynamic event is accompanied by several changes in the rheological blood properties (*Ehrly*, 1975), it has been purposed that an improvement in the disturbed flow properties of blood could result in a beneficial effect in the circulation of the affected areas.

Accordingly, the purpose of this study was to investigate the modifications induced by exercise in the peripheral blood flow and other blood parameters in 40 patients with occlusive atherosclerosis of the lower limbs, and to compare the results with those obtained after one month of oral treatment with pentoxifylline.

Materials and methods

Forty male patients ranging in age from 49 to 67 years and affected by peripheral arterial insufficiency of the lower limbs were included in the study. The diagnosis was established on the basis of impedance plethysmographic recordings as well as arteriography. The impedance plethysmographic tracings were recorded in the affected limb while the subjects lay in the supine position. Simultaneously, blood samples were taken from the radial artery and from a vein of the ischemic area. Subsequently, an exercise test was performed on a bicycle ergometer until the occurrence of pain in the limb. Two minutes later, new plethysmographic tracings were recorded and blood samples were taken. The entire study was repeated after one month of oral treatment with pentoxifylline administered at the dosage of 600/800 mg daily and the patients performed the same work load as under control condition.

In order to quantify the changes of the plethysmographic waves, the Jantsch's index (Jantsch, 1958) was calculated in five consecutive waves and then averaged. The pO2 values were calculated on the arterial and venous blood in 10 patients and the artero-venous difference of pO2 (Δ A$-$V pO2) was estimated. Plasma osmolarity was evaluated on the venous blood samples. Plasma fibrinogen and hematocrit were evaluated on the venous blood only at rest. Statistical analysis was performed by standard techniques (*Snedecor and Cochran*, 1967).

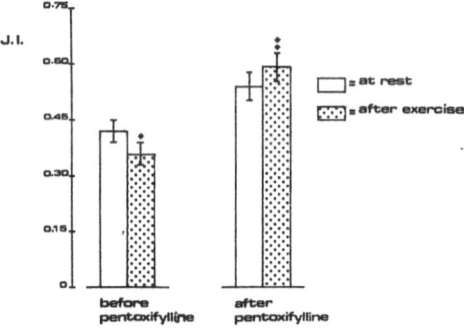

Fig. 1. Changes of Jantsch's index induced by exercise before and after pentoxifylline. * = p < 0.01 ** = p < 0.001.

EFFECT OF PENTOXIFYLLINE ON ΔA-VpO2

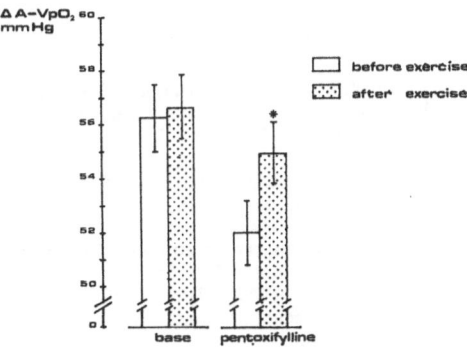

Fig. 2. Changes in oxygen artero-venous difference induced by exercise before and after pentoxifylline. * = p < 0.05.

Results

Before pentoxifylline administration, exercise induced a significant reduction in the blood flow of the affected limb. Actually, Jantsch's index decreased from 0.42 ± 0.03 to 0.36 ± 0.03 (p < 0.01). No

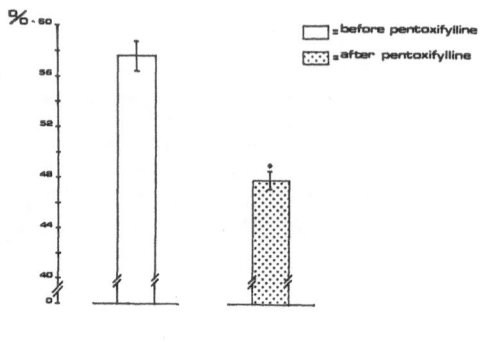

EFFECT OF PENTOXIFYLLINE ON PLASMA FIBRINOGEN CONCENTRATION

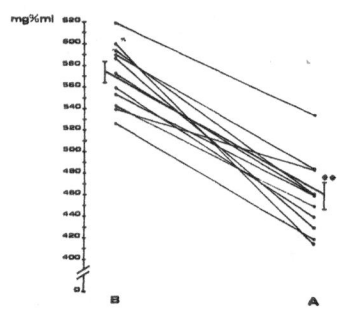

Fig. 3. Changes in hematocrit (upper panel) and plasma fibrinogen concentration (lower panel) after one month of oral treatment with pentoxifylline. B = before treatment; A = after treatment. * = p < 0.001.

changes in plasma osmolarity and $\Delta A - V$ pO2 were observed after physical stress.

Following treatment, Jantsch's index rose, after exercise, from 0.54 ± 0.04 to 0.59 ± 0.04 (p < 0.001) (Fig. 1), this indicating an increase in blood flow to the affected area. Moreover, it has been noted that only four patients presented claudicatio after treatment. $\Delta A - V$ pO2 rose from 52.3 ± 2.3 to 55.1 ± 2.2 mm Hg (p < 0.05) (Fig. 2), while plasma osmolarity did not change.

Plasma fibrinogen concentration decreased from 571.9 ± 9.7 to 475.9 ± 11.4 mg % ml (p < 0.001) after pentoxifylline treatment. Hematocrit too decreased from 57.3 ± 1.14% to 54.6 ± 0.92% (p < 0.001. These two parameters were evaluated only at rest (Fig. 3).

Discussion

Although vasodilators have been commonly employed in the treatment of obstructive vascular diseases, the evidence of their therapeutic efficacy is questionable (*Hansteen and Lorentsen*, 1974). Therefore, the possibilities of new approaches to the treatment of peripheral arterial insufficiency have been recently explored. In particular, the importance of rheological properties of blood in the vascular bed of the ischemic region has been underlined. Actually, elevated blood osmolarity and viscosity have been demonstrated in the poststenotic area during intermittent claudication (*Ehrly*, 1975).

REFERENCES

1. *Ehrly, A. M. (1975):* The effect of pentoxifylline on the flow properties of hyperosmolar blood. I.R.C.S. Med. Sci. 3, 465.
2. *Grigoleit, A. G., Lehroch, F. Muller, R. (1973):* Diabetic angiopathy and blood viscosity. Acta diabet. lat. 10, 1311.
3. *Hansteen, V. and Lorentsen, E. (1974):* Vasodilator drugs in the treatment of peripheral arterial insufficiency. Acta Med. Scand. 556, 3.
4. *Jantsch, M. (1958)* Zur Answeitung des Peripheren Rheogramms. Wiener Med. Wschr. 45, 1004.
5. *Olivari, N. und Olivari, B. (1975):* Beeinflussung der Lappendurchblutung und Nekroserate nach Verschiebeschwenkplastik durch Pentoxifyllin und Dextran 40. Arzneim.-Forsch. 25, 745.
6. *Snedecor, G. W., Cochran, W. G. (1967):* Statistical methods. Iowa, Iowa University Press.
7. *Zetterquist, S. (1968):* Muscle and skin clearance of antipyrine from exercising ischemic legs before and after vasodilator trials. Acta Med. Scand. 183, 487.

G. B., *Istituto di Patologia Medica, II Policlinico, Università di Napoli, Via S. Pansini 5, 80131 Napoli, Italy*

EFFECT OF BENCYCLANE, PENTOXIFYLLINE, AND VINCAMINE ON CEREBRAL VASCULAR RESISTANCE IN RABBITS

P. VAUPEL and H. HUTTEN

Institute of Physiology, University of Mainz, Mainz, F.R.G.

Introduction

The application of vasoactive drugs in order to improve cerebral blood flow is a commonly used but often disputed therapeutical procedure. Numerous studies have attempted to determine the effectiveness of these substances both clinically and experimentally whereby a large number of methods has been employed. The results concerning the effects on cerebral blood flow are, in part, contradictory. This study is designed to test the effectiveness of Bencyclane, Pentoxifylline and Vincamine on cerebral vascular resistance whereby the influences caused by eventual side effects of the drugs are for the most part eliminated.

Materials and methods

Experiments were performed on a total of 50 New Zealand rabbits of both sexes (2.1—4.6 kg BW, normal acid- base balance, superficial anaesthesia induced with ketamine and maintained with urethane, tracheotomy tube). Cerebral vascular resistance (CVR = perfusion pressure divided by cerebral blood flow CBF) before and after administration of the drugs into both internal carotid (i.c.) arteries was determined by using a decoupling extracorporeal bypass system (*Hutten and Vaupel*, 1977). This system consists mainly of a roller pump with pressure- independent output and a heat- exchanger (Fig. 1). Blood was taken from the abdominal aorta through a catheter in a femoral artery and reinfused into both i. c. arteries. At the site of reinfusion, Bencyclane-hydrogenfumarate (Be), Pentoxifylline (Pe), and Vincamine- monohydrogentartrate (Vi) were added to the blood (0.5 to 0.6 mg/ml blood), and the perfusion pressure was measured continuously. The total injection volume was 0.1—0.2 ml for both i. c. arteries. The maximum decrease of CVR (Δ CVR) after application of the drugs was calculated as a percentual decrease from initial CVR values before administration of the vasoactive drugs. In addi-

tion, the duration of the acute CVR- decrease (t) and the planimetric value of the area (A) above the curve of the perfusion pressure (PD) and under the prolongation of the initial level was calculated from the original graphs (Fig. 2). This area is the most relevant parameter as it takes into account both the extent and the duration of the decrease in CVR. Values for A are expressed in $kPa.min^2/ml$.

The effects of some solvents or vehicles (distilled water, isotonic NaCl solution, 0.7% NaCl + 0.1% NaOH in distilled water, propanediol, polyethylene glycols) were also examined in order to exclude unspecific or hemodilutional effects. The following parameters were monitored throughout all experiments: mean arterial blood pressure in the abdominal aorta (SD), ECG, heart rate (HF), respiratory rate (AF), tidal volume (V_T), respiratory gas parameters

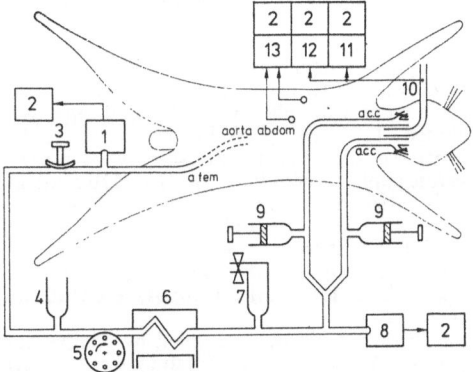

Fig. 1. Experimental device for determination of cerebral vascular resistance in rabbits using an extracorporeal bypass system.
1 = Statham pressure transducer (arterial pressure in the abdominal aorta), 2 = recorder, 3 = adjustable resistor, 4 = pressure equalizer, 5 = roller pump with pressure- independent output, 6 = heat exchanger, 7 = bubble trap, 8 = Statham pressure transducer (perfusion pressure), 9 = precision syringes, 10 = tracheotomy tube with microthermistor, 11 = bridge connection and amplifier, 12 = 13 = time-frequency- converter.

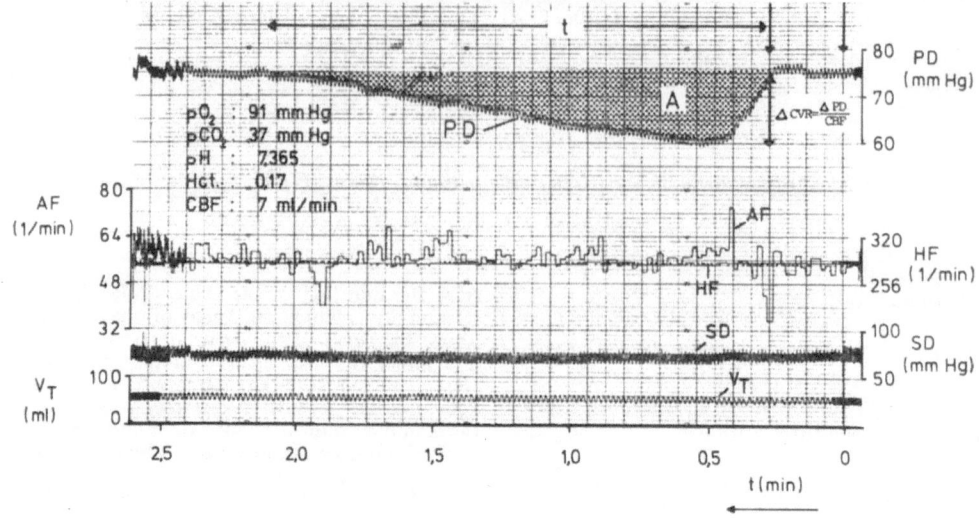

Fig. 2. Original graph showing relevant parameters after drug application. The time of application of the drug is marked by arrows.
PD = perfusion pressure, HF = heart rate, AF = respiratory rate, V_T = tidal volume. At constant cerebral flow rate, the decrease of PD is a direct indicator for the drop of CVR (ΔCVR = ΔPD/CBF). t = duration of the acute CVR−decrease, A = area above the curve of the perfusion pressure and under the prolongation of the initial level.

in the arterial blood (pO_2, pCO_2), pH, hematocrit, and hemoglobin concentration. Since a long-lasting non-pulsatile flow leads to a distinct rise in cerebral vascular resistance (*Held et al.*, 1971), during all experiments pulsatile perfusion pressure, whose frequency and amplitude are in accordance with physiological conditions, was chosen. The mean perfusion pressure was adjusted so that normal pressures were present before application of the drugs (70−110 mmHg).

In order to investigate the effects of the drugs on cerebral vessels not only under normal physiological conditions, 38 experiments were performed on additional rabbits whose cerebral vessels had low parietal tonus, i. e., during acidosis.

Statistical significance is studied by comparison with the Wilcoxon-Mann-Whitney test (U test). Mean values are given $\pm$SEM.

Results

While the application of solvents or vehicles into both i.c. arteries (0.1 − 0.2 ml per application) has no measurable effect on CVR, all drugs used in these experiments show an acute vasodilatory effect in the rabbit brain. The results obtained after i.c. administration of a dose of 0.5 to 0.6 mg/ml blood of the different substances

are summarized in Table I. The heart rate, tidal volume, respiratory rate and mean arterial blood pressure in the abdominal aorta are not modified systematically by the drugs when they are injected into both i.c. arteries at the chosen doses.

In order to investigate the effects of the drugs on partially dilated cerebral vessels experiments were performed on animals during acidosis (mean arterial pH = 7.065) Under these conditions of respiratory or non- respiratory acidosis the cerebral vessels have low parietal tonus; the cerebral vascular resistance decreases to about 90% of the values in non- acidotic rabbits. When Bencyclane, the most effective vasodilatory drug among the substances tested, is applied at comparable doses, the maximum drop of CVR after application of the drug and the planimetric value of the area are slightly increased as compared with data obtained at a normal acidobasic balance (ΔCVR = 24.3 $\pm$ 1.3%, A = 1.0 $\pm$ $\pm$ 0.2 kPa . min^2/ml). There is a pronounced enhancement in the duration of the acute CVR- decrease (t = 4.2 $\pm$ 0.4

Table I. Relevant data from measurements of CVR changes in the rabbit cerebral circulation after intracarotid injection of vasodilatory substances. N = number of animals, n = number of measurements (1 mmHg = 0.133 kPa)

	Bencyclane	Vincamine	Pentoxifylline
N	23	15	12
n	44	52	35
pO_2 (mmHg)	103 ± 3	107 ± 4	95 ± 2
pCO_2 (mmHg)	30 ± 1	26 ± 2	26 ± 1
pH	7.31 ± 0.01	7.31 ± 0.01	7.37 ± 0.01
Hct	0.33 ± 0.01	0.31 ± 0.01	0.31 ± 0.01
CBF (ml/min)	6.2 ± 0.2	5.6 ± 0.1	5.7 ± 0.2
CVR (kPa . min/ml)	1.9 ± 0.1	1.8 ± 0.1	1.9 ± 0.1
dose (mg/ml)	0.54 ± 0.04	0.53 ± 0.02	0.56 ± 0.04
Δ CVR (%)	21.3 ± 1.4	18.0 ± 0.8	12.9 ± 1.2●
T (min)	3.2 ± 0.3	1.8 ± 0.2●●	1.1 ± 0.2●●
A (kPa . min^2/ml)	0.8 ± 0.1	0.3 ●●	0.1 ●●

● $p < 0.005$, ●● $p < 0.0001$ as compared to BENCYCLANE values.
Values are means ±SEM

min, $p < 0.05$). From these results it can be concluded that the intensity, and above all the duration of the Bencyclane effects, have increased in cerebral acidosis. Products which primarily enhance flow in diseased areas must decrease CVR more strongly during acidosis than under normal conditions. Their minor activity in healthy regions can preclude any intracerebral steal (*Cosnier et al.*, 1977). If the acidotic brain of the rabbits shows some similarities with the ischemic human brain during cerebral circulatory insufficiency, this pattern may also be true for patients.

Conclusions

(1) All drugs used in these experiments show a vasodilatory effect. (2) The extent and the duration of these effects are different and vary with the drug. (3) Among the drugs tested, Bencyclane is the most powerful vasoactive substance. (4) vasodilatory effect of Bencyclane is increased during acidosis as compared with normal conditions. This fact may imply that a supplementary vasodilation is possible in ischemic areas thereby precluding an intracerebral steal.

REFERENCES

Cosnier, D., Cheucle, M., Rispat, G., Streichenberger, G.: Influence of hypercapnia on the cerebrovascular activities of some drugs used in the treatment of cerebral ischemia. Drug. Res. 27, 1566 (1977).
Held, K., Niedermayer, W., Gottstein, U.: Die Hirndurchblutung bei nicht pulsierender Perfusion. Z. Kreislaufforsch. 60, 336 (1971).
Hutten, H., Vaupel, P.: Der Einfluss von Bencyclan auf den zerebralen Gefässwiderstand bei normalem und gestörtem Säure- Basen-Status. Med. Welt (N. F.) 28, 1567 (1977).

P. V., Institute of Physiology, University of Mainz, Saarstrasse 21, D-6500 Mainz, F.R.G.

DOUBLE-BLIND TRIAL WITH BENZYCLANE IN PATIENTS WITH PERIPHERAL ARTERIAL DISEASE

V. VIDEČNIK

3rd Department of Internal Diseases, Medical Centre, Ljubljana, Yugoslavia

Introduction

In spite of great progress achieved in the field of angiology, surgical treatment in chronic peripheral arteriopathies is adequate in only 50% of all cases or less. Systemic application of pure vasodilators is not recommended (*Nielssen*, 1977; *Heidrich*, 1978); because of the steal phenomenon ("borrowing-lending-phenomenon") and following lessened blood flow in the ischemic areas (*Hänsgen*, 1977). Intra-arterial application of vasodilators having a short-lived effect is therefore recommended.

Today, those preparations are interesting which affect rheological properties of blood at the level of microcirculation (*Ehrly*, 1976). They lower serum fibrinogen, thereby decreasing blood viscosity; they preserve the flexibility of erythrocytes in hypoxic areas, and inhibit aggregation of platelets and of erythrocytes. Such a preparation is also benzyclane which has a direct spasmolytic effect on arterial walls and also inhibits aggregation and adhesivity of platelets. Besides, it preserves the flexibility of erythrocytes (*Ehrly*, 1974) and decreases blood viscosity. Used systemically, it does not lower blood pressure. Up to now, the preparation has been clinically assessed in almost 8.000 patients in various countries, predominantly in double-blind trials. In our clinical study the same method was used.

Patients and methods

The study included 38 patients with stable disturbances of circulation in the lower limbs. All patients belonged to stage II, according to Fontaine. Testing was carried out in 31 outpatients. The characteristics of our groups of patients are shown in Table I. The control group was given xantinol nicotinate, predominantly for ethical reasons. The distribution of samples was randomized. Both preparations were given as pills in doses of 600 mg daily for 3 months. The following parameters were observed: a) Subjective 'troubles as paresthesies, feeling of cold, claudication distance; b) Objective examinations: the walking test on a treadmill, Ratschow's test, systemic blood pressure, mechanical oscillography, and acral photopletysmography. Beside these examinations we followed also: ECG, examination of the fundus, chest X-ray, haemogram, coagulation examinations as thromboplastin time (Quick), recalcification time, fibrinolysis time (Bukhel), spontaneous aggregation of platelets, cholesterol, triglycerides, and transaminases.

The following parameters were statistically assessed: 1) Anamnestic data on claudication distance (in metres); 2) The walking test on a treadmill (in minutes); 3) Mechanical oscillography (indexes in mm on the thigh, calf and instep); 4) Photopletysmogram of the toes (amplitude in centimeters and crest time in seconds); 5) Fibrinolytic activity (in minutes).

Table I. Walkig test-treadmil painless distance in minutes: A — group received Benzyclan B — control group received Xantinol nicotinate

	GROUP $\overline{1}$ BENZYCLANE	CONTROL / GROUP	STATISTICAL SIGNIFICANCE
NUMBER	14	17	
AGE - $\overline{x}$	58,5	57,9	N
SEX - $\overline{x}$ male	13	15	N
female	1	2	N
CLAUDICAT TIME BEFORETESTING - $\overline{x}$	4,17	3,67	N
DURATION OF SYMPTOMS - $\overline{x}$ (years)	1,3	1,8	N

Tabel $\overline{1}$ presenting homogenity of both groups

Results

1) Four patients in the benzyclane group (consisting of 14 patients) reported no more claudication after treatment. In other patients this distance was substantially lengthened; the difference is statistically significant ($P < 0.05$). No significant difference was detected in the control group. 2) A lengthening of the distance was found in both groups, the difference being statistically significant in both. Arithmetic means in both preparations differ significantly in favour of benzyclane 3) No significant difference in oscillometric indexes was observed in either preparation. 4) The difference in the arithmetic mean of amplitudes obtained by acral photopletysmography is significant before and after treatment in both preparations, whereas there are no significant differences in the crest time. 5) No significant difference between fibrinolytic activity before and after treatment was found for either preparation. Equally, in all other examinations mentioned above there were no differences in either preparation. In no case treatment had to be discontinued due to side effects.

Discussion

Clinical evaluation of the efficacy of drugs in the treatment of chronic peripheral arteriopathies is always difficult, and only a double-blind trial can objectify the results of therapy. In our study, however, evaluation is made even more difficult by the use of a vasoactive substance in the control group, not of placebo. In all clinical studies, great significance is attributed to the lengthening of the claudication distance. We observed it in both preparations, with a significant difference in arithmetic means in favour of benzyclane. Many of our patients practised active walking at home. The combination of active training with drug therapy improves the clinical effect (Heidrich, 1978), but renders it more difficult to assess the efficacy of a preparation. The use of more subtle non-invasive angiologic methods would surely better objectify the success of therapy. Spontaneous aggregation in vitro (Breddin) is not an adequate method for observing the efficacy of antiaggregation therapy, which is probably the reason why we found no changes in the aggregability of platelets.

REFERENCES

Ehrly A. M. (1976): Improvement of the flow properties of blood: a new therapeutical approach in occlusive arterial disease. Angiology 27, 188.

Heidrich, H. (1978): Konservative Therapie peripherer arterieller Verschlusskrankheiten. Münch. Med. Wochenschr. 120, 23.

Hänsgen, K. et al. (1977): Untersuchungen zum Borrowing-Lending-Phänomen unter den Bedingungen einer intraarteriell induzierten Vasodilatation. Z. Kardiol. 66, 511.

Nielsen, P. E. et al. (1976): Intra-arterial infusion of prostaglandin E1 in normal subjects and in patients with peripheral arterial disease. Scand. J. Clin. Lab. Invest. 36, 633.

V. V., 3rd Department of Internal Diseases, Medical Centre, Ljubljana, Yugoslavia

SIGNIFICANCE OF ANTHOCYANINS IN THE TREATMENT OF PERIPHERAL VASCULAR DISEASES

A. NUTI, S. B. CURRI, C. VITTORI and M. LAMPERTICO

Angiological Division of the S. Maria Nuova Hospital,
Florence-Center of Molecular Biology, Milano and 2nd Medical
Division of the General Hospital, Saronno, Italy

The involvement of the microvessels and particularly of the blood flow regulating structures (arterio-venous anastomoses and blocking arterioles in arteriosclerotic peripheral vascular diseases has been outlined in these last years (1, 2). The AVA of the finger-tip and of the hallux ball are shortened, the whole glomic organ is upset and smaller; its connective capsule trends to fuse with the dermal fibrous tissue and the layers of the myo-epitheloid cells (m. e. cells) show various degrees of regressive alterations (centripetal sclerosis). The AVA's lumen remains apparently unaffected in the first stages of the arteriosclerotic damage; in the further stages or in cases complicated with hypertension the lumen is permanently open, as a rigid canal, or on the contrary narrowed or completely obliterated (3): AVA's "hyperstomy", or "hypostomy" and "astomy", see (4). The capillary bed, besides the interdependence between fine structure the microvessels wall and the biochemical constitution of the pericapillary ground substance sheath (5) show the well known pathological features, related to the changed haemodynamic situation. It can be assumed that in the arteriosclerotic involvement of macrocirculation in the limbs, also the microcirculation play a role of primary importance. In fact, some symptoms such as throphic alterations and phaenomena of districtual ischemia with pain, paresthesia etc. cannot be attributed only to parietal lesions of larger arteries, but probably also to the compromised microcirculatory blood flow as suggested for the macrophlebopathies (6). A therapeutic assay with some of the so-called "capillary-protective" substances seems to be justified. From among them high dosed anthocyanins (equivalent to 25% anthocyanidins, (7) have been selected because of their significant vasoprotective and antiinflammatory activity (8, 9, 10).

Materials and methods

42 male patients, aged 39—84 years, with severe arteriosclerotic vascular disease of the lower limbs were treated with a daily dosis of 480 mg of anthocyanins orally for 40 days. Before the treatment, 76.2% showed claudicatio, 54.8% trophic lesions, 54.8% paresthesia, 69% cold sensation on the legs and 52% modifications of the lower limbs skin colour. 73.8% had severe pain. All the patients were submitted to the common angiological and humoral tests before, during and after the treatment.

Results

No modification has been found in the arterial blood supply in the lower limbs. A vasodilatatory action of the drug can be excluded. The plasma triglycerides level shows in significant variations (mean $155,51 \pm 10.37$ before and 161.73 ± 9.82 mg % after the treatment). Plasma cholesterol level show a trend to a slight decrease, although statistically significant ($t = 2.47 - P < 0.05$). On the contrary, the clinical symptoms which can be related to the microcirculatory situation and to the tissue-vascular relationship show statistically significant modifications, summarized in Table I.

Discussion

A correct evaluation of our findings present remarkable difficulties. Antho-

572

Table I. Modifications induced by high dosed anthocyanosides on some symptoms of arteriosclerotic peripheral vascular diseases of the lower limbs.

Symptom	Presence in %	Means before (°) the treatment	Means after the treatment (°)	Student's t	Significance
Claudicatio	76.2	1.55 ± 0.17	0.59 ± 0.10	2.68	$P < 0.05$
Trophic lesions	54.8	1.00 ± 0.16	0.45 ± 0.12	5.03	$P < 0.001$
Pain	73.8	1.55 ± 0.18	0.14 ± 0.05	8.4	$P < 0.001$
Paresthesia	54.8	0.78 ± 0.13	0.07 ± 0.04	5.54	$P < 0.001$
Cold sensation	69.0	1.28 ± 0.17	1.28 ± 0.17	7.84	$P < 0.001$
Skin colour	52.4	0.86 ± 0.15	0.14 ± 0.05	5.75	$P < 0.001$

(°) The intensity of the single symptoms was expressed as arbitrary units from 0 to 3

cyanins are known to have a peculiar affinity for the endothelial cells of the capillaries (11) and for some constituents of the cell membrane (12). The aglycones of the anthocyanins form complexes "in vitro" with the main phospholipidic components of the cell membrane, phosphatidylcholine and phosphatidylethanolamine (12). Biochemical and morpho-histochemical observations have shown an increase of the biosynthetic patterns of the ground substance glycosamino-glycans (9).

Our data emphasize the possibility of a direct action of anthocyanins on the capillary-tissue exchanges, without any influence on vasomotility.

REFERENCES

1. *Curri, S. B.* (1968): "Fisiopatologia del circolo preterminale delle dita", Piccin ed., Padova.
2. *Curri, S. B.* (1972): "The diagnostic significance of the finger-tip biopsy in microangiopathies — Pathology of arteriovenous anastomoses and preterminal circulation", Bibl. Anat. 11, 310—316.
3. *Scelsi, R., Rosso, R. Caspa, L., Scelsi, M, and Mosca, L.* (1976): "Morphology of arteriolo-venular anastomoses in hallux ball in health and various diseases", Bioch. exp. Biol. 12, 139—147.
4. *Tischendorf, F. and Curri, S. B.* (1974/75): "Senile Involution of arterio-venous Anastomoses (after Bioptic and Autoptic Examination of the Human Finger-tip), Bioch. exp. Biol. 11, 207—228.
5. *Curri, S. B.* (1977): Regional differences in the relationship between vessels and tissues: importance of glycosaminoglycans", Bioch. exp. Biol. (in press).
6. *Mian, E.* (1977): "Microangiology in the macrophlebopathies", Bioch. exp. Biol. (in press).
7. *Bombardelli, E., Bonati, A., Gabetta, B., Mar-*

tinelli, E. M., Mustich, G. and Danieli, B. (1976): "Gas liquid chromatographic and mass spectrometric identification of anthocyanidines", J. Chromat. 120, 115—122.
8. *Lietti, A., Cristoni, A. and Picci, M. (1976):* "Studies on Vaccinium myrtillus anthocyanosides. I. Vasoprotective and antiinflammatory activity" Arzneim. Forsch. (Drug Res.) 26, 829—832.
9. *Mian, E., Curri, S. B., Lietti, A. and Bombardelli, E. (1976):* "Antocianosidi e parete dei microvasi, nuovi aspetti sul modo di azione dell'effetto protettivo nelle sindromi da abnorme fragilità capillare", Min. Med. 67, 3565—3581.
10. *Ghiringhelli, C., Gregoratti, L. and Marastoni, F.* (1978): "Attività capillarotropa di antocianosidi ad alto dosaggio nella stasi da flebopatia", Min. Cardioangiol. (in press).
11. *Piovella, C.* (1978): unpublished results.
12. *Curri, S. B. and Bombardelli, E.* (1975): "Antocianosidi, sostanza fondamentale del connettivo e correlazioni istangiche" 46 nd Riun. Sci. Soc. It. Angiologia, Salsomaggiore, 14—16 nov.

A. N., Lungarno Colombo, 44; 50136 Florence, Italy

AN APPROACH TO THE INDIVIDUALIZATION
OF PHENPROCOUMON THERAPY

K. O. HAUSTEIN, W. BARTHEL and G. VOGEL

*Section of Clinical Pharmacology of the Institute of Pharmacology
and Toxicology and Department of Medicine, Medical Academy Erfurt,
Erfurt, G.D.R.*

Introduction

The use of phenprocoumon (PPC) for prophylaxis of thromboembolic disorders is very complicated because of its long elimination half-life ($t_{0.5}$) and the small therapeutically useful range of prothrombin-complex synthesis blocking efficacy. On the one hand the inappropriate use of the drug includes the danger of cumulation and thus the occurrence of bleeding, on the other hand, the risk of thrombosis in-

Dose (mg)

Quick Value (%)

Time after Administration (d)

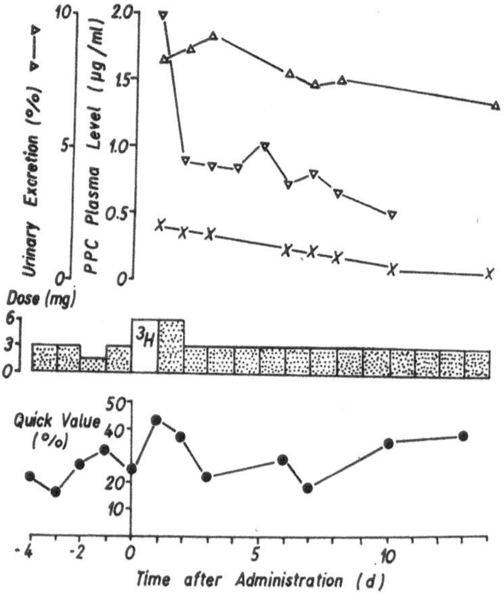

Fig. 1. Time course of total plasma concentration ( ) and of prothrombin-complex activity during PPC treatment (dotted columns) in an inpatient. On the first day, ^{3}H-PPC (open column) was administered and on the following days, radioactivity of plasma (x) and activity excreted in urine (in % of administered dose), were measured.

creases. Furthermore, interactions of PPC with additionally administered drugs as well as genetic differences in the irritability of the phytomenadion-PPC interaction are well known.

The aim of this investigation was to develop a method for the individualization of drug dosage during long-term treatment with PPC. In previous studies correlations between the mean daily dose of PPC and the plasma level or the Quick value were found (*Haustein, et al.*, 1975). In spite of correlations, the deviations from the regression line were too wide to use the results for evaluation of maintenance doses (D_E) instead of coagulation tests in the clinic.

Following our conception, $t_{0.5}$ of PPC represents the most essential parameter for the extent of PPC intake necessary to depress the coagulation potential to a suitable antithrombotic level. We estimated the individual $t_{0.5}$ during continous long-term treatment with Falithrom[R] tablets. Determinations were performed by administration of the drug in its tritiated form (^{3}H-PPC) as a single dose and by measurement of the rate of disappearance of radioactivity in plasma within the following 2 weeks.

Results

In a first investigation, on one day of PPC treatment 10 female and male inpatients of the Department of Medicine took per os instead of Falithrom[R] maintenance dose, 6 mg ^{3}H-PPC (118 – 124 μCi). During the observation period, radioactivity and total PPC plasma content (*Rich-*

574

ter, 1976) as well as Quick value were estimated. Taking into account the decrease in radioactivity, the area under plasma concentration/time curve from $t=0$ to $t=$infinity (AUC) was calculated by dividing the extrapolated concentration (c_0) by the apparent firstorder elimination constant (k_e) after solution of the integral

$$\text{AUC} = {}^{t \,=\, \infty}_{t \,=\, 0} \, c_0 \cdot e^{-k_e t} \, dt \, .$$

(Equ. 1)

The graphical estimation of c_0 became possible assuming an absorption percentage of neerly 100 per cent (*Seiler and Duckert*, 1968).

A typical regimen is demonstrated in Fig. 1. The patient took PPC for several weeks and his Quick value was lowered to the therapeutically useful range. The radioactivity of plasma declined, the total PPC level, however, did not decrease. The Quick value remained in therapeutically useful limits. Attemps to correlate D_E administered to 10 patients to their individual $t_{0.5}$ or to k_e did not lead to satisfactory results because of deviations from the regression line. A closer relationship was found between the mean D_E (x, in mg per kg b.w.) and AUC. Between both parameters, the following exponential function was calculated:

$$\text{AUC} = 3.37 + 8.90 \cdot e^{-0.052x} \, .$$

(Equ. 2)

In a second investigation, 19 anticoagulated male and female outpatients between the age of 21 and 69 years, underwent the same procedure. After a single intake of 100 µCi ^{3}H-PPC, plasma radioactivity was measured 1, 5, 8 and 15 days after intake. The regression line was estimated by the method of least squares. By extrapolation at $t = 0$ the radioactivity in the equilibrium state (c_0) was evaluated.

A relationship was found between the values of AUC and those of total body clearance (Cl_{tot}), as demonstrated in Fig. 2. The slope of the curve confirms the

general rule that AUC is reversely proportional to Cl_{tot}. According to our investigations, D_E is equivalent to that PPC dose which is eliminated within the interval T from the volume of distribution (V_d) by Cl_{tot}. D_E is defined by

$$D_E = V_d \cdot k_e \cdot c_0 \cdot T \quad \text{(Equ. 3)}$$

and after substituting $V^d = D_0/c_0$, equation 3 becomes

$$D_E = D_0 \cdot k_e \cdot T \, . \quad \text{(Equ. 4)}$$

Discussion

In case of the known initial dose (D_0) or of the known PPC plasma level in the equilibrium of distribution c_0, D_E can be calculated for any interval T. Thus, D_E can be estimated by the use of D_0 as well as a relevant PPC plasma concentration under the conditions of steady state.

In literature, data have been recommended for both methods. An initial dose of 0.3 mg PPC per kg b.w. causes a total block of the synthesis of prothrombincomplex (*Christke et al.*, 1973). Plasma

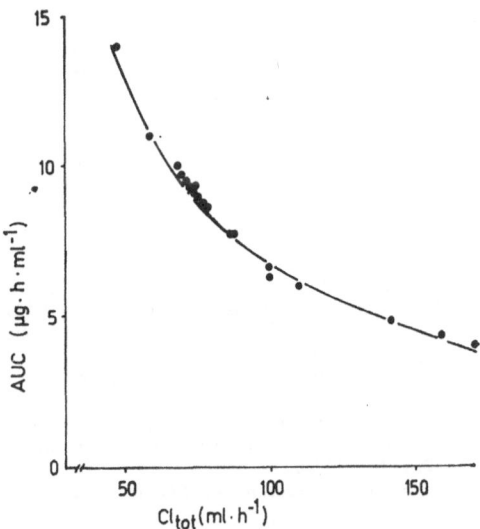

Fig. 2. Correlations between area under curve (AUC) and the total body clearance (Cl_{tot}) in 19 anticoagulated patients after a single dose of ^{3}H-PPC instead of PPC (Falithrom$^{(R)}$).

concentrations of $1-2$ µg PPC per ml depress the prothrombin synthesis by 50 percent (*Husted and Andreasen*, 1977) and the Quick value to $20-40$ percent (*Haustein et al.*, 1975). Taking $D_0 = 0.3$ mg per kg and $c_0 = 1$ µg per ml as a basis for calculation of D_E according to Equs. 3 and 4, values are obtained which only in some patients are in good agreement with the administered dose (Table I).

Since in our studies PPC was used alone, combination effects on its pharmacokinetic behaviour were neglected. The effect of phytomenadion on the pharmacokinetics of PPC is not yet known. Therefore, further investigations have to be done to clarify the influence of the phytomenadion

metabolism on the kinetic behaviour of PPC.

Conclusions

1. Simultaneous administration of ^{3}H-PPC during long-term treatment with PPC allows an estimation of the pharmacokinetics of ^{3}H-PPC as if PPC had not been administered.

2. A high correlation between the pharmacokinetic parameters (^{3}H-PPC) and the required D_E of PPC necessary to maintain therapeutically suitable levels was found.

3. We consider the procedure to be a method to improve long-term treatment with anticoagulants.

Table I. Comparison of the administered and calculated maintenance doses[1] of PPC in 10 anticoagulated outpatients and the Quick value[2]

Patient	Administered D_E	Calculated D_E on the basis of		Quick value (%)
		$D_0 = 0.3$ mg/kg	$c_0 = 1$ µg/ml	
G.H.	18	28.9	21.5	30
A.H.	31	24.3	20.4	$38-43$
H.A.	33	34.8	30.9	$31-57$
K.G.	38	27.5	21.6	$33-100$
W.R.	40	34.7	21.6	30
G.H.	50	43.3	35.2	30
E.F.	19	30.0	42.6	30
W.S.	15	39.0	38.0	$42-64$
P.M.	25	22.0	17.0	30
A.M.	34	44.3	46.7	$68-88$

[1] Values in µg per kg body weight.
[2] Quick values obtained from 4 determinations during the observation period.

REFERENCES

Christke, H. W., Gross, R., Hilger, H. H., Oette, K., v. Smekal, P., Knabe, M., Kray, D. (1973): Pharmakokinetische Untersuchungen zur Phenprocoumon (Marcumar)-Resistenz. Verh. Dtsch. Ges. inn. Med. 79, 1311–1314.

Haustein, K.-O., Richter, M., Vogel, G. (1975): Zur Optimierung einer Langzeitbehandlung mit Phenprocoumon. Dtsch. Gesundh.-wesen 30, 1514–1518.

Husted, S., Andreasen, F. (1977): Individual

variation in the response to phenprocoumon. Europ. J. clin. Pharmacol. 11, 351–358.

Richter, M. (1976): Zur fluorimetrischen Bestimmung von Phenprocoumon im Blutplasma. Zbl. Pharm. 115, 611–614.

Seiler, K., Duckert, F. (1968): Properties of 3-(1-phenyl-propyl)-4-oxycoumarin (Marcoumar(R)) in the plasma when tested in normal cases and under the influence of drugs. Thrombos. Diathes. haemorrh. (Stuttg.) 19, 389–396.

K. O. H., Inst. Pharmacol., Toxicol. Medical Academy, Erfurt, DDR 506 Erfurt, G.D.R.

CONTROL OF THERAPY IN PATIENTS WITH CHRONIC ISCHEMIC DISEASE OF THE EXTREMITIES BY MEASURING THE LOCAL OXYGEN PRESSURE

J. HAUSS, K. SCHÖNLEBEN, U. SPIEGEL and M. KESSLER

Surgical University Clinic Münster, Department of General Surgery,
Münster — Max-Planck-Institute of Systemphysiology, Dortmund, F.R.G.

Aims

It is well known that in modern highly developed countries most people, i.e. about 50 per cent, die of some kind of disturbance of arterial circulation.

The methods used until now for investigation in the clinic and also for controlling the effect of therapy are not very accurate, because most of them are based on subjective findings. The main aim of these investigations was therefore to find objective parameters for diagnostical orientation and for controlling the effect of our surgical or pharmalogical therapy, and to get important hints about the situation of the microcirculation, whose quality is decisive for the survival of critically ill patients.

Methods

The measurements were carried out in 68 patients using the oxygen-multiwire-surface-electrode, which was developed by *Kessler* and *Lübbers*.

We chose the musculus quadriceps femoris as test-organ. A 1—2 cm wide incision of the skin and the muscular fascia is necessary, 15 cm above the proximal patella edge. The electrode can be held in position on the muscular surface nearly without any weight. We registered the local pO_2 tension in the form of histograms.

Results

Figure 1 shows one typical finding when we compared our preoperative and postoperative measurements. The histogram written before the operation was taken while the patient was resting in bed and it shows a mean value of 31.25 mm HG (Fig. 1).

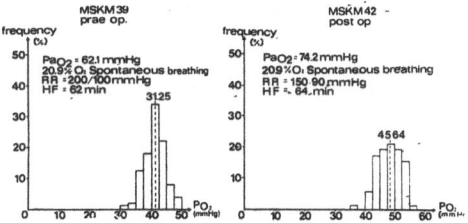

Fig. 1.

The configuration is normal, but compared with a histogram of the musculus tibialis anterior in healthy persons taken with a different method using needle electrodes, as has been first demonstrated by Kunze in 1967, it is significantly shifted to the right.

The postoperative histogram shows another slight shift to the right, which means that the local oxygen pressure increased. This result was not unexpected. What was surprising was the effect of some drugs we use in the intensive care unit. For example at the beginning of these in-

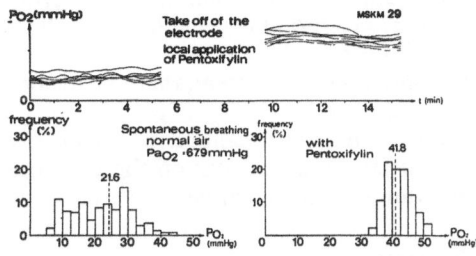

Fig. 2. The effect of local application of Pentoxifylin. Continuous registration and histograms (below).

vestigations the effect of Pentoxifylin on the local pO_2 was studied. Pentoxifylin is said to have a blood flow promoting effect, resulting from a reduction in blood viscosity and an increase in red blood cell flexibility. Apart from these effects, the reduced tendendy of platelet aggregation may also be advantageous.

Some drops of Pentoxifylin, which is usually added to an infusion, were put locally on the surface of the muscle (Fig .2).

The comparison of the pO_2-histograms showed an obvious increase in the local oxygen supply after application of this drug which does not contain any substance causing hyperemia. In the upper part of the illustration, the continuous registration of the 8 wires of the electrode is demon-

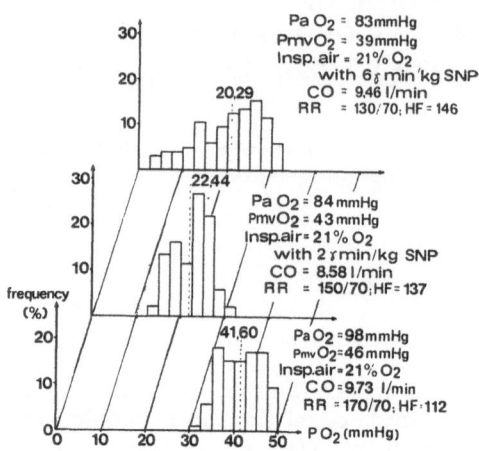

Fig. 4. Downward trend of local pO_2-tension under different dosages of SNP. Below: Histogram without SNP.

(SNP) to get a controlled hypotension. SNP diminished blood pressure gradually in a patient who got SNP because of a critical blood pressure rise after a vascular operation (Fig. 4).

Altogether 48 mg SNP were applied within 3 hours, a very low therapeutic dosage, far below the assigned toxic dosage. The wanted therapeutic effect was soon obtained, the other parameters did not show threatening reactions. Acidosis in the blood analysis was not observed. Nevertheless we found a decrease in local pO_2 tension dependent on the dosage. Al-

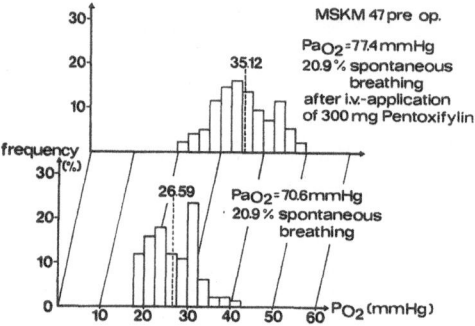

Fig. 3. Histogram before (below) and after (above) intravenous application of 300 mg Pentoxifylin.

strated. This finding was controlled in a series of 12 patients (Fig. 3).

Also other substances in some more series were tested: for example vasopressin, dopamin, human albumin, the "drug" oxygen, glucose and laevulose as volume substitution in hypovolemic patients for nitroprusside. At present, there is no comparable method making it possible to get a qualitative and quantitative analysis of the effects of these drugs on the microcirculation in different organs.

Example

There are different indications for the application of sodium-nitroprusside

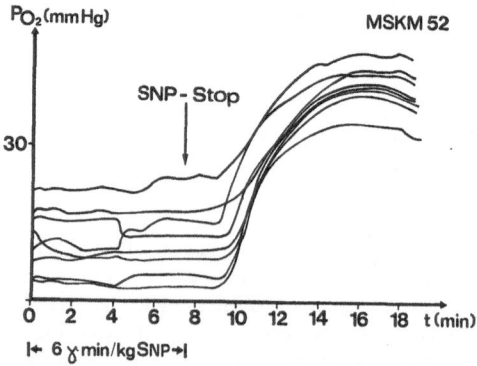

Fig. 5. After stopping SNP-application, the local oxygen supply recovers within a few minutes.

578

though the decrease in this range did not cause local anoxia, we obtained a result which was unknown until now. We have only hypothetic ideas about this effect of SNP. Is it a redistribution of blood volume or a toxic effect, which causes the diminution of pO_2 tension in sceletal muscle? Or does the SNP induced vasodilatation cause a change of the oxygen transport to the tissue?

Figure 5 shows how fast the SNP-induced effects on the sceletal muscle disappear.

It is important for clinicians to have a method for direct control of therapy during clinical treatment.

J. H., University Clinic of Surgery, Dept. AA. Surgery, Westring 3, D-4400 Münster, F.R.G.

STUDY ON LONG-TERM TREATMENT WITH ANTICOAGULANTS OF ATHEROSCLEROSIS OBLITERANS

H. HEINE, H. SCHMIDT, L. HEINEMANN, C. NORDEN,
J. SCHOLZE and H. MACH

*Central Institute for Heart and Blood Circulation Research,
Academy of Sciences, Berlin, G.D.R.*

We have been carrying on research into the long-term prognosis of arteriosclerosis obliterans for years and have observed more than 1800 patients with an average control interval of 6 years (2−20 years).

SURVIVAL RATES

AC - anticoagulant therapy

C - control

N - age standardized

    GDR - population

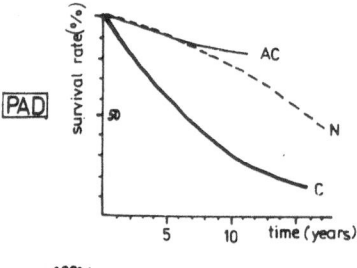

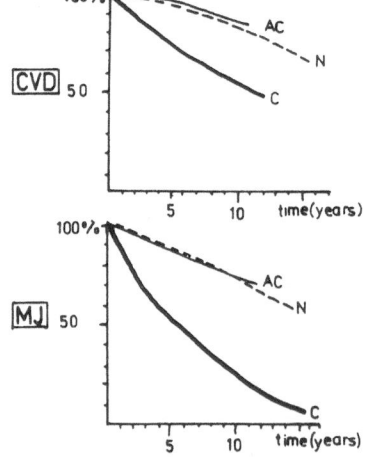

Fig. 1.

We analysed three groups patients with cerebrovascular disease (7 years, n = 331), patients with acute myocardial infarction (5 years, n = 257) and patients with peripheral arteriosclerosis (7 years, n = 1193): The prognosis quo ad vitam is especially bad in peripheral (63% died) und coronary arteriosclerosis (57% died), better in extracranial CVD (24% died).

We made long term therapy tests using oral anticoagulants (n = 556) compared with control groups (n = 1188). Long-term angiographic controls were performed in 182 patients after 2, 5 and 7 years (i.e. more than 1000 peripheral angiograms) with a mean control interval of 5 years. There are no significant differences between the anticoagulant- and control-groups in the three subgroups regarding to age, degree of severity, type of obliteration and cardiovascular diseases.

The lethality rate in patients with PAD, CVD and after MI using long-term-anticoagulant-therapy is much lower than in the control groups.

The yearly survival rates make this clear (Fig. 1). For example, only 32% inpatients with peripheral arteriosclerosis using anticoagulants against 63% in the control group died, corresponding to a yearly death rate of 4 and 11%.

We found an improvement in the prognosis using angicoagulant-therapy not only in patients with arteriosclerosis obliterans without risk factors but also in combinations with other cardiovascular diseases or risk factors. We observe a distinct effect of the anticoagulant-therapy in long-term-periods.

We also observed a lesser myocardial in-

Long-term anticoagulant therapy

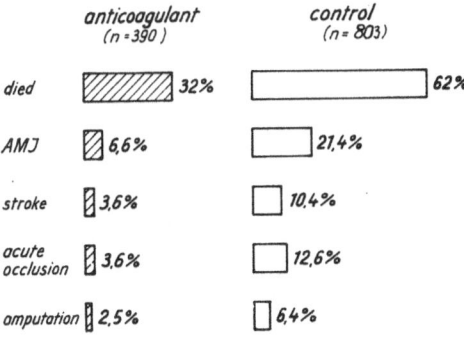

Fig. 2.

whereas 22% complications when the therapy was interrupted and 33% complications after the therapy was broken off. The number of significant bleeding when using anticoagulants is relatively small. Bleeding lead to a stoppage of the anticoagulant therapy in a very small percentage. This, however, does not constitute a serious objection to this effective form of therapy.

A long-term follow up survey of oral anticoagulant therapy in patients with atherosclerosis obliterans shows:
– improved survival rate
– decreased cardiovascular (thromboembolic) complication-rate
– decreased clinical impairment
– delayed angiographic progression
– improved rehabilitation

farction and stroke incidence when using long-term anticoagulant therapy (Fig. 2). We also found similar results in the other sub-groups. We observed a statisticaly lesser progression of the obliterations and the stenosis controlling repeated angiograms during 2, 5 and 7 years.

In the pelvis and thigh region then is always a more progressive trend of oblitera tions than in the more distal parts (Fig. 3). Stenoses remained significantly more often unchanged when using anticoagulants in contrast to the control group. The longer the anticoagulants were used, the more was this effect noticed.

In summary, we emphasize that according to our opinion long-term anticoagulant therapy is the most intense progression postponing therapy today available in arteriosclerosis obliterans.

The quality of the therapy influences the danger of thromboembolic complications. We experienced 12% complications during 25.272 patient-therapy-months

•*Long-term anticoagulant therapy*•.
Angiographic progression and type of obliteration

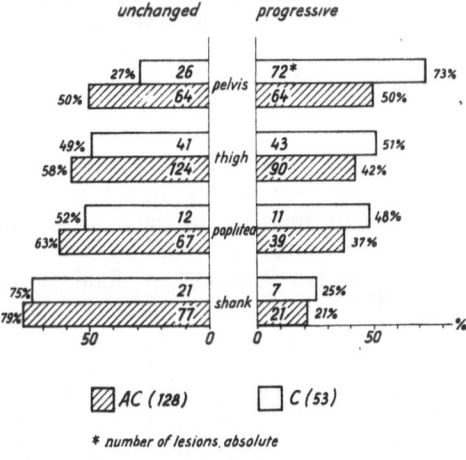

Fig. 3.

H. H., Central Institute for Heart and Bld. Circulation Res., Berlin. G.D.R.

581

TREATMENT FOR LYMPHEDEMA OF THE EXTREMITIES

A. SCHIRGER and J. A. SPITTELL, Jr.

Mayo Clinic and Mayo Foundation Rochester, U.S.A.

The purpose of this presentation is to reiterate the principles and guidelines of medical treatment for lymphedema. I shall not dwell on the differentiation of lymphedema from other disorders that may present as swelling of the arm or leg. And because both idiopathic and secondary lymphedema are treated by the same principles and with the same modalities, I shall not emphasize points of distinction between the types. What I shall offer is an account of the practices my colleagues and I employ in management of edema at the Mayo Clinic. This will be given under five headings: mobilization of fluid, maintenance of the edema-free state, control of infection, general supportive measures, and surgical intervention and possibility of malignancy.

1. *Mobilization of Fluid.* The cardinal principle of medical therapy for lymphedema is to reduce the size of the extremity as much as possible by medical means alone. This is accomplished by mobilization of the lymphedematous fluid in the extracellular tissue spaces of the extremity. According to our experience, for this phase of therapy to be maximally effective, the patient should be hospitalized. In the hospital a specially designed sling, elevating the affected extremity to a 45-degree angle, facilitates fluid removal and contributes directly to patient comfort. Such a sling elevates only the affected extremity, whether leg or arm; and in application to the leg, particularly, it obviates discomfort that would result from jackknifing the bed or flexing both hips and back unnecessarily.

While the patient is remaining in bed with the affected extremity elevated, administration of furosemide in doses of 40 to 80 mg daily will hasten mobilization of fluid from the limb. If a thiazide diuretic is employed during this stage, a baseline serum potassium value should have been obtained and periodic monitoring of the serum potassium is in order, particularly in patients prone to cardiac arrhythmiasl Although we have never seen clinica. thromboembolism during the period of bed rest and diuresis, prudence requires serious consideration of small doses of heparin as prophylaxis in those individuals at increased risk - for example, a patient with obstructive lymphedema due to adenocarcinoma of the prostate who is receiving synthetic estrogen therapy. In such circumstances, it is our practice to administer 5.000 to 10.000 units of heparin subcutaneously every 12 hours during the period while the patient is confined to bed. The time required to obtain maximum drainage of lymphedematous fluid from the extremity is different in different patients. Generally, however, one can predict that 48 to 72 hours will suffice and that continued elevation of the extremity and administration of diuretics will bring little additional benefit.

2. *Maintenance of Edema-Free State.* Once a lymphedematous leg has been reduced to its normal size, or as close to that as possible, it is measured for an appropriate form of elastic support. It is important that this be done with the papatient still supine, so that the benefit achieved by fluid removal will not be lost. The elastic support most often employed by members of our group is a made-to-measure special elastic stocking. After the appropriate measurements have been made, the patient should remain in bed until the stocking arrives from the manufacturer which, at our institution, is within 48 to 72 hours. Under the supervision of a knowledgeable and experienced nurse,

and preferably with the physician present, the stocking is then tried by the patient. Many elderly patients, because of other infirmities, have difficulty in applying a snugly fitting elastic stocking. They must have help from another person, or the physician must order a stocking with a zipper, which is now obtainable.

As a rule, we have not employed various pneumatic pumping devices for mobilizing fluid in lymphedema of the lower extremities. In postmastectomy lymphedema of the arm, however, a pneumatic device may indeed prove to be useful. For this problem Stillwell (of our institution) also has described a long-term program that can be carried out at home after adequate instruction. It consists of manual massage, periodic exercise, elevation of the extremity, and adequate bandaging.

Long-term control of lymphedema has been aided greatly by the introduction of oral diuretic drugs, particularly thiazides. We have been in the habit of prescribing hydrochlorothiazide, 25 mg, and triamterene, 50 mg, once or twice daily for 3 days of each week, such as Monday, Wednesday, and Thursday. Some patients require daily administration. Whether a thiazide is being administered every day or every second day, the serum potassium should be checked periodically.

3. *Control of Infection.* Recurrent lymphangitis and cellulitis should be treated with appropriate antibiotic therapy. For patients not sensitive to penicillin, we prescribe long-term antibiotic prophylaxis - usually benzathine penicillin G (Bicillin), 1,200.000 units intramuscularly once a month or penicillin V, 250 mg orally four times daily for 1 week of each month. Patients sensitive to penicillin usually respond satisfactorily to erythromycin, 250 mg orally four times daily for 1 week out of each month. Fungal infection is treated with topical application of clotrimazole (Latrimin) 1% cream or with miconazole nitrate (MicaTin) 2% lotion or cream. Significant trichophytosis may need — in addition to the local treatment — systemic antifungal therapy utilizing ultra-microsized griseofulvin in doses of 125 mg twice daily over a period of several weeks or months.

4. *Supportive Measures.* An integral part of medical treatment of lymphedema is emotional support and counselling. The patient and his family need both. Only a physician has the objective knowledge and the training to fulfill these needs. When lymphedema is first diagnosed, a brief discussion of its nature, course, and implications will help to avoid misconceptions. If the patient is a minor, one will need to alleviate the anxiety and concern of the parents, which might be transmitted to the youngster. It has been our practice to discuss the nature of the problem with the parents and the child, frankly in objective terms, and to present an optimistic view of how the swelling can be controlled, emphasizing not only the possibility but the need of maintaining a full and active life.

A number of patients of pediatric age whom we have followed into their teens and early adulthood have been able to maintain a normal and active life, including participation in carefully selected sports, both recreational and competitive. We find that informing the child and the family of these possibilities alleviates much of the unspoken fear and concern that may arise when lymphedema — which appears as a deformity — first occurs in the arm or leg of a child. Of the various forms of sport, we have encouraged particularly swimming during the summertime. Several of our patients were able to have swimming pools built in their own backyards and so could proceed with normal physical development while at the same time benefiting from the hydrostatic pressure on the edematous extremity, a preferred substitute for an elastic stocking.

The concerns of female patients in their late teens or early twenties often revolve around pregnancy. Two specific questions commonly arise — will the pregnancy aggravate the swelling, and will the offspring be afflicted with lymphedema? Although usually, in the absence of a positive family history, one can answer the second question reassuringly, we should admit frankly that, indeed, there may be some aggravation of the swelling during pregnancy. In general, however, this has not led us to discourage pregnancy in patients afflicted with lymphedema. One can use the prospects of the pregnancy as a stimulus for improved compliance with the previously outlined lymphedema regimen.

5. *Surgical Intervention and Possibility of Malignancy.* Not least important in medical treatment for lymphedema is recognition of the time for elective surgery. There are reasons for delaying this as much as possible; but even so, surgical

consultation should be obtained whenever one has the feeling that, despite satisfactory compliance by the patient, adequate control of the swelling is not being achieved.

Finally, any physician undertaking treatment for lymphedema on a long-term basis should be alert for the complication of lymphangiosarcoma. Although this is more common with postmastectomy lymphedema (a Stewart-Treves syndrome), its occurrence in patients with idiopathic lymphedema should not be forgotten. Invariably, in the cases we have seen, recognition of this condition has been delayed by insufficiency of awareness by the patient, the family, and the physician. However much we would prefer not to impose an additional burden by imparting knowledge about potential malignancy in the lymphedematous limb, a brief warning to bring any change in the appearance of the extremity or its skin promptly to the physician will go a long way in avoiding delay in the diagnosis of this dreaded complication.

A. S., Mayo Clinic, 200 First St. Southwest, Rochester, Minnesota 55901, U.S.A.

ASPIRIN IN THE PROPHYLAXIS OF ARTERIOVASCULAR DISEASES IN CARDIAC INFARCTION

D. LOEW

Katernbergerstrasse 255, 5600 Wuppertal 1, F.R.G.

Since 1971 we, together with the various teams in Germany, Austria and Norway, have studied the prophylactic value of antiaggregating substances in obliterative angiopathies.

The therapeutic recommendation of acetyl salicylic acid (ASA) as an aggregation inhibitor is based on the involvement of the blood platelets in the thrombogenesis and on the interaction of ASA between the blood platelets and the vessel wall. In the meantime, the following have become generally recognized adhesion and aggregation of blood platelets to foreign surfaces, endothelial desquamation, in particular to collagen of the type III and the release of procoagulatory factors.

In studies of miniature pigs reflecting the risk factors for obliterative arteriopathy in man was showed that blood platelets were detectable on the endothelia of different arteries after local stimulation with ice and adrenaline as well as after systematic stimulation with cholesterol or cigarette smoke. According to more recent biochemical findings the prostaglandins are responsible for the adhesion of the blood platelets to the vessel walls. This theory is based on the different metabolisations of arachidonic acid in the blood platelets and in the vessel walls. Thus, in the blood platelets the platelet aggregating and vasoconstricting Thromboxan A_2 is produced from the instable intermediate products, the cyclic endoperoxides PGG_2 and PGH_2. In contrast, from the same intermediate product in the vessel walls a potent antagonist, prostacyclin PGI_2, is synthesized which has antiaggregating and vasodilatory effects.

Peripheral angiopathies: Here, the percutaneous recanalisation of arterial obliterations according to *Dotter* and the thrombo-arteriectomy offered themselves as suitable models. Using the first method, the inner walls of the arteries are traumatized due to the opening of the stenosis. Such exposures of the inner arterial walls are greater after thrombo-arteriectomy. In a controlled study on 177 patients *Zeitler* et al. determined in lower hemorrhagic risks that after administration of ASA practically the same number of thrombotic re-closures occurred as after the combination of ASA and anticoagulants (Table I). In a double blind study *Ehresmann* treated 428 patients, with either ASA or

Table I. Clinical studies with ASA in peripheral angiopathy

Author	Indications	n	vascular complication/therapy
Zeitler et al. 1973	Percutaneous recanalisation	196	21.1% anticoagulant 6.7% anticoag. + ASA 4.6% ASA
Ehresmann et al. 1977	Endarteriectomy or Bypass	428	22.0% placebo 11.2% ASA
Bollinger et al. 1978	Endarteriectomy	90	38.0% anticoagulant 18.0% ASA + Dipyridamol
Linke and *Loew* 1973	Vascular complication % 1 year	150	13.0% vasodilator 7.3% ASA 4.5% anticoagulant
Hess et al. 1976	Vascular complication % 2 years	299	23.4% placebo 14.9% ASA 12.2% anticoagulant

585

placebo for 1 year. The patients were subjected to follow-up checks at 3 monthly intervals. When one considers the uncomplicated cases, one sees that the operative improvement of the influx and eflux alone achieved a marked improvement in the initial Fontaine stage from on average 2.5 to 1.1. The results for both groups did not differ within the first 12 months. Altogether a total of 71 re-occlusions occurred. Of these 24 (11%) occurred in the ASA group and 47 (22%) in the placebo group. The statistical assessment showed a significant reduction in the number of re-occlusion after ASA. Recently similar positive results after thrombo-arteriectomy are reported by *Bollinger*. As is known from other substances the clinical testing of ASA to prevent new arterial closures in patients with manifested obliterative arteriopathy proved difficult. The main causes were insufficient co-operation of the patients during these long-term studies which require a minimum observation period of 2 years, insufficient definition of the test models, standstill in chronic processes alone due to the removal of risk factors or spontaneous remissions, interaction with other drugs as well as a considerable amount of technical monitoring equipment, in many instances with disturbing test methods. Despite the criticisms of such studies, the results should be accepted when certain conditions are fullfilled such as the method is accurately planned and the study is correctly carried out. In a long-term study on patients with stage II peripheral arteriopathy according to Fontaine *Linke* and *Loew* compared the effect of vasodilators, ASA and phenprocoumon. The yearly rate for vascular complications under vasodilators was 13.0%, under ASA 7.3%, and under anticoagulants 4.5% (Table I). *Hess* et al (14) reported similar results. In a 2 year double blind study on patients with manifested obliterative angiopathy the percentage of vascular complications occurring under placebo was 23.4%, under ASA 14.9% and under anticoagulants 12.2% (Table I).

Cerebrovascular angiopathy: Early signs of a stroke with persistant neurological deficiencies are usually transitory, ischaemic attacks (TIA). Among the mechanisms which released such transitory, cerebrovascular dysfunctions are disturbed cardiac rhythm, hypotensive or hypertensive crises, functional compression of the vertebral artery during rotation or reclining of the head as well as microembolisms which originate from the carotid artery. In 1973 *Dyken* first reported on the protective effect of ASA to prevent TIA. The different therapeutic methods were compared in a follow-up study. Significantly fewer fatalities occurred under ASA (3%) than under anticoagulants (17%). The results of further prospective studies carried out by *Fields, Barnett* and *Reuther* are now available (Table II). In the first 6 months of the study carried out by *Fields* significantly unfavourable outcomes occurred under ASA (19.2%) than under placebo (44.2%). In the study carried out by *Barnett* Sulfinpyrazon was ineffective. Under ASA, significantly fewer fatalities, strokes and TIA's were observed than under placebo. In the investigations carried out by *Reuther* when the attacks originated from the carotid artery also significantly fewer TIA's occurred under ASA (6.6%) than under placebo (50.0%) (Table II).

Cardiovascular angiopathy: In a controlled study on 163 patients with artificial

Table II. Clinical studies with ASA in cerebral ischaemia

Author	End point	n	Frequency
Dyken 1977	Death	658	17.0% anticoagulant 7.0% surgery 3.0% ASA
Fields 1977	Mortality, cerebral infarction Retinal infarction Stroke mortality	178	44.2U placebo 19.2% ASA
Reuther and *Dorndorf* 1977	TIA, cerebral infarction carotid type	31	50.0% placebo 6.6% ASA
	vertebro-basilar type	27	38.6% placebo 35.7% ASA

Table III. Clinical studies with ASA in coronary cardiac diseases

Study	End point	n	Frequency
B.C.D.S.P. 1974/77	Myocardial infarction	11.909	4.1% control 0.9% ASA
M.R.C. 1974	Mortality	1.126	10.9% placebo 8.3% ASA
C.D.P.A. 1976	Coronary deaths	1.529	8.3% placebo 5.8% ASA
G.A.M.I.S. 1977	Fatal myocardial infarction Sudden death Survived re-infarction	946	12.0% placebo 10.0% anticoagulant 7.6% ASA

cardiac valves *Sullivan* et al studied the incidence of thrombo-embolisms under anticoagulants alone or after a combination with 400 mg dipyridamol/day. Within one year, significantly fewer thrombo-embolisms occurred in the dipyridamol group (1.3%) than in the anticoagulant group (14.3%). *Dale* et al carried out a similar control study on patients having *Starr-Edwards*-prostheses. In the group receiving anticoagulants + ASA having an index of 1.76 (incidence/100 patients/year) significantly fewer thrombo-embolisms occurred than under the monotherapy with anticoagulants (index 9.32). In a further pilot study on patients having aortic ball valves the combination therapy with ASA was superior to that of ASA alone (incidence-index 14.5).

The first report on the protective effect of ASA as a prophylactic against re-infarction originates from *Craven* in 1955. This information remained unconsidered until in 1974 *Jick* from the "Bostoner Collaborative Drug Surveillance-Group" published similar results. From the regular registration of the drug-intake of hospitalized patients it was established that the relative risk of an acute myocardial infarction in "Aspirin-Users" as opposed to "Non-Users" is approx. 0.2.

In one of the more recent investigations the myocardial infarction incidence in "Aspirin-Users" was 0.9% as opposed to 4.1% for "Non-Users" (table 3). The first prospective multicentre re-infarction study with ASA was carried out by M.R.C. in 1970. In 1974 *Elwood* reported that with the aid of ASA (8.3%) the myocardial mortality was reduced by approx. 25% compared with placebo (11%) (Table III). In the meantime, a further prospective study that of the "Coronary Drug Project Aspirin" (CDPA) is available. 52 American clinics took part in this study. 1529 patients were treated either with ASA or placebo. The observation period after the myocardial infarction was between 10–23 months. In the ASA group the total mortality was 5.8% and in the placebo group 8.3%. As in the M.R.C. study ASA reduced the mortality by 30% (Table III). In the "German-Austrian-Myocardial-Infarction-Study" (G.A.M.I.S.) 946 patients received either placebo or Phenprocoumon or ASA for two years after a myocardial infarction (24). The frequency of fatal myocardial infarctions, sudden death and survived re-infarctions was 7.6% in the ASA group, 10.0% under anticoagulants and 12.0% under placebo. The reduction of approx. 37% in cardiovascular complications compares favourably with the results of the M.R.C. and C.D.P.A. studies.

D. L., Katernbergerstr. 255, 5600 Wuppertal1, F.R.G.

ANTICOAGULANT PROPHYLAXIS AND THROMBOLYTIC THERAPY FOR THROMBOEMBOLIC COMPLICATIONS OF ANGIOGRAPHY

G. LEONE and P. G. FALAPPA

Department of Internal Medicine and Department of Radiology
Catholic University of Sacred Heart, Rome, Italy

The reported incidence of thrombo-embolic complications of arterial catheterization is generally less than 2% whether such procedures are performed for cardiac catheterization or for angiography in peripheral vascular disease (*McGraw* 1963 *Barnes et al.* 1977). Emboli are derived from deposition of platelet aggregates and fibrin meshwork on the catheter and guide wire. In fact all available commercial plastic catheter are thrombogenic if exposed in vivo to blood stream (*Durst et al.* 1974). The degree of thrombogenity does not vary greatly although some catheters appear to be more thrombogenic than others; only benzalkonium-heparin coating prevents thrombus formation on catheters for one hour (*Durst et al.* 1974). But at present for practical reasons systemic anticoagulation with heparin or simple flushing with heparinized saline through a catheter are more frequently used to prevent clot deposition (*Anderson* 1974). The introduction of heparin reduced but did not cancelled the thromboembolic complications and simultaneously has increased postangiography bleeding complications (*McGraw* 1963 *Anderson et al.* 1974). In this comunication we report our experience in the treatment of thromboembolic complications in more than a thousand angiographies. In two cases of embolization we used with success a potent thrombolytic agent the urokinase, the plasminogen activator isolated by urine (*Fletcher et al.* 1965 *Bizzi et al.* 1976).

Methods

From February 1973 to April 1978 thousand and one hundred patients were submitted to diagnostic angiographic procedures in the Radio-logy Department of the Catholic University in Rome. 40% of diagnostic angiography was performed for peripheral arterial occlusive disease of the lower extremities, 15% for suspected renal vascular disease, 10% for coronary disease, 35% for miscellaneous abdominal disease. All patients submitted to angiographic examination were evaluated regarding to coagulation parameters (Activated Partial Thromboplastin Time (APTT), Prothrombin Time (PT), Bleeding Time, Platelet Count). Patients with abnormal coagulation tests (APTT > 50 sec, PT > 20 sec, Platelet count < 100.000/mmc, were not treated with systemic anticoagulation. All the other patients (more than 90%) were submitted, shortly before the angiography, to systemic anticoagulation with heparin and during the examination to local flushing with heparinized saline (Heparin 5000 Units/1000 ml).

Results and discussion

With our heparinization schedule a sufficient systemic anticoagulaticn was achieved in almost all patients; at the end of the angiographic examination the Activated Partial Thromboplastin Time

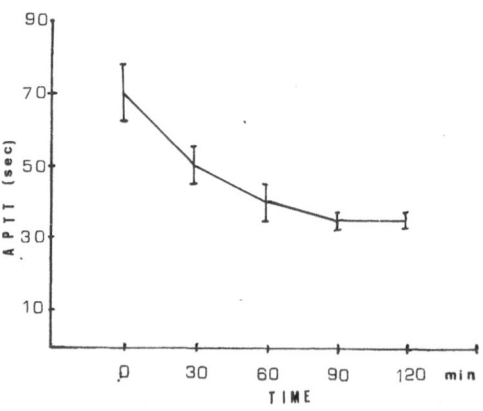

Fig. 1. Activated Partial Thromboplastin Time at the end (Time 0) of the angiographic examination. APTT returns to normal within an hour.

(APTT) ranges from 60 to 80 seconds and returns to normal within an hour (Fig. 1) Bleeding complications were minimal and limited to local hematoma. Thromboembolic complications based on patients symptoms and pulse deficits were observed in three patients of whom two underwent transfemoral angiography for lower extremity arterial occlusive disease, and the third for suspected renal vascular disease (Fig. 2). In two cases thrombolytic therapy with urokinase was promptly instituted and in both complete dissolution of the thrombus was obtained (Fig. 3). 200.000 CTA units of urokinase were immediately administered for local infusion

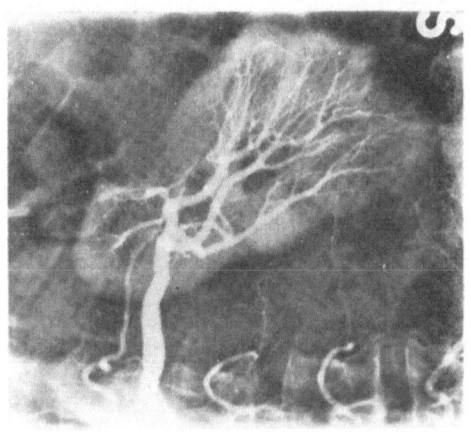

Fig. 3. Complete thrombus dissolution after six hours of urokinase thrombolytic therapy.

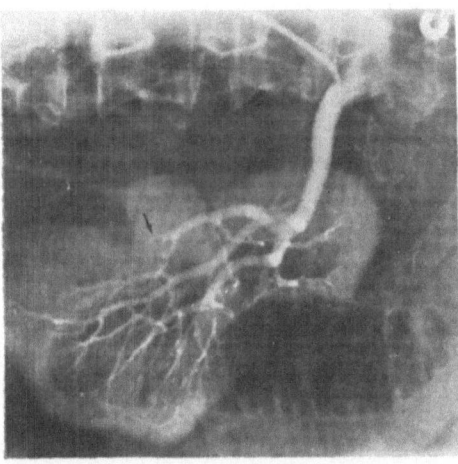

Fig. 2. The occlusion of the lower branch of renal artery (arrow) was not present in the previous aortography.

and soon after catheter removal further 250.000 units/h were administered by continuous general infusion for six hours.

After urokinase suspension anticoagulant treatment with continuous heparin infusion was instituted.

No bleeding complication was observed and local haematoma were very well controlled by careful compression.

In conclusion our experience suggests that a general anticoagulation with a initial low dose of heparin associated with local flushing of heparinized saline prevents in most cases thromboembolic complications of angiographic procedures without an increase in bleeding complications: thrombolytic therapy could be considered in every case of thromboembolism.

REFERENCES

Anderson G. H., Gianturco C., Wallace S. et al. (1974): "Anticoagulation technique for angiography". Radiology III, 573—576.

Barnes R. W., Slaymaker E. E., Hahn F. J. Y. (1977): "Thromboembolic complications of angiography for peripheral arterial disease: Prospective assesment by Doppler ultrasound". Radiology 122, 459—461.

Bizzi B., Leone G., Accorrà F. (1976): "Pretreatment with heparin in thrombolytic therapy with urokinase". Haemostasis 5, 147 to 154.

Durst S., Leslie J., Moore R., Aplatz K. (1974): A comparison of the thrombogenicity of commercially available catheters". Radiology, 113, 599—600.

Fletcher A. P., Alkiaersig N., Sherry S. et al. (1965): "The development of urokinase as a thrombolytic agent. Maintenance of a sustained thrombolytic state in man by its intravenous infusion". J. Lab. Clin. Med. 65, 713—731.

McGraw J. Y. (1963): "Arteriography of peripheral vessels: a review with report of complications". Angiology 14, 306—318.

G. L., Istituto di Clinica Medica Università Cattolica del Sacro Cuore Roma, Largo Gemelli 6, Italy

INTRA-ARTERIAL INFUSION OF MIDDLE DOSES OF UROKINASE IN OBLITERATIVE ATHEROSCLEROSIS OF THE LOWER LIMBS

M. TESI, L. CARAMELLI and A. BORGIOLI

Department of Angiology, Main Regional Hospital of S. Maria Nuova, Florence, Italy

Urokinase (Uk) is a direct activator of plasminogen (plg) discovered in urine in 1947 by *MacFarlane and Pilling* in England and identified by *Sobel et al.* in 1952 in the U.S.A.

The activation of plasminogen (plg) to plasmin (pl) by means of cleavage of the lysil-serine bond and of the argynil-methionine bond of the plg molecule. Various researchers have isolated different molecular forms of plg; for this reason, we can speak of the microheterogenity of plg. However, the two principle molecules are those of plg with terminal HN_2-glutamic acid at 93.000 mw, and plg with terminal lysine (or valine) at 81.000 mw.

The stages of conversion from plg to pl by Uk activation, appear mainly in two in steps (*Rickli,* 1975).

First stage. This includes the detachment from the plg molecule of the peptide part, of small mw which includes the terminal NH_2-glutamic acid. The intermediate compound, with high mw and non-homogenous terminal, remains unchanged; sometimes this terminal is NH_2-serine, or methionine, or valine, or lysine. However, cleavage takes place mainly on the lysil-serine bond in positions $63-64$, and argynil-methionine in positions $68-69$.

Second stage. From the intermediate compound the heavy chain polypeptide with non-homogeneous terminal, and the light-chain polypeptide with NH_2-valine terminal are formed. These two peptides show enzymatic activity, i.e., they are the molecule of plasmin (pl), one heavy-chain-type.

Fibrinolysis and middle doses of Uk.

The treatment of acute vascular occlusions with Uk is known, and the dosages used in controlled clinical trials have become practically stan therefore have only partial data, we shall present some preliminary results concerning lysis standardized according to the American dosage going back to the first clinical work of *Sherry* (1969), to the trials of *Hyers* (1971), of *Bell* (1977), of *Duckert* (1977) etc.

Our intention, instead, has been that of studying the action of middle doses of Uk, administered by arterial perfusion directly to the affected region, repeated once a day for 20 days, in chronic arteriopathies of the lower limbs.

Research Methodology. In 16 arteriopathic patients with chronic obliteration at the femoral level, the following tests have been made:

1) Regional basal venous and arterial lysis. Tests have been made on blood taken from the femoral vein and from the femoral artery of the affected zone.

2) Administration of Uk. In the femoral artery, i.e. in the artery afferent to the affected region, we have carried out an arterial perfusion of 200.000 U.I. of Uk in 30 minutes.

3) Regional activated venous and arterial lysis. After finishing the perfusion, we again evaluated the lysis in the blood drawn from the femoral vein and from the femoral artery of the same zone.

4) Regional lysis of upper limb. In order to evaluate the fibrinolytic condition of a zone which was not injected, expressive of the general lysis values, we have evaluated the lysis of blood, drawn from the brachial vein and from the brachial artery at the end of the perfusion.

All tests were made at the first, and at the twentieth perfusion of Uk.

In addition to the euglobulin lysis time test, the following tests were performed on each sample of arterial and venous blood (6 samples in all): Plasminogen, Fibrinogen, Fibrin/Fibrinogen Degradation Products, Partial Thromboplastin Time, Prothrombin Time, Thrombin Time, Factor VIII (Procoagulant and Immunological), Platelet Count, Platelet Aggregation (from ADP, Adrenalin, Ristocetin).

These experiments included also angiografic examinations before and after treatment with Uk, and clinical remarks.

Results

The euglobulin-lysis time for which we present the data, represents the average of 16 cases.

First perfusion of Uk.

1) Regional basal venous and arterial lysis

Before beginning treatment with Uk, the venous and arterial lysis of the lower limb zone struck by arterial obliteration, measured respectively in the femoral venous and arterial blood, lasted both 370 minutes (Figure 1).

2) Regional activated venous and arterial lysis

After the infusion of 200.000 U.I. of Uk made over a period of 30 minutes in the femoral artery, i.e., in the artery afferent to the affected zone, the femoral venous lysis was observed to be diminished amounting to 150 minutes. The femoral arterial lysis too, was lower than the basal lysis 290 minutes. It should be noted that the values of the femoral venous lysis (150 minutes), express the activation of the region of the lower limb, as they are evaluated in the blood flowing back from the perfused zone affected by obliterating arteriopathy. (Figure 1).

3) Regional lysis of upper limb

Lysis of a district not affected by the injection, expressive as already stated, of the ysis values of the organism in general, was

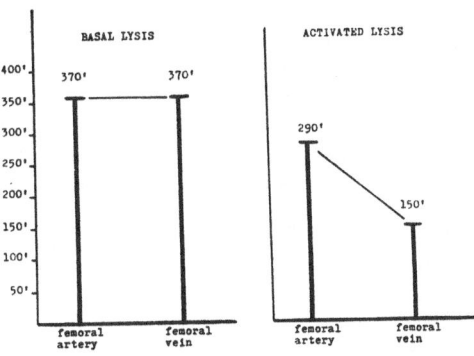

Fig. 1. Uk action on the lower leg's lysis, affected by the chronic femoral obliteration. The Uk is injected in the femoral artery of the affected zone, at the rate of 200.000 U. I./30 minutes. First perfusion.

determined at the end of the infusion. Brachial venous lysis time was found to be 290 minutes. Brachial arterial lysis took 240 minutes.

Twentieth perfusion of Uk

1) Regional basal venous and arterial lysis

At the twentieth perfusion of Uk, the values of the basal femoral venous lysis, and those of the basal femoral arterial lysis were observed to be equal to those of the first infusion, both 370 minutes (Figure 2).

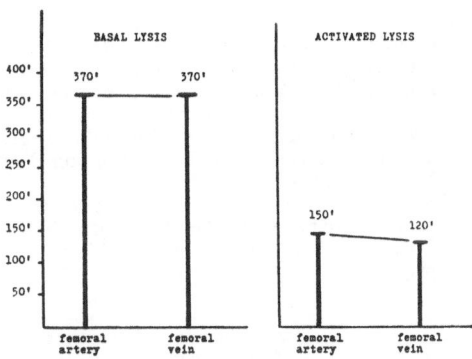

Fig. 2. Uk action on the lower leg's lysis, affected by the chronic femoral obliteration. The Uk is injected in the femoral artery of the affected zone, at the rate 200.000 U.I./30 minutes. 20th perfusion.

2) Regional activated venous and arterial lysis

After the twentieth perfusion of Uk, the femoral venous lysis was again observed to be diminished in respect the basal value, being of 120 minutes. Also the femoral arterial lysis was considerably lower, being 150 minutes. Therefore at the twentieth perfusion, it was not only the blood flowing back from the injected zone (femoral venous blood) which showed a notable activation of lysis in comparison with basal values; but also the femoral arterial blood coming from the heart was shown to be activated almost in the same measure as the former (Figure 2).

3) Regional lysis of the upper limb.

Evaluation of the lysis of a region not affected by injection, representing the lysis values of the organism in general, was effected after the twentieth perfusion. Brachial venous lysis took 130 minutes. Brachial arterial lysis lasted 160 minutes.

It may be stated consenquently that the perfusion of middle doses of Uk in the artery, activated the lysis of the injected territory also by repeated daily administration for 20 days.

General lysis too, is activated, as shown by the values of arterial femoral lysis after infusion, and the values of brachial venous and arterial lysis always after infusion. This activation is even more intense after the twentieth administration of Uk.

As regards the results of the other tests, we are still in the course of experimentation and not yet ready to present final data. However, a few trends have emerged, of which we can give very provisional synthesis only:

a) Plasminogen — Slight reductions were observed after Uk.

b) Fibrinogen — Slightly diminished.

c) FDP — Do not seem to very significantly.

d) Factor VIII — Both procoagulant and immunological factor have shown variations in only one case.

e) PTT, Prothrombin Time, Thrombin Time, Platelet Count and Aggregation — Variations have not been observed.

f) Angiographic Findings — These were invenstigated only in a few cases; re-channelling was not observed.

g) Clinical Findings — Remarkable improvement was observed during the treatment, both as regards the general symptomotology of the arterial disease, and as regards gangrene when such was present.

REFERENCES

Bell W. R. (1977): Urokinase in the treatment of pulmonary thromboemboli. By "Thrombosis and Urokinase" Academic Press, London New York S. Francisco, pag. 153

Duckert F. (1977): Urokinase treatment in myocardial infarction. By "Thrombosis and Urokinase", Academic Press, London New York S. Francisco, pag. 217.

Hyers T. M. (1971): Urokinase in the treatment of pulmonary embolism. By "Thrombolytic Therapy", Shattauer, Stuttgart New York, pag. 165.

MacFralane R. G., Pilling J. (1947): Fibrinolytic activity of normal urine, Nature, 159, 779.

Rickli E. E. (1975): The activation mechanism of human plasminogen. Thromb. Diath. Haemorrh., 34, 367.

Sobel G. W., Mohler S. R., Jones N. W., Dowdy A. B., Guest M. M. (1952): Urokinase an activator of plasma profibrinolysin extracted from urine. Am. J. Physiol., 171, 768.

Sherry S. (1969): Thrombolysis by urokinase. J. Atheroscl. Res., 9, 1.

M. T., Department of Angiology Main Regional Hospital of S. Maria Nuova Florence, Italy 50129

EXPERIENCE WITH UROKINASE IN OLDER PHLEBOTHROMBOSIS

G. TRÜBESTEIN, K. GLÄNZER, TH. BRECHT, G. FRICKE,
D. HERMANUTZ and F. ETZEL

Department of Internal Medicine, Department of Radiology,
Department of Experimental Haematology and Blood Transfusion
University of Bonn, F.R.G.

So far the use of fibrinolytic therapy in phlebothrombosis has seemed to be restricted to 1 to 6 day old thromboses (*Hess* 1967; *Robertson* 1971). Recently, however, there has been an increasing number of reports of fibrinolytic therapy in thromboses older than 6 days by using urokinase as well as streptokinase (*Tilsner*, 1974).

Study: Urokinase – heparin treatment was administered to 16 patients with thromboses of the subclavian, the femoral and the iliac veins. 3 patients had an occlusion of the subclavian veins and 13 patients an occlusion of the femoral and/or the pelvic veins. The age of the thromboses of the subclavian veins lay between 6 and 16 days, the age of the thromboses of the

Table I. Urokinase treated patients

Patient	Occlusion	Age (d)	Urokinase (d)	Success
T.G.*	V. subclavia	16	2	+
L.I.	V. subclavia	6	4	+
M.J.*	V. subclavia	14	5	+
H.K.*	V. iliaca/fem. Tibial V.	15	8	(+)
H.G.*	V. femoralis Tibial V.	18	10	(+)
T.R.	V. iliaca V. femoralis	12	16	(+)
S.G.*	V. iliaca/fem. Tibial V.	15	42	(+)
H.R.	V. iliaca/fem. Tibial V.	28	20	(+)
D.U.	V. iliaca/fem.	12	18	(+)
Z.F.*	V. iliaca/fem. Tibial V.	42	14	+
G.T.	Tibial V.	5	7	+
H.H.	V. poplitea Tibial V.	7	6	(+)
H.H.*	V. iliaca/fem. Tibial V.	21	7	(+)
B.M.*	V. iliaca/fem. Tibial V.	8	9	(+)
G.M.*	V. iliaca/fem. Tibial V.	6	4	−
P.St.	V. iliaca/fem. Tibial V.	18	12	−

* pretreated with streptokinase

femoral and iliac veins between 5 and 42 days. The duration of treatment was between 2 and 20 days. In the case of one patient with an extensive thrombosis of the tibial femoral and iliac veins the therapy lasted 42 days including 2 short interruptions on account of bleeding. 9 patients had already been pretreated with streptokinase.

Indications: The indication for an urokinase therapy was determined on the one hand by contra-indications against streptokinase especially when a streptokinase therapy shortly preceded or the antistreptokinase titer lay over 1.000.000 units, and on the other hand by previous unsuccessful streptokinase treatment of extensive thromboses which would lead to a severe postthrombotic syndrome.

Dosages: After an initial dose of 100.000 IU UK/10 min, 11 patients received an

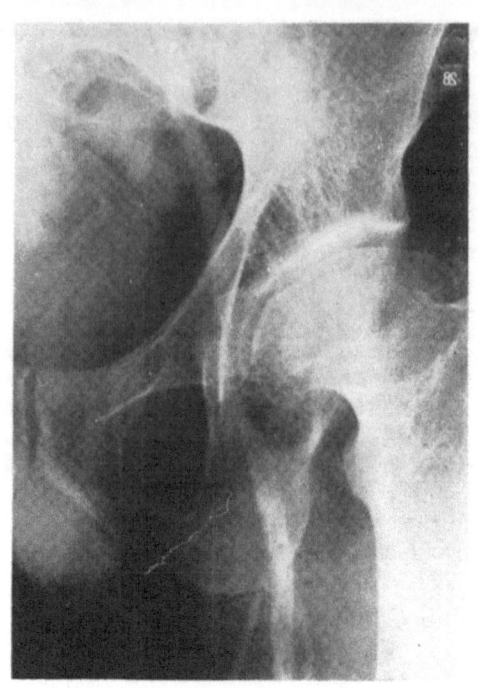

Fig. 1b. Control phlebography after a 5 day unsuccessful streptokinase therapy and a 5 day following urokinase therapy. Patency of the iliac vein and recanalisation of the femoral vein.

average dose of 1.000.000 IU UK/24 h, and 5 patients 2.000.000 IU UK/24 h. From the very beginning heparin was given in a dose of 500 – 1.000 IU/h and later on adjusted so that the thrombin time was between 30 and 60 seconds.

Laboratory controls: For control of the lysis therapy we daily determined the blood count, the urinalysis, the thrombelastogram, the fibrinogen and the thrombin time as well as the reptilasis time as a not heparin influenced parameter of the fibrin and fibrinogen degradation products. The single factor determination (factor II, X, V, VII, VIII) and the determination of plasminogen, antithrombin III, alpha-I-antitrypsin, alpha-II-macroglobulin and the fibrin and fibrinogen degradation products were performed at a later date.

Therapy controls: Before starting the fibrinolytic therapy a phlebography was

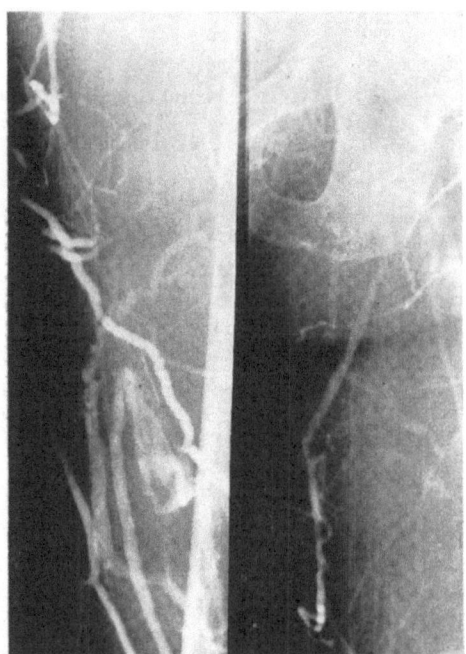

Fig. 1a. Phlebogram of a 32 year old patient (H. H.) with a 3 week old leg and pelvic thrombosis. Complete occlusion of the femoral and the iliac veins; poor collateral net.

carried out on all patients. The first phlebography controls were carried out after 2 to 5 days depending on the clinical findings.

Side effects: As a result of previous i.m. injections one patient developed painful gluteal hematoma under the highly dosed urokinase therapeutic scheme, which required discontinuation of the fibrinolytic therapy. An other patient twice developed a strong bleeding from the uterus post partum whereby a temporary reduction of the dose was necessary. The last patient had a strong bleeding in the right shoulded which also required discontinuation of the fibrinolytic therapy. In contrary to streptokinase early reactions, temperature, or a rise of transminases did not occur.

Results: All venous occlusions could be completely or partly re-opened. The 3 occluded subclavian veins became patent after 2, 4 and 5 days of urokinase therapy. The 6 week old leg and pelvic phlebothrombosis as well as the 5 day old tibial phlebothrombosis could be dissolved completely after an urokinase therapy of 14 days and 7 days respectively. With 9 of the remaining 11 patients a partial recanalisation could be achieved. Two patients treated with this form of therapy for 10 and 12 days respectively showed only a recanalisation of the popliteal vein and a recanalisation of the tibial veins but no patency of the femoral or the iliac veins as the other patients.

Discussion: The results imply that it was possible to dissolve partially and in some cases completely, several week old phlebothromboses with a longer urokinase therapy. The complication rate was relatively small in this form of administration. Specific side-effects as those we know from the streptokinase therapy did not occur. Our results are similar to those of *Tilsner* who achieved complete (30%) and partial (24%) recanalisation with a combined streptokinase-urokinase-heparin therapy in venous occlusions older than 1 week. No binding statement can be made about

the effectiveness of both the dosage schemata. As far as was comparable the 5 patients treated with the higher dosed scheme did not show better results. Our experiences with altogether 30 patients treated with urokinase have only proved that with the highly dosed urokinase therapy there is a pronounced decrease of the fibrinogen, the plasminogen and a clear prolongation of the reptilasis time as a result of the increased fibrin and fibrinogen split prcducts whereas with the lower dosed scheme the plasminogen and the fibrinogen lie in the lower normal range and the reptilasis time is only slightly prolonged on account of only a small increase in split products. Contrary to a standard streptokinase therapy with 100.000 IU/h even the higher dosed urokinase scheme results in less marked changes of the fibrinolytic system.

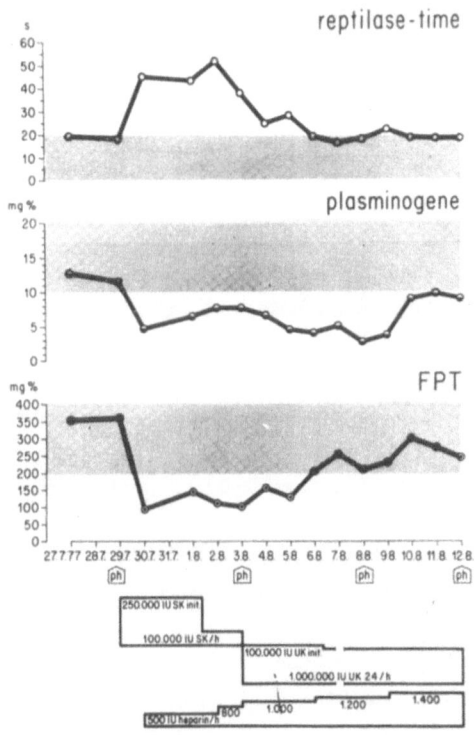

Fig. 2. Therapeutic scheme of the patient (H. H.) with the following parameters: thrombin time, plasminogen and fibrinogen.

In conclusion we can state that a successful therapy is still possible in older venous thromboses or an amelioration of the sequelae of the postthrombotic syndrome with a combined urokinase-heparin therapy. At present the indication for a urokinase therapy is restricted for us due to the high costs. Therefore, we generally administer urokinase only to young patients with an extensive peripheral venous occlusion with whom fibrinolytic therapy of longer than 4 days can be expected, and in the case of contra-indications against streptokinase as fibrinolytic agent. We have now started a multicentric, randomized study to prove which dosages should be given to get good results.

REFERENCES

Hess, H.: Indikationen, Erfolgsaussichten und Komplikationen der Thrombolytischen Therapie mit Streptokinase. In: Hess, H. (Hrsg.): Thrombolytische Therapie. (Schattauer: Stuttgart 1967).

Robertson, B. R.: Thrombolytic treatment with streptokinase. In: Haeger, K. (ed.): Thrombosis and Embolism. (Huber: Bern 1971).
Tilsner, V.: Spätlysen von Venenthrombosen. VASA 3, 458, 1974.

G. T., Medizinische Universitäts-Poliklinik, Wilhelmstr. 35—37, 53 Bonn, F.R.G.

EXPERIMENTAL HOMOCYSTEINEMIA AND THROMBOEMBOLISM ACTION OF TICLOPIDINE

O. PEPIN, B. LACAZE and J. C. FERRAND

Parcor R. & D., Toulouse, France

Homocysteine metabolism abnormality due to a deficiency of cystathionine synthease has been reported in man in 1962 (1). The phenotype being arteriosclerosis and vascular thrombosis. In addition, human atherosclerosis damage is complicated with thromboembolic disorders at a late stage. To evaluate the activity of a new antiaggregating agent, Ticlopidine (5), two experimental models reproducing these types of human disease have been used.

Model 1: Experimental homocysteinemia has been induced in white New-Zealand rabbits by I. P. injection of high doses of methionine, a sulfur-containing amino acid taking part in the homocysteine synthesis.

Material and methods

3 batches
— Control batch: 5 animals — 10 ml/kg/d of methionine in 5% glucose solution subcutaneously and 10 ml/d of distilled water orally.
— Methionine batch: 10 animals — 80 mg/kg/d of methionine in 5% glucose solution subcutaneously and 10 ml/d of distilled water orally.
— Methionine + Ticlopidine batch: 10 animals — 80 mg/kg/d of methionine in 5% glucose solution subcutaneously and 50 mg/kg/d of ticlopidine in distilled water orally.
Trial duration: 60 days
The last day, a blood sample has been taken from all the animals by cardiac puncture.
. The platelet aggregation has been measured by a technique using total blood (3).
. Various coagulation parameters have been measured as well as fibrinogen level.
. Sulfur-containing amino acids have been investigated in the urine by thir layer chromatography.
. The animals were bled to death and autopsied. Various organs were taken for histological examination.

Results

Venous thromboses, as seen during the preliminary tests on animals dead during experimentation were not found in this study. No spontaneous death, even after massive doses of methionine was specially noted.

Autopsy

— In some animals of each batch: a focal damage of the aortic wall, morphology being a calcified media with elastolysis.
— In all the animals of the methionine batch: venous stasis, passive congestion of the liver, thrombosis obliterans of the right ventricle (Fig. 1).
— Macroscopic examination: normal in all control animals.
— One animal of the Ticlopidine batch had a small thrombus in the right heart but the others, a normal ventricle lumen (Fig. 1).
The microscopic examination of the ventricular thrombi revealed a non organized

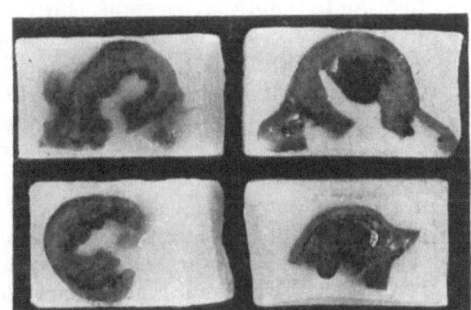

Fig. 1. Ticlopidine activity (in aggregation test)
a) Right ventricle thrombosis (animals treated by methionine 80 mg/kg/d).
b) Normal right ventricle (animals pretreated by Ticlopidine 50 mg/kg/d).

Table I. Methionine surcharge in rabbit.

	Howell time sec.	Prothrombin time sec.	Thrombin time sec.	Cephaline time sec.	Fibrinogen level g/l	Aggregation index after 1 mn 30	after 3 mn
Samples (3)	205 ±18	5.9 ±0.1	15.0 ±0.1	19.8 ±1.3	4.02 ±0.10	0.19 ±0.01	0.17 ±0.03
Methionine (6)	252 ±46	7.1 ±1.2	15.0 ±0.6	25.7 ±4.0	4.86 ±0.42	0.16 ±0.03	0.19 ±0.03
Ticlopidine + Methionine (9)	221 ±16	6.1 ±0.1	15.0 ±0.7	20.3 ±0.9	5.47 ±0.61	0.34* ±0.04	0.51** ±0.05

* p < 0.10; ** p < 0.02.

mixed thrombus of recent and agonal onset.

The biochemical tests showed no modification of coagulation factors. Aggregation results showed Ticlopidine activity (Table I.)

In the urine, intermediary compounds of the methionine metabolism were found to be between methionine and homocysteine.

Discussions

— Wall lesions seen in this study have no special significance, as they are common spontaneous lesions in the rabbit. Loss of endothelium and proliferation of smooth muscle cells were not seen. In order to obtain such lesions, is would be better to give continuous lower doses of methionine rather than medium or massive doses, as we did.

— Furthermore, the absence of death, the acute hepatic changes due to stasis, the no organization of the thrombus, the unmodified coagulation parameters are infavour of a recent onset of the thrombosis. The thrombosis would result from a thrombophilic state of the methionine loaded animals and from a lesion of ventricular endothelium, produced by the cardiac puncture. The evident inhibition of this phenomenon in the animals loaded with methionine but treated by an antiaggregating agent prompts us to investigate more thoroughly this experimental model.

Model 2:

Materials and methods

Atherosclerosis at a late stage has been induced in 20 rabbits, by alternating normal and cholesterol rich diet during 8 months. Through the synergism of blood hypercoagulability (administration od Russel viper venom 150 μg/kg/I. P. for two days) and hypertension (hypertensin 20 μg/kg/I. P. for two days), the thrombosis has been induced as a complication of the calcified plaque.

Half of the animals have been pre-treated for 10 days, before setting of thrombosis with 50 mg Ticlopidine/kg/d orally. The third day after the induction of the thrombosis, the animals were killed and various organs taken for examination.

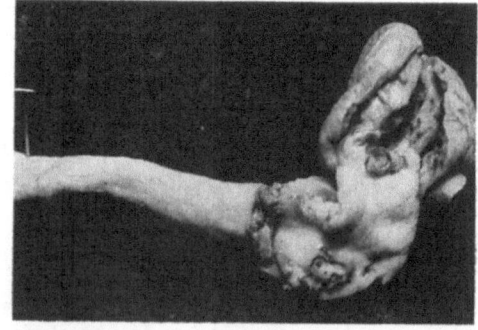

Fig. 2. Mural thrombosis of aorta.

Results

- All the animals showed advanced atherosclerotic and stenosed pulmonary, renal, and coronary arteries.
- A difference was noted between control and treated batches, as far as thromboembolic disorders are concerned.

In the control batch:
- Mural thrombosis of the aorta in a few animals (Fig. 2).
- The presence of small aggregates of platelets and leucocytes on the surface of the fibrous plaques.
- Confluent foci of myocardial necrosis.
- Platelet aggregates, occlusive thrombi in the pulmonary vessels with alteration of the pulmonary parenchyma.
- Renal infarction and bilateral cortical necrosis.
- Haemorrhagic suffusion with homogenization necrosis in the intestine.

The massive mural thrombosis, the disseminated intravascular coagulation with complications of tissular necrosis and its haemorrhagic syndrome due to a consumption coagulopathy, as seen in the atherosclerotic control animals were singificantly inhibited in the atherosclerotic animals pre-treated by Ticlopidine, an antiaggregation agent.

REFERENCES

1. *Carson N. A. J., Cusworth D. C.,* (1963): Homocystinuria: a new inborn error of metabolism associated with mental deficiency, Arch. Dis. Child., 38: 425—436.
2. *Constantinides P.,* (1965): Experimental atherosclerosis. Elsevier, Amsterdam, London, New-York. 158 p.
3. *Ferrand J. C., Gaich C., Gully D., Dumas A.,* (1978): Evaluation de l'effet antiagrégant de la Ticlopidine sur sang total., Scéance Soc. Biol. Toulouse.
4. *McCully K. S., Wilson R. B.,* (1975): Homocystéine. Theory of arteriosclerosis., Ather., 22, 215—227.
5. *Podesta M., Aubert D., Ferrand J. C.,* (1974): Contribution à l'étude pharmacologigue de thienopyridines et d'analogues furanniques., Eur. J. Med. Chem., 9, (5), 487—490.

O. P., Parcor R. & D., Département Recherche et Développement, 195, route d'Espagne, 31024 Toulouse-Cedex, France

DEHYDROEPIANDROSTERONE — A NEW CORONARY PAIN RELIEVING FACTOR. IN VITRO AND IN VIVO REDUCTION OF OXYGEN CONSUMPTION

J. ŠONKA, F. KÖLBEL, J. HAMPL, J. HILGERTOVÁ
and J. KRATOCHVÍL

*Laboratory for Endocrinology and Metabolism, Faculty of General Medicine,
Charles University, Prague, Czechoslovakia*

Fassati et al. reported in 1970 a coronary pain releaving effect of dehydroepiandrosterone sulphate (DHEA-S) administered to patients with a stabilized angina pectoris. All patients receiving 40 mg of DHEA-S in coated tablets twice a day reported a reduction of pain attacks leading to a decrease of the amount of self-administered nitroglycerin. As no substantial changes in coronary blood flow were observed in comparison to some other organs in dehydroepiandrosterone (DHEA treated rats (*Kapitola et al.*, 1972), the *in vitro* and *in vivo* effects of DHEA or DHEA-S on oxygen consumption were studied in rats.

Rat heart mitochondria or rat liver mitochondria in state 3 according to Chance were incubated with growing concentrations of DHEA, DHEA-S, progesterone, etiocholanolone, testosterone, estrone, pregnenolone and cholesterol. Oxygen consumption was measured by using of the Clark electrode. DHEA with the substrate citrate, alfa-ketoglutarate, malate or pyruvate inhibited oxygen consumption. No inhibition was obtained with sucinate. Alfa-ketoglutarate was used as a substrate in experiments represented in Fig. 1. The most effective inhibition of respiration was obtained with equimolar concentrations of progesterone and DHEA no inhibition was observed in the case of DHEA-S or cholesterol.

The effect of DHEA on some NAD-dependent dehydrogenases was therefore studied. DHEA had no inhibitory effect on the dehydrogenases of alfa-ketoglutarate, beta-hydroxybutyrate or lactate. DHEA is a potent inhibitor of glucose 6-phosphate dehydrogenase, but this NADP dependent enzyme does not lead to oxygen consumption (*Šonka*, 1976).

On the other hand, DHEA reduced oxygen consumption of electron transporting particles (ETP) obtained from

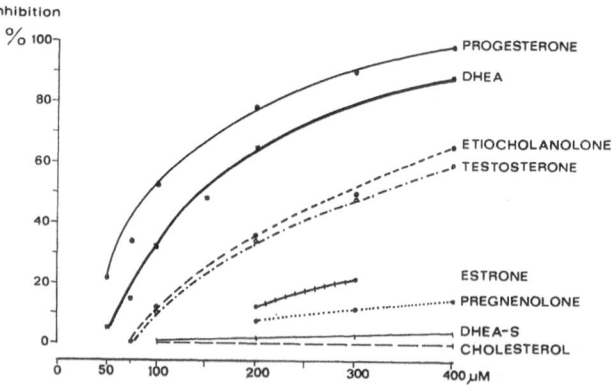

Effect of steroids on O_2 consumption in intact rat heart mitochondria

Fig. 1. Effect of several steroid on oxygen consumption in intact rat heart mitochondria.

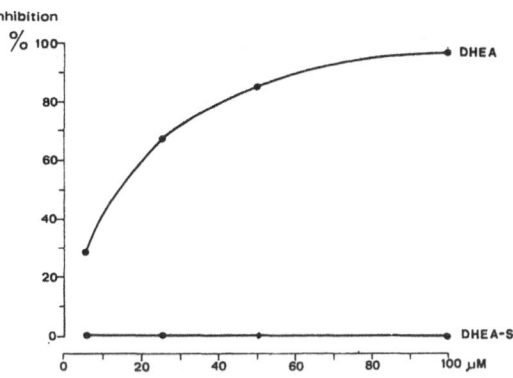

Fig. 2. Effect of DHEA and DHEA-S on NADH oxidase activity. Electron transporting particles of rat heart muscle mitochondria.

rat heart mitochondria, incubated with NADH. DHEA-S was ineffective (Fig. 2). It may be assumed from these experiments that the DHEA mediated inhibition of mitochondria respiration is located at site 1 of the respiratory chain (Fig. 3).

To see if this inhibitory effect of DHEA is also manifest in vivo, whole body oxygen consumption in rats was measured in the Spirolyt apparatus. DHEA at a dose of 50 mg/kg was injected intraperitoneally to male adult rats. Oxygen consumption was measured 1, 9, 17 and 49 hours after DHEA administration to groups of 10 rats. In comparison to controls with an injected solvent, a decrease of oxygen consumption was observed at intervals of 1, 9 and 17 h after DHEA administration. The major decrease of oxygen uptake (by about 20%) was observed 9 h after DHEA administration. No significant decrease was obtained if only 5 mg DHEA per kg were administered at this critical time interval. Oral administration of 25 mg DHEA/kg for 6 days was also ineffective.

These inhibitory effects of DHEA on oxygen consumption led us to reinvestigate the pain relieving effect of this steroid in angina pectoris. In a double blind test, where each patient with a stabilized coro-

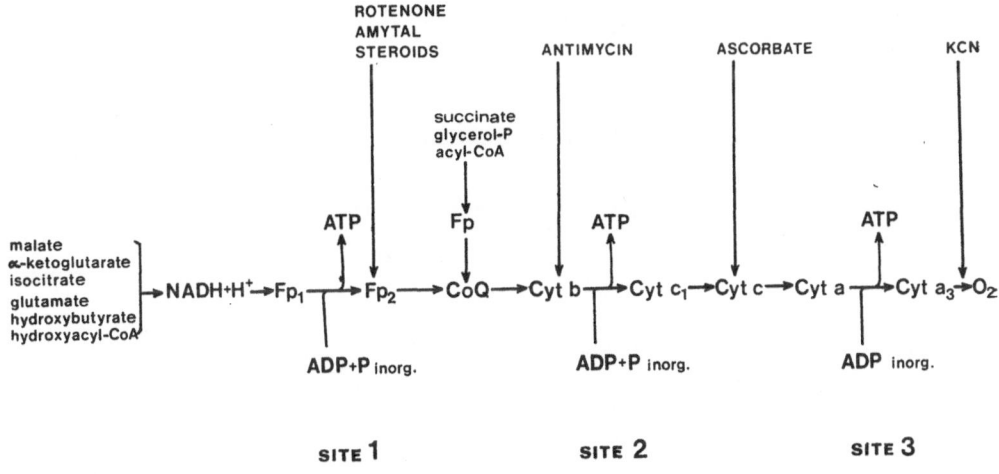

Fig. 3. Respiratory chain. DHEA mediated inhibition at site 1.

nary syndrome was randomly administered 80 mg DHEA-S a day for a month, followed by a month of placebo or vice versa, out of 16 patients, only 4 had an undoubtedly good response to DHEA, in 7 subjects the effect of placebo and of DHEA-S could not be differentiated while in 5 patients no relief was observed.

To summarize, the observed effects of DHEA on oxygen consumption and the clinical response to DHEA-S administration to patients with angina pectoris support further investigation which is expected to clarify the conditions under which DHEA would bring more profit to patients with ischemic heart disease.

REFERENCES

Fassati, P., Fassati, M., Šonka, J., Lešenský, K. (1970): Dehydroepiandrosterone sulphate — a new approach to some cases of angina pectoris therapy. Agressologie, 11, 421—426.

Kapitola, J., Šonka, J., Kölbel, F., Schüllerová, M. (1972): Hemodynamic effects of dehydro-epiandrosterone in rats. Agressologie 13, 247 to 251.

Šonka, J. (1976): Dehydroepiandrosterone — metabolic effects. Acta Universitatis Carolinae Med., Monographia LXXI, Prague 1976, pp. 171.

J. Š., Laboratory for Endocrinology and Metabolism, U nemocnice 1,128 21 Prague, Czechoslovakia

CLINICAL ANTIHYPERTENSIVE ACTIVITY OF ISF 2123

R. PELLEGRINI and M. CARNOVALI

ISF Medical Department-Trezzano S/N Milan, Italy

Chemical structure

ISF 2123 (propildazine) is a 3-hydrazino-pyridazine derivative (*Pifferi et al.*, 1975; *Pinza et al.*, 1975) which has the following structure:

Main pharmacological and toxicological features

Pharmacological research carried out in normotensive and hypertensive animals has shown that propildazine by administered oral and i.v. route has a marked hypotensive effect which is five to thirteen times that of hydralazine (depending on the animal species and the administration route). Other studies have demonstrated that like hydralazine, propildazine reduces the peripheral vascular resistance and increases the femoral, coronary and renal flow. It does not have any α-receptors blocking, sympatholytic or ganglioplegic effect, and its acute and chronic toxicity is several times lower than that of hydralazine (*Carpi et al.*, 1974; *Carpi and Dorigotti*, 1974; *Dorigotti et al.*, 1976).

Clinical pilot trials

11 different investigators (*Pellegrini and Abbondati*, 1976) studied a total of 380 subjects (mostly out-patients) with essential hypertension and diastolic pressure over 95 mm Hg after at least a week of wash-out. 99 patients were treated for 28 days with 4.5 to 12 mg/day; the other patients were treated for shorter periods, with doses varying from 0.5 to 18 mg/day.

The product was given in tablets by oral route, no other drugs being concurrently administered. A decrease in diastolic pressure by at least 10% and/or a diminution of the mean pressure by at least 15 mm Hg was regarded as a significant effect. The findings relative to the antihypertensive action of propildazine with the exclusion of other drugs given alone are summarised in the following table:

- marked but gradual antihypertensive effect already significant within the first week of treatment in about 40% of the cases;
- in highly responsive patients, favourable effects on BP could be obtained even at a dose of 3 mg/day;
- at doses ranging from 3 to 12 mg/day, favourable results were obtained in 60−80% of the cases, according to the different investigators.

Routine laboratory testing of blood and urine, performed before and after treatment, did not reveal any abnormality. The relatively more frequent side effects were tachycardia, headache and dizziness. These side effects were generally mild and transient.

Comparison with hydralazine

In a double blind trial 18 hypertensive out patients were treated for 4 weeks with 3 to 9 mg/day of propildazine versus 50 mg/day of hydralazine. The results obtained demonstrated that at the doses used propildazine has an antihypertensive effect which is higher or at least equal to that of hydralazine.

Another double blind trial (*Garagnani et al.*, 1977) compared the antihypertensive effect of 9 mg/day of propildazine versus

75 mg/day of hydralazine in 28 patients. The action of the two compounds administered for 4 weeks, showed to be similar. Thus, at equal doses, propildazine is five to eight times more active than hydralazine.

Comparison and association with beta-blocking agent

A study (*Garagnani et al.*, 1977) on 21 patients has shown that 9 mg/day of propildazine has a higher antihypertensive effect than 7.5 mg of pindolol. It has also been observed that associating the two drugs at the above-mentioned doses produces a synergistic effect and a mean decrease of diastolic pressure by 19%.

Association with diuretic and beta-blocking agent

20 patients with severe hypertension unsatisfactorily treated with chlorthalidone,

100 mg/day on alternate days combined with 120–160 mg/day of propranolol and/or a sympatholytic agent, were studied (*Angelino and Lavezzaro*, 1978). Adding 4.5–9 mg/day of propildazine led to a mean decrease by 22 mm Hg of the diastolic pressure.

Conclusions

Propildazine (ISF 2123) has a marked antihypertensive activity at doses much below the ones commonly used for hydralazine with a tolerance equal to, if not better than that of hydralazine.

In cases of severe arterial hypertension the association of propildazine with a diuretic and/or beta-blocking agent provides an even better control of the blood pressure and, above all, appreciably reduces or even eliminates the characteristic side-effects which accompany all hydralazine-like peripheral vasodilators.

REFERENCES

Angelino P. F. and Lavezzaro G. (1978): Propildazine hydrochloride combined with a diuretic and a beta-blocker in the treatment of severe hypertension, 5th Scientific Meeting of International Society of Hypertension, Paris, June 12–14.

Carpi C. and Dorigotti L. (1974): Antihypertensive activity of a new 3-hydrazino-pyridazine derivative: ISF 2123. Proc. British and Italian Pharmacological Societies, Bristol, September 11–13.

Dorigotti L., Rolandi R., Carpi C. (1976): A new antihypertensive compound: 3-hydrazino-6-(2-hydroxypropylmethylamino) pyridazine dihydrochloride (ISF 2123). Pharm. Res. Com., 8, 295.

Garagnani A., Faggioli M., Lama G. (1977): Ricerche cliniche pilota sulla propildazina (ISF 2123) e sue associazioni nel l'ipertensione essenziale. Arch. Med. Int., 29, 273.

Pellegrini R. and Abbondati G. (1976): Characteristics and clinical effects of ISF 2123, a new antihypertensive agent. Proc. 10th Int. Congress of Angiology, Tokyo, August 30—Sept, 3.

Pifferi G., Parravicini F., Carpi C., Dorigotti L. (1975): Synthesis and antihypertensive properties of new 3-hydrazinopyridazine derivatives. J. Med. Chem., 18, 741.

Pinza M., Parravicini F., Pifferi G. (1975): Synthesis of antihypertensive 3-hydrazinopyridazines and derivatives. XI Rencontres Internationales de Chimie Therapeutique, Montpellier, September 10—12.

R. P., ISF. Medical Dept., Via Leonardo da Vinci 1, Trezzano S/N Milano, Italy

THE INFLUENCE OF L-ASCORBIC ACID ON HYPERLIPEMIA IN MATURITY-ONSET DIABETES MELLITUS

E. GINTER, B. ŽDICHYNEC, O. HOLZEROVÁ, I. POLÁČEK,
O. ČERNÁ, L. OZDÍN, F. HRUBÁ and V. NOVÁKOVÁ

Institute of Nutrition, Bratislava; Regional Institute of National Health, Počátky; Institute of Clinical and Experimental Medicine, Prague, Czechoslovakia

An enhanced rate of endogenous cholesterol formation was found in subjects with uncontrolled maturity-onset diabetes mellitus. A state of chronic vitamin C deficiency is often reported in diabetic patients. Experimentally induced diabetes provokes an ascorbate deficiency, a slowed down cholesterol catabolism, hypercholesterolemia and an augmentation of the size of a rapidly exchanging cholesterol pool. A marginal chronic vitamin C deficiency creates similar disorders in experimental animals, as it slows down the rate of cholesterol transformation in to bile acids (*Ginter*, 1973). Ascorbate is required for a normal course of the rate-limiting re-action of this process, 7α-hydroxylation of cholesterol (*Ginter*, 1975; *Björkhem and Kallner*, 1976). Hence, the metabolic situation in many diabetics probably corresponds to the scheme

sexes were selected, aged predominantly between 50 and 60 years, with repeatedly determined hypercholesterolemia (above 7 mM per 1). Towards the end of the winter period (march 1977), fasting concentrations of vitamin C in blood and leucocytes were determined. During the same period, the same parameters were determined in a matched group of 85 healthy blood donors. A significantly lower vitamin C concentration has been found in the blood and particulary in the leucocytes of diabetics than in controls. This points to a lowered availability of ascorbate for storage in the tissues of diabetics.

From the diabetic group, 48 permanently hypercholesterolemic outpatients with metabolically stabilized maturity-onset diabetes were selected. The patients were kept on a diabetic diet, without insulin, oral diabetic drugs or any other

$$\begin{array}{ccc} \text{DIABETES} & \text{TISSUE ASCORBATE} \\ \text{MELLITUS} & \text{DEFICIENCY} \\ \downarrow & \downarrow \\ \text{Acetate} \rightarrow \text{Cholesterol} \dashv \mapsto 7\alpha \text{ OH-Cholesterol} \end{array}$$

Bile acids from which it ensues that the cause of the frequent occurence of hypercholesterolemia in diabetes resides in the imbalance between the rate of synthesis and catabolism of cholesterol. As high doses of ascorbic acid tend to enhance cholesterol catabolism in experimental animals (*Ginter*, 1975), this study has been designed to ascertain whether ascorbate could be utilized to depress hypercholesterolemia in diabetes mellitus.

From a group of 658 diabetic outpatients, 127 stabilized diabetics of either

drugs affecting lipid metabolism. In march 1977, fasting values of serum cholesterol, triglycerides, vitamin C and immunoreactive insulin were determined. In a test designed as double-blind experiment, 35 subjects received 500 mg ascorbic acid per day (Celascon effervescens Spofa), and 13 had placebo. The same parameters as at the start were determined after 6 and 12 months.

Daily administration of ascorbic acid led to a substantial increase of ascorbemia, a striking decline of cholesterolemia and a moderate, though statistically significant decline of triglyceridemia after 6 and 12 months. The decline of cholesterolemia was of clinical interest in the majority of the patients. After one year of ascorbic acid administration, cholesterolemia dropped in 60% of the patients dropped minimally by 40 mg %. In about one-third of the patients, vitamin C proved without effect. In the group receiving placebo the serum lipid levels remained unchanged. Immunoreactive insulin level in the fasting serum was not affected by ascorbate. It thus seems plausible to assume that the mechanism of hypolipemic action of ascorbate was not conditioned by its effect on the secretion or turnover of insulin.

The mechanism of the hypocholesterolemic action of ascorbate is probably as follows: the extremely low ascorbate values found in leucocytes permit to presume very low ascorbate levels also in the diabetic liver. Long-term administration of ascorbic acid led to an enhanced ascorbate concentration in the liver, resulting in an enhanced cholesterol catabolism. An improvement of the imbalance between the synthesis of endogenous cholesterol and its transformation in to bile acids led in a long-term experiment to a decrease of cholesterol circulating in the blood. The mechanism of a moderate hypotriglyceridemic action of ascorbate may perhaps be related to the lipolytic systems whose activity is depressed in both experimental and human diabetes. High doses of ascorbate were found to stimulate postheparin lipolytic activity of plasma in monkeys and guinea pigs.

These data underline the necessity of monitoring the vitamin C status in diabetic patients and in case the values are low, to increase the intake of vitamin C. The dose of ascorbic acid used in the present experiment (500 mg per day) cannot be considered as extremely high in hypercholesterolemic diabetics, for both hypercholesterolemia and diabetes mellitus lay enhanced claims of the organism on vitamin C.

REFERENCES

Björkhem, I., Kallner, A. (1976): Hepatic 7α-hydroxylation of cholesterol in ascorbate-deficient and ascorbate supplemented guinea pigs. J. Lipid Res. 17, 360—365.
Ginter, E. (1973): Cholesterol: vitamin C controls its transformation to bile acis. Science 179, 702—704.
Ginter, E. (1975): Ascorbic acid in cholesterol and bile acid metabolism. Ann. N. Y. Acad. Sci. 258, 410—421.

E. G., Institute of Nutrition, Bratislava, Czechoslovakia

MULTICENTER TRIAL WITH TIADENOL IN PRIMARY HYPERLIPIDEMIAS

G. CREPALDI, G. BRIANI, U. SENIN, U. MONTAGUTI,
A. CAPURSO and A. BONDIOLI

Italian "Lipid Clinics" of Padua, Perugia, Bologna, Bari and Milan, Italy

Tiadenol, (bis-hydroxyethylthio-1,10 decane) is a new hypolipidemic drug. Its mechanism of action, though not completely understood, seems to be similar to that of clofibrate (Debray et al. 1972; Rousselet and Clenet, 1972; Martin and Feldman, 1974). Some reports indicate that the maximum therapeutic effect of this drug is obtained when using a daily dose of 1200 to 3400 mg per os (Assous et al. 1972).

This paper reports the results of a multicenter trial investigating the effects of this drug on serum lipids of hyperlipoproteinemic patients.

Materials and methods

This trial was carried out in 5 Italian "Lipid Clinics" (Milan, Padua, Bologna, Perugia, Bari). 53 hyperlipoproteinemic patients (37 males and 16 females) with ages ranging between 19 and 63 years were studied. All of the patients presented primary hyperlipoproteinemia, in almost all cases familial. The hyperlipoproteinemia, typed on the basis of the WHO classification (Beaumont et al., 1970) fell into 3 groups:

Type IIa: 20 cases (8 males and 12 females)
Type IIb: 11 cases (10 males and 1 female)
Type IV: 22 cases (19 males and 3 females)
45 days before the beginning of treatment the patients were instructed to follow an isocaloric diet formulated on the basis of each subject's typing. 2.4 g of tiadenol, subdivided into 3 daily doses was administered to these patients for 5 months. Biochemical and clinical controls were carried out every other week during the pretreatment period and every month during the trial with the active drug. At each control, serum cholesterol and triglyceride levels as well as plasma glucose, serum uric acid, and transaminase were determined. Body weight, blood pressure and possible liver enlargement or other possible side effects were checked. Plasma urea, creatinine, bilirubin, serum proteins (total, albumin and globulin) prothrombin time, blood cell count, haemoglobin, and urine analysis were analyzed at the beginning and at the end of treatment. T_3 (triiodothyronine) and T_4 (tetraiodothyronine) were determined before the onset of treatment.

Serum cholesterol and triglyceride variations were expressed in Δ mg/dl of decrement or increment from basal values. The statistical evaluation of the results was carried out using the Student's two tailed "t" test for paired data.

The trial was begun in April 1977 and ended in September 1977 in all 5 Lipid Clinics.

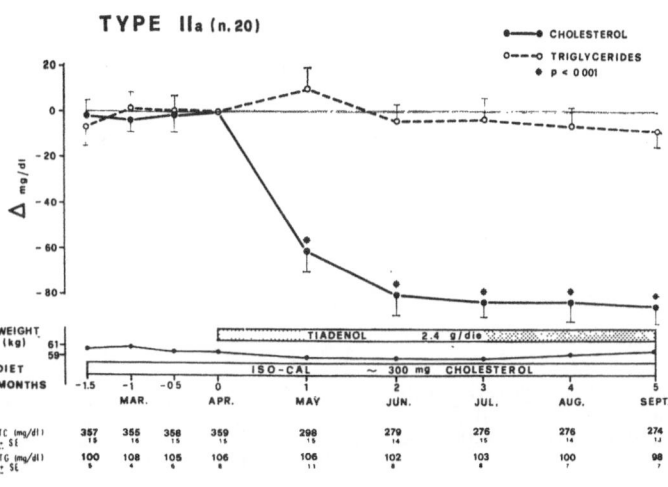

Fig. 1. Mean serum cholesterol and triglyceride values and decrement (Δ) in mg/dl in patients with Type IIa.

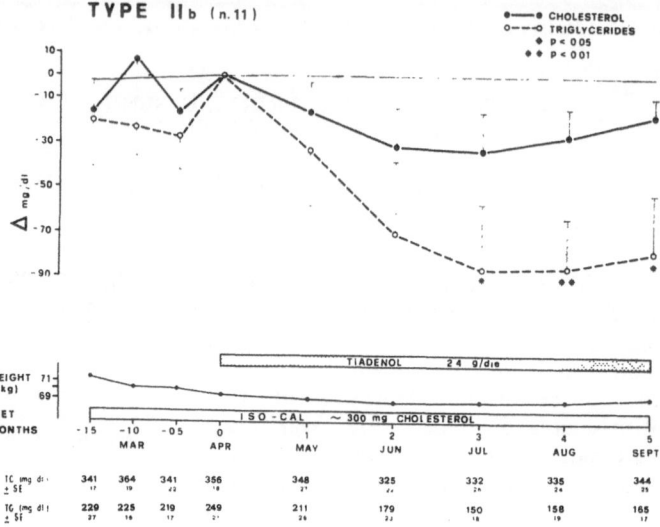

Fig. 2. Mean serum cholesterol and triglyceride values and decrement (Δ) in mg/dl in patients with Type IIb.

Results

In Type IIa (Fig. 1) a significant decrement in cholesterol levels from the mean basal value (359 ± 15) was evident after the first month of treatment. This decrement was constant throughout the trial. Triglyceride values were, however, normal (106 ± 8) and did not vary.

In Type IIb (Fig. 2), the decrement of cholesterol from the mean basal value (356 ± 18) was not significant during the 5 months treatment period. Triglycerides, on the other hand, underwent a significant decrease at the 3rd, 4th, and 5th months (34% at the end of the trial) of treatment.

In Type IV (Fig. 3), a slightly significant cholesterol decrement and a highly significant reduction in triglycerides was observed.

No significant variations were observed in serum uric acid levels or in the other parameters studied.

On the whole, the drug was well tolerated. Ten patients presented mild gastrointestinal disturbances (pyrosis, epigastralgia, meteorism, constipation).

A transitory increase in the transminase

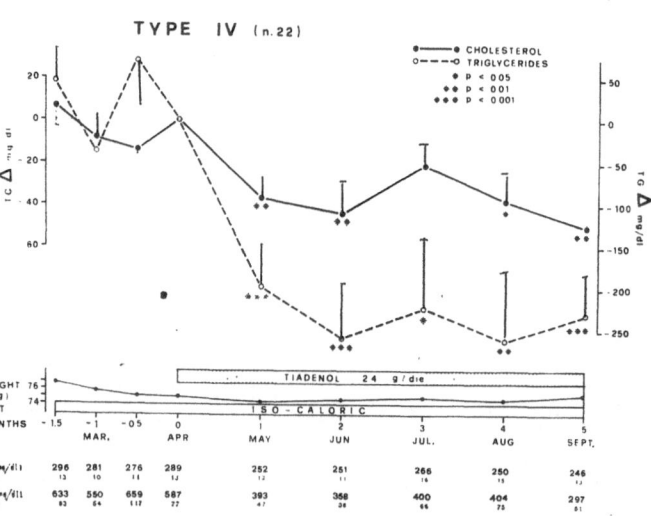

Fig. 3. Mean serum cholesterol and triglyceride values and decrement (Δ) in mg/dl in patients with Type IV.

608

was noted in 14 out of the 53 patients. These values normalized spontaneously during the treatment period.

A slight liver enlargement was observed in two patients.

Treatment was discontinued in one case (not included in our case report) because of haematologic alterations (anemia, leucopenia) which subsided when treatment was suspended.

Discussion

The pharmacological effect of the drug seems to be different in the various types of hyperlipoproteinemia.

In Type IIa, the drug provoked a highly significant hypocholesterolemic effect. The mean decrease (22%) observed in our patients was higher than that previously reported by Rouffy and Loeper (1972) and Briani et al. (1976) but was nearly the same as that recently reported by Rouffy (1975) and Baggio et al. (1977). According to our results, tiadenol seems to be more effective than clofibrate in lowering cholesterol levels in Type IIa patients.

The drug's hypocholesterolemic effect is evident after the first few weeks of treatment. In Type IIa this striking hypocholesterolemic effect was likely due, according to Baggio et al. (1977), prevalently to a reduction in LDL cholesterol. Moreover, tiadenol does not affect triglyceride values in Type IIa nor does it modify the composition of the VLDL.

No significant variation in serum cholesterol was observed in the Type IIb patients. These data are very similar to those reported by Rouffy and Leoper (1972) who studied the same type of patient. In fact, these authors showed similar hypocholesterolemic (6%) and hypotriglyceridemic (25%) effects.

In Type IV patients the hypolipidemic effect of the drug was very striking, with a mean triglyceride decrease of 39%. The hypocholesterolemic effect was inferior (17%).

In conclusion, the results obtained show that tiadenol is particularly useful in lowering cholesterol levels in Type IIa patients. It is also effective in reducing triglyceride levels in Type IV subjects. Nevertheless, it does not seem to be very useful in the treatment of Type IIb patients.

REFERENCES

Assous, E., Pougeot, M., Nadau, J., Tartary, G., Henry, M., Duteil, J. (1972): Etude d'un nouvel hypolipidémiant, le bis (hydroxy-ethil-thio) 1—10 décane: LL 1558. Thérapie, 22, 395—411.

Baggio, G., Briani, G., Martini, S., Fellin, R., Crepaldi, G. (1977): Effect of Tiadenol on serum lipoprotein concentrations in familial hypercholesterolemia. International Conference on Atherosclerosis, Milan — November 9—12.

Beaumont, J., Carlson, L. A., Cooper, G., Fefjar, Z., Fredrickson, D. S., Strassler, T. (1970]: Classification of hyperlipidaemias and hyperlipoproteinemias. Bull. World Health Organization 43, 891—908.

Briani, G., Balestrieri, P., Baggio, G., Baiocchi, M. R., Manzato, E., Fellin R., Crepaldi G. (1976): Trattamento delle iperlipoproteinemie primitive con Tiadenol, un nuovo farmaco ipolipidemizzante. Giorn. Arterioscl. 1, 39—51.

Debray, Ch., Vaille, Ch., Roze, Cl., M. Ile Souchard (1972): Action d'un hypolipidémisant, le bis (hydroxy-ethil-thio) 1—10 décane sur la cholèrese chez le rat. Thérapie, 27, 423—432.

Martin, E., Feldman, G. (1974): Etude histologique et ultrastructurale du foie chez le rat après administration subaigue d'un nouvel agent hypolipedémiant, le bis (hydroxy-ethyl-thio) 1—10 décane. Pathologie-Biologie, 22 — II: 179—188.

Rouffy, J. (1975): Effets hypolipidémisants et tolerance biologique du Fonlipol. Thérapie, 30, 815—823.

Rouffy, J., M. Ile Loeper, L. (1972): Effets hypolipidémiants du bis (hydroxy-2-ethil-thio) 1—10 décane (LL 1558) a partir de 77 observations d'hyperlipidémie essentielle. Thérapie, 27, 433—444.

Rousselet, F., Clenet, M. (1972): Etude d'un hypolipidémiant le bis (hydroxy-etyl-thio) 1 to 10 décane: (LL 1558). Thérapie, 27, 413—422.

G. C., Dept. of Intern. Med.. Div. of Gerontology Policlinic, Via Giustiniani 2, 35 100 Padova, Italy

MODERN DRUG TREATMENT OF HYPERCHOLESTEROLEMIA

R. MORDASINI, W. RIESEN and H. P. GURTNER

Section of Cardiology, Department of Internal Medicine and Lipid Research Laboratory, University of Berne, Switzerland

The significance of hyperlipoproteinemia as a major risk factor of cardiovascular disease has been clearly demonstrated by recent epidemiological studies. In these studies, however, it was also shown that only part of the atherogenity of a lipid disorder can be defined by the measurement of total cholesterol and triglycerides, as the atherogenic effect varies widely among the individual lipoprotein fractions. Decreased HDL levels (usually determined by the HDL-cholesterol content) represent the most important risk factor, followed by increased LDL concentrations. The correlations between increased concentrations of triglyceride-rich lipoproteins and the incidence of cardiovascular complications are less well defined (*Gordon et al.*, 1977, *Salel et al.*, 1977).

Therefore the evaluation of the effectiveness of a cholesterol-lowering treatment requires, in additon to the measurement of lipid concentrations in the whole serum, determination of the LDL- and HDL-cholesterol content.

By means of a fat-modified, low-cholesterol diet, which has to precede any drug treatment, the serum cholesterol concentration can with the presently available nutrition be reduced only by about 10% (*Schlierf et al.*, 1978). New regimen such as soya protein and fibre diets are being tested and promise greater effectiveness of cholesterol-lowering dietary treatment (Table I.) (*Sirtori et al.*, 1977). At present, however, the reduction of increased cholesterol levels resulting from dietary measures alone is generally insufficient. Thus, the administration of cholesterol-lowering drugs becomes very often indispensable.

Numerous substances have been tested in cholesterol-lowering drug therapy; only few of them are considered standard medications. These substances are summarized in Table 1 with regard to their effect on LDL- and HDL-cholesterol content. Apart from their lipid-lowering effect, however, some other – often neglected – aspects must be considered in the application of these drugs, i.e. questions concerning their compatibility, side effects and costs, because lipid-lowering drug treatment means long-term or even life-long treatment.

All absorbable cholesterol-lowering drugs produce considerable side effects; the most frequent of them are summarized in Table II. Non-absorbable substances are more favorable (sitosterol, anion exchange resins). When applied correctly, they have only harmless gastrointestinal side-effects.

In order to determine the effectiveness, side-effects and subjective tolerance of some of the standard substances in cholesterol-lowering therapy we have successively studied β-pyridylcarbinol (900 mg per day) clofibrate (1.5 g per day) and the anion exchange resin colestipol (20 g per

Table I. Current cholesterol lowering agents with their effects on LDL- and HDL-cholesterol levels

Usual cholesterol lowering drugs

substance	dose/day	effect on LDL-chol. and HDL-chol.	
β-Pyridylcarbinol (nicotinic acid)	900-1200mg (~3g)	~ -15%	-
anion exchange resins (colestipol, colestyramine)	10-30g	~ -20-25%	-
d-thyroxin	4-8mg	~ -15-20%	-
sitosterin	10-20g	~ -15%	-
clofibrate	1.5-20g	~ -10%	-

Table II. Frequent side effects of current hypo-cholesterolemic drugs

Side effects of cholesterol lowering drugs

substance	side effects
ß-Pyridylcarbinol (nicotinic acid)	flush, nausea, diarrhea
anion exchange resins	gastroint. discomfort, constipation
d-thyroxin	tachycardia, angina pectoris, insomnia
sitosterin	constipation
clofibrate	nausea, interaction with cumarin-anticoagulants, myopathy, gall stones

day) in 30 patients with primary Type IIa hyperlipoproteinemia. As some of the patients suffered from coronary heart disease, D-thyroxine was not administered in this study. All the patients had been under controlled isocaloric dietary treatment for at least 6 months before the beginning of the study; their adherence to the diet had been controlled in short intervals. Other medications which might influence lipo-protein metabolism were discontinued 4 weeks before starting the therapy. All three substances were tested in a double-blind cross-over study; controls were carried out every month.

Combined with dietary treatment, the cholesterol-lowering effect of the anion exchange resin colestipol was markedly superior to that of ß-pyridylcarbinol and especially to that of clofibrate (Fig. 1). With a 10% reduction of increased total and LDL-cholesterol levels, clofibrate was of only minimal therapeutical relevance; the result of ß-pyridylcarbinol was slightly better. HDL-cholesterol levels were not changed by the tested substances. Also with regard to subjective and objective side effects, the anion exchange resin (no serious side-effects) was better tolerated than the other two drugs; under ß-pyridyl-carbinol, the therapy had to be discontinued in three cases (diarrhea, pruritus), under clofibrate in one case (colics in cholelithiasis).

Thus, the present study confirms the introductory statements on the effectiveness and side-effects of the commonly applied cholesterol-lowering drugs. It shows that the anion exchange resins are at present the most effective cholesterol-lowering medication. When applied correctly (twice a day dissolved in juice strictly taken at the meals) the side effects of such a therapy are negligible. In serious cases of hypercholesterolemia the anion exchange resins can be combined with clofibrate or nicotinic acid derivatives which makes it possible to further improve the cholesterol-lowering effect.

Numerous new cholesterol-lowering substances are at present subject to tests and part of them are already being applied on a large scale. In this context especially substances related to clofibrate i.e. procetophene and bezafibrate as well as the synthetic antioxydant probucol have to be mentioned.

The discussion of the significance of cholesterol-lowering dietary treatment is still going on (*Mann* 1977). However we think that it is justified (*Klose et al.* 1978). In our opinion dietary treatment remains the basis of a reasonable cholesterol-lowering treatment especially with regard to possible improvements (fiber diets). Drug therapy alone cannot at present fully replace dietary treatment.

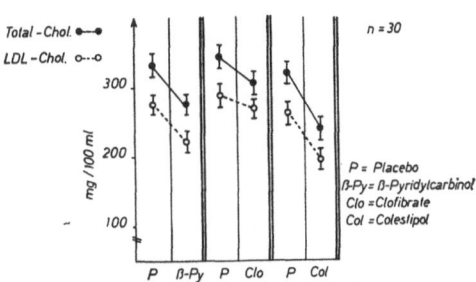

Patients with primary hyperlipoproteinaemia type IIa

Total-Chol. ●–●
LDL-Chol. ○--○

n = 30

P = Placebo
ß-Py = ß-Pyridylcarbinol
Clo = Clofibrate
Col = Colestipol

Fig. 1. Decrease of total- and LDL-cholesterol after a 6 weeks treatment with ß-Pyridylcarbinol (900 mg daily), Clofibrate (1,5 g daily) and Colestipol (20 g daily) in 30 patients with primary hyperlipoproteinemia of type IIa (details in the text).

611

REFERENCES

1. *Gordon T., Castelli W., Hjotrland M. C., Kannel W. B., Dawber T. R.:* High density lipoprotein as a protective factor against coronary heart disease. Amer. J. Med. 62, 707 (1977).
2. *Klose G., Mordasini R., Middelhoff G., Augustin J., Greten H.:* Medikamentöse Behandlung primärer Hyperlipoproteinämien. Klin. Wschr. 56, 99 (1978).
3. *Mann G.:* Diet-heart: end of an era. New Engl. J. Med. 297, 644 (1977).
4. *Mordasini R.:* Therapie der Hyperlipoproteinämien- wann? wie? Schweiz. med. Wschr. 108, 113 (1978).
5. *Mordasini R., Twelsick F., Oster P., Schellenberg B., Raetzer H., Heuck C. C., Schlierf G.:* Eine vergleichende Untersuchung von Cole-styramin und Colestipol bei Kindern und Heranwachsenden mit familiärer Hypercholesterinämie. Monatsschrift für Kinderheilkunde (in press).
6. *Salel A., Fong A., Zelis R., Miller R., Borhani N., Mason D.:* Accuracy of numerical coronary profile. New Engl. J. Med. 296, 1447 (1977).
7. *Schlierf G., Vogel G., Heuck C. et al.:* Zur Diättherapie der familiären Hypercholesterinämie bei Kindern und Jugendlichen. Monatsschrift Kinderheilkunde (in press).
8. *Sirtori C., Agradi E., Conti F., Mantero O.:* Soybean-protein diet in the treatment of type II hyperlipoproteinemia. Lancet I, 275 (1977).

R. M., Section of Cardiology, Department of Internal Medicine, University of Berne, Berne 3010, Switzerland

THE PRESENT POSITION OF CLOFIBRATE

A. HART

Medical Adviser ICI Limited, Pharmaceuticals Division, Medical Dept.
Macclesfield, Cheshire and Physician Salford Royal Hospital, Lancashire, U.K.

Clofibrate ('Atromid'-S) has been in clinical use as a hypolipidaemic agent for over fifteen years. However, its detailed properties and their relationship to its therapeutic effects have only more recently been evaluated.

It has five major effects:
Reduction in elevated cholesterol
triglyceride
fibrinogen
Increased fibrinolysis
Reduction in platelet adhesiveness

Early clinical trials concentrated solely on its lipid-lowering properties and the relationship between elevated lipids and ischaemic heart disease was the predominant influence in investigations. Insufficient account was taken of other risk factors in the simplistic application of the lipid hypothesis to atherosclerosis pathogenesis.

Increasingly it has been realised that a drug having several effects within the framework of a multifactorial disease process cannot be evaluated solely in respect of one risk factor, such as serum cholesterol.

Not all risk factors implicated in atherosclerosis development show a positive association and several workers have drawn attention to the negative correlation between high density lipoprotein levels and Ischaemic Heart Disease incidence, (1, 2).

The Edinburgh/Stockholm study further emphasised this and showed that the Edinburgh high risk men differ in many risk parameters from the more favoured Stockholm population. (3).

Long-term prospective studies have the inevitable draw-back that in their planning, little account can be taken of the advancing body of knowledge.

It is thus hardly surprising that much of the recent work with clofibrate has been concerned with demonstrating whether or not benefit is derived from giving the drug to patients with established disease.

The most exciting work relates to the demonstration that some atherosclerotic lesions are reversible, i.e. capable of regressing, in association with successful modification of some risk factors by clofibrate therapy. This possibility was suspected in studies using non-invasive techniques of evaluation, (7). Confirmation was only achieved by trials of clofibrate treatment with monitoring by serial angiography (8 and 9) Apart from lipid reduction (both cholesterol and triglyceride) control of elevated diastolic blood pressure has also been shown to correlate with regression of atherosclerotic lesions (10). Thus control of lipid elevation may not be solely responsible for the regression of some atherosclerotic lesions seen in patients treated with clofibrate.

A reciprocal rise of circulating high density lipoprotein (HDL) has been observed when the elevated very low density lipoprotein (VLDL) fraction is lowered by clofibrate therapy, (11).

Plasma fibrinogen elevation has been associated with poor prognosis (12) and reduction of this parameter by the administration of clofibrate may also be of importance in reducing atherosclerosis.

Theories relating lipid deposition to high density lipoprotein (HDL) function and fibrinogen level and fibrin deposition (1, 13), fit well with the known spectrum of activity of clofibrate.

Recently a further benefit of reducing elevated plasma fibrinogen has been demonstrated with patients with cerebrovascular disease and reduced cerebral blood flow. Using xenon isotope perfusion techniques, significant improvement in cerebral blood flow has been demonstrated in association with reducing elevated plasma fibrinogen by clofibrate therapy (14).

Improvement in platelet adhesiveness has not yet been critically evaluated in relation to therapy for atherosclerosis.

Collectively available studies emphasise that clofibrate needs to be used as part of a therapeutic approach to a multifactorial disease. The advice relating to therapy must be at an individual level and include control of all the pertinant risk factors. It is likely that a 15% reduction in cholesterol will be of more help to a heavy smoker who is hypertensive if these are also controlled.

Any therapy should also be evaluated in terms of its potential dangers, especially if long-term therapy may be contemplated. The incidence of the major side-effect of clofibrate treatment, 'gallstones', is small and compare well with dietary regime therapy (15, 16). In both instances increased biliary excretion of cholesterol is responsible and this, within the framework of a population already having a higher risk of gallstones and atherosclerosis. Other side-effects are largely minor and of rare occurrence and resolve on withdrawal of the drug.

Serial liver biopsy studies and the long-term large clinical experience have confirmed the relatively high margin of safety for clofibrate administration. Clofibrate, as a lipid reducing agent, both for cholesterol and triglyceride, should be considered after a reasonable trial of diet (in a dose of one and a half to 2 G's daily).

In resistant hypercholesterolaemia, it may usefully be given in conjunction with other agents, eg: cholestyramine.

Administration of clofibrate can be expected to produce, in the majority of patients, a return towards normal in chronically elevated plasma fibrinogen and an improvement in platelet adhesiveness. Lipoprotein lipase activity and glucose utilisation have also been reported to be improved.

It is not clear which individual property or combination confers the therapeutic benefit observed in those patients who respond to clofibrate. However, we now have greater encouragement to use a more active approach in patients with established atherosclerosis and extend its use in correcting known risk factors.

REFERENCES

1. *Miller, G. J. and Miller, N. E. (1975):* Lancet, i 16—19.
2. *Gordon, T., Castelli, W. P., Hjortland, M. J. (1977):* Amer. J. Med. 62, 707—714.
3. *Logan, R. L. et al. (1978):* Lancet i, 949—954.
4. *Oliver, M. F., Dewar, J. A. et al. (1971):* B. M. J. 4, 767—784.
5. *Oliver, M. F., Dewar, J. A. et al. (1975):* JAMA 231, (4) 360—381.
6. *Krasno, L. (1972):* JAMA 219, 845—851.
7. *Zelis, R. et al. (1970):* J. Clin. Invest. 49, 1007—1015.
8. *Basta, L. L. et al. (1976):* Amer. J. Med. 61 (3) 420—423.
9. *Blankenhorn, D. H. (1977):* Ann. Int. Med. 86, (2) 139—146.
10. *Sanmarco, E., (1976):* Circulation, 53 & 54, Suppl. II, 11—140.
11. *Wilson, D. and Less, R.,* J. Clin. Invest. Vol. 51, 1051—1072.
12. *Dormandy, J. A. et al. (1973):* M.B.J. ii, 576—581.
13. *Smith, E. B. and Smith, R. H. (1976):* Early Changes in Aortic Intima. Atherosclerosis Review, Vol. 1, New York Raven Press, E. R. Paoletti and Gotto.
14. *Thomas, D. and Marshall, J.:* Private communication — National Hospital for Nervous Diseases, Queens Square, London.
15. *CDP Research Group (1977):* New Eng. J. Med. 296, 19, 1185—1190.
16. *Sturderant, R. A., Pearce, M. L. and Dayton, S. (1973):* New Eng. J. Med. 288, 1, 24—27.

A. H., Medical Dept. Macclesfield, Cheshire and Physician Salford Royal Hospital, Lancashire, U.K.

BETA BLOCKERS AND LIPID METABOLISM

J. F. ENGLAND, A. HUA and J. SHAW

University Department of Medicine, The Royal Melbourne Hospital, Victoria, Australia

Beta adrenoreceptor blocking drugs are rapidly becoming the most commonly used agents in the long term management of patients with asymptomatic essential hypertension. Despite effective control of hypertension, there still remains a high, progressive incidence of coronary artery disease. The aim of this clinical study was to evaluate lipid and glucose metabolism after four drugs of differing relative beta one receptor blockade, "cardioselectivity", were used in conjunction with a thiazide diuretic to control elevated blood pressure.

Methods

The initial therapy for all 18 patients with WHO Grade I or II Essential Hypertension was Chlorothiazide 500 mg given twice a day. Later a beta blocker was added in addition to the diuretic, initially as a dose finding study with both Propranolol (160 or 240 mg) and Pindolol (15 or 30 mg) for blood pressure control. After 6 months 13 women and 5 men of mean age 45 years (with an age range of 16 to 60 years) entered the double blind phase, where all the Propranolol or Pindolol or a set 100 mg of Atenolol was given as a single morning dose. A randomised block design was used with 4 weeks active beta blocker therapy, followed by a 2 week placebo wash-out period before the next active therapy. At the completion of this study 17 of the patients entered a single blind comparison of placebo and 100 mg Metoprolol. Tablet counting was performed throughout the double blind study and compliance to the fasting conditions of the blood tests could be checked by any disparity in the insulin and glucose levels.

At regular intervals each patient fasted from 10.00 p.m. the night before and (for the relevant three patients) abstained from smoking and alcohol, and subsequently blood samples were taken at the same time of day, 24 hours after the last beta blocker dose was consumed. All patients were aware of the value of weight reduction, but no attempts were made throughout the study to introduce dietary modifications. The plasma triglyceride levels were measured by a Boehringer enzymatic method.

Results

There were significant falls in both lying and standing blood pressure with each beta blocker employed when compared to the preceding placebo phase (see figure).

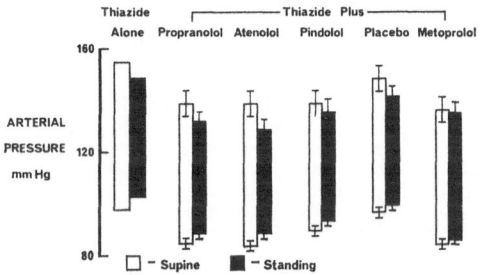

Fig. 1. Supine and Standing Blood Pressures for 18 patients on once a day beta blocker therapy for essential hypertension.

The results of fasting lipids for each treatment phase are shown in Table I. There were elevations in the fasting triglycerides at the end of all 1 month beta blocker therapy phases when compared to placebo. The triglyceride elevation was significant for all drugs (Paired T Test < <0.05) but maximal for the new beta one selective drug Atenolol. The influence of

Table 1. Fasting Lipid Results on once a day beta blocker therapy (mean and S.E.)

		MEAN RESULTS FOR 17 PATIENTS			
	PLACEBO	ATENOLOL	PINDOLOL	PROPRANOLOL	METOPROLOL
TRIGLYCERIDES	1.35	2.19*	1.73*	1.85*	1.79*
(MMOL/L)	± 0.11	± 0.44	± 0.19	± 0.28	± 0.22
CHOLESTEROL	5.5	5.6	5.8	5.7	5.6
(MMOL/L)	± 0.21	± 0.33	± 0.28	± 0.27	± 0.22

* P 0.05 BY PAIRED T-TEST

615

diet was not prominent as the fasting cholesterol levels remained unchanged.

The largest drug induced increments in triglyceride levels were observed in those patients with pre-existing elevated levels, whilst on placebo and thiazide diuretic. These patients were potentially Type IV hyperlipidaemia patients under the Fredrickson classification, with associated asymptomatic hyperuricaemia. The patients with this susceptible metabolic profile constituted one thrid of the patient group selected for the double blind study.

At the same time as the lipid studies separate samples were taken for blood glucose and hormone assays. The results are shown in Table II. The fasting immunoreactive pancreatic glucagon was suppressed with each beta blocker, in many instances to the limit of sensitivity of the assay. Glucose and insulin levels remained unchanged.

Discussion

Many studies involving patients with mild hypertension have demonstrated a rise in triglyceride levels with thiazide diuretics alone. (*Ames and Hill* 1976). In this study there was baseline therapy of one gram of chlorothiazide a day to which was added a placebo or beta blocker. It is likely that the beta blocker elevations in triglycerides are merely an additive effect upon a metabolic process already initiated by the thiazide diuretic.

The significance of the suppression of fasting immunoreactive glucagon is un-

Table 2. Fasting Blood Sugar, Insulin and Glucagon Levels on once a day beta blocker therapy (mean and S.E.)

MEAN RESULTS FOR 17 PATIENTS

	PLACEBO	ATENOLOL	PINDOLOL	PROPRANOLOL	METOPPOLOL
BLOOD GLUCOSE (MMOL/L)	4.3 ± 0.21	4.1 ± 0.16	4.0 ± 0.11	4.1 ± 0.15	4.1 ± 0.15
FASTING INSULIN (M U/L)	12.2 ± 0.86	12.5 ± 1.65	11.8 ± 0.89	12.4 ± 1.21	13.3 ± 1.38
FASTING GLUCAGON (PG/ML PLASMA)	62 ± 10	24[*] ± 4	28[*] ± 4	29[*] ± 5	31[*] ± 5

[*]$P < 0.005$ STUDENTS T-TEST

certain and in this clinical study it is not possible to link the triglyceride elevation with glucagon suppression. A hepatic role is suggested as Fredrickson Type 4 patients had the largest induced increments in triglycerides.

Elevations in triglyceride levels have been reported for patients on Metoprolol, who had not been on beta blockers previously (*Waal-Manning* 1976). Other studies have noted no change in absolute lipid levels, but alterations in lipoprotein composition with Propranolol therapy have been reported with an increase in lipids of very low-density lipoprotein and a decrease in lipids of both low-density and high density lipoprotein.

The clinical relevance of a long term alteration in triglyceride levels remains to be studied in large epidemiology studies. However, the benefit of lowering blood pressure may be offset by these changes in lipid metabolism in the overall clinical assessment of coronary risk factors in the patient with essential hypertension.

REFERENCES

Ames R. P. and Hill P. (1976): Elevation of Serum Lipid Levels during Diuretic Therapy of Hypertension. Am. J. Med. 61, 748—757.
Tanaka N., Sakaguchi S., Oshige K., Niimura T. and Kanehisa T. (1976): Effect of Chronic Administration of Propranolol on Lipoprotein Composition. Metabolism 25, 1071—75.
Waal-Manning H. (1976): Metabolic Effects of Beta-Adrenoreceptor blockers. Drugs 11, 1: 121—126.

J. F. E. Katoomba Medical Centre, New South Wales, 2780 Australia

BLOOD VISCOSITY IN PRIMARY HYPERLIPOPROTEINEMIA UNDER HYPOLIPIDEMIC THERAPY

H. R. ARNTZ, H. LEONHARDT, H. R. DREYKLUFT
and R. INGEROWSKI

Clinic of Medicine, Free University Berlin— West

Patients with primary hyperlipoproteinemia (HL) of type IIa (n = 20), IIb (n = 15) and IV (n = 22) were treated with clofibrate (2 × 1 g/die), bezafibrate (3 × 200 mg/die) and gemfibrozil (3 × 400 mg/die) for 8−10 weeks. Subgroups of patients received all 3 substances (n = 9), whereas a major collective received either 2 (n = 33) or only a single (n = 15) drug. The groups where thus not fully comparable. In addition to determining lipids and lipoproteins by preprarative ultracentrifugation and polyanionic precipitation (for methods see Ref.) before and after therapy, rheological blood parameters were also obtained: kinematic plasma and serum viscosity in an Ubbelohde-capillary-viscometer (*Mayer et al.*, 1966), the apparent whole blood visc. at shear rates 46 sec.$^{-1}$ and 115 sec.$^{-1}$ in a Wells-Brookfield-platecone-viscometer (*Schmid-Schönbein*, 1976; *Schmid-Schönbein*, 1971). The relative apparent blood visc. was calculated from the quotient of plasma visc. and apparent blood visc. The erythrocyte flexibility was tested by means of a filtration technique (*Schmid-Schönbein*, 1976). These rheological characteristics are elevated in patients with HL, depending on the type and degree of HL (*Leonhardt et al.*, 1977; *Leonhardt et al.*, 1978).

Results

Table I gives a survey of changes in lipids and lipoproteins after therapy. Significant reductions were noted with all 3 drugs. Differences in efficacy are marked in the

Table I. Effect of bezafibrate, clofibrate and gemfibrozil on lipid and lipoprotein concentration (in mg%) in primary hyperlipoproteinemia

HL Type	Gemfibrozil (3 × 400 mg/die)		Clofibrate (2 × 1 g/die)		Bezafibrate (3 × 200 mg/die)	
	Type II (a + b) n = 12	Type IV n = 10	Type II (a + b) n = 19	Type IV n = 10	Type II (a + b) n = 15	Type IV n = 12
Total-Triglycerides	(135) −42*	(355) −131*	(144) −46*	(473) −142*	(158) −36*	(367) −123.5*
VLDL-Total Lipids	(146) −72*	(421) −145	(141) −59*	(562) −184*	(131) −37*	(430) −128*
Total Cholesterol	(320) −44*	(282) −33	(356) −56*	(278) +12	(350) −58*	(287) −32*
LDL-Total Lipids	(466) −85*	(263) +21*	(463) −81*	(264) +74*	(507) −107*	(338) −25*

(Median values of changes of lipid and lipoprotein concentrations for each group after therapy. In parenthesis: median values of initial lipid concentrations. VLDL/LDL-total lipids = sum of VLDL/LDL-triglycerides, cholesterol and phosphatides. * = significance 2α 0.05 (Wilcoxon-Test for matched pairs)).

Table II. Effect of bezafibrate, clofibrate and gemfibrozil on rheological parameters in primary hyperlipoproteinemia

HL Type		Gemfibrozil (3 × 400 mg/die)		Clofibrate (2 × 1 g/die)		Bezafibrate (3 × 200 mg/die)	
		Type II (a + b)	Type IV	Type II (a + b)	Type IV	Type II (a + b)	Type IV
Plasmaviscosity (sec.)		(192.8) +3.3	(193.6) −2.1	(192.6) −5.7*	(191.6) −8.1*	(195.5) −9.9*	(192.5) −8.2
Serumviscosity (sec.)		(175.2) +1.5	(174.2) −4.3*	(177.6) −3.8*	(173.4) −5.7*	(175.6) −7.1*	(174.0) −4.9*
apparent whole blood viscosity	46 sec.$^{-1}$	(5.7) −0.2	(5.7) +0.1	(5.7) −0.2	(5.7) −0.5*	(5.5) −0.1	(5.6) −0.5*
at shear rate (cps)	115 sec.$^{-1}$	(4.6) +0.1	(4.6) +0.1	(5.0) −0.3	(4.6) −0.2	(5.1) −0.1	(4.6) −0.2
relative apparent whole blood viscosity	46 sec.$^{-1}$	(4.04) −0.21	(4.32) +0.01	(3.97) −0.05	(4.04) +0.01	(3.97) +0.11	(4.03) −0.09
at shear rate	115 sec.$^{-1}$	(3.13) −0.11	(3.25) +0.15	(3.51) −0.12	(3.26) −0.17	(3.56) +0.09	(3.23) −0.03
Erythrocyteflexibility (sec.)		(43.6) −2.1	(45.1) +3.7	(48.1) −7.6	(43.1) −0.1	(56.4) −12.0	(42.7) −4.0

The table gives the median values of reduction or increase of the rheological parameters for each group after therapy. In parenthesis: median values of the parameters before therapy. * = significance 2α 0.05 (Wilcoxon-Test for matched pairs).

LDL-fraction, the LDL being reduced in all groups by bezafibrate, whereas increasing LDL were registered Table II in type IV with clofibrate and gemfibrozil. Table II summarizes the rheological results. The erythrocyte flexibility remained unchanged with all 3 drugs as well as the relative apparent blood visc. The apparent blood visc. was improved only in type IV at shear rate 46 sec.$^{-1}$ but not with gemfi-

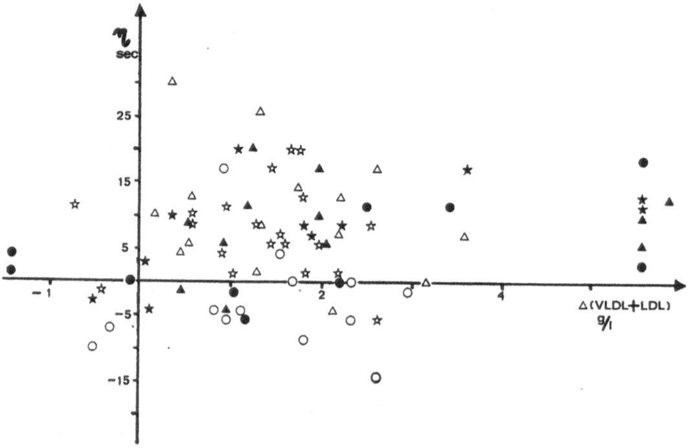

Fig. 1. Relation between change in plasma viscosity and change in lipoprotein concentrations under clofibrate (*), bezafibrate (∇) and gemfibrozil (○) — therapy.

The difference in plasma viscosity before and after therapy is plotted against the difference in the sum of VLDL- and LDL-lipoprotein concentrations (lipid fraction) (closed symbols: Type II a + b; open symbols: Type IV)

brozil. The serum and plasma visc. was diminished by bezafibrate and clofibrate in all groups, whereas gemfibrozil reduced only the serum visc. in type IV. The relationship between changes in the lipoprotein concentrations and changes in visc. is shown in figure 1 for the case of plasma visc. A qualitative correlation is apparent.

Discussion

Serum and plasma visc. is diminished in all groups by clofibrate and bezafibrate treatment. Gemfibrozil has an effect only on serum visc. in type IV. The reduction of visc. runs parallel to the lowering of lipoproteins. It should be noted, however, that the different lipoprotein fractions possess varying effects with respect to visc. (*Leonhardt et al.*, 1977). The whole blood visc. remains constant, except for the apparent blood visc. at shear rate 46 sec.$^{-1}$ in type IV. The relative apparent blood visc. was completely unchanged. This may be due to the lack of red blood cell aggregating properties of lipoproteins in contrast to e.g. fibrinogen. Furthermore the unchanged red blood cell flexibility may play a role. The lipid lowering efficacy of bezafibrate and clofibrate is qualitati-

vely and quantitatively similar to the results listed in the literature (*Carlson et al.*, 1974; *Olsson et al.*, 1977), whereas we found gemfibrozil to be less effective than previously reported (*Vessby et al.*, 1976). The superiority of bezafibrate is seen best in the reduction of the LDL-lipoprotein-fraction in type II and IV. In the latter type bezafibrate reduces the LDL, whereas clofibrate and gemfibrozil therapy leads to a significant increase in LDL-total lipids.

A direct comparison of the drug effects between the different groups is, however, only possible to a limited degree, since the individual group of patients are not completely identical (which can be seen from the varying "starting values"). Our results, therefore, should be interpreted as follows: 1. Hypolipidemic drugs may reduce pathologically elevated blood visc. in HL. The improvement of blood rheology may lead to a better organ perfusion by better flow conditions. 2. There appears to be a correlation between the antilipidemic drug-effects and its ability to reduce visc. 3. The effects of hypolipidemic agents on blood rheology should be included in their pharmacological assessment.

REFERENCES

Carlson, L. A., Olsson, A. G. et al. in: Schettler, G., Weizel, A. (Edtrs.) (1974): Atherosclerosis III. Springer Verlag Berlin, Heidelberg, New York.
Schettler, G., Weizel, A. (Edtrs.)) (1976): Handbuch der inneren Medizin, Vol. 7, Part 4., Fettstoffwechsel. Springer Verlag Berlin, Heidelberg, New York.
Leonhardt, H., Arntz, H.-R. (1978): Blutviskosität und Erythrozytenflexibilität bei primären Hyperlipoproteinämien. Klin. Wschr., 56, 271.
Leonhardt, H., Arntz, H.-R. et al. (1977): Studies in plasma viscosity in primary hyperlipoproteinemia. Atherosclerosis 28, 29.
Mayer, G. A., Fridrich, J. et al. (1966): Plasma

components and blood viscosity. Biorheology 3, 177.
Olsson, A. G., Rössner, S. et al. (1977): Effect of BM 15075 on lipoprotein concentrations in different types of hyperlipoproteinemia. Atherosclerosis 27, 279.
Schmid-Schönbein, H. (1971): Normale Fließeigenschaften des Blutes und deren krankhafte Veränderungen. Schweiz. Med. Wschr., 101, 1766.
Schmid-Schönbein, H. (1976): Microrheology of erythrocytes, blood rheology and the distribution of blood flow in microcirculation. Int. Rev. Physiol.: Cardiovascular Physiology II, Vol. 9, 1.

H. R. A., Med. Klinik, Klinikum Steglitz, Freie Univ., Berlin— West

THE EFFECT OF TRIMEPRANOL ON SEROTONIN RELEASE AND THROMBOCYTE AGGREGATION IN THE RAT

R. NOSÁL

Institute of Experimental Pharmacology, Slovak Academy of Sciences, Bratislava, Czechoslovakia

Introduction

Many drugs among them beta-adrenergic blocking drugs stabilize cell membranes by non-specific mechanism (*Langslet*, 1970). They affect serotonin transport across the membranes of human blood platelets (*Lemmer et al.*, 1972) and protect human erythrocytes against hypotonic hemolysis (*Wiethold et al.*, 1973). Trimepranol (TMP) = 1-(2,3,5-trimethyl-4-acetophenoxy)-3-isopropylamino-2-propanol) is widely used in the treatment of angina pectoris and arrhythmias. In our studies we investigated the effect of TMP on serotonin release from isolated or platelet rich plasma (PRP) and on the aggregation of thrombocytes both isolated or in plasma. The reason for selecting rats was to compare the effect of TMP on thrombocytes with those on mast cells as far as both amines (histamine and serotonin) play an important role in several pathological mechanisms in the organism.

Methods

Thrombocytes were isolated from rat blood by differential centrifugation. For aggregation studies a heparin-citrate mixture was used, for 5-HT release a chelating mixture was taken as anticoagulant. Aggregation of isolated or PRP was measured photometrically. Mast cells were isolated from rat pleural and peritoneal cavities (*Thon and Uvnäs*, 1967). Serotonin and histamine release was measured spectrofluorometrically.

Results

Figure 1 demonstrates the dose-response curves for serotonin release from isolated rat thrombocytes after 5, 15, 30 and 60 minutes with TMP at 37 °C. As evident,

TMP induced significant 5-HT release and linear relationship occurred between the TMP concentration and 5-HT release. On the contrary we did not observe any histamine release from mast cells after the same concentration of TMP. The uptake of labelled serotonin was inhibited in isolated thrombocytes with increased concentration of TMP (10^{-5} to 10^{-3} M) similarly as has been shown for other beta-blockers. During the incubation of PRP with TMP (10^{-3} M) significant release cf 5-HT oc-

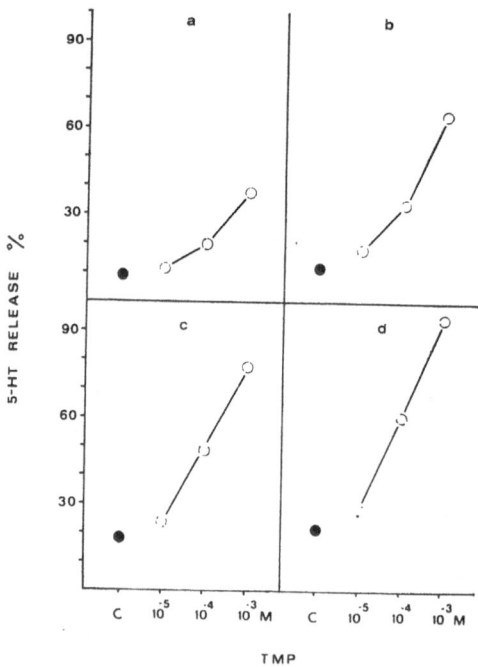

Fig. 1. Dose-response curves for 5-HT release from isolated rat thrombocytes at 5(a), 15(b), 30(c) and 60(d) min with trimepranol (TMP) at 37 °C. Each point of the curves represents the mean of 5 experiments. C = control.

620

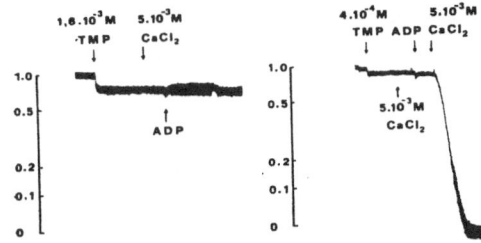

Fig. 2. The effect of TMP, ADP (3×10^{-5} M) and calcium ions on aggregation of isolated rat thrombocytes.

curred after 15 and 30 min of incubation.

TMP blocked aggregation of isolated thrombocytes induced by ADP (3×10^{-5} M) and calcium ions. With lower concentration of TMP the aggregation started only if calcium ions were in abundance (Fig. 2).

The ADP-induced aggregation of PRP treated with TMP (Fig. 3) was time-dependent. If the lag period between TMP and ADP addition was shorter than 2 min incomplete aggregation developed. This could be terminated by calcium ions. Prolonging the lag period to 5 min resulted in complete inhibition of aggregation. This effect of TMP was reversed by calcium ions.

Discussion

Trimepranol induced serotonin release from PRP as well as from isolated rat thrombocytes in a dose dependent way. This was not found for isolated rat mast

cells storing histamine in similar way (*Anderson et al.*, 1974). In equimolar concentration TMP blocked amine uptake in both cells. The difference in the release and uptake of amines due to beta-blockers has not yet been explained and could be a result of specific changes induced in the membrane structure as shown for erythrocytes (*Godin et al.*, 1976). If the aggregation of thrombocytes should be followed by release reaction of seortonin, this was not shown for TMP. In a concentration which released serotonin from PRP or isolated thrombocytes TMP blocked the aggregation induced by ADP. In PRP only calcium ions reversed the inhibitory effect of TMP. This could be either due to the displacement of TMP bound to active sites in thrombocytes or due to activation of mechanisms that trigger the aggregation process.

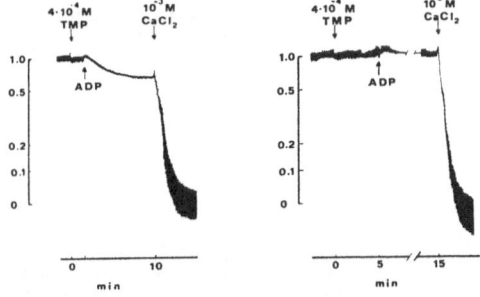

Fig. 3. Time-dependent trimepranol (TMP) inhibition of rat PRP aggregation induced with ADP (3×10^{-5} M) and calcium ions.

REFERENCES

Anderson, P., Slorach, S. A., Uvnäs, B. (1974): 5-HT storage in rat and rabbit blood platelets. Acta physiol. scand. 90, 522—532.
Godin, D. V., Ng, T. W., Tuchek, J..M. (1976): Studies of the interaction of propranolol with erythrocyte membranes. Biochim. Biophys. Acta 436, 757—773.
Langslet, A. (1970): Membrane stabilization and cardiac effect of d, l-propanolol, d-propranolol and chlorpromazine. Europ. J. Pharmacol. 13, 6—14.
Lemmer, B., Wiethold, G., Hellenbrecht, D., Bak,

I. J., Grobecker, H. (1972): Human blood platelets as cellular model for investigation of membrane active drugs: Naunyn-Schmied. Arch. Pharmacol. 275, 299—313.
Thon, I. L., Uvnäs, B. (1967): Degranulation and histamine release. Acta physiol. scand. 71, 303—315.
Wiethold, G., Hellenbrecht, D., Lemmer, B., Palm, D. (1973): Membrane effects of beta-adrenergic blocking agents. Biochem. Pharmacol. 22, 1437 to 1449.

R. N., Inst. Exper. Pharmacol. Slovak Academy of Sciences, 881 05 Bratislava 1, Czechoslovakia

ANTIHYPERTENSIVE ACTION OF TRIMEPRANOL AND TRIMEPRANOL COMBINED WITH SALTUCIN

Z. MODR and J. ŠEDIVÝ

Clinical Pharmacology Research Centre of the Institute for Clinical and Experimental Medicine, Prague and Department of Pharmacology, Faculty of Medicine, Charles University, Prague, Czechoslovakia

Trimepranol (metipranolol) has been used since 1971 in the treatment of patients with angina pectoris and other manifestations of ischaemic heart disease, tachyarrhythmias and thyrotoxicosis. Its daily doses averaged 20–40 mg.

Several clinical studies dealt with the antihypertensive effect of Trimepranol in patients with essential or renal hypertension (1, 2, 3, 4). In 1976, an open multicentral clinical trial involving a high number of patients was carried out to evaluate the antihypertensive effect of Trimepranol alone or combined with a saluretic butizide (Saltucin). The trial of a uniform lay-out was performed in the Federal Republic of Germany and in Czechoslovakia.

In Czechoslovakia, 90 men and 95 women, both out-and inpatients, with essential or renal hypertension (casual blood pressure over 160/90 mm Hg at repeated measurement), unresponsive to earlier therapy and without contraindication for beta-sympatholytic treatment were included in the trial. Its schedule is presented on Fig. 1. After a 2-week observation period without any antihypertensive treatment, the patients were randomized in two groups: one group received increasing doses of Trimepranol while the other group was given Trimepranol and Saltucin combined. Blood pressure and heart rate were measured once a week in recumbent, sitting, and standing positions, in every case repeatedly 3 times. Complaints and tolerance of the drug(s) were recorded, too. A 15% decrease of systolic blood pressure in relation to the initial value during one week of treatment was considered as criterion of antihypertensive efficacy. When the

WEEK	−2	−1	0	1	2	3	4
Group T (mg/day)	0	0	T 2×20	T 2×40	T 3×40	T 3×40	
Group TS (mg/day)	0	0	T 2×20 + S 1×2.5	T 2×40 + S 2×2.5	T 3×40 + S 3×2.5	T 3×40 + S 3×2.5	

T = TRIMEPRANOL
TS = TRIMEPRANOL + SALTUCIN

Fig. 1. Plan of clinical evaluation of the effectiveness of Trimepranol and its combination with Saltucin in hypertonics.

criterion was fulfilled after the initial dose 20 mg of Trimepranol (plus 2.5 mg Saltucin, respectively), the same dose was given also in the second week of the treatment. If blood pressure failed to decrease the

Group		n	before	after	
T	BP recumbent	86	179/107	153/94	***
	HR "	86	78	66	
T	BP standing	86	175/110	152/97	***
	HR "	86	87	69	
TS	BP recumbent	96	183/109	154/94	***
	HR "	96	81	67	
TS	BP standing	96	181/113	148/98	***
	HR "	96	87	70	

*** $p < 0.001$

Fig. 2. Mean values of blood pressure and heart rate of patients before treatment and after termination of the trial.

dose was doubled or trebled during the subsequent weeks. The highest administered daily dose was 120 mg Trimepranol or 120 mg Trimepranol plus 7.5 mg Saltucin, respectively. The whole observation period lasted 6 weeks.

Mean values of blood pressure and heart rate of patients before the treatment and after the termination of the trial are summarized in Fig. 2. The relatively rough criterion of the blood pressure decrease was fulfilled in $35-40\%$ patients with a dose 40 mg Trimepranol (day when measured in the recumbent position (Fig. 3). The effect was evident after a week of treatment. With the increasing doses the percentage of patients fulfilling the criterion was remarkably higher in the group of patients receiving the combination of Trimepranol with Saltucin ($77\% : 58\%$ up to dose 80 mg and $90\% : 71\%$ up to dose 120 mg). The rest of the patients (29% in a group of Trimepranol and 10% in a group of drugs' combination) did not fulfill the criterion even with a daily dose 120 mg Trimepranol. No difference between both groups in respect to sex, type, and phase of hypertension could be proved. Age- and sex related normalization of systolic (and diastolic) blood pressure was achieved in $43-45\%$ ($34-39\%$) of patients without any significant difference between the groups.

The tolerance of drugs was characterized in 90% of patients as good, no postural hypotension was observed during the treatment. The medication was discontinued due to side effects in 3 cases (1.6% of all patients): In the group of Trimepranol, one patient suffered from permanent headache, weekness, and vertigo with bradycardia 46 BPM; in the group of combination, a marked dyspnoea with bronchospastic chest findings was found in one patient and palpitations appeared in another one. All these symptoms disappeared spontaneously after the withdrawing of the drugs. Approximately 1/3 of patients in both groups experienced light side effects.

It may be concluded, that Trimepranol in small doses either alone or in combination with Saltucin, is an effective agent in the treatment of mild and moderate hypertension.

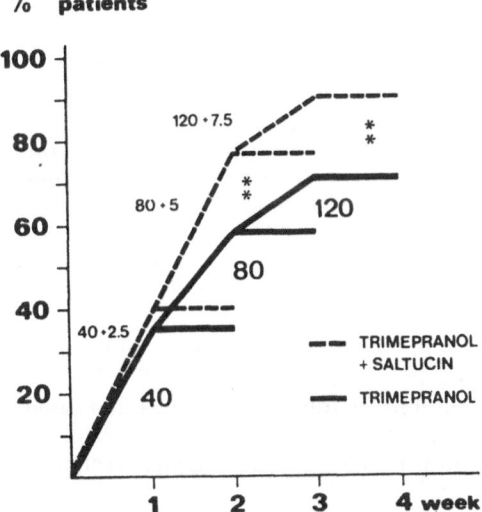

% patients

Fig. 3. Percentage of hypertonics who met the criterion of effectiveness in the recumbent position after $40-120$ mg Trimepranol per day (Group T) or after $40-120$ mg Trimepranol plus $2.5-7.5$ mg Saltucin (Group TS). xx $p < 0.01$.

REFERENCES

1. *Jounela, A. J., Pentikäinen, P. J., Neuvonen, P. J.* (1978): Antihypertensive effect of trimepranol, a new beta-blocking agent. Int. J. clin. Pharmacol. 16, 183—188.
2. *Schweers, A., Glocke, M. (1977):* Verlaufsbeobachtung bei Dauertherapie in der Praxis mit Torrat[R]. Archiv Boehringer.
3. *Slabý, A., Došková, M., Jirák, J., Pavlát, J.,* *Urbánek, J., Reisenauer, R. (1975):* Dlouhodobé léčení kolísavé hraniční hypertense Trimepranolem a jeho vliv na plasmatickou reninovou aktivitu. Sbor. lék. 77, 107—111.
4. *Stříbrná, J., Nádvorníková, H., Žofková, I.* (1975): Zkušenosti s antihypertenzivním účinkem methypranolu (Trimepranol Spofa). Farmakoterap. zprávy Spofa 21, 11—20.

Z. M., IKEM, Vídeňská 800, 140 00 Prague 4, Czechoslovakia

HYPERLIPEMIC EFFECT OF BETA-BLOCKING AGENTS IN EXPERIMENTAL ATHEROSCLEROSIS

J. REINIŠOVÁ, D. HORÁKOVÁ, A. KLIMEŠOVÁ and K. GORIČAN

Laboratory of Protein Metabolism and Angiological Laboratory,
Faculty of General Medicine, Charles University, Prague, Czechoslovakia

Long-term administration of beta-blocking agents (trimepranol or propranolol) to cocks and rabbits fed a cholesterol diet was associated with a significant increase of serum lipids (1, 2, 3). On the other hand, several authors observed decreased values of e. g. cholesterol and triacylglycerols of serum when beta-blockers were applied without a high fat diet (4). The question is whether the hyperlipemic effect of beta-blockers in combination with a cholesterol diet is of fundamental importance for the development of atherosclerotic changes. In our paper we tried to contribute to the study of this problem.

In the experiments we used 60 cocks and 40 rabbits. The animals were divided into four groups:

1. Standard diet
2. Standard diet supplemented by beta-blockers (at a ratio of 15 miligrams of TMP or 30 miligrams of PPL to 100 g of the feed)
3. Cholesterol diet (2 g of cholesterol and 5 g of germ oil to 100 g of the feed)
4. Cholesterol diet together with beta-blockers (15 miligrams of TMP or 30 miligrams of PPL 100 g of the feed)

Abbreviations: C = controls, TMP = trimepranol group, PPL = propranolol, CH = cholesterol fed group, CH + TMP = cholesterol fed group with trimepranol.

At the beginning, after the first and second month of the experiment, the content of total lipids, cholesterol, triacylglycerols, phospholipids and sphingomyelin in serum or tissues was determined. Fractions of cholesterol esters and phospholipids were estimated using thin-layer chromatographic methods. Tissue samples were obtained by autopsy after the two months' experiment and subjected to biochemical and histological examination. In Table I the influence of TMP on the amount of total serum lipids and cholesterol after the two months' experiment is shown. A significantly higher increase in total serum lipids as well as serum cholesterol was observed in cholesterol fed animals treated with TMP.

Table I. The values of total lipids and cholesterol in serum of cocks and rabbits after two months' experiment

		C	TMP	CH	CH + TMP
COCKS	Total lipids mg/100 ml	211 (±26)	198 (±35)	839 (±417)	1511 (±430)
	Total cholesterol mg/100 ml	131 (±17)	135 (±10)	1126 (±560)	2072 (±599)
RABBITS	Total lipids mg/100 ml	88 (±8)	82 (±14)	1927 (±140)	3484 (±729)
	Total cholesterol mg/100 ml	37 (±5)	43 (±5)	2136 (±145)	3376 (±546)

Values in parenthesis = standard error of the mean

Table II. The values of total phospholipids and sphingomyelin in serum of cocks and rabbits after two months' experiment

		C	TMP	CH	CH + TMP
COCKS	Total phospholipids mg/100 ml	143.0 (±25)	142.2 (±25)	259.9 (±102)	377.7 (±103)
	Sphingomyelin mg/100 ml	29.6 (±2.3)	34.5 (±1.7)	131.6 (±16.3)	199.4 (±14.3)
RABBITS	Total phospholipids mg/100 ml	61.3 (±3.2)	56.0 (±4.0)	872.0 (±74.8)	1216.0 (±174.9)
	Sphingomyelin mg/100 ml	5.7 (±0.37)	6.9 (±1.5)	236.4 (±13.1)	366.0 (±44.8)

Values in parenthesis = standard error of the mean

The determination of serum triacylglycerols showed analogous results. In cholesterol fed cocks treated with TMP a significant rise from 218 ± 107 (CH-group) to 404 ± 128 mg/100 ml (CH + TMP group) of serum was determined. Similar but statistically not significant changes were found in rabbits.

In Table II a similar picture is evidenced as to serum phospholipids and sphingomyelin. TMP in combination with a cholesterol diet significantly influenced the amount of phospholipids and sphingomyelin.

In the composition of the spectrum of the individual major serum phospholipids there are no substantial differences between the control and TMP groups either in cocks or in rabbits. A cholesterol diet however causes considerable changes in the spectrum of phospholipids in both animals. This was especially observed in the increase of sphingomyelin and to a certain extent of phosphatidylcholine. TMP induced a further significant increase in the amounts of both these phospholipids.

When free and esterified cholesterol were analysed chromatografically a considerable elevation in both fractions was observed after feeding cholesterol in combination with TMP.

However, the composition of the fractions of cholesterol esters was not changed considerably through beta-blockers. This was influenced by the cholesterol feeding itself which was demonstrated in the increased percentage of the monoenic fraction by about 15% as compared with the control group.

The cholesterol content of the liver in experimental animals fed on a standard diet increased only slightly after administration of TMP. In animals fed a cholesterol diet the effect of beta-blockers was reversed and a decreased cholesterol content was observed in both cocks and rabbits. In cocks this difference was statistically significant.

Interesting results were found in the aorta. In cholesterol fed rabbits TMP significantly decreased the amount of total lipids as well as cholesterol and phospholipids (Fig. 1).

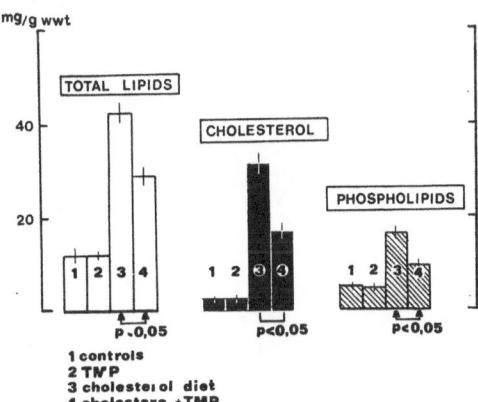

Fig. 1. Lipids in rabbit aorta after trimepranol treatment. Arrows indicate statistical significance.

The two months' experiments with cholesterol fed cocks and rabbits confirmed that beta-blocking agents promote alimentary lipemia. Similarly as TMP, PPL stimulated lipid accumulation in serum which was characterized by considerably higher total serum lipids, cholesterol, triacylglycerols and phospholipids (including sphingomyelin).

Probably one of the factors stimulating lipid accumulation in the serum is a reduced permeability of the vascular wall which develops when the action of catecholamines on the vascular tissue is inhibited (5). This agrees with the lower lipid level found in the aorta of rabbits fed a cholesterol diet and supplemented with TMP as contrasted with the animals without beta-blockers. According to the morphological findings the degree of experimental atherosclerosis was not elevated in spite of increased serum lipid accumulation due to beta-blockers action. Using beta-blockers the atherogenic effect of a high-fat cholesterol diet can be limited to a certain extent, even when the serum lipid concentration attains abnormal high values.

REFERENCES

1. *Barboriak, J. J., Friedberg, H. D.: (1973)* Propranolol ahd hypertriglyceridemia: Atherosclerosis, 17, p. 31—35.
2. *Barboriak, J. J., Meade, R. C., Owenby, J., Stiglitz, R. A.: (1967)* Blockers of free fatty acid release and postprandial lipemia. Arch. int. Pharmacodyn., 176, p. 249.
3. *Wexler, B. C.: (1973)* Protective effects of propranolol on isoproterenol-induced myocardial infarction in arteriosclerotic and non-arteriosclerotic rats. Atherosclerosis, 18, p. 11.
4. *Whittington-Coleman, P. J., Carrier, O. Jr., Douglas, B. H.: (1973)* The effects of propranolol on cholesterol-induced atheromatous lesions. Atherosclerosis, 18, 1973, p. 337.
5. *Reiniš, Z., Lojda, Z., Heyrovský, A., Horáková, D., Reisenauer, R.: (1976)* Effect of beta-blocking agents in experimental atherosclerosis of cocks. Rev. Czechoslov. Med., 22, 1976, p. 117.

J. R., Laboratory of Protein Metabolism, U nemocnice 5, 120 00 Prague 1, Czechoslovakia

METIPRANOLOL AND SEVERAL OTHER BETA-BLOCKING AGENTS — A COMPARATIVE PHARMACOLOGICAL STUDY

M. VANĚČEK, V. TRČKA, I. HELFERT and SVĚTLA MÁCOVÁ

Research Institute for Pharmacy and Biochemistry, Prague, Czechoslovakia

Metipranolol (MP), 1(2,3,5-trimethyl-4--acetoxyphenoxy)-3-isopropylamino-2-prc-panol, Trimepranol — SPOFA, has been introduced into current clinical practice in Czechoslovakia in 1972 (*Bergmann and Horák*, 1970).

To demonstrate the position of MP among the other most frequently used preparations, we compared it with a series of beta-blocking drugs from various pharmacological aspects. In anaesthetized cats as criterion of anti-isoprenaline effect on the heart rate and diastolic blood pressure we chose the minimal effective dose that significantly lowered the response to isoprenaline of the heart rate and diastolic pressure. The results were expressed in terms of relative efficacy values, accepting MP as standard with efficacy equalling unity.

The relationship of the blocking efficacies of tested drugs on isoprenaline-induced tachycardia and the drop in diastolic blood pressure, expressed as quotient, indicates the ratio of the effects on beta$_1$ — cardiac — and beta$_2$ — vascular receptors. The pertinent quotients summarized in Table I show marked differences between some blockers. MP belongs to the group of substances with relatively higher effect on cardiac than peripheral receptors.

An important criterion of clinical acceptability of beta-blockers is their effect upon spontaneous myocardial contractility, which effect should be minimal. For this reason we tested MP for its negative inotropic activity by several procedures in various animal species (Table II). In electrically stimulated isolated cat papillary muscle the relative effective doses, halving the contraction of the preparation, were determined. It was found that the negative inotropic activity of MP was almost one eighth of that of propranolol and likewise lower than the activities of oxprenolol and alprenolol. In isolated, spontaneously beating guinea-pig atria similar findings were obtained both after applica-

Table I. Relative ratio of anti-isoprenaline activity on the diastolic blood pressure to the anti-isoprenaline activity on the heart rate in anaesthetized cats

Drug	Ratio
Practolol	0.6
Atenolol	0.8
Talinolol	0.8
Metipranolol	1.0
Tolamolol	1.0
Timolol	2.1
Pindolol	3.0
Alprenolol	5.0
Oxprenolol	5.5
Propranolol	12.0

Table II. Relative negative inotropic activity

	Meti-pranolol	Propra-nolol	Oxpre-nolol	Alpre-nolol	Pindolol
Electrically stimulated cat papillary muscle	1	7.8	2.0	4.1	—
Spontaneously beating guinea-pig atria					
at 10% heart rate decrease	1	2.2	2.0	2.5	1.8
at 25% blockade of isoprenaline tachycardia	1	2.0	2.0	2.4	1.7
Perfused spontaneously beating guinea-pig hearts	1	5.0	2.0	5.0	—
Electrically stimulated rabbit left atria	1	2.3	—	—	1.8

tion of beta-blockers reducing the basal heart rate by 10% and in 25% blockade of isoprenaline-induced tachycardia.

Another criterion was the reduction of amplitude of isolated guinea-pig heart, perfused for 10 min with a beta-blocker in concentration reducing the heart rate to 50 per cent. In this test the substances compared with MP likewise exhibited higher negative inotropic activities (Table II).

Higher relative negative inotropic activities of propranolol and pindolol, in comparison with MP, were also found in electrostimulated rabbit atria (Table II).

Isoprenaline-enhanced myocardial contractility can be blocked in vitro (Trčka et al., 1979) as well as in vivo. In dogs under pentobarbital anaesthesia, in which the contractility was assessed from the derivative of left ventricular pressure with respect to time, the increase in contractility induced by isoprenaline was blocked by 0.3 mg.kg^{-1} of MP i. v., and by 10 mg . . kg^{-1} of practolol. The dose 1.2 mg.kg^{-1} of propranolol was without significant effect in this respect.

A comparison of these findings of relative negative inotropic activities with the anti-isoprenaline activities shown in Tab. III, suggests that our findings do not indicate any parallel between the inotropic and chronotropic activities of beta-blockers. Although in the modification of contractility by some of the drugs compared also other factors than the simple effect upon myocardial beta-receptors may participate, the findings discussed do not seem to indicate that chronotropic and inotropic beta-receptors would be identical. A recent study of a series of agonists, however, leads to the conclusion that both

types of receptors are identical (Lumley and Broadley, 1977).

Our findings of relative anti-isoprenaline efficacies on the heart rate of ten beta-blockers tested on anaesthetized cats do roughly correlate with their average therapeutic daily doses (Table III). The first three most effective substances, pindolol, timolol, and metipranolol are currently administered in doses one-tenth times as high as the doses of the preparations less effective in animal experiments.

Table III. Comparison of relative anti-isoprenaline activity on the heart rate of anaesthetized cats and recommended human daily doses of 10 beta-blockers

Drug	Relative beta-blocking activity on the heart	Therapeutic daily dose mg
Pindolol	4.0	15—30
Timolol	1.2	20—30
Metipranolol	1.0	20—40
Oxprenolol	0.5	80—240
Alprenolol	0.5	100—300
Propranolol	0.25	80—240
Atenolol	0.25	100—300
Tolamolol	0.1	300—900
Talinolol	0.05	100—300
Practolol	0.05	200—600

When a beta-blocker is being chosen for therapeutic application, then, besides its effect on myocardial beta-receptors and the much discussed cardioselectivity, its antihypertensive efficacy, pharmacokinetic factors etc., also its direct effect on myocardial contractility should be considered. Substances exerting a major negative inotropic effect may, at higher dosage levels, unfavourably affect the cardiac performance.

REFERENCES

Bergmann, K., Horák, O. (1970): Trimepranol, a new czechoslovak sympatholytic blocking agent. Čas. lék. čes. 109, 473—476.
Lumley, P., Broadle, K. J. (1977): Evidence from agonist and antagonist studies to suggest that beta₁-adrenoceptors subserving the posi-

tive inotropic and chronotropic responses of the heart do not belong to two separate subgroups. J. Pharm. Pharmac. 29, 598—604.
Trčka, V., Vaněček, M., Helfert, I., Mácová, S. (1979): Pharmacology of Trimepranol (metipranolol). This collection, p. 638.

V. T., Research Institute for Pharmacy and Biochemistry, Kouřimská 17, 130 00 Praha 3, Czechoslovakia

PINDOLOL: A PHARMACOKINETIC COMPARISON WITH OTHER BETA-ADRENOCEPTOR BLOCKING AGENTS

J. MEIER

Biopharmaceutical Department Sandoz, Basle, Switzerland

Obviously beta-blockers are drugs which have and will be used in long-term treatment and, therefore, the question of their longterm efficacy and safety has been of great interest and concern.

The relation between the pharmacokinetics of the beta-adrenoceptor blocking agents and their effects has been established, e. g. in exercise induced tachycardia [1, 2] and for the antihypertensive effect [3].

Chemically, the beta-adrenoceptor blocking agents carry in all but two cases (sotalol and timolol) the isopropylaminopropoxy side chain, a major element for their pharmacological and therapeutic activity and an aromatic group which is different for each drug. This group which could be called modulator of the pharmacological activity also determines the pharmacokinetic properties of these drugs. This is illustrated by the observation that the most lipophilic beta-blockers (like alprenolol, propranolol, metoprolol) are com-pletely metabolized in the liver, and show shorter half-lives whereas those of lower lipophilicity (like practolol or sotalol) are mainly excreted via the kidney and have a longer half-life. The volume of distribution increases also with increasing lipophilicity of the drug.

As illustrated in Table I [4], all beta-blockers (with the exception of acebutolol and atenolol) are absorbed completely. However the extent of their bioavailability differs strongly due to the variations in the ability of the liver to extract and metabolize the drugs during the first transport from the gastrointestinal tract into the general circulation. This phenomenon, which is called first-pass effect, shows important variations with practolol and pindolol having a negligible first-pass effect as against a first-pass effect of 60% for propranolol, 90% for alprenolol, 50% for metoprolol and 30 to 50% for oxprenolol.

Two parameters, the hepatic extraction

Table I. Pharmacokinetic parameters of β-blockers which are different

β-blocker	Daily dose mg	Absorption, % of dose	First-pass effect %	Bioavailability oral %	Urinary excretion parent drug %	Accumulation of plasma levels Liver disease	Accumulation of plasma levels Renal failure
Acebutolol	300	50	—	$\simeq 50$	< 35	—	Yes
Alprenolol	400	90	$\simeq 90*)$	$\simeq 10*)$	< 1	—	—
Atenolol	200	50	$\leqq 15$	$\geqq 40$	$\simeq 40$	—	Yes
Metoprolol	300	> 95	$\simeq 50$	$\simeq 50$	$\simeq 3$	—	—
Oxprenolol	160	$70 - 95$	$30 - 50$	$24 - 60$	$2 - 5$	—	—
Pindolol	15	> 95	13	87	$\simeq 40$	No	No
Practolol	400	> 95	0	100	> 90	No	Yes
Propranolol	300	> 90	$\simeq 60*)$	$30*)$	< 1	Yes	Yes
Sotalol	240	> 75	$\leqq 15$	$\geqq 60$	$\simeq 60$	—	Yes
Timolol	30	> 90	—	—	$\simeq 20$	—	No

*) Dose dependent ——→ nonlinear pharmacokinetics.

ratio and the hepatic blood flow, contribute to the unpredictability of plasma levels in the beta-blockers with high hepatic clearance in the following ways.

First, the hepatic extraction and metabolism of a beta-blocker may be saturated by an increase in dose leading to a more than proportional increase in plasma concentration. This phenomenon is important for propranolol and alprenolol, whereas plasma pindolol levels rise in porportion to the oral dose, the bioavailability being independent of the dose [4].

Second, a reduction in hepatic blood flow with advancing age, in cardiac insufficiency or liver cirrhosis or as a consequence of chronic beta-blocker administration, will reduce hepatic metabolization and, therefore, produce higher plasma levels and longer half-lives in beta-blockers with intense hepatic clearance.

The disadvantage of a strong first-pass effect is, therefore, not only the lower availability after oral administration which can be compensated by higher dosage, but also the resulting unpredictable larger biological, individual variation in the plasma levels and drug response.

There are wide differences between the 10 drugs as to how they are cleared (Fig. 1, [4]).

Practolol and atenolol, for instance, are almost completely cleared by the kidneys. In kidney impairment, therefore, the dosage has to be reduced; otherwise a considerable drug accumulation in the organism might occur due to the much smaller elimination constant [6, 7].

On the other hand, the beta-blockers alprenolol, propranolol, metoprolol and oxprenolol are almost completely eliminated by hepatic metabolism. In this case, it could be shown that the clearance decreased with increasing impairment in liver function [8]. Pindolol and probably also timolol are the "happy medium drugs" [4] which are cleared partly by the kidneys and partly by the liver. An impairment of liver or kidney function cannot be so critical theoretically.

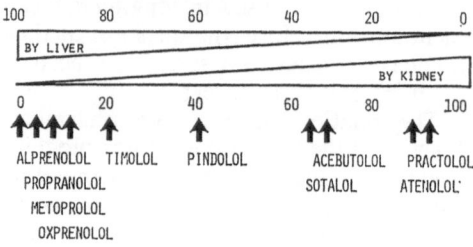

Fig. 1. Clearance of β-adrenoceptor blocking agents.

For pindolol it could be shown in various published pharmacokinetic experiments [9, 10, 11] that the dosage regimen is not critical in patients with renal or hepatic [11] impairment.

Taking the most prolonged half-life value found in one paper dealing with renal function impairment [10] the usual value is prolonged by a factor of 1.4 as against a factor of 4 for atenolol and acebutolol, 6.6 for practolol and 6 for sotalol (Table II).

Interestingly enough, even propranolol which is cleared mainly by hepatic metabolism, has shown much higher plasma levels in patients with renal impairment or terminal uremia [12, 13]. This has been

Table II. Eliminations half-lives of some β-blockers in patients with renal impairment

	With renal impairment	Normal subjects	Factor of increase
Practolol	60—100 hours	5—13 hours	6.6
Sotalol	42 hours	6—8 hours	6
Atenolol	22 hours	5 hours	4
Acetutolol	12 hours	3 hours	4
PINDOLOL	5 hours	3—4 hours	1.4

related either to a change in first-pass effect or in the volume of distribution of propranolol in these patients.

The pharmacokinetic comparison shows that pindolol has some relevant advantages. Due to the moderate metabolism, a negligible first-pass effect results which yields a high oral bioavailability and leads to predictable plasma concentrations with small variability (single and multiple dosing, volunteers and patients, with and without concomitant food). As a result of the balanced clearance by the liver and the kidney, and probably some compensating factors, no accumulation of pindolol has to be expected in patients with partial liver or kidney impairment. Therefore, apart from having the lowest daily dosage of the beta-blockers studies, administration of pindolol is less likely to be critical in patients with partial renal or hepatic insufficiency.

REFERENCES

1. *Johnsson, G. and Regårdh, C. G.: (1976):* Clinical Pharmacokinetics 1, 233—263.
2. *McAinsh J.: (1977):* Postgraduate Med. J. Suppl. 53, 3, 74—78.
3. *Weiss, Y. A., Loria, Y., Safar, M. E., Lavène, D. E., Simon A. C., Georges, D. R., Milliez, P. L.: (1977):* Curr. Ther. Res. 21, 644—655
4. *Meier, J.: (1977):* Current Med. Res. Opin. 4, Suppl. 5, 31—38.
5. *Bobik, A., Jennings, G., Korner, P. I.: (1977):* Med. J. Aust., No. 2 (Spec. Suppl.) 3—5.
6. *Bodem, G., Grieser, H., Eichelbaum, M., Gugler R.: (1976):* Europ. J. Clin. Pharmacol. 7, 249—252
7. *Baker, L, R., Kaye, C. M., Kumana, C. R.: (1974):* Int. J. Clin. Pharmacol. 10 (2), 136—158
8. *Branch, R. A., James, J., Read, A. E.: (1975):* Brit. J. Clin. Pharmacol., 2, 183P,
9. *Ohnhaus, E. E., Nüesch, E., Meier, J., Kalberer, F.: (1974):* Europ. J. Clin. Pharmacol. 7, 25—29
10. *Chau, N. P., Weiss, Y. A., Safar, M. E., Lavène, D. E., Georges, R., Milliez, P. L.: (1977):* Clin. Pharmacol. Ther. 22, 605—610
11. *Ohnhaus, E. E., Münch, U., Meier, J (1976):* Schweiz. Med. Wochenschr. 106, 1748—1750
12. *Bianchetti, G., Graziani, G., Brancaccio, D., Morganti, A. Leonetti, G., Manfrin, M., Sega, R., Gomeni, R., Ponticelli, C., and Morselli, P. L.: (1976):* Clin. Pharmacokinetics 1. 373—384
13. *Lowenthal, D. T., Briggs, W. A., Gibson, T. P., Nelson, H., Cirksena, W. J.: (1974):* Clin. Pharmacol. Therap. 16, 761—768

J. M., Sandoz Ltd., 4002 Basle, Schwitzerland

THE ANTIHYPERTENSIVE AND ANTIARRHYTHMIC EFFECT OF PINDOLOL

J. POKORNÝ, A. HEYROVSKÝ, V. BAZIKA and J. TIŠEROVÁ

Laboratory of Angiology, IVth Medical Clinic, Prague, Czechoslovakia

The aim of the present study was to evaluate, above all, the antihypertensive effect of pindolol alone or in combination with diuretics and then to discuss the reduction of pulse rate and also arrhythmias after oral administration of pindolol at the end of exercise.

Among the various types of antiarrhythmic agents now available, beta-adrenoreceptor blocking drugs have attained a definite place in clinical cardiology. There exists evidence that this class of drugs exert their clinically observed antiarrhythmic activity by antagonizing the actions of catecholamines on automaticity and conduction. It is possible that some extracardiac effects of beta-blocking agents in particular blockade of the mobilization of fatty acids by catecholamines, could contribute to their antiarrhythmic action; however at present this remains highly speculative and is under investigation in several laboratories including our own.

From the clinical point of view, beta-blocking agents have equipped physicians with a rational approach to treat the various types of arrhythmias especially when they are induced by exercise. In our study exercise-induced tachycardia was chosen because it was thought to be more closely related to the physiological beta-adrenoreceptor stimulation occurring in normal life. The degree of beta-blockade was assessed by measuring the blood pressure and pulse rate in recumbent position in the morning before the morning dose of the drug.

Thirty five outpatients in an age-range between 35 and 50 years with essential or renal hypertension were recruited for this part of study. We have chosen to study men within a narrow age span in order to minimize any influence of age and sex on the variables studied.

After a washout period of two weeks (for eliminating the effects of eventually previously administered drugs) during which the patients received one placebo tablet daily, the treatment commenced with 15 mg pindolol, given daily in the morning for 3 weeks (period 1). If the response was satisfactory, this was followed by 15 mg pindolol only during the period 2 which lasted two weeks. In patients in whom the response after the first 3 weeks was unsatisfactory, 7.5 mg pindolol was added at noon. Thereafter the non-responders received 30 mg pindolol daily (15 mg in the morning and 15 mg in the afternoon) in the third period lasting two weeks again. However, 8 patients in whom a satisfactory response was still not obtained were given 15 mg pindolol and 5 mg clopamide twice a day successfully (Fig. 1). A completely satisfactory response to treatment was defined as a systolic pressure maintained at 140 torr and diastolic pressure of not more than 95 torr. According to these criteria 27 out of 35 cases were treated satisfactorily with pindolol alone. Of these 27 patients, the majority (20) belonged to WHO stage 1. and 7 to WHO stage 2. As mentioned above, in 8 patients we did not attain a fall in systolic blood pressure to 140 torr or in dias-

BLOOD PRESSURE		SIDE EFFECTS	
VERY GOOD	27	29	NONE
GOOD	6	4	FEW
SUFFICIENT	2	2	MANY

TAB.I   EFFECT OF PINDOLOL IN 35 PATIENTS WITH HYPERTENSION

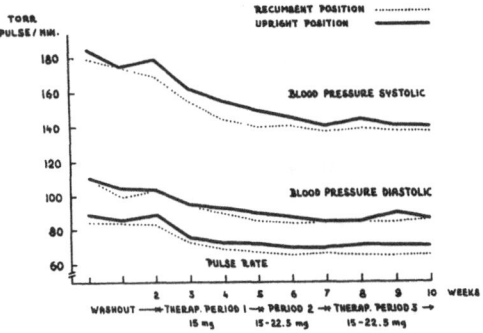

EFFECT OF PINDOLOL ON BLOOD PRESSURE AND PULSE RATE

Fig. 1.

tolic blood pressure to 95 torr. However, as compared to the placebo period, they showed a significant fall both in systolic and diastolic blood pressure ($2p < 0.01$). Out of these 8 patients, 6 belonged to WHO stage 2 and 2 of them to stage 1. Only patients with a systolic pressure 170 and diastolic pressure 100 torr and more at the end of a run-in (washout) period were included in the study. During the trial, no other drugs were administered.

Fig. 2 shows that not only blood pressure but also the heart rate were markedly reduced after administration of 15 mg pindolol:

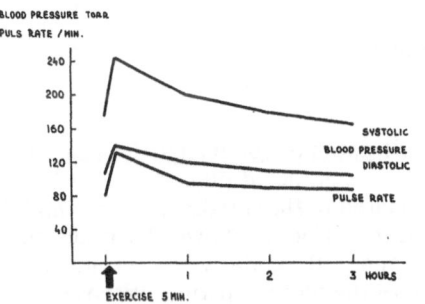

INHIBITION OF EXERCISE - INDUCED HYPERTENSION AND ARRYTHMIA BY PINDOLOL ADMINISTERED ORALLY (15 mg)

Fig. 2.

As we know, another method to evaluate the beta-receptor blockade is to compare the heart rate and blood pressure during physical exercise before and after a administration of the drug. Five of our hypertensives (men) exercised on a bicycle ergometer with a work load of 100 W for 5 min. This produced a mean increase in systolic blood pressure to 235 torr and in the heart rate to 140 beats/min. This heart rate and blood pressure increase at the end of exercise were lowered within one hour after oral administration of 15 mg pindolol (given immediately after exercise) on the average to 90 beats/min, to 165 torr of systolic blood pressure and 110 torr of diastolic blood pressure. It maximally dropped, to 86 beats/min, to 155 torr of systolic blood pressure and 100 torr of diastolic blood pressure on the range after 3 hours. However, increased pulse rate and hypertension induced by exercise without pindolol lasted twice as long.

As regards the duration of pindolol action we found that one dose daily is sufficient and practically as effective in controlling high blood pressure as 3 doses a day. Pindolol and nearly all beta-blocking drugs as well have been found to increase exercise tolerance and to have a prophylactic utility in the treatment of angina pectoris. Furthermore, in the treatment of hypertension and angina pectoris or arrhythmias beta-blocking agents may have a double advantage.

We are far from pretending that drug treatment with beta-blockers is the only approach to the problem of hypertension therapy. Nevertheless, treatment with beta-blocking agents is part of the total therapeutical approach to the patient suffering from hypertension. In conclusion we can also claim that the beneficial effects of beta-adrenoreceptor blocking drugs in the treatment of hypertension, arrythmias and angina pectoris are now well established.

J. P., Lab. of Angiology, 128 08 Prague 2, U nemocnice 2, Czechoslovakia

ANTIHYPERTENSIVE EFFECT OF PINDOLOL (VISKEN) AND A COMBINATION OF PINDOLOL AND CLOPAMIDE (BRINALDIX) IN MODERATE HYPERTENSION

ESTHER TÖRÖK, M. WAGNER and M. ERDÉLYI

Hungarian Institute of Cardiology, Division of Clinical Pharmacology, Budapest, Hungary

We previously found Visken at a dose of 30 mg (15 – 45 mg) daily to control blood pressure (BP) in more than half the patients with moderate hypertension without causing bradycardia or cardiodepressive action. However, BP control could be obtained only with higher than 15 mg of Visken in the majority of the patients.

The aim of the present study was

1. to compare the antihypertensive effect of Visken 10 mg when used alone and in combination with saluretic clopamide (Brinaldix), 5 mg,

2. to determine the effects when doubling the doses of the drugs,

3. to evaluate the side effects of the combination.

Patients and methods

Twelve outpatients entered the trial. The 9 women and 3 men, aged 51 (29 – 64) years had essential hypertension of moderate severity as estimated by the criteria of the Veterans Administration Cooperative Study (1960). The average known duration of hypertension was 11 ± 8 years.

Table I.

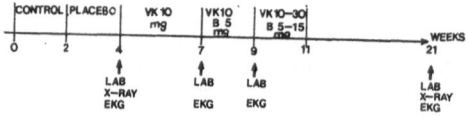

PATIENTS AND SCHEME OF VISKEN + BRINALDIX STUDY

NUMBER OF PATIENTS: 12
AGE: 51 ± 10/29 – 64/YEARS
SEX: M: 3 F: 9
STADE OF HYPERTENSION
WHO II: 8 WHO III: 4
/ VETERANS: 8 – 15 SCORES

DURATION OF HYPERTENSION 11 ± 8 YEARS
DURATION OF THE STUDY 21 ± 5 WEEKS

EVERY WEEK:
BLOOD PRESSURE AND HEART RATE

A single blind study (Table I.) was conducted over a period of 21 ± 5 weeks and consisted of a two week period without medication two weeks on a placebo, three weeks on Visken, 10 mg, fourteen weeks on a combination of Visken 10 mg and Brinaldix 5 mg daily augmented every other week until BP normalized (diastolic BP 95 mmHg in patients aged over 40 years and 90 mmHg under 40 years) or a maximum dose of Visken 30 mg and Brinaldix, 15 mg daily was reached. 10 mg tablet of Visken and 5 mg tablet of Brinaldix were used. Visken, 10 mg, then the combination of Visken, 10 mg plus Brinaldix, 5 mg, were administered in a once a day dosage. Where it was indicated, the doses of the Visken plus Brinaldix combination were increased at a ratio of 2 : 1.

The patients were seen every week throughout the trial, when the severity of symptoms, eventual side effects, BP and heart rate were recorded in the supine, sitting and standing position. At the end of the placebo period and after each two week interval detailed laboratory tests were performed. At the beginning and end of the trial a 12 lead ECG and heart volume measurement, using the formula L × B × D × 0.4 were done. Statistical methods: paired "t" test and the Wilcoxon test were used.

Results

All patients completed the trial. There was no significant difference in BP values measured in the standing, sitting and lying position. Fig. 1. shows the mean sitting BP and HR of the whole group. At the end of the placebo period, BP rose insignificantly from 163/101 to 167/107 mm Hg. Visken alone, 10 mg daily produced no change in mean BP, whereas the combination of Visken, 10 mg plus Brinaldix, 5 mg caused an appreciable fall in systolic and diastolic BP from 167 ± 13 (107 ± to 144 ± 15) 96 ± 7 mm Hg. These changes were significant when compared with placebo or Visken alone (p < 0.01). The heart

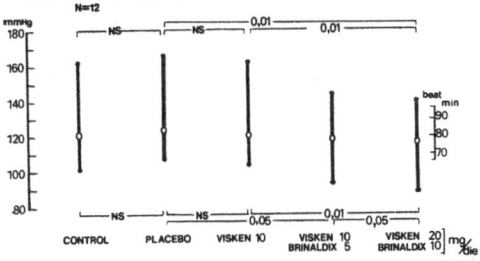

CHANGES IN BLOOD PRESSURE AND HEART RATE
DURING THE VISKEN BRINALDIX STUDY

Fig. 1.

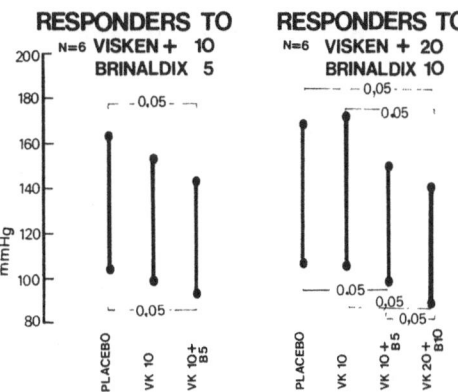

Fig. 2.

rate was significantly reduced from 84 ± 8 to 76 ± 8 beats/min with the higher doses of the combination (p < 0.05).

Treatment with the combination led to a good BP control in 11 out of 12 patients (Table II.). In six out of them this was achieved with the smaller doses of the combination. In six patients only higher doses were effective. No difference could be found between the two groups regarding age and pretreatment BP (Fig. 2.). Once the optimum doses had been reached,

Table II.

INDIVIDUAL BLOOD PRESSURE RESPONSES TO TREATMENT WITH VISKEN + BRINALDIX

DIAST BP mmHg	PLACEBO	TREATMENT VK + B
90	0	8
95	0	3
100	3	1
105	5	0
110	2	0
120	2	0

rapid onset of action was seen and BP remained well controlled over the subsequent phase of the trial. Once a day dosage was effective in patients receiving the smaller doses of the combination. At the end of the treatment period, the heart volume index showed a small but significant decrease from 690 ± 40 to 638 ± 30 ml/m^2 (p < 0.05). ECG showed no change. A small but significant decrease in serum potassium, chloride, creatinine and an increase in serum uric acid and blood sugar were observed (in all instances p < 0.05).

After initiating treatment with Brinaldix, 5 mg daily one patient showed a serum potassium value of 3.3 mE/1 and one patient developed a value of 3.4 mE/1 on Brinaldix, 15 mg daily. In both cases serum potassium values increased spontaneously. At the end of the trial no patient showed values for serum potassium less than 3.8 mE/1. No side effects were encountered.

REFERENCES

Collins, I. S., King, I. W. (1972): Pindolol (Visken, LB 46), a new treatment for hypertension; report of a multicentric open study. Curr. ther. Res. 14: 185—194.

Thorpe, P. (1972): A controlled study of pindolol (Visken) in hypertension. Med. J. Aust. ii: 306—309.

E. T., [Hungarian Institute of Cardiology, H-1450 Budapest P.O. Box. 88, Hungary

DOES BETA BLOCKADE AFFECT BLOOD FLOW TO THE LIMBS?

D. L. CLEMENT

*Department of Cardiology, Section of Hypertension,
University Hospital, Gent, Belgium*

Intermittent claudication and vaso-spastic signs are reported as side effects of non-selective beta blockade (*Conway*, 1975; *Marshall et al.*, 1976; *Rodger et al.*, 1976). If these side effects are due to beta block-ade of the vessels, selective beta-1-blockers might prevent these symptoms. However, direct information concerning this aspect in man is scarce (*Johnson*, 1975; *Van Herwaarden et al.*, 1977). Therefore, in the present work, isoproterenol dose-response curves on muscle blood flow were made before and after selective (metoprolol) and nonselective beta blockade (propranolol).

Patients and methods

Experiments were performed on nine patients with moderate essential hypertension. All anti-hypertensive treatment was withdrawn at least two weeks before the first test was done.

The patients were lying quietly on a couch; blood pressure was measured in the right arm. Blood flow was determined with an EG-triggered venous occlusion plethysmograph (Periflow, Janssen) in the left calf.

Isoproterenol was infused I. V. at a dose of $2-10 \,\mu g/min$ before and after administration of one beta blocker and one week later before and after the other beta blocker. The choice of giving metoprolol (10 mg total dose) or propra-nolol (5 mg total dose) was made at random to the double-blind test.

Results

The increase in the heart rate with iso-proterenol is significantly more inhibited by propranolol than by metoprolol; the latter shifts the dose-response curve to the right but much less than propranolol.

The increase in systolic blood pressure with isoproterenol is completely abolished by metoprolol and to a lesser degree by propranolol. On the contrary, the decrease in diastolic blood pressure with isoprote-renol is much more inhibited by propra-nolol than by metoprolol. As a result, pulse pressure is inhibited by both blockers but significantly more by propranolol than by metoprolol ($p < 0.01$).

The increase in calf blood flow with isoproterenol is significantly more inhi-bited by propranolol than by metoprolol. The latter shifts the curve to the right, but it remains significantly closer to the control than after propranolol. The same conclu-sions can be made even when the results are expressed as absolute or relative flow values and also in terms of calculated vas-cular resistance.

Discussion

The data demonstrate that in hyperten-sive patients there is a quantitative dif-ference in the beta blocking properties of propranolol and metoprolol as assessed from the dose response curve to isoprote-renol. The decrease in diastolic blood pressure and the increase in the heart rate with isoproterenol are significantly less in-hibited by metoprolol than by propranolol. It is likely that this difference is due to a different degree of beta blockade at the level of the vascular receptors, since the increase in calf blood flow isoproterenol is significantly less depressed by meto-prolol than by propranolol. These results suggest that the vascular response to sym-pathetic stimulation is significantly less affected after beta blockade with meto-prolol than after beta blockade with pro-pranolol.

636

REFERENCES

Clement, D. L., (1977): Blood pressure variability in hospitalized patients. Acta Clin. Belgica 32, 163—167.

Clement, D. L., (1977): Effect of Beta-Adrenergic Blockade on Blood Pressure Variation in Patients with Moderate Hypertension. Europ. J. Clin. Pharmacol. 11, 325—327.

Conway, J. (1975): Beta adrenergic blockade and hypertension. Modern Trends in Cardiology — 3; Butterworths, 376—403.

Johnsson, G., (1975): Influence of metoprolol and propranolol on hemodynamic effects induced by adrenaline and physical work. Acta Pharmacol. Toxicol. 36, Suppl. V, 59 to 68.

Marshall, A. J., Roberts, C. J. C., Barritt, D. W. (1976): Raynaud's phenomenon as side effect of beta-blockers in hypertension. Brit. Med. J. 1, 1498—1499.

Rodger, J. C., Sheldon, C. D., Lerski, R. A., Livingstone W. R., (1976): Intermittent claudication complicating beta-blockade. Brit. Med. J. 1, 1125.

Van Herwaarden, C. L. A., Fennis, J. F. M., Binkhorst, R. A., Van't Laar, A., (1977): Haemodynamic effect of adrenaline during treatment of hypertensive patients with propranolol and metoprolol. Europ. J. of Clin. Pharmacol. 12, 397—402.

D. L. C., Dept. of Cardiovascular Diseases, De Pintelaan 135, B-9000 Gent, Belgium

PHARMACOLOGY AND PHARMAKOKINETICS OF TRIMEPRANOL (SYMPOSIUM)

EXPERIMENTAL PHARMACOLOGY

V. TRČKA, M. VANĚČEK, I. HELFERT and S. MÁCOVÁ

Research Institute of Pharmacy and Biochemistry, Prague, Czechoslovakia

Thanks to their good therapeutic effects, beta-blockers have became a valuable component of cardiovascular therapy. At present, more than ten preparations of this type are used clinically.

In Czechoslovakia, besides other beta-blocking drugs, the original Czechoslovak preparation Trimepranol (INN metipranolol) has been used for almost ten years. This substance, 1-(2,3,5-trimethyl-4-acetoxyphenoxy)-3-isopropylamino-2-propanol- is protected by several domestic (*Bláha et al.*, 1968) and many foreign patents. It is now also marketed by Boehringer Mannheim as Disorat and, in combination with Saltucin (butizid), as Torrat in the FRG.

The position of metipranolol (MP) among other most frequently used beta-blocking drugs is described elsewhere in this collection (*Trčka et al.*, 1979). In the present paper some other aspects of the effects of MP are discussed.

An example of the fundamental effects and activity of MP is the data on anaesthetized cats, summarized in Tab. 1. To simplify the comparison, the results are expressed in terms of relative efficacy values, using MP as a standard with efficacy equalling unity. The minimal effective doses producing statistically significant effects were chosen as criteria of the activity. Table I shows that, with the exception of pindolol, every drug tested exerted a lower effect on the basal heart rate and a lower antagonizing effect on isoprenaline-induced tachycardia than MP.

Table I. Relative activity of 6 beta-blocking agents in anaesthetized cats and guinea pigs and in isolated guinea-pig trachea

	Meti-pranolol	Propra-nolol	Oxpre-nolol	Alpre-nolol	Pindo-lol	Practo-lol
Cats						
Basal heart rate	1.0	0.25	0.2	0.2	3.0	0.005
Anti-isoprenaline activity on heart rate	1.0	0.25	0.5	0.5	4.0	0.05
Anti-isoprenaline activity on diastolic pressure	1.0	2.5	2.5	2.0	12.0	0.03
Guinea pigs						
Ratio of relative anti-isoprenaline activity on isolated trachea to anti-isoprenaline activity on the heart rate	1.0	8.0	2.2	2.5	1.5	0.35

The blocking effect of MP on isoprenaline-induced lowering of diastolic blood pressure was weaker in comparison with the other agents, with the exception of practolol. A relatively weaker blockade of beta$_2$ — receptors by MP had been also proved in guinea pigs. The quotient expressing the relationship between the anti-isoprenaline effects of MP on isolated guinea-pig trachea and on the heart rate is one eigth that of propranolol (Tab. I).

Among clinicists apprehension is felt concerning the lowering effect of beta-blockers on myocardial contractility. Individual agents, however, differ considerably in this respect. After doses equally effective on the heart rate, that is 0.3 mg. .kg^{-1} of MP and 1.2 mg.kg^{-1} of propranolol i.v. (Tab. II), a significant difference was found in dogs in the decrease in cardiac output. After MP the decrease in cardiac output was caused solely by a deceleration of the heart rate. The pulse volume increased after MP, but decreased after propranolol.

Table II. Effect of metipranolol (0.3 mg . kg^{-1} i.v.) and propranolol (1.2 mg . kg^{-1} i.v.) on the cardiac output and other circulatory parameters in anaesthetized dogs expressed in per cent of the initial values

	Metipranolol M (s_M)	Propranolol M (s_M)
Cardiac output	83 (3.2)	60 (3.7)*
Pulse volume	19 (5.1)	−14 (6.9)*
Mean transit time	145 (7.1)	190 (13.7)*
Peripheral resistence	109 (8.7)	162 (9.3)*
Central blood volume	112 (5.6)	108 (10.6)
Mean arterial pressure	90 (5.7)	94 (3.7)
Heart rate	69 (2.2)	71 (2.9)

* statistically significantly different from metipranolol (p > 0.05)

The isoprenaline-induced increase in myocardial contractility is reliably blocked by MP both *in vitro* and *in vivo*. The antagonism to isoprenaline in electrically stimulated isolated rabbit left atria (Tab. III) may serve as an example.

The antiarrhythmic activity of MP has been demonstrated in a great variety of tests. As a example, its effect on the functional refractory phase in comparison with other agents is given in Table III.

In conscious spontaneously hypertensive rats with hypertension over 200 torr, a combination of MP with chlorthalidone

Table III. Anti-isoprenaline activity and activity on functional refractory phase in isolated electrically stimulated rabbit left atria

	Anti-isoprenaline activity pA$_2$	Activity on functional refractory phase EC 50 M . ml^{-1}
Pindolol	10.73	$1.4 \cdot 10^{-9}$
Metipranolol	10.06	$1.6 \cdot 10^{-8}$
Tolamolol	10.03	$1.0 \cdot 10^{-7}$
Timolol	9.97	$5.0 \cdot 10^{-7}$
Propranolol	9.75	$2.6 \cdot 10^{-8}$
Atenolol	8.94	$1.6 \cdot 10^{-6}$

and dihydroergocrystine caused a profound drop in blood pressure with a maximum 6 hours after oral administration. A slight decrease in blood pressure after administration of this combination was also observed in normotensive monkeys.

In the light of pharmacological findings, of which only a selection is presented here, MP belongs to the group of most effective blockers (*Trčka et al.* 1979). It possesses a certain degree of cardioselectivity. It differs from other beta-blocking agents particularly in its very low effect on spontaneous myocardial contractility. In this relatively lower negative inotropic activity of MP, also described elsewhere in this collection (*Trčka et al.* 1979), together with its high beta-blocking and antiarrhythmic activities, we see an argument favouring the application of MP in an attempt to test the suggestion by Z. Fejfar, namely, to administer a beta-blocker in the early stage of developing myocardial infarction as a first-aid measure before the arrival of a mobile coronary unit.

REFERENCES

Bláha, L., Weichet, J., Hodrová, J., Trčka, V. (1968): Czechoslovak patent No. 128 471 and No. 143 069.

Trčka, V., Vaněček, M., Helfert, I., Mácová, S. (1979): Metipranolol and several other beta-blocking agents — a comparative pharmacological study. This collection, p. 627.

V. T., Research Institute for Pharmacy and Biochemistry Kouřimská 17, 130 00 Praha 3 Czechoslovakia

EFFECTS ON CARDIAC FUNCTION IN DOG

M. VRÁNA, Z. FEJFAR, I. VANĚK, L. HEJHAL and Z. WINTER

Cardiovascular Research Centre of the Institute for Clinical and Experimental Medicine, Prague 146 22, Czechoslovakia

The effect of Trimepranol (metripranolol) on heart frequency, ventricular fibrillation and left ventricular performance has been compared with surgical denervation of the heart.

Methods

Acute experiments were performed on mongrel dogs in pentobarbital anaesthesia. Other experiments were also carried out on nonanaesthetized dogs trained in running exercise. Tendency to ventricular fibrillation was assessed from the level of ventricular fibrillation threshold. Short series of 400 msec alternating current impulses were induced at increasing intensity into the apex of the right ventricle of anaesthetized dogs at 8 sec intervals via a catheterization electrode. Increasing the stimulating current first elicited premature ventricular contractions, then produced ventricular tachycardia and finally resulted in ventricular fibrillation. The current intensity at which ventricular fibrillation sets in has been called the ventricular fibrillation threshold (VFT).

Ischemic damage to the left ventricle was produced by ligature of the anterior descending branch of the left coronary artery in open chest dog preparations. Ventricular pump function was investigated during increasing loading pressure in the right auricle. (1) Surgical sympathetic denervation of the heart was performed by bilateral extirpation of the stellate and thoracic ganglia to the level of Th 5. The effect of denervation was studied in acute experiments and in dogs 6 to 18 months after the denervation.

The drugs were dosed as follows: Trimepranol 0.3 mg/kg b. w. and Pentobarbital 20 mg/kg b. w.

Results

Heart frequency

Trimepranol injected intravenously into dogs with pentobarbital anaesthesia reduces the heart frequency by about 30%. A similar decrease was observed after cardiac denervation by excision of the right

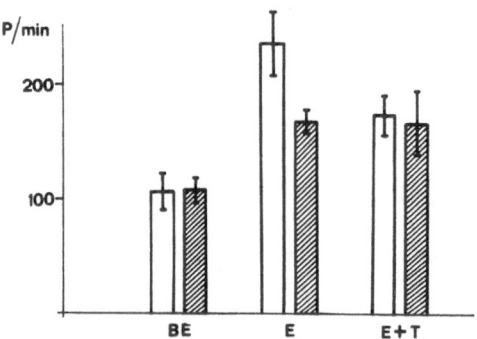

Fig. 1. Changes in the heart frequency (P) of unanaesthetized dogs before (BE), during running exercise (E) and under the combined effect of Trimepranol and exercise (E + T). Open and shaded columns relate to dogs prior and after sympathetic denervation, respectively.

but not the left stellate ganglion. Heart frequency in the non-anaesthetized dogs at rest did not change significantly either after heart denervation or after Trimepranol (Fig. 1). Exercise (E), Trimepranol or cardiac denervation or the two combined (E + T) reduced heart frequency by 28% versus control values prior to surgical or pharmacological treatment.

Ventricular fibrillation

There was an abrupt fall in VFT in the first phase after Harris (2). Trimepranol was found to be capable not only of preventing a decrease but, on the contrary, of eliciting a multiple increase in VFT. A similar rise in VFT was also seen in animals treated 15 min following the ligation of the artery. (Fig. 2)

Ventricular performance

If cardiac performance is increased by sympathetic activation (e.g. by pentobarbital anaesthesia or exercise) it tends to decrease both by the application of Trimepranol and surgical denervation. If there is no sympathetic activation, cardiac performance does not change after Trimepranol is applied. (Fig. 3)

Conclusion

The effect of Trimepranol on heart frequency, ventricular fibrillation and heart performance is comparable to the effect of sympathetic denervation of the heart. Trimepranol produces a conspicuous rise in ventricular fibrillation threshold in ischemic hearts. This observation confirms the antifibrillation effect of Trimepranol. Ventricular pump function de-

creases after Trimepranol due to its suppressive effect on sympathetic heart innervation. Therefore overall heart performance is decreased in all animals with primary elevated sympathetic heart activation.

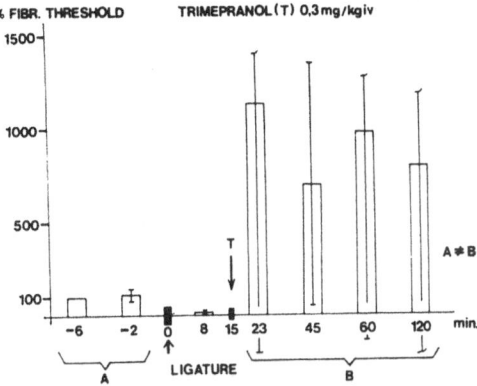

Fig. 2. Relative fibrillation threshold of animal hearts with ischemic damage under pentobarbital anaesthesia. Trimepranol brings about a substantial threshold increase even when applied 15 minutes following coronary artery ligation.

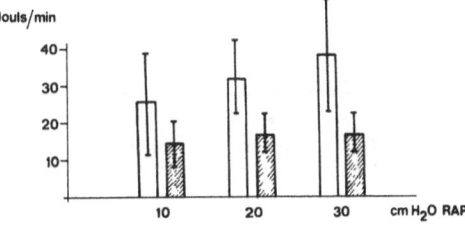

Fig. 3. Heart performance prior (white columns) and after (shaded columns) sympathetic denervation responding to various loading pressure in the right auricle (RAP). 10 cm H_2O equals approximately 1 kPa.

REFERENCES

1. *Guyton A. C.:* Determination of cardiac output by equating venous return curves with cardiac response curves. Physiol. Rev. 35, 1955, pp. 123—129.

2. *Harris A. S. et al.:* Ventricular ectopic rhythms and ventricular fibrillation following cardiac sympathectomy and coronary occlusion. Amer. J. Physiol. 165, 1951, pp. 505 to 512.

M. V. Cardiovascular Research Centre, IKEM, Vídeňská 800, 146 22 Prague 4, Czechoslovakia

PHARMACOKINETICS AND EFFECTS ON HEART ACTION IN MAN

O. MAYER, V. ČEPELÁK, J. VITOUŠ and J. POTMĚŠIL

Dept. of Clinical Pharmacology and Clinic of Medicine, Faculty Hospital, Plzeň, Czechoslovakia

Our present report concerns a study comparing the kinetic properties of metipranolol (Trimepranol) with its cardiac β-blocking effects in healthy volunteers.

Trimepranol (TMP) was determined by a gas chromatographic technique as an active metabolite desacetyltrimepranol. The plasma levels, reached after a single oral dose of 40 mg trimepranol, were followed. In this part of the study, conventional linear regression methods were used for evaluation of the pharmacokinetic constants (Table I.).

The absorption rate of TMP from the gastrointestinal tract appeared surprisingly rapid and corresponded to a half-life of 18 minutes, or in another group of probands (not included in Tab. I.) to only 9 minutes. This finding suggests that absorption of TMP starts in the stomach. The elimination rate of TMP correspdnded to 4 hours when applying a one-compartment model. In case of a two-compartment model (not included in Tab. I.), the faster constant α, corresponding to a half-life of

	n	k_a (min⁻¹)	$t_{1/2}$ a (min)	k_e (min⁻¹)	$t_{1/2}$ (min)	C_{max} (ng/ml)	t_{max} (min)	S (ng.min.ml⁻¹)
$\bar{x}$	13	0.0621	18	0.0075	249	95	60	33350
s_x		0.0067	2	0.0058	70	13	13	7882
min		0.0138	3	0.0009	19	80	20	3045
max		0.2440	50	0.0366	706	214	150	80320

Tab. I. Pharmocokinetic parameters derived from single oral dose of trimepranol (40 mg). k_a, absorption rate constant; $t_{1/2}$ a, half-life of absorption; k_e, elimination rate constant; $t_{1/2}$, half-life of elimination; C_{max}, peak plasma concentration; t_{max}, time of peak plasma concentration; S, area under plasma concentration curve, calculated to infinity. All values are given as $\bar{x} \pm s_{\bar{x}}$.

21 minutes, and the slower constant β, corresponding to a half-life of approximately 4 hours, were distinguished. The peak plasma concentration (C_{max}) was found at the level of 95 ng/ml. The area under plasma concentration curve (S) varied considerably, suggesting that the bioavailability displays interindividual variations.

We attempted to establish whether the rapid absorption from GIT was associated with the rapid onset of a pharmacodynamic effect. For this purpose the dynamics of the antiisoprenaline effect of TMP (40 mg again dosed orally) was followed. Both before and at various intervals after TMP administration, intravenous doses of isoprenaline were titrated. A rapid onset of this effect during the first 20 minutes was demonstrated; the peak effect was observed between the 2nd and 3rd hour, the necessary effective doses of isoprenaline being 15 to 20 fold higher when compared with the premedication dose (before the TMP administration). As late as after 10 hours, the antiisoprenaline effect of TMP was still present.

The resting heart rate was not influenced to a considerable degree by the above dose of TMP. The maximum bradycardia was observed from 2−2.5 hours after the administration (the heart rate reduction corresponded to 10%), and the initial value was resumed 8 hours after ingestion of TMP. The effect of TMP appeared more pronounced on the exercise tachycardia, evoked by a load of 1.5 W/kg on a bicycle ergometer. Development of the β-blocking effect on the exercise tachycardia was observed as early as 25 minutes after TMP administration, when the heart rate increased by 25 bpm less than before ingestion of TMP; the peak effect was observed after 2.5 hour, and the tachycardic response remained reduced 8 hours after TMP administration.

The correlation between the plasma levels of TMP and its pharmacodynamic effects was also investigated after repetitive administration, i.e. in 20 mg doses administered orally twice daily, at the relatively long intervals of 12 hours. A tendency to stabilization of the plasma concentration at the level of 60 ng/ml was evident from the 3rd day of repetitive administration. When the medication was terminated on the 7th day, TMP disappeared from the plasma with a short half-life of 2.5 hours. Both the rest heart rate and the exercise tachycardia were measured under the same conditions. (Fig. 1). A reduction of the rest heart rate to the value of 50−60 bpm was found without major fluctuations throughout the followed period. A very standard response was also obtained after repetitive exercise on the bicycle ergometer. The heart rate values were always 30−40 bpm lower than the initial values before the first dose of TMP. From the results presented it can be derived that the pharmacodynamic action of TMP is not subject to such short-term variations as the TMP plasma levels.

In our study we also followed an additional problem, i.e. the TMP-atropine interaction during its absorption from

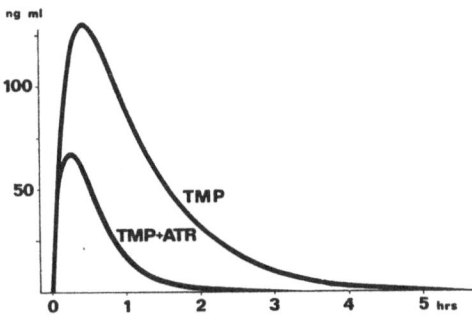

Fig. 2. Plasma trimepranol concentrations following oral administration of 40 mg trimepranol alone or in combination with 1 mg atropine. The summary curves are characterized by the mean values of the absorption and elimination constants and those of areas under the plasmatic concentration curves, $n = 10$.

GIT. A single oral dose of 40 mg TMP with 1 mg atropine was administered. After the single TMP administration, the areas under the plasma concentration curves as well as the other pharmacokinetic constants were larger in 8 out of 10 cases. (In this case the calculations were made by a more exact iteration method.) For a simple illustration in Fig. 2 depicts a summary curve characterized by mean values of the absorption and elimination constants and those of areas under the plasmatic concentration curves. It is clearly evident that the bioavailability of the sole TMP was better than in combination with atropine.

In conclusion, TMP is a potent β-blocking agent, whose reliable effect may be expected even after dosages lower than those so far recommended. The β-blocking effect persists even though TMP disappears from the central compartment, namely, in the case of a single administration as late as 10 hours after ingestion, while still longer in the case of repetitive administration. A peculiar property of TMP occur is its rapid absorption from the digestive tract, accompanied at the same time by a rapid start of the β-blocking effect.

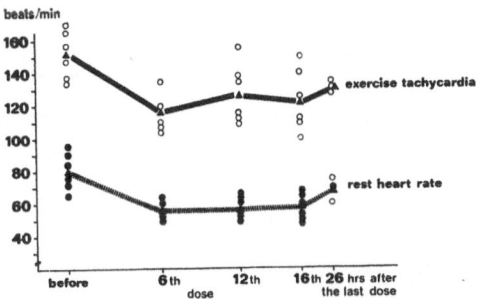

Fig. 1. Changes in rest heart rate and exercise tachycardia following repeated oral dosing with trimepranol (20 mg every 12 hours for 8 days), $n = 6$.

O. M. Dept. Clin. Pharm., Faculty Hospital, 300 00 Plzeň, Czechoslovakia

K. DIETMANN

Boehringer, Mannheim, F.R.G.

The therapeutical effectiveness and the safety of drugs can be enhanced if special knowledge on pharmacokinetics and pharmacodynamics is available. Among other beta blockers metipranolol (M) is used increasingly in Czechoslovakia and West Germany. For optimal use of this potent drug, pharmacokinetics and pharmacodynamics have been evaluated. Plasma concentrations have been measured in 20 healthy volunteers after a single oral dose of 40 mg M/subject. M is rapidly metabolized to desacetyl-M. This first and active metabolite has been analyzed by a special gaschromatic analytical procedure. In another study the plasma concentration after i. v. administration of 10 mg M/subject was measured. Mean values of pharmacokinetic parameters after oral administration are: absorption half-life 5 min, distribution half-life 20 min, half-life of elimination 2.5 h life-time 15 min, peak concentration time 40 min, peak concentration 75 microgram/liter. In Figure 1 a comparison is given between plasma concentration curves of desacetyl-M after oral administration of 40 mg M and after i. v. infusion of 10 mg M. Besides a graphical analysis we were able to calculate pharmacokinetic data using a specially developed computer program. In this way we were able to confirm our first assumption that the elimination of desacetyl-M from the blood follows first-order kinetics and that

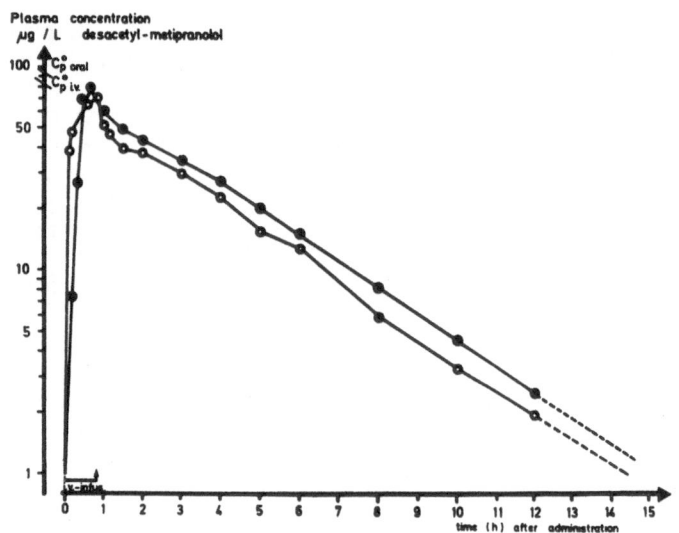

Fig. 1

the pharmacokinetics are compatible with a two-compartment model.

By graphical analysis we were able to obtain the theoretical drug concentration at time zero, i. e. the hypothetical drug concentration at this time obtained by back-extrapolation of the K_{el} slope to the ordinate. These values are useful for further calculations of the distribution volume and the dose intervals. We calculated an

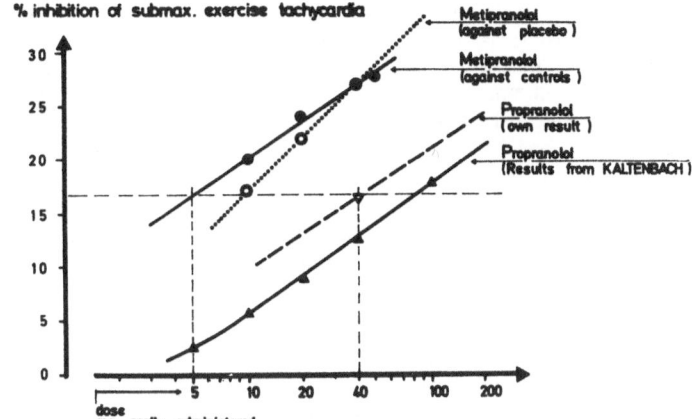

% inhibition of submax. exercise tachycardia

Metipranolol (against placebo)

Metipranolol (against controls)

Propranolol (own result)

Propranolol (Results from KALTENBACH)

dose mg orally administered

Fig. 2.

apparent distribution volume of 120 liter.

Using the trapezoid rule and the calculation of the end of the area under the curve with the help of the elimination rate constant we can compare the two areas under the curves after intravenous and oral administration (Fig. 1). Taking into account the two different doses, we calculated a bioavailability of desacetyl-M from M-tablets (Disorat[(R)]) of nearly 30%. We assume that a "first pass" effect is responsible for the diminished bioavailability of desacetyl-M after oral administration of M, an effect well known with other beta-blockers such as propranolol (P) and metoprolol.

For comparison of pharmacokinetic and pharmacodynamic behaviour of M we conducted a controlled double blind trial in healthy subjects comparing 3 oral doses of M with a placebo and 40 mg P. Beta blockade was assessed by measuring the inhibition of intrinsic beta sympathetic drive increased by a standardized submaximal exercise test on a bicycle ergometer. Maximum inhibition of exercise tachycardia with 10, 20 and 40 mg M or 40 mg P were 20, 25 and 27% or 16%. Inhibition declined linearly with time. Duration of effects were dose dependent 8, 10 and 12 h after 10, 20 and 40 mg M and 7 h after 40 mg P. In Fig. 2 the dose-dependent inhibition of tachycardia is given for the different orally administered doses of M

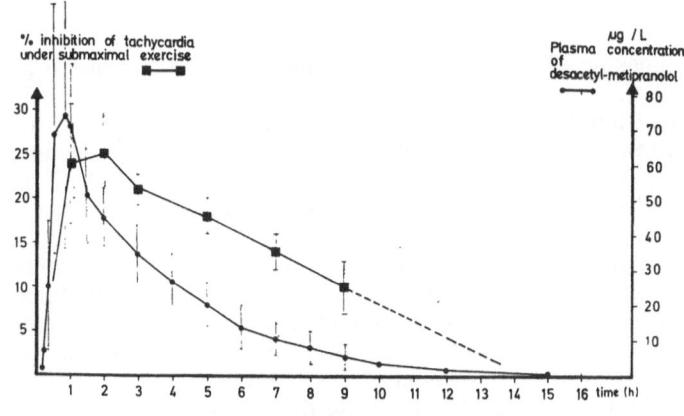

% inhibition of tachycardia under submaximal exercise

Plasma concentration of desacetyl-metipranolol µg/L

Fig. 3.

Time course of plasmaconcentration and effect after 40 mg metipranolol orally. Mean values ; N = 20

and for P. In this figure we plotted our results together with those from *Kaltenbach* From the graph in Fig. 2 we can calculate the mean equieffective dose relationship between M and P to be 1 : 6. This relationship has been confirmed in a trial on patients with angina pectoris by *Kaltenbach*.

Fig. 3 shows time curves of plasma concentration and effect after oral administration of 40 mg M. From these results we took the values of plasma concentration at the exercise times and plotted them logarithmically against a linear scale for the

relationship between concentration and effect. This limits the value of determination of plasma concentrations in adjustment of the therapeutic dose. In selected patients with poor therapeutic response and in those with impaired liver or renal function, determination of plasma concentration may be useful.

By graphical extrapolation of the concentration-effect slope in Fig. 4 we obtain a mean concentration of 3.2 micrograms/liter for a 5 to 10% inhibition of exercise-induced tachycardia, as indicated by the dotted line. We assume that this degree of

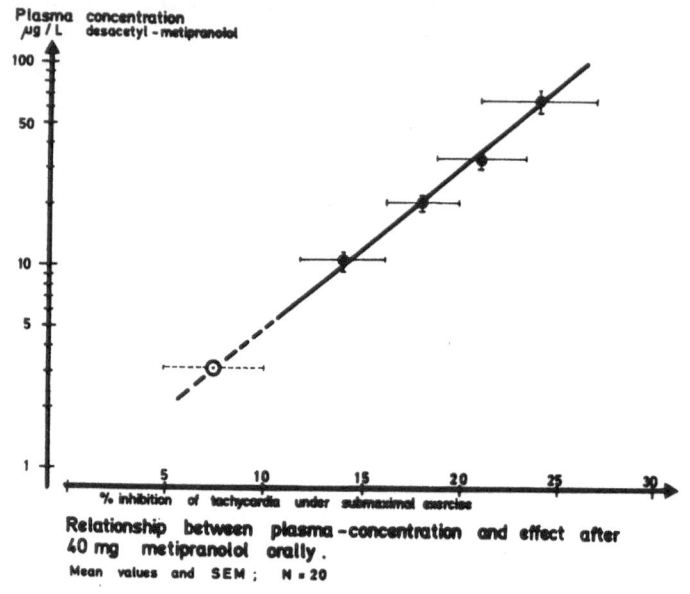

Fig. 4.

blocking effect at the different times (Fig. 4). These plots have been taken after distribution of desacetyl-M in the body. From this graphical analysis we can conclude that, on an average, the blocking effect of M is linearly related to the logarithm of the plasma concentration of desacetyl-M, as found for different beta-blockers studied, both in the acute and steady state situation. In spite of this relationship, it is difficult to predict from the mean data the individual plasma concentration, necessary for a certain degree of effect, because there exist marked interindividual differences in the slope of the

inhibition is a strong effect, in spite of the work load being very high. We know from clinical experience that even low physical stress can induce an unphysiologically high sympathetic drive to the heart in pathological cases, for instance in angina pectoris. Therefore, we can expect that the above-mentioned plasma concentration effectively enhances tolerance to physical stress in patients. We would like to define this plasma concentration as the "mimum effect concentration".

With he help of the minimum effect concentration, the hypothetical concentration at time zero for the administered dose and the elimination rate constant we can calculate the dose interval T that ensures the minimum effect concentration. Resolution of this calculation leads to a time of 12.5 hours. This calculation was able to confirm the previously established dose-dependent duration of effect by extrapolation of pharmacodynamic data. These calculations and results are only valid on an average. For the therapeutical use of M we can recommend a twice a day dose regimen.

K. D., Boehringer, Mannheim, GmbH, D 6800 Mannheim 31, F.R.G.

RENOVASCULAR HYPERTENSION

RENAL ARTERIAL FIBRODYSPLASIA AND SPECTRUM
OF THE STRUCTURAL CHANGES OF HUMAN ISCHAEMIC KIDNEY

P. T. SCARPELLI, S. PELLEGRINI-FAUSSONE, A. M. CICIANI,
R. SPROVIERO, A. PASSALEVA, S. LAMANNA and D. TURINI

School of Medicine, University of Florence, Italy

Since earlier researches on experimental Goldblatt hypertension the stenotic kidney was generally found to be free from changes due to substained chronic increase of arterial blood pressure. This kidney has been called "protected" when compared to the contralateral which, instead, completely bears the injury of systemic hypertension. In some animals, like rats, the difference in the pathomorphologic picture of the two kidneys is particularly evident. The characteristic structural changes of the "untouched" kidney are represented by areas of arteriolar necrosis surrounded by an inflammatory reaction, while in "clamped" kidney, tubular atrophy without arteriolar lesions is predominant. Few studies on stenotic human kidney revealed different degrees of glomerular damage, tubular atrophy, interstitial fibrosis and hyperplasia of juxta-glomerular apparatus.

Moreover arteriosclerotic changes of segmental and arcuate arteries and a fibroelastic thickening of small arteries were described. Fibrinoid necrosis was rarely or not at all found in renal vessels beyond the stenosis, when clinically malignant hypertension is present. This fact has been considered to prove the protective effect of the stenosis.

The purpose of this work is to review the morphological changes of human ischaemic kidney, based on light and electron microscopy and immunohistochemical studies.

Materials and methods

Renal specimens from 16 patients affected by various degrees of renal vascular disease and from 3 patients with a complete occlusion of renal artery were obtained by nephrectomy or surgical biopsy. Specimens from 5 patinets with essential malignant hypertension were also used for comparison. Tissue samples for light micro-

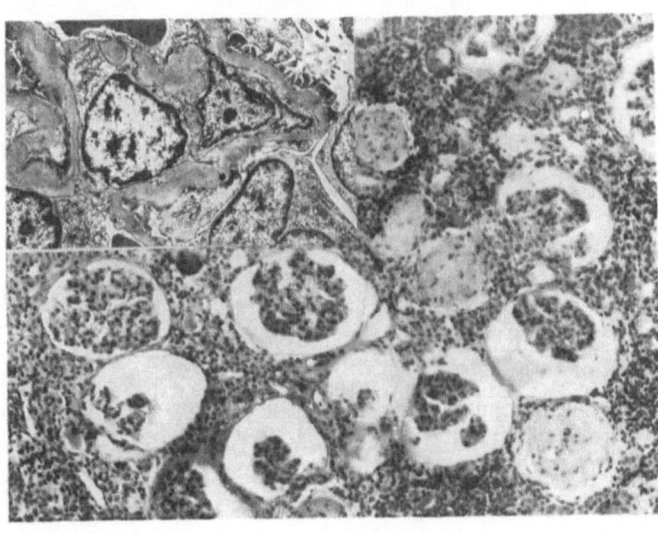

Fig. 1. Various degrees of glomerular damage. HE (×770) Inset: irregular thickening of glomerular basement membrane. E. M. (×4800).

scopy (L. M.) were fixed in Bouin's liquid and stained with heamatoxylin-eosin (HE), Periodic Acid Schiff (PAS) and Mallory-Azan (MA); for electron microscopy (E. M.) other fragments were fixed in osmium tetroxide and observed at a Siemens Elmiskop IA E. M. Tissue samples for immunofluorescence studies were processed with fluorescein-labeled anti-sera against immunoglobulins, beta-1C-globulin (C_3) and fibrinogen.

Results

Glomeruli: At L. M. various degrees of glomerular involvement up to obsolescence are observed. Glomerular size varies considerably: in the same area abnormally large, completely hyaline small and quite normal glomeruli can be found. Generally, capillary loops are decreased in number, collapsed and narrowed. With PAS stain the collapse is recognizable by wrinkling of glomerular B. M. The capsular space is often expanded and becomes filled with slight PAS+ material. Capsular B.M. appears thickened and splitted in PAS and MA stained sections. In the hyalinized glomeruli, the Bowman's space contains material organized in several layers, among which fibrocytic-like cells are found. At E.M. glomerular B. M. is occasionally thickened and wrinkled, moreover podocytes show a focal fusion of "foot processes" (Fig. 1).

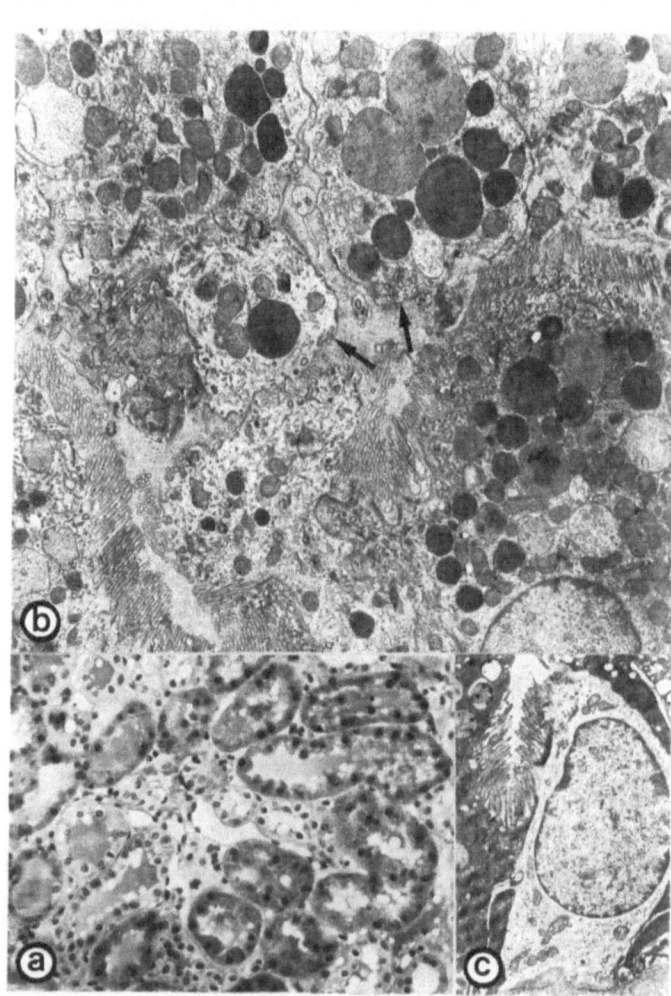

Fig. 2. a) Epithelial tubular atrophy. HE ($\times 650$), b) Tubular cells filled with lysosomes and apical blebs (arrows). E. M. ($\times 7000$), c) A regenerating tubular cell. E. M. ($\times 4800$).

Tubules: At L.M. areas of normal tubules are mixed with areas of complete atrophy, thus tubules cannot be always identified, their lumens are expanded and filled with eosinophilic and PAS+ material. When several contiguous nephrons have tubular casts, a "thyroid-like" picture can be observed. At E.M. occasionally a cytoplasmatic swelling is particularly pronounced in the apical region of cell, where the cytoplasm bulges bleb-like into the lumen. Sometimes indifferentiated regenerating epithelial tubular cells can be found (Fig. 2).

Vasa: Different types and degrees of degenerative vascular lesions are observed; hyaline arteriolosclerosis, musculo-mucoid intimal hyperplasia, "onion-skin" appearance of arterioles and rarely fibrinoid necrosis (Fig. 3). The musculo-mucoid intimal hyperplasia is characterized by an intimal thickening due to circumferentially oriented spindle cells, that are confirmed to be smooth muscle cells at E.M. The small arteries display "onion-bulb-like" splitting for the elical course of the PAS+ material and myocytes.

Juxta-glomerular apparatus: The juxta-glomerular apparatus appears hyperplastic but with few specific granules. In the walls of arterioles metaplasic changes of smooth muscle cells can be observed.

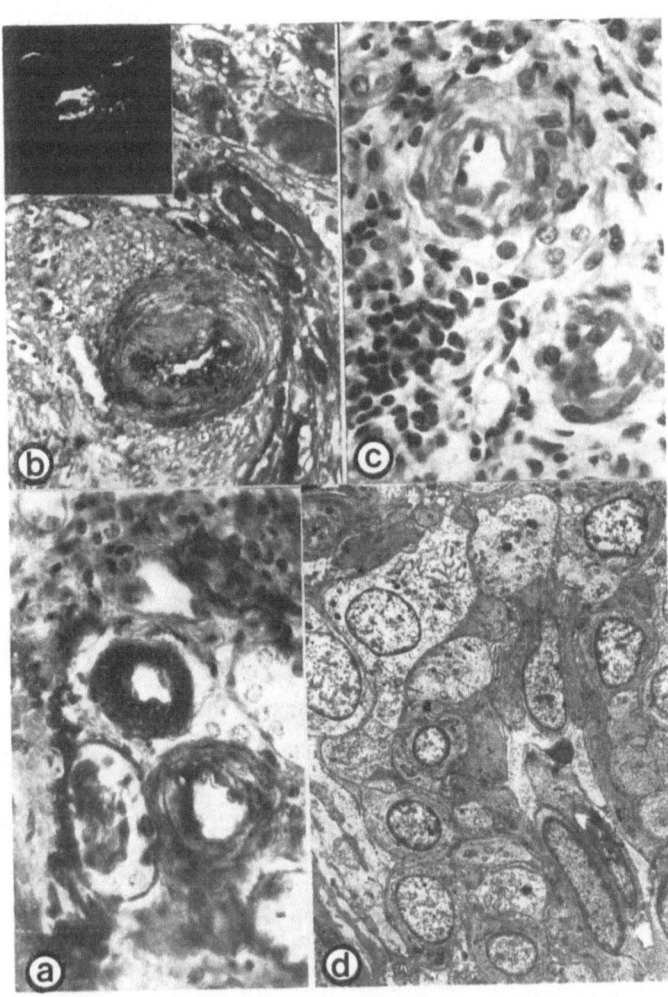

Fig. 3. Various types of vascular lesions: a) PAS (×650); b) PAS (×270); c) HE (×650), d) Hyperplasia of juxta-glomerular apparatus with few specific granules. E.M. (×2100); Inset: an arteriole with localization of C_3 in its wall (Fluorescent anti-C_3, ×180).

Immunofluorescence studies failed to reveal deposits of immunoglobulins, complement and fibrinogen on the walls of the main stenotic and intrarenal arteries. In all the 5 cases of malignant hypertension isolated finely granular deposits of C_3 in the thickened wall of arterioles and occasionally in the glomerular tufts were found. These deposits were found in the walls of arterioles only in one case of ischaemic kidney.

Discussion

Our findings show that the morphological lesions of the ischaemic kidney due to a chronic decrease of blood flow do not differ from lesions of essential malignant hypertension. The pathogenesis of structural changes of intrarenal arteries, as arteriolosclerosis, musculo-mucoid intimal hyperplasia, "onion-skin" thickening, is not completely known. It was suggested in some cases the stenosis is not a sufficient protection against the effects of increased blood pressure. However, this hypothesis is somewhat in contrast with the fact that some of our patients had a relatively moderate increase of blood pressure. On the other hand, there are other pathological condi ions, e.g. sclerodermia, which present the same renal changes even without high blood pressure. Thus it seems likely that changes are secondary to ischaemia or to ischaemia eventually together with a dyspla ic tendency extended to intrarenal vasculature.

The possible role of an immunological mechanism, based mainly on the finding of deposits of immunoglobulins, complement and fibrin on the walls of vessels, was suggested by Paronetto (1965) for the renal lesions of malignant hypertension and more recently by Dornfeld and Kaufmann (1975) for renal artery dysplasia. In our studies we found deposits of C_3 in all the 5 cases of malignant hypertension, but only once in the ischaemic kidney of reno-vascular hypertensive patients.

P. T. S., Istituto di Clinica Medica Generale e Terapia Medica (II), Cattedra di Semeiotica Medica, Università di Firenze, Italy

ANGIOGRAPHIC FINDINGS IN HYPERTENSION

H. J. MAURER, K. ARNTZ and M. JUNG

Dept. of Radiology, St. Josef-Hosp., Acad. Teaching Hosp.
of the University, Heidelberg and Inst. a. Clin. of Med. Radiology,
University, Düsseldorf, F.R.G.

Hypertension represents an important risk factor in cardiovascular disease. Two statements may illustrate this statement: 1) 2 Mio pat. with hypertension are known in the FR Germany (*Zeitler*, 1976). 2) Investigations in the USA have shown manifest hypertension in men older than 16 years in 5% and older than 20 years in up to 10% (*Heyden*, 1975).

Diagnosis of hypertension is mostly more or less by chance except on occasion of screening investigations (*Heyden*, 1975; *Widmer et al.*, 1976). Aetiology of hypertension is rarely single-factorial, but generally multi-factorial. The difficulty in disclosing the different factors is very high: On an average 70%−85% of most collectives are listed under "essential hypertension". But due to intensified investigation programs these disturbing unsatisfying numbers have been reduced to 45.5% (*Losse*, 1968) or 37.5% (*Robertson et al.*, 1962). The investigation program of hypertension has to include aortorenography as a standard method. Nevertheless, according to our knowledge and experience aortorenography is used relatively rarely in Central Europe especially if clinical or/and biochemical data do not indicate a vascular factor. Furthermore, aortorenography is applied mainly only to look for stenosis of A. renalis, whereas other anatomical, morphological and/or functional changes are more or less neglected. Therefore, we wish to demonstrate some further findings in patients with hypertension.

Table I. The angle between the aorta and renal artery

	right		left	
	n	∢°	n	∢°
Healthy	107	109.4°	107	104.5°
Hypertensives	63	111.4°	67	103.0°

Materials and methods

In the study of 334 aortorenovasographies the findings of 75 patients with hypertension were analyzed and compared with those of patients without pathological findings or other renal diseases.

No differentiation was made between males and females due to the relatively small number of cases. The majority of our patients was older than 30 years. The following items were investigated: angle of origin from the aorta (Table I), course of A. renalis (Table II (a) straight, (b) only one angle (toward cranial), (c) double or more S-shaped, number of arteries per kidney, except aberrant arteries, renal size, breadth of parenchyma, flow rate of contrast medium.

Result

In 16 of 75 patients (19.5%) accesory arteries were found.

The frequency of the different courses (Table II) due to right and left kidney

Table II. The course of renal arteries with respect to sides and types (according to Arntz and Jung) (R = right, L = left)

Type	n	(a) n	(a) %	(b) n	(b) %	(c) n	(c) %	
Healthy	107	74	69.2	17	15.9	16	14.9	R
	107	62	58	38	35.5	7	6.5	L
Hypertensives	70	44	62.9	16	22.9	16	14.2	R
	70	35	50	24	34.3	11	15.5	L

Table III. The width of parenchyme in the right and left kidney

| | right | | | | | | left | | | | | |
| | cranial | | medial | | caudal | | cranial | | medial | | caudal | |
	n	mm	n	mm	n	mm	n	mm	n	mm	n	mm
Healthy	51	32	48	25	47	31	48	31	50	24	49	31
Hypertensives	13	35	13	27	12	32	7	31	8	23	8	32

shows type (b) most frequent at right, type (c) at left kidney in comparison to the control group. The pooled types (b) and (c) are more frequent for each kidney in patients with hypertension than in the control groups. This is also evident in the pooled values of both kidneys: 43.6% - 36.4%.

Kidney size is bigger by 9.5% for the right and 4.5% for the left kidney compared with the control group. The breadth of parenchyma (Table II) measured at 3 points shows absolute values slightly greater in patients with hypertension than in the control group.

The flow rate determination was based on measurement's by Olsson: 8−10 sec. in normal kidneys. 30 of our 76 patients had flow rate of both kidneys within this time limit, 26 of 27 of the left and 4 of 76 of the right kidney alone. Prolonged flow rates were found in both kidneys in 15 of 76 patients. Thus the flow rate is extended in more than half of our patients. In only 1 patient was the flow rate shortened to 3 sec.; histological investigation showed an arterionephrosclerosis.

Atheromatic stenoses of A. renalis were found in only 10 patients of our group. Nevertheless, the findings for these patients did not differ from those for the whole hypertension group.

Discussion

Anatomical as well functional studies should be carried out in aorto-renographies in addition to morphological investigations in patients with hypertension. Regrettably, comparison with other authors' findings is difficult or impossible because of the very different techniques used. Nevertheless, anatomical, morphological and functional facts must be investigated in as much detail as possible to obtain more data enabling better diagnostic evidence.

In spite of very small differences in the angle between the aorta and aa. renales compared to that of the controls this fact should be investigated experimentally with regard to flow dynamics. According to haemodynamic studies (*Müller-Mohnseen et al.*), very small changes in this angle can have important consequences for the arterial wall and its metabolism.

The course or the renal artery changes as a result of aging from a straight to a more or less S-like shape. Nevertheless, the frequency of bent and S-shaped arteries in patients with hypertension is remarkable compared with the control group. Further investigation should deal with this change which could be primary and, therefore, could lead to development of hypertension. If secondary it would be without etiological and therapeutic importance. Follow-up studies of young patients with hypertension may give more evidence.

Multiple renal arteries are discussed as an important etiological factor in hypertension (*Bönner et al.*, *Elias, Maurer, Robertson et al.*). The angle of origin of these arteries is about 90° or less resulting in serious consequences for the arterial wall of these arteries (*Müller-Mohnsesn*). In our hypertension group a peculiar frequency does not exist; it is less than in the *Robertson et al.* group (48%). Nevertheless, this problem seems to require further investigation.

In hypertension the right kidney shows a slightly broader parenchyma than the left but this difference is very small. We did not find attenuation with regard to contracted kidney either generalized nor localized. Flow rates in patients with hypertension were prolonged in more than 50% of the cases studied.

The purpose of all vasographic investigations must be to collect as much data as possible. Beyond the usual investigation it is possible to demonstrate anatomical and morphological functional factors. But the differences found must be studied further in larger groups than ours to obtain more acurrate information, for instance if the enlargement (hypertrophy?) of the kidney in hypertension is correct, the dependence on stage, duration or other factors (compare with Halpern). At least one important factor with regard to prophylaxis: Hypertension develops in about 15% of cases after blunt lower thoracic and/or abdominal trauma (Maurer). Therefore, these traumatized patients should be investigated very carefully particular cases angiographic (Maurer) and followed up carefully.

Only if we obtain more information on as many factors as possible in hypertension it will be possible to develop better prevention and therapy.

REFERENCES

Bönner, G., H. Dreesbach, A. Helber u. W. Kaufmann (1978): Hypertonus und multiple Nierenarterien. Dtsch. med. Wschr. 103, 345—349.

Heyden, S.: Risikofaktor Hypertonie. Beiträge zur Epidemiologie und Therapie der Hypertonie. Boehringer, Mannheim 1975.

Müller-Mohnssen, H. (1976): Experimental Results to the Deposition Hypothesis of Atherosclerosis. Thrombosis Res. 8, 553—566.

Olsson, O.: Renal Angiography, in: Abrams, H. L. (Ed.) Angiography; Little, Brown a. Comp., Boston/Mass. 1971.

Zeitler, E.: Eröffnungsansprache, in: Zeitler, E. (Hrsg.): Hypertonie, Risikofakotr in der Angiologie. Witzstrock, Baden-Baden, Brüssel, Köln 1976.

Zeitler, E.: Röntgendiagnostik bei renaler Hypertonie, in: Kröpelin, Traute (Hrsg.): Pathologie und Radiologie von Hochdruck- und Nierenerkrankungen; Thieme, Stuttgart 1977.

H. J. M., Slevogtstr. 10, D-6908 Wiesloch, F.R.G.

DIURNAL RHYTHM OF ELECTROLYTE EXCRETION AND SURGICAL MANAGEMENT OF RENOVASCULAR HYPERTENSION

JARMILA STŘÍBRNÁ, V. BRODAN, P. FIRT, J. HEJNAL,
K. DRÁB and L. HEJHAL

Institute for Clinical and Experimental Medicine, Praha, Czechoslovakia

In this study we attempted to establish whether the disturbed rhythm of renal Na and water excretion is reversible following successful surgical treatment.

Materials and methods

The diurnal rhythm before and after surgery was studied in 27 patients with RVH (in 8 patients several times). The blood pressure (BP) was monitored indirectly in the sitting position and urine collected at 3 hour intervals for 24 hours, starting at 6 a. m. Blood samples were collected only in the morning. A control group of 20 normotensive volunteers was examined in the same manner. All examinations were performed during hospitalization; intake of food and liquids as well as daytime activity were not restricted. The change in urine flow, excreted amount of Na and K and calculated C_{cr} and the excretion fraction of water $(V/C_{cr}) . 100$, Na $(C_{Na}/C_{cr}) . 100$ and K $(C_K/C_{cr}) . 100$ were recorded.

Depending on the effect of surgery, patients with RVH were divided into three groups. Group 1 — "cured", diastolic BP without medical therapy was 94 mm Hg or less. Group 2 — "improved", diastolic BP was less than 95 mm Hg with the same or less intense therapy than preoperatively, or at least 15% lower without medication. Group 3 — "failure", this group also included patients with restenosis or obstruction of by-passes and one patients in whom the renal artery was desected free from fibrous band. Results were evaluated by cosinore analysis according Halberg and by the pair T-test and nonpair F—T test.

Results

The mean values and amplitudes (A), i.e. half of the difference between the maximum and minimum of the oscillations, appear in the Table. Figures 1 and 2 show changes in the excretion fraction of Na and water during 24 hours.

Group 1 — "cured hypertension":

After surgery the mean C_{Na}/C_{cr} value increased significantly, while A % decreased. The curve of the diurnal rhythm is similar to that of the control group (Fig. 1). No significant deviations were

Table I. Diastolic blood pressure and renal function in normotensive controls and 3 groups of hypertensive patients

n group		diast. BP mm Hg mean A	$C_{cr.}$ ml/min mean A	V ml/3 h mean A	$U_{Na} V$ mekv/3 h mean A	$U_K V$ mekv/3 h mean A	$\frac{V . 100}{C_{cr}}$ % mean A	$\frac{C_{Na} .}{C_{cr}}$ % mean A	$\frac{C_K . 100}{C_{cr}}$ % mean A
20 control		76 4.0	111 17.1	172 79	25.3 11.5	6.6 3.9	0.86 0.31	0.89 0.33	8.1 4.1
17 cured	before	102 5.7	90 11.6	158 77	18.8 8.9	5.6 1.7	0.99 0.48	0.78 0.33	8.3 2.2
	after	83 7.0	89 14.7	167 72	20.7 7.8	5.5 1.9	1.06 0.43	0.97 0.30	8.4 2.7
19 improved	before	121 8.9	78 11.0	188 90	17.1 8.8	5.8 1.8	1.52 0.75	0.84 0.42	10.5 2.5
	after	97 7.1	74 10.9	187 50	16.7 5.8	5.6 1.9	1.56 0.52	0.92 0.33	11.9 4.4
12 failure	before	111 7.4	77 10.2	198 102	16.8 10.5	5.8 1.8	1.53 0.79	0.88 0.51	10.8 2.4
	after	111 7.1	78 11.7	194 69	17.7 6.4	5.3 1.8	1.69 0.71	0.98 0.31	10.5 2.9

Mean values and amplitudes (A) of urine flow (V), sodium ($U_{Na} V$) and potassium excretion ($U_K V$), excretion fraction of water (V/C_{cr}), sodium (C_{Na}/C_{cr}) and potassium (C_K/C_{cr}) before and after surgery.

recorded in parameters V/3 hours and V/C_{cr}. The mean C_K/C_{cr} gave significantly lower A and A% than controls both before and after surgery. The C_{cr} value was significantly higher after surgery than the corresponding value in the "improved" group.

Group 2 — "improved hypertension": This group showed the highest BP values before surgery. The preoperative curve of the diurnal C_{Na}/C_{cr} rhythm was greatly disturbed. After surgery the curve came closer to the control one. Nevertheless, the deviation from normal biorhythm remained more pronounced than in the "cured" group (Fig. 1). The mean V/C_{cr} value was significantly higher both before and after surgery compared with controls (Fig. 2). Surgical management improved the increase in A and A% of the V/C_{cr} mean values. Its pre-operatively delayed acrophase (17.3 hours) shifted post-operatively to 12.7 hours. Improved hypertension failed to affect the low A and A % of the mean C_K/C_{cr} value.

Group 3 — "failure" to affect hypertension:

Changes in the diurnal rhythm of Na and water excretion fractions resembled the changes in the "improved" patients before surgery (Fig. 1 and Fig. 2). Post-

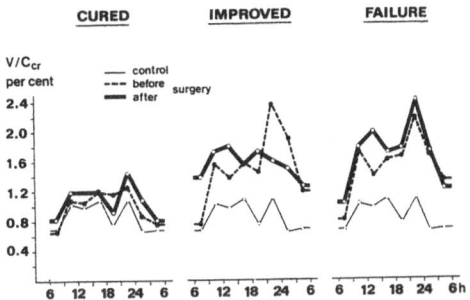

Fig. 2. Diurnal rhythm of water excretion fraction (mean values of V/C_{cr}) in normotensive controls and in 3 groups of hypertensive patients.

operative findings remained unchanged, which documented the influence of hypertension on this diurnal rhythm.

Conclusions

Patients with more severe renovascular hypertension and lower glomerular filtration rate value (C_{cr}), even at the bottom of normal values, showed more pronounced irregularity in diurnal rhythm of renal Na excretion and poorer prognosis for surgical management. In patients with "cured" hypertension the disturbance of Na excretion rhythm was post-operatively reversible and was not followed by changes in water excretion rhythm. In patients with "improved" hypertension a pronounced irregularity in water excretion, evidently due to greater disturbed diurnal rhythm of Na excretion, was found. Both rhythms displayed amelioration after successfull operation. Neither of these two patient groups displayed significant changes in glomerular filtration rate values due to the effect of surgery. These data and unaffected irregularities in patients with surgery "failure" suggest that severity of hypertension affects the biorhythm of renal Na excretion more than glomerular filtration rate values. The fact that surgery had no influence on the disturbed rhythm of K excretion in any of the patient group remains unexplained.

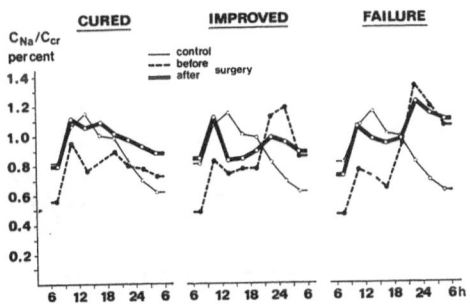

Fig. 1. Diurnal rhythm of sodium excretion fraction (mean values of C_{Na}/C_{cr}) in normotensive controls and in patients with renovascular hypertension before and after surgery. Patients with hypertension are divided into 3 groups according to the effect of surgery.

J. S., IKEM, Vídeňská 800, 146 22 Prague 4, Czechoslovakia

RENOVASCULAR HYPERTENSION IN TAKAYASU'S ARTERITIS

S. YONEDA, T. NUKADA, T. TAKANO, K. TANAKA
and M. IMAIZUMI

*Department of Internal Medicine, Osaka University Medical School,
Osaka, Japan*

Introduction

Takayasu's arteritis includes wide varieties of manifestations which are caused by inflammatory lesions of unknown etiology. Arterial involvement is localized in the arteries of elastic type, that is, the aorta and its main branches, and the pulmonary arteries. The renal artery is frequently involved and hypertension is consequently observed clinically.

Hypertension is an important risk factor in cerebrovascular disease and cardiac failure. Cerebrovascular disease and cardiac failure account for the high incidence of fatality in Takayasu's arteritis.

This study was concerned with impairment of organ circulation and the hemodynamic characteristics in hypertension with renal artery disease caused by Takayasu's arteritis.

Materials and methods

This study was based on data obtained from 33 patients with Takayasu's arteritis diagnosed by physical and laboratory examinations and aortographies. Twenty-two patients were normotensive and 11 patients were hypertensive. Patients with aortic regurgitation were excluded. Hemodynamic investigation was performed in 7 hypertensive and 6 normotensive patients and all hypertensive patients had renal arterial lesions.

The diagnosis of renovascular hypertension was based on the angiographic findings of renal artery stenosis.

The criteria for hypertension was decided as followed: systolic ≥ 150 mm Hg and/or diastolic ≥ 90 mm Hg; if there was stenotic or occlusive lesion in the arteries of the right arm, the blood pressure in the other extremity was accepted.

Severity of organ damage was estimated by clinical data obtained in five prognostic indices: arterial blood pressure, optic fundi and cardiac, cerebral and renal complications.

Cardiac output measured by the RISA dilution method and by an external counter sited over the precordium. The dilution curve obtained was analyzed by the MacIntyre technique. The total peripheral resistance (TPR) was calculated as the ratio of the mean arterial pressure to cardiac output. Blood volume was calculated from volume of distribution of RISA.

Results and disscussion

1. Severity of organ damage

Fig. 1 indicated the relationship between the severity index of 22 normotensive patients (open circles) and 11 hypertensive patients (solid circles) and the duration after the onset. No correlation was found in normotensive patients. However, there

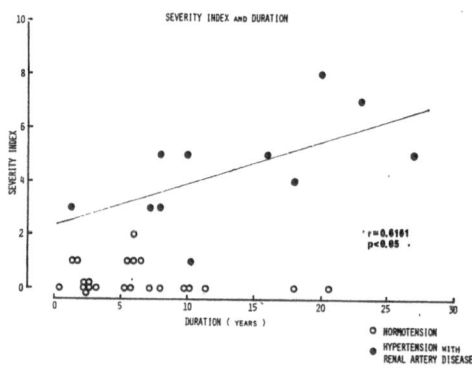

Fig. 1. Relationship between severity index and duration after onset in 22 normotensive and 11 hypertensive patients. Direct and significant correlation was found in the hypertensive group.

was a significant direct correlation in hypertensive patients ($p < 0.05$). It is well known that in hypertensive patients the organic damage advances in proportion to the duration of blood pressure elevation. It was indicated that the patients with

Table I. Hemodynamic Parameters in Cases with Takayasu's Arteritis

Hemodynamic Parameters	Normotensives (n = 6)	Hypertensives (n = 7)
MABP (mmHg)*	81 ± 3	125 ± 15
Blood Volume (ml/cm)	23.5 ± 2.6	26.5 ± 2.9
Cardiac Index (ml/min . m²)	3680 ± 570	3856 ± 1036
TPR Index (dynes sec./cm⁵ m²)	880 ± 98	1382 ± 759

MABP: Mean Arterial Blood Pressure
TPR Index: Total Peripheral Resistance Index
* $p < 0.001$

hypertension in Takayasu's arteritis also have poor prognosis.

2. Hemodynamic parameters

Mean arterial blood pressure (MABP) was significantly higher in 7 hypertensive patients than in 6 normotensive patients ($p < 0.001$). There were no significant differences in blood volume, cardiac index and TPR index in the 2 groups. The average values were higher in the hypertensive group than in the normotensive group (Table I).

A significant inverse correlation between cardiac index and MABP was found in the hypertensive group ($p < 0.02$, Table II). Among the hypertensive patients, MABP was directly correlated with the TPR index ($p < 0.01$, Table II). No correlation was found between the blood volume and MABP in hypertensive and normotensive groups. However, there was a tendency of negative correlation between the blood volume and MABP (Table II).

Dustan (1972) and *Tarazi* (1973) confirmed that in hypertensive patients with renal artery disease of the fibrosing and atherosclerotic types, MABP was significantly and directly correlated with cardiac index and TPR, and was significantly and inversely correlated with plasma volume.

The cardiac index was a low value in two hypertensive patients with long duration, although there was no relationship in normotensive and hypertensive groups between the cardiac index and the duration after the onset. This was the same result as in renovascular hypertension reported previously (*Tarazi* 1973).

It may be concluded that the hypertension with renal artery disease caused by Takayasu's arteritis has some of the same hemodynamic changes as that of the other etiologies.

Table II. Relationship of Mean Arterial Blood Pressure to Cardiac Index, Total Peripheral Resistance Index and Blood Volume in Different Groups of Takayasu's Arteritis

Blood Pressure (mm Hg)	Cardiac Index		TPR Index		Blood Volume	
	r	P	r	P	r	P
A. Hypertension with Renal Artery Disease (7 patients)						
MABP	−0.873	0.02	0.913	0.01	−0.625	NS
B. Normotension (6 patients)						
MABP	0.141	NS	0.050	NS	0.767	NS

MABP: Mean Arterial Blood Pressure
TPR Index: Total Peripheral Resistance Index

S. Y., Dept. of Internal Medicine, Osaka University, Fukushima, Osaka 553, Japan

THERMAL DIAGNOSIS OF PERIPHERAL VASCULAR RESISTANCE IN ARTERIAL AND ESPECIALLY RENOVASCULAR HYPERTENSION

F. KADEŘÁVEK, J. STŘÍBRNÁ, J. POLÁK and M. KULHAVÁ

Institute for Clinical and Experimental Medicine, Prague, Czechoslovakia

Hypertension is, as a rule, attributed to disturbed regulation of the peripheral arteries and arterioles (*McMichael*, 1975). Because of the high number of vasoconstrictive nerve receptors and large vascular network, the skin is of great importance haemodynamically. The dynamics of skin vascular resistance may contribute to our understanding of the pathogenetic mechanisms of hypertension and possibilities of their management. One of the tools for studying these processes is clinical thermometry.

In this paper we analyse the effect of selected vasoactive drugs on vascular resistance of the skin in patients with arterial and especially renovascular hypertension. We have tested the effect of nicotinamide, which is a model vasodilator with a near selective action on the skin area, and methypranol, a new Czechoslovak beta-adrenolytic drug, because it is also used as an antihypertensive; prazosin is used for the fast onset of its alpha-adrenolytic effects and favourable antihypertensive action.

Methods and materials

We measured the skin temperature at eight sites on the body, as well as sublingual and room temperatures. The room temperature was maintained constant automatically. The intensity of the thermoregulatory blood flow is determined from outer and inner temperature gradients. The indicator of thermoregulatory vascular resistance is the ratio of the mean arterial pressure and the intensity of the thermoregulatory blood flow.

The measurements are perfomed thermo-electrically for 120 minutes on pre-acclimatised patients in the supine position. Temperatures are taken every three minutes. Heart rate (f) and arterial pressure on the arm using indirect auscultation were recorded at the onset of measurements and then at 30, 42, 60, 90 and 120 minutes.

Tablets of the tested drugs were administered immediately before the start of measurement, intravenous solutions at 31 minutes.

We examined altogether 60 patients divided into six groups of 10 patients each. Their mean age was 45.8 ± 11.0 years. Twenty-seven patients suffered from renovascular, seven from renal and twenty-six from essential hypertension. In 10 patients stage I, in 35 stage II and in 15 stage III were involved. In terms of etiology and functional stage, the groups did not show marked differences in incidence. This was not true of the group of patients examined at low temperature which included a much higher percentage of individuals with essential hypertension.

Results

Neopeviton (nicotinamide)

An intravenous dose of 5 ml solution elicited and abrupt but transitory increase in the intensity of thermoregulatory blood flow (I_{bf}) with a simultaneous decrease in arterial pressure (P_s, P_d). This resulted in a marked decrease in thermoregulatory

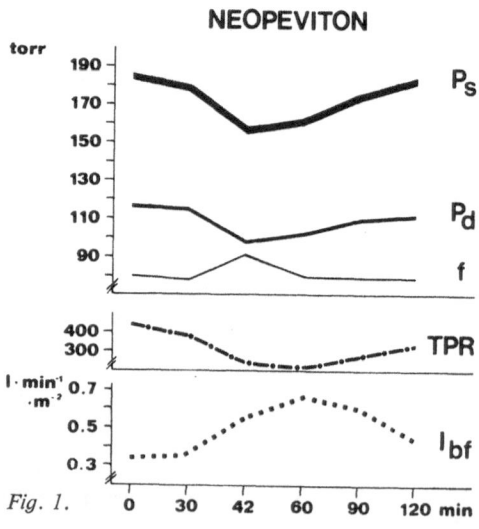

Fig. 1.

vascular resistance (TPR) (Fig. 1). At low temperatures, the resistance was much higher and the response lower and of shorter duration.

Trimepranol (methypranol)

One mg intravenous Trimepranol led to a slow increase in the thermoregulatory vascular resistance, which was significant from the 90th minute within 42 minutes od administration (Fig. 2). This change was accompanied by a corresponding course of both pressures and a reverse course of intensity of the thermoregulatory blood flow. Though minor, the changes were a significant reflection of the different initial trends.
Eighty mg Trimepranol given orally elicited similar changes, but the statistical significance shifted to 120 minutes.

Thirty-one minutes after 40 mg of oral Trimepranol and 5 ml intravenous Neopeviton were administered effect of Neopeviton predominated, which makes it difficult to specify the effect of Trimepranol. A conspicuous feature was the distinctly lower heart rate level. Owing to its tendency to induce collapse it was necessary to administer Neopeviton with greater than usual care.

Trimepranol evoked a pronounced slow-down in heart rate lasting 43 minutes irrespective of the route of administration.

Minipress (prazosin)

Oral administration of 1 mg Minipress was followed by a minor but between 42 and 60 minutes statistically significant decrease of thermoregulatory resistance with a corresponding pressure decrease and a moderate increase in the thermoregulatory blood flow (Fig. 3). This was followed by a reverse but statistically significant course after 120 minutes.

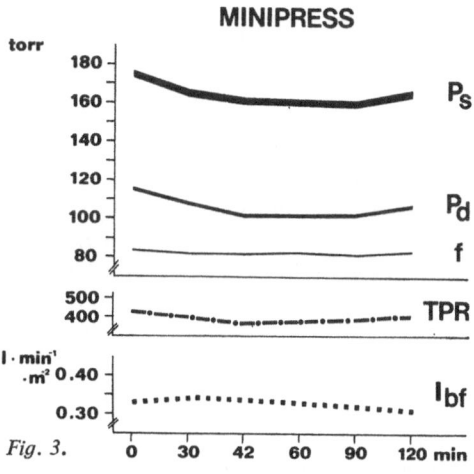

Fig. 3.

Conclusion

Thermal diagnosis of peripheral vascular resistance in the skin based on clinical thermometry is suited for assesing even relatively discreet effects of antihypertensive drugs on the pathogenetic mechanisms of systemic hypertension. Nicotinamide and prazosin are assumed to have a similar effect on the skin. There was a transitory decrease in thermoregulatory resistance associated with a decrease in arterial pressure and increase in skin circulation. Methypranol had a reverse effect. Combined with nicotinamide, its effect manifested itself mainly by lower heart rate than after Neopeviton alone. This combination was not well tolerated by the patients.

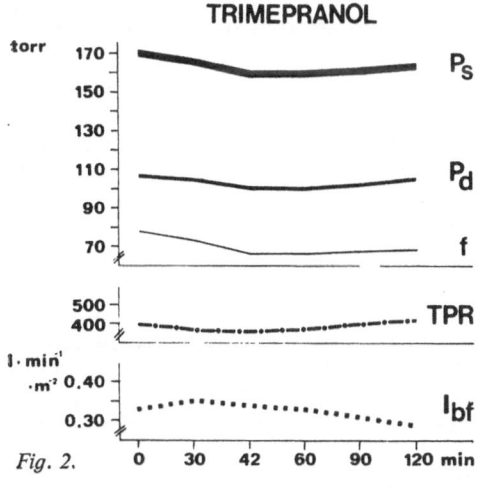

Fig. 2.

F. K., IKEM, Vídeňská 800, 146 22 Prague, Czechoslovakia

EXPERIENCE IN EX-SITU REPAIR OF RENAL ARTERY STENOSIS

D. TURINI, C. SELLI, G. NICITA, C. FIORELLI and P. T. SCARPELLI

Departments of Urology and Internal Medicine, University of Florence, Italy

Over a period of 6 years we performed 17 renal autotransplantations for surgical treatment of renovascular hypertension. All patients presented with diastolic hypertension and had been evaluated with rapid-sequence IVP, angiography and PRA from the renal veins. There were 5 males and 12 females ranging in age from 29 to 48 years. Renal artery stenosis was unilateral in 16 cases (14 right, 2 left) and bilateral in one case: the cause of stenosis was in 10 cases fibromuscular hyperplasia, in 6 cases atherosclerosis and in one case a paraganglioma compressing the renal artery. One case presented an associated cyst and uretero-pelvic junction obstruction. In 14 cases we used a midline transpertitoneal incision, in 3 an extraperitoneal approach.

The kidney was removed under hemodilution and hyperdiuresis (*Gelin*, 1971) and perfused with lactated Ringer's solution at a temperature of 4° C., with the addition of xylocain and heparin, in continuous gravity flow at a mean pressure of 150 cm/H$_2$O. The ureter was resected only once. In 16 cases, vascular reconstruction was performed using autologous segments of the hypogastric artery while we used only once a segment of the saphenous vein. Mean cold ischemia time was 80 minutes. The kidneys were autotransplanted to the ipsilateral iliac vessels. We often used flexible metallic dilators to improve the diameter of arterial branches, and as stents to facilitate the performance of the anastomoses in 6−0 Prolene. In the 7 more recent cases we preferred to detach completely the hypogastric artery from its origin, to perform an accurate reconstruction of the branches of the renal artery and to reimplant the proximal part of the hypogastric artery end-to-side to the common iliac artery. This technique, though involving one additional vascular suture, allows a more accurate repair of multiple lesions.

Complete follow-up has been obtained in all patients, with periods ranging from 6 months to 6 years. Fifteen patients have become normotensive completely between 2 and 6 weeks after the procedure, while 2 still require anti-hypertensive drugs. Postoperative IVP and angiography have demonstrated good renal function in 14 cases, while in 3 we observed graft thrombosis.

Case report

A 42-year-old woman hypertensive from 5 years, presented at IVP a right hydronephrosis and a small upper pole cyst; the left kidney was rather small and pyelonephritic (Fig. A). Angiography demonstrated fibromuscular hyperplasia of the right renal artery, causing stenosis of the main trunk up to its bifurcation (Fig. B). Plasma renin activity from the renal veins showed a lateralization to the right side. At surgery the kidney was removed from the iliac fossa the two branches of the artery were anastomosed to the hypogastric artery; two renal veins were present and they were both anastomosed end-to-side to the common iliac vein. Subsequently a dismembered pyeloplasty was performed and the cyst was marsupialized. An IVP 3 months postoperatively demonstrated good simultaneous elimination, and absence of right hydronephrosis (Fig. C). This case shows that autotransplantation can be used for simultaneous treatment of multiple renal lesions which can concur in causing hypertension.

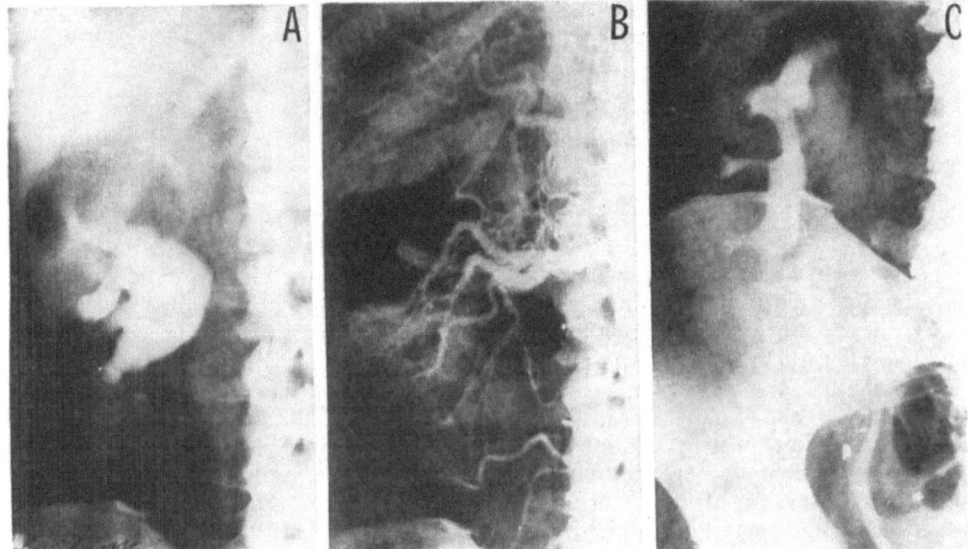

Discussion

Autogenous arterial grafts are today increasingly used for the treatment of renal artery stenosis (*Novick*, 1977) since they have a low failure rate, while it has become evident that saphenous veins become stenosed and more often dilated when used for arterial by pass operations (*Dean* 1974 *Stanley*, 1973).

Extracorporeal kidney repair allows us to perform more accurate anastomoses without time problems when compared to traditional in-situ techniques. This kind of reconstruction is mainly used in fibromuscular hyperplasia, which often extends to the branches of the renal artery, making traditional repair hazardous or impossible.

Autotransplantation can also be performed for the correction of atherosclerotic lesions (Diethelm, 1975), particularly when the atheroma extends to the bifurcations, since it is easier to perform an endarterectomy on the isolated kidney.

Continuous perfusion allows a better dissection of the arterial branches which are distended, and a repair of the anastomotic leaks, increasing when necessary the pressure of the fluid.

We can conclude that ex-situ repair of renal artery stenosis is a reasonably safe and efficient procedure, which has extended the range of reparative surgery for renovascular hypertension and we are sure that in future it will be used on a wider scale.

REFERENCES

Gelin G. E., Claes G., Gustaffson A. and Storm B. (1971): Total bloodlessness for extracorporeal organ repair. Rev. Surg. 28, 305.

Novick A. C., Stewart B. H. and Straffon R. A. (1977): Autogenous arterial grafts for the treatment of renal artery stenosis. J. Urol. 118, 919.

Dean R. H., Wilson J. P., Burrogh H. and Foster J. H. (1974): Saphenous vein aorto-renal by-pass grafts: serial arteriographic study. Ann. Surg. 180, 469.

Stanley J. C., Ernst C. B. and Fry W. J. (1973): Fate of 100 aortorenal vein grafts: characteristics of late graft expansion, aneurysmal dilatation and stenosis. Surgery 74, 931.

Diethelm A. G., Wattie W. J., Sterling W. A. and Tauxe W. N. (1975): Renal autotransplantation using hypothermic storage and pulsatile perfusion. J. Urol. 113, 755.

D. T., Dept. of Urology, University of Florence, Viale Pieraccini 18, Florence, Italy

OUR OPINION ON DISPUTABLE PROBLEMS
OF VASORENAL HYPERTENSION TREATMENT

A. A. SPIRIDONOV

Bakulev Institute, Moscow, U.S.S.R.

In this work the following problems of vasorenal hypertension are discussed:

1. What per cent of patients with vasorenal hypertension is found among hypertensive patients?

2. What per cent of patients with vasorenal hypertension must be operated on?

3. What per cent of nephrectomies is carried out for vasorenal hypertension?

4. What diagnostic test is decisive in the selection of indications for an operation: angiography or plasma renin activity?

5. Which method of renal arterial reconstruction is the operation of choice?

At the Bakulev Institute of Cardiovascular Surgery 3,834 patients with elevated arterial pressure were examined and 1,175 patients with preliminary diagnosis of renovascular hypertension were hospitalized. In 666 patients the diagnosis of vasorenal hypertension was confirmed during examination. Thus, vasorenal hypertension was revealed in 16% of the examined patients and in 56% of hypertensive patients examined at the Institute.

According to summary data by Maxwell (1972) in the USA, 57% of patients with vasorenal hypertension were operated on and 43% were treated therapeutically. Our surgical material averages 84% and in the last years it has increased from 56% to 96%. Our radicalism can be explained by the following factors: firstly, postoperative mortality amounts to 2.2% among patients with isolated renal arterial stenosis; secondly, late survival among comparable age groups of operated and nonoperated patients with vasorenal hypertension clearly shows (Shapiro, 1976) the advantage of the surgical method. Mortality in the group of operated patients is only 9% and 40% in the group of non-operated patients. Finally, in case of renal arterial stenosis, arterial hypertension is a compensatory reaction directed to normalization of circulation in the kidneys. The elevated arterial pressure helps the kidneys to maintain normal or subnormal function and size for a long period of time. Therefore, in cases of renal arterial stenosis measures aimed at a decrease in the systemic pressure are not pathogenetically sound. Conservative treatment is of symptomatic character, its efficacy is temporary and only delays the date of radical surgery. It is possible to compare hypotensive therapy for renal arterial stenosis and analgetics and narcotics used for ischemia and the pain syndrome secondary to occlusive lesions of the limb arteries.

Surgical treatment of patients with renovascular hypertension should be performed at the specialized vascular departments. Operations in the general department or in nephrological clinics result in a high per cent of primary nephrectomy. We performed nephrectomy on 16% of patients with renovascular hypertension. At the same time the number of nephrectomies at the best nephrological clinic of the U.S.S.R. amounts to 50% (E. B. Maso, 1974).

Angiography of the kidneys is a final diagnostic test used for the selection of indications for an operation. Absolute figures of plasma renin activity in the renal venous blood cannot be a criterium for selection of patients for an operation, as the elevated reninemia is seen only in 32% of our patients. In 22% of patients renin activity is normal and in 46% it is decreased. The diagnostic value of this index lies in the revealed correlation of indices of the plasma renin activity in both kid-

Table I. Aetiology of renal arterial disease

Author	Year	Aetiology in %			
		athero-sclerosis	arteritis	fibro-muscular dysplasia	Others*
De Bakey	1968	83	—	13	4
Bookstein	1975	63	—	32	5
Knjasev M. D.	1974	64	9	27	—
Lopatkin N. A.	1975	44	14	31	—
The Bakulev Institute	1978	39	22	15	24

* Other renal vascular diseases are: thrombosis, embolism, trauma, retroperitoneal fibrosis, aneurysm, hypoplasia, extravasal factors of compression

neys. If this ratio is above 1.4, the operative prognosis is considered to be favourable.

In contrast to results published by foreign authors, in 22% of our patients renal arterial stenosis was due to non-specific aorto-arteritis and those patients were the most serious cases. In addition, 55% of our patients have renal arterial stenosis of unilateral isolated character. In 45% of patients were found associated lesions of the contralateral renal artery and of arteries in other sites: aortic arch branches, visceral branches, abdominal aorta and limb extremities. Therefore, one third of operations is of complex reconstructive character with simultaneous reconstruction of other arteries and the aorta.

The type of reconstructive operation depends on the etiology of the process. In case of the atherosclerotic stenosis of the renal artery transaortic endarterectomy is the prefered operation; in cases of fibromuscular dysplasia we perform resection of the renal artery in combination with venous autoplasty or with replantation into the aorta. We prefer distal anastomosis with the renal artery, which is oblique and of the end-to-end type. Allotransplantation is carried out only in cases of associated lesion of the aorta and its

Table II. Per cent of isolated and associated renal arterial reconstructions dependent on aetiology of the stenosing process

Aetiology of stenosis	Isolated reconstruction	Associated reconstruction
Atherosclerosis	65%	35%
Arteritis	38%	62%
Fibromuscular dysplasia	100%	
Total	66%	34%

branches and is combined with simultaneous plastic procedures.

We do not use any methods of "kidney protection" during an operation: neither regional perfusion nor external renal hypothermia.

This summarizes our approach to surgical treatment of patients with vasorenal hypertension elaborated during a 15-year period of investigations into this area of vascular surgery.

Table III. Main types of renal arterial reconstruction

Transaortic endarterectomy	44%
Resection and autoplasty	22%
Resection and alloplasty	21%
Others	13%

A. A. S., Bakulev Institute of Cardiovascular Surgery, Moscow, U.S.S.R,

SURGICAL CORRECTION OF MALIGNANT HYPERTENSION BY MEANS OF RENAL ARTERY RECONSTRUCTION

S. ZELLOS, A. TRIANTAFILIDIS, E. MASOURIDOU and I. KABOUKAS

Department of Vascular and Thoracic Surgery, Metaxas Memorial Hospital, Piraeus, Greece

From the department of thoracic and vascular surgery of Diagnostic and therapeutic institute "Metaxas memorial hospital" Piraeus more than 100 patients were investigated and treated for renal hypertension. The majority of these patients were given a clinical trial for the control of the blood pressure by means of standard drugs. In a selected group of 10 patients it was found necessary to adopt surgical correction of the renovascular disorder because of failure of the medical treatment. During the same period more than 300 patients underwent a variety of arterial reconstruction operations. The purpose of this paper is to demonstrate that surgical treatment is an effective method in controlling malignant hypertension when medical drug therapy has failed.

Materials and methods

The age and sex of the 10 patients with renal artery obstruction are given in Table I.

Table I. Age and sex in 10 patients with renal artery obstruction

AGE (RY)	31—40	41—50	51—60
Females	1	2	1
Males		2	4
Total			10

The reasons which led these patients to submit to clinical and laboratory investigations fall into 3 categories.
1) Accidental finding of high blood pressure 200–300 systolic or 130–150 diastolic.4 patients.
2) Symptomatology, headache precordial pain and irritability. 5 patients.
3) Sudden rise of the blood pressure from 160 to 220 in one patient.

All patients on admission and after thorough examination are referred for ECG, chest-X-ray and blood samples to a laboratory test. Table II shows the lab findings in our series. Renogram, renal and suprarenal scan, pyelogram and determination of renin levels both at rest and on exertion and renovascular angiography are indispensable in making the diagnosis and placing the indication for surgical correction of the anomaly. We prefer to perform the angiography using the translumbar technique

Table II. Laboratory tests in 10 patients with renovascular hypertention

	1	2	3	4	5	6	7	8	9	10
B.U.N.	0.33	0.35	0.40	0.27	0.38	0.39	0.40	0.37	0.39	0.38
Creatinine	0.87	0.67	0.85	0.84	0.78	0.83	0.75	0.82	0.79	0.83
ECG	+	+	+	+	+	+	+	+	+	+
Regitine	—	—	—	—	—	—	—	—	—	—
Ca	9	10	10.5	10	9.5	10.5	10	10.5	9.8	10.5
Scot	13 m	12	14	15	13	12	13	14	15	14
SGPT	3.5	3.7	3.8	3.6	3.9	3.8	3.9	3.6	3.8	3.7
Blood volume	4286	5000	5500	5300	4950	4980	5100	5500	5000	5200
Plasma volume	2486	2560	2890	2750	2500	2480	2750	3000	2850	2890
Na urine 24 hours (meq)	75	78	80	79	80	85	79	87	83	81

Table III. Plasma renin levels before and after surgery blood pressure levels before and after surgery in 10 patients with renovascular hypertension

Before surgery	1	2	3	4	5	6	7	8	9	10
Plasma renin at rest	2.26	2.15	2.20	2.25	2.10	2.65	2.20	2.25	2.15	2.10
And after exertion	2.26	4.75	5.1	2.75	2.45	5.3	2.60	4.85	5.2	2.45
Post operative levels	2.26	2.15	5.3	2.10	2.05	2.65	2.15	2.10	2.10	2.05
Before surgery Blood pressure	250/150	220/130	220/130	250/140	260/145	240/135	250/135	230/130	245/145	255/150
Post-operative levels	130/75	220/130	140/70	130/75	140/80	145/78	120/65	135/67	145/75	150/85

and when indicated we insert a catheter in the aorta descendens through the left axilliary artery.

The angio-findings were those of a localised obstruction due to atherosclerosis in all but two. The exception was a lady of 41 with segmental obstruction of the RT renal artery and an aneurysm formation. And a man of 47 with obstruction of the renal RT upper artery just proximal to the aorta by embolus due to clot formation inside the lumen of the aorta.

We prefer to use the anterior abdominal approach. It is well accepted now that for atherosclerotic occlusions of the renal artery, the anterior approach must be employed because it permits good inspection of both kidneys, adequate exposure of the proximal renal vessels and easy access to the aorta.

The object of the surgical reconstruction is to restore adequate blood flow to the ischaemic kidney. Various techniques have been used in several vascular centers with success. Of these the most popular are the thromboendarterectomy, excision of the stenosed segment and end to end anastomosis, by-pass procedures by means of venous or Dacron graft splenorenal anastomosis on the left side or RE implantation of the renal artery in a new selected site of the aorta.

In 7 cases we used thromboendarterectomy with vein patch. In one patient we removed the aneurysm as well as the atheroma and then used reconstruction with vein patch.

In another patient we employed a vein by-pass prosthesis from the aorta to the renal artery and on the last patient we opened the aorta and removed the atheroma and clot formation in the proximal part of the renal artery closed to the aorta.

Results

The results have been excellent in 7 patients, who are now with normal blood pressure. In two patients there is considerable improvement but drug dependent normalization of the blood pressure. The patient with aortorenal vein graft was a failure. He had a smooth post-operative cure with normal blood pressure and was discharged home. Almost a month later he had to be re-admitted because of sudden rise of his blood pressure to the pre-operative levels. A translumbar aortography demonstrated complete closure of the graft and filling of the lower part of the kidney by the second lower artery. As we mentioned before the pre-operative catheter angiography demonstrated two separate arteries suplying the RT kidney independently. Summarizing:

1. 10 previously unreported cases of malignant hypertension due to renal artery obstruction are reported.
2. All patients were diagnosed by standard diagnostic methods including translumbar angiography.
3. Evidence is given that renal artery reconstruction effectively controls and normalizes the blood pressure when medical drugs have failed.

S. Z., 26 Aristippou Str., Athens, Greece

CURRENT STATUS OF SURGICAL MANAGEMENT OF RENOVASCULAR HYPERTENSION

J. HEJNAL, P. FIRT, J. STŘÍBRNÁ, L. HEJHAL, K. DRÁB,
Z. ROTNÁGLOVÁ and I. ŽOFKOVÁ

Institute for Clinical and Experimental Medicine, Praha, Czechoslovakia

Surgical management of renovascular hypertension has become a routine procedure in vascular surgery. The progress made in surgical techniques and tactics assure safety of the operation and long term patency of the reconstruction. In contrast, the diagnosis and, above all, proportionately accurate prognosis of the results as regards the effect of the reconstruction on hypertension still have many shortcomings.

The first is our limited knowledge on the incidence of renovascular hypertension. Its prevalence in the hypertensive population is reflected only in estimates which put it between 5 to 15%. But, in terms of absolute figures, even the lowest estimate represents thousands of patients to whom an operation might bring a complete cure or a substantial improvement.

For the purposes of diagnosis, the present methods can be divided into screening and indication methods. The first include primarily isotope nephrography and elimination urography with special emphasis on the wash-out effect. They are valuable mainly if the results are positive. Most important among the indication methods is vascular renography. If performed appropriately, it is a reliable method for evaluating the morphology of the renal arteries and their main branches. Marked renal artery stenosis need not necessarily be a causal factor in hypertension. Other methods such as separate examination of renal functions and determination of plasma renin concentrations are therefore required for a functional evaluation. Before a patient is indicated for surgery the results of at least two of the above investigations must be positive; we also consider the results of screenig tests. It is helpful to determine the number of points of patients score for indicating the operation. For example, if a patient scores at least 6 points he is indicated for operation. If he scores 8 or more points, the operation is thought to carry a good prognosis (Tab. I).

Tab. I.

Results	—	+	++
Angiography	0	2	4
Split renal function	0	1	2
Renin tests	0	1	2
Urography	0	0.5	1
Isotope nephrography	0	0.5	1

Indicated for operation . . . . 6 points
Good prognosis. . . . . <8 points

Apart from hypertension, the impending loss of kidney function due to extreme sevire stenosis can also be an indication for operation. An absolute indication is severe bilateral involvement with impendig renal failure. Obviously, a parenchymatous disease such as chronic pyelonephritis or glomerulonephritis greatly reduces the prospects for a favourable outcome of the operation, though they need not necessarily contraindicate it. The initially wide range of proposed reconstruction techniques has narrowed. Just as in other spheres of vascular surgery, use of a bypass has emerged as a superior technique. We think that end-to-end anastomosis of the distal end of the graft and the renal artery is most advantagenous because of its simplicity, safety and better haemodynamics. End-to-side anastcmosis in this area is of little value because a new reconstruction is almost always impossible if the graft becomes occluded. Venous patch plasty should be performed only in children with fibromuscular narrowing. Measurements of the flow rate before and after reconstruction is an inherent and essential part of the reconstruction procedure.

The material used for the bypass merits great attention. Our clinical experience and experimental studies speak distinctly in favour of artificial prostheses in adults. Long-term follow-up has shown them to yield good results at the high flow rates prevailing in the renal artery. Vein grafts tend to aneurysmal dilatation and late complications in most patients. If it is absolutely necessary to use a vein, which is

Tab. II.

	No.	%	
371 adults .... Hosp. mortality 1%			
280 long-term follow-up			
Cured	142	51	
Improved	87	31	82
Failures	51	18	18
Total	280	100	

occasionally the case with brittle small-calibre arteries afflicted with fibromuscular stenosis and in children, we place the vein graft in a very loose, thin artificial prosthesis.

The following tables show the results in our operated patients. Of the 371 adults, arteriosclerotic stenosis was involved in 88%, fibromuscular in 8% and other causes of renal artery narrowing in 4%.

In the group of 35 children up to 16 years of age fibromuscular stenosis was present in 94% and other causes in 6%. The types of reconstruction included a bypass in 86%, endarterectomy in 4%, patch plasty in 4% and another technique of arterial repair in 3%. Three % required nephrectomy.

Four of our patients, i. e. 1%, died. Of the 280 adults who appeared for periodic follow-up examinations 82% showed a distinct improvement postoperatively, and of these 51% were normotensive without medication. The operation brought no relief to 18%. (Tab. II)

None of our young operated patients died. Of the 35 children 96% improved significantly after the operation and 70% were normotensive without medication. The operation produced no results in 4%. (Tab. III).

In summing up I should like to point out that surgical management of renovascular hypertension is by no means a closed subject and above all its diagnosis is important. Many failures are undoubtedly due to the use of an unsuitable type of reconstruction or imperfect technique. Nonetheless, surgical management helps us to handle a grave health problem such as hypertension and its complications even at this stage of development.

Tab. III.

	No.	%	
35 children .... Hosp. mortality 0			
31 long-term follow-up			
Cured	22	70	
Improved	8	26	96
Failures	1	4	4
Total	31	100	

P. F., IKEM, Vídeňská 800, 146 22 Prague 4, Czechoslovakia

VENOUS ALLOGRAFTS FOR ARTERIOVENOUS FISTULAS IN HAEMODIALYSIS

MARCELA KESTLEROVÁ, V. KOČANDRLE, J. VRUBEL and J. HEJNAL

Institute for Clinical and Experimental Medicine, Prague, Czechoslovakia

Introduction

The progress in dialysis and renal transplantation permits effective treatment and long-term survival in patients with irreversible renal failure. An important condition for a successful long-term treatment of these patients is the creation of an adequate vascular access for repeated haemodialysis. In most cases, subcutaneous arteriovenous (A—V) fistulas by means of the patient's own veins proved suitable (*Brescia et al.*, 1966, *Kočandrle and Kestlerová*, 1973) and permitted repeated connection of patients to an artificial kidney. However, their life span is limited; in many patients with systemic disease or with impaired or primary hypoplastic veins A—V fistulas cannot be created. Therefore, various vascular prostheses are used for A—V fistulas.

We have been concerned with the methods of connecting patients to artificial kidneys since 1966. Since 1973 we have used vein allografts for A—V fistulas whenever the routine vascular access is exhausted or has failed. This communication describes our experience with vein allografts.

Methods

From 1973 through May 1978 we created 32 A—V fistulas for haemodialysis using vein allografts in a group of 30 patients with irreversible renal failure.

The vein allografts were obtained from patients with primary varicose veins of the lower limbs who were indicated for removal of the great or small saphenous vein. When removed, the veins were washed out with Ringer's lactate solution and immersed in Gross' preservation solution (*Gross and Bill*, 1949). This is an aqueous polyion solution containing glucose, antibiotics, human AB serum and phenol red, which is an indicator of pH 7.4. The vein grafts were stored at 2—4 °C in a refrigerator for up to 6 weeks. Before transplantation the grafts were trimmed. We selected the most suitable segment, ligated all the tributaries and, if necessary, sutured lacerations from stripping Compatibility in ABO blood groups was the criterion for selecting veins for transplantation. The grafts were transplanted to the arm. Depending on the condition of the recepient's vessels, we placed them in the forearm between the radial or ulnar arteries and a patent cubital vein, or in the upper arm. Arteriography of the right forearm (Fig. 1) shows filling of the vein graft between the radial artery and me-

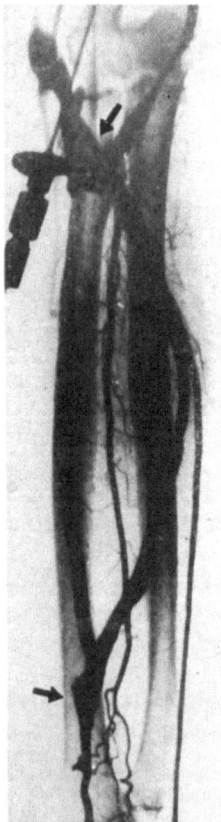

Fig. 1. Arteriography of the right forearm. Vein allograft anastomosed end-to-side to the artery (→) and end-to-side to the cephalic vein (←) is filled from the radial artery.

dian cubital vein. At the time of examination, this A—V fistula was used for a total of 170 haemodialyses. The vein graft has un ven edges due cicatrization of the wall aftererepeated punctures. So far, the patient has undergone over 250 dialyses via the same fistula which is, still patent after 2 1/2 years. On the upper arm the grafts were placed between the brachial artery and brachial or cephalic vein. The arteriogram (Fig.2) shows filling of the vein graft on the left arm placed between the brachial artery and cephalic vein. We examined the fistula 4 months after its construction and 2 months after it was used for heamodialysis. After 16 months the fistula used for 120 haemodialyses is still patent.

Results

Three cases of early thrombosis, 2 of which have been successfully reopened by thrombectomy. were the only severe complications in 32 A—V fistulas created through vein allografts. Six late occlusions of the fistulas were mostly due to late thrombosis of various origin. Major risks in graft patency are compression by hae-

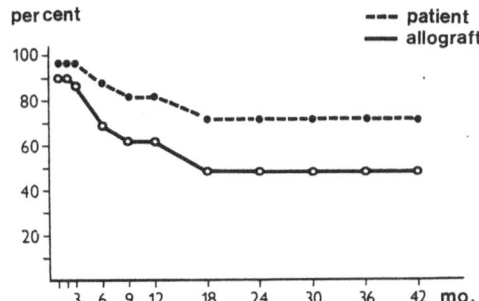

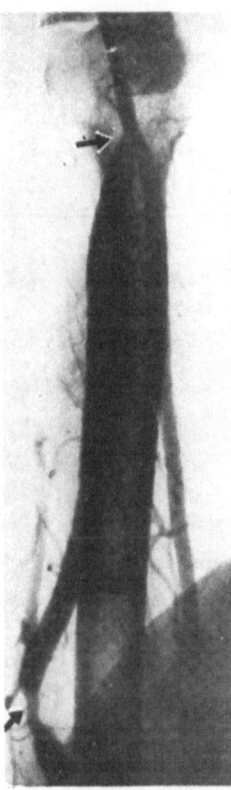

Fig. 2. Arteriography of the left arm. Vein allograft anastomosed end-to-side to the artery (←) and end-to-side to the cephalic vein (↙) is filled from the brachial artery.

Fig. 3. Cumulative patient survival and cumulative vein allograft patency.

matoma due to faulty puncture techniques and prolonged hypotension. Medication applied to the fistula resulted in occlusion as late as 5 months after its creation. After 4 months, changes in the venous wall transformed the graft into a fibrous cord. Twenty five fistulas (78%) remained patent for a prolonged period of time. At present, cumulative patency based on the statistical "life table" method averages 3 1/2 years in 48% of the fistulas (Fig. 3).

Discussion

According to the literature, the venous wall has a low antigenicity and the vein does not usually show more severe signs of rejection (*Schwartz et al.*, 1967). Our patients who received ABO compatible grafts and no immunosuppressive drugs exhibited no signs of vein rejection.

Complications requiring reoperation occurred in 9% of our patients. *Ahmed et al.*, using frozen vein allografts, reported a 10% complication rate in spite of preventive Heparin administration. Other veinprostheses such as modified bovine xenografts or microporous expanded polytetrafluoroethylene (PTFE) are reported to cause complications in 46 to 67% of patients. They include infections, false aneurysms, ruptures and bleeding (*Mohaideen et al.*, *Butler et al.*, 1977). These complications never occurred in our group.

Conclusion

Vein allografts for A—V fistulas for repeated haemodialysis proved suitable in

673

all tested cases. Cold storage in the Gross solution keeps the venous wall viable for a long time and permits use of the grafts as required. They can be punctured soon after operation. Allografts spare the patient's own leg veins or replace them. Their advantage lies in easy availability, low cost, long-term patency and low complication rate.

REFERENCES

Ahmed, N., DiScala, V., Nielsen, E., Le Veen, H. H., Piccone, V. A. (1976): Brachial artery to brachial vein preserved vein allograft for hemodialysis. J. Cardiovasc. Surg. 17, 483 to 488.

Brescia, M. J., Cimino, J. E., Appel, K., Hurwich, B. J. (1966): Chronic hemodialysis using venipuncture and surgically created arteriovenous fistula. New Engl. J. Med. 275, 1089—1092.

Butler, H. G., Baker, L. D., Johnson, J. M. (1977): Vascular access for chronic hemodialysis. Polytetrafluoroethylene (PTFE) versus bovine heterograft. Amer. J. Surg. 134, 791 to 793.

Gross, R. E., Bill, A. H. (1949): Methods for preservation and transplantation of arterial grafts. Surg. Gynecol. Obstet. 88, 689—701.

Kočandrle, V., Kestlerová, M. (1973): Arteriovenous shunt for hemodialysis in patients before and after kidney transplantation. Rozhl. Chir. 52, 195—200.

Mohaideen, A. H., Mendivil, J., Avram, M. M., Mainzer, R. A. (1977): Arteriovenous access utilizing modified bovine arterial grafts for hemodialysis. Ann. Surg. 186, 643—651.

Schwartz, S. I., Kutner, F. R., Neistadt, A. (1967): Antigenicity of homografted veins. Surgery 61, 471—477.

M. K., Olbrachtova 1045, 146 00 Prague 4, Czechoslovakia

CORONARY CIRCULATION

ANOMALOUS CORONARY ARTERIES

J. F. GUNNING, N. P. MADIGAN, H. C. SMITH,
R. E. VLIETSTRA and E. R. FULTON

*Mayo Clinic, Rochester Minnesota, U.S.A. and Royal North Shore
Hospital, Sydney, Australia*

Although rare, anomalous origin and course of the coronary arteries, is being seen with increasing frequency because of the increasing number of selective coronary angiograms being performed. The incidence in the only other series reported was 0.83%. Since an individual investigator's experience with unusual anatomic variants would be expected to be small, we decided to review our experience.

Materials and methods

A review of selective coronary angiograms performed at the Mayo Clinic during the period November 1, 1970 to April 1, 1977 showed that 46 had anomalous origin or course of the coronary arteries. During this period 6.640 selective coronary angiograms were performed in the adult cardiac catheterization laboratory at this institution. Patients undergoing cardiac catheterization for complex congenital heart disease were excluded as we wished to consider only the experience which might be expected by investigators performing coronary angiograms for the usual indications in adults. Selective coronary angiograms were performed by either a right brachial artery cutdown using a Sones No. 8 catheter (30 cases) or percutaneous transfemoral approach with Judkins preformed cardiac catheter (18 cases) in the first instance. Coronary cine angiograms were recorded at 30 and 60 frames/sec. on either 16 mm or 35 mm film and in some instances on 105 mm film, in multiple views. Biplane left ventricular angiograms were obtained prior to the coronary artery injections. The mean age of the 46 patients (33 males, 13 females) was 52.9 years (range 23–73 years) at the time of the cardiac catheterization. Twenty-nine patients had coronary angiograms because of symptoms of typical angina or previous infarction. Eight were studied because of atypical chest pain. Seven had valvular heart disease, all of which was predominant aortic stenosis. Two had suspected cardiomyopathy.

Results

The incidence of anomalous coronary artery anatomy was 0.69%, representing 46 of 6640 coronary angiograms performed.

The anomalies found were subdivided as follows: Group 1, anomalous coronary artery origin (32 cases). Group 2, Separate ostia for coronary artery branches (8 cases). Group 3, Absent coronary arteries (6 cases).

1a. The commonest abnormality (50% or 16 cases) in Group 1 was for the circumflex artery to arise from either the right aortic sinus, with separate ostia in 3, or proximal right coronary artery. In all cases the circumflex artery passed retroaortically.

1b. There were 7 examples of the right coronary artery arising from the left sinus. The right coronary artery arose at a separate orifice and passed between aorta and pulmonary artery.

1c. The left anterior descending arose from right coronary artery or right cusp in only two cases and passed anterior to the pulmonary artery in both cases.

1d. Single right cusp supplied all three coronary arteries in six cases. In one case the left anterior descending passed between aorta and pulmonary artery and circumflex posterior to aorta. In two cases left main coronary artery passed anterior to pulmonary artery before dividing, and in one case left main coronary artery passed posterior to aorta before dividing. In two cases left main coronary artery passed between aorta and pulmonary artery.

1e. Left anterior descending arose from non coronary sinus.

In Group 2 there were separate ostia for circumflex and left anterior descending coronary arteries in 6 cases. Separate ostia for right coronary artery and conus branch caused technical problems in two cases.

This anomaly is much more frequent at pathological studies and was not analyzed in detail regarding incidence. This nevertheless, can present significant clinical problems, particularly to the less experienced angiographer who might interpret the conus artery as a diminutive right coronary artery in patients with a dominant left coronary system.

In Group 3 the left anterior descending coronary artery was absent in five cases and the right coronary artery absent in one. When the anterior descending artery was absent it was represented by large septal and diagonal branches with no vessel in the distal anterior interventricular groove.

Significant obstructive coronary artery disease was present in 36 of the 46 coronary artery trees studied. In 27 of the 32 cases where the coronary artery took an unusual course, because of anomalous aortic cusp origin, there was significant coronary artery disease in the anomalous segment. In all but 6 of these 27 cases, where there was significant obstruction somewhere in the coronary tree, there was significant obstruction in this aberrantly coursing artery segment. In two cases the only significant obstruction to the coronary tree was in the aberrantly coursing artery segment.

Technical difficulties were encountered during catheterisation because of the unusual anatomy, and in seven cases recatherisation was performed because of inadequate visualization at the initial investigation. In all these cases the initial study was performed via the brachial artery and the second via the femoral artery. The total time required for each initial investigation averaged 84.3 minutes (range 40−225 minutes) with fluoroscopy time of 16.1 minutes (range 6−37.5 minutes).

REFERENCE

Chaitman, B. R., Lesperance, J., Saltiel, J. and Bourassa, M. G. (1976): Clinical, Angiographic and Haemodynamic Findings in Patients with Anomalous Origin of the Coronary Arteries. Circulation 53, 122.

J. F. G., Royal North Shore Hospital, Sydney, NSW 2065, Australia

CORONARY CIRCULATION ON THE VENOUS SIDE IN THE HUMAN HEART WITH THE SPECIAL REFERENCES TO THE VENAE CORDIS MINIMAE

EWA PAKALSKA and B. GOŁĄB

Department of Normal Anatomy, IBM Medical Academy in Lodz, Poland

The venous side of the coronary circulation is particularly important not only in physiology and pathology but also after arterialization of the coronary veins (*Moll*, 1977). Previous investigations connected with the venae cordis minimae (thebesian veins) and with venous vascularization of the myocardium of the left ventricle (LV) after ligation of the coronary arteries (*Pakalska*, 1977; *Ratajczyk-Pakalska*, 1974), have shown a greater number of cardiac veins (also thebesian veins) in the myocardium of the ventricles in those hearts where atherosclerotic lesions in the coronary arteries were present. The purpose of this study was to investigate the venous side of the coronary circulation using the technique of microangiography.

Materials and methods

The study material consisted of 10 hearts from human bodies (6 men and 4 women) aged 18—42 years. The causes of death were diseases of other organs, but in 4 cases distinct atherosclerotic lesions in the coronary arteries were present. The cardiac veins were injected with Micropaque under a pressure of 60 to 100 mm Hg. After the fixation of the hearts, cross sections at about 1000 μm thickness were prepared and then radiographs were taken and inspected with a microscope at 10 to 25 magnification.

Results and discussion

Inspection of transverse slices of the walls of the ventricles has shown three zones of venous vascularization, viz.: the external — epicardial zone containing thin, about 1 mm external layer of the free walls of the LV, the medial — subepicardial, the thickest zone, which together with the external zone consists of about 2/3 thickness of the walls of the LV and interventricular septum (IS), the internal — subendocardial zone which contains the rest of the walls of the LV and IS facing this ventricle.

Some other investigators, among them *Grayson et al.* (1974) distinguished only two zones: the external — subepicardial and internal — subendocardial.

Moreover, we have observed that uniform venous filling in all zones of the walls of the ventricles depends on the pressure used to inject the examined veins. A pressure below 50 mm Hg fills only the veins of the external and medial zones, whereas pressures up to 80 mm Hg filled the veins in all the zones.

The previous and present studies have shown (*Pakalska*, 1977) that good filling of the walls of LV depends on the functional phase of the heart. If LV stopped in systole, the venous filling of the internal

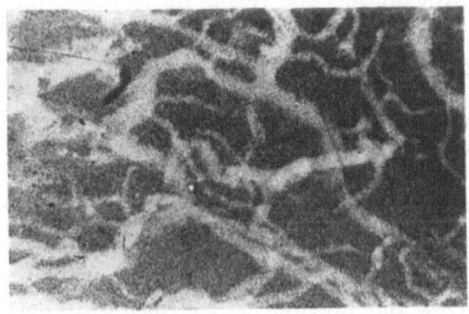

Fig. 1. Microangiograph of 800 μm-thick cross section of the anterior wall of the left ventricle. Venous network (situated in the medial — subepicardial zone) is clearly demonstrated (× 28.3). A human heart with the atherosclerotic lesions in the coronary arteries.

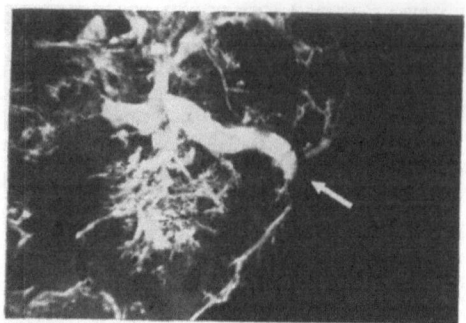

Fig. 2. Microangiograph of 1000 μm-thick cross section of the interventricular septum .Arboriform — thebesian vein is opening into the left ventricle marked by arrow (×10). A human heart with the atherosclerotic lesions in the coronary arteries.

— endocardial zone became more difficult (needed higher pressure and sometimes was impossible).

In the walls of the right ventricle (RV) only two zones of venous vascularization were observed, viz.: the external — epicardial zone (as in the walls of LV) containing thin, about 1 mm part of the most peripheral layer of the walls of RV, and the internal zone containing the whole thickness of RV if compared with LV, which in thickness equaled to both, the medial — subepicardial and the internal — subendocardial zones.

The use of lower pressure (about 50 mm Hg) to inject the veins in the walls of RV, brought only contrast in the larger cardiac veins. The pressure higher than 80 mm Hg filled all the veins of RV walls.

It was noticed that the small veins in the epicardial zone of the both ventricles were connected together by simple connections.

The largest veins were situated in the peripheral layer of the medial zone. The tertiary and quaternary tributaries of these veins composed a characteristic venous network which has been identified with the previously described intramuscular venous plexus (Pakalska, 1970).

Among minute vessels of the subendocardial zone larger vessels were noticed. Because of their size and connections with lumen of the ventricles we recognized them as the thebesian veins. Moreover, we also found in both ventricles of the human heart different types of thebesian vein shape (arboriform, sinuous, canaliculated) which Esperanca-Pina (1975) recognized only in the dog's heart RV. Because of atypical connections and the lengths (about 15 mm) of the veins connecting larger veins of the medial zone with the lumen of the ventricles we have termed them as "connecting — thebesian veins".

Comparison of two groups of studied hearts (normal and atherosclerotic) showed some differences. In the hearts with atherosclerotic lesions in the coronary arteries we observed more rich venous vascularization in all zones, particularly in the internal zone, than in normal hearts.

We are quite aware that the number of examined hearts was too small for the final conclusions, and that the problem need further investigation, but our present results connected with a greater number of the small veins and also of thebesian veins in the atherosclerotic hearts are in agreement with the previous observations of Pakalska (1977) and Samojlowa (1970).

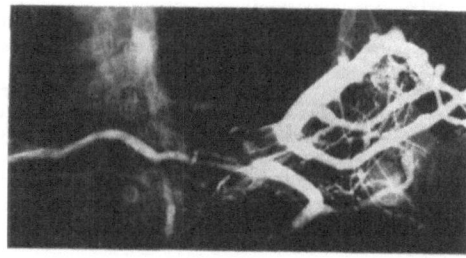

Fig. 3. Microangiograph of 1000 μm-thick cross section of the interventricular septum close to the anterior wall of the right ventricle (normal human heart). Connecting — thebesian vein opening into the right ventricle marked by arrow (×10).

REFERENCES

Esperanca Pina, Correira M., O'Neill J. G. (1975): Morphological study on the thebesian veins of the right cavities of the heart in the dog. Acta Anat. (Basel), 92, 310—320.

Grayson J., Davidson J. W., Fitzgerald-Finch A., Scott C. (1974): The functional morphology of the coronary microcirculation in the dog. Microvasc. Res., 8, 20—43.

Moll J. W., Dziatkowiak A., Rybiński K., Edelman M., Ratajczyk-Pakalska E. (1973): Arterialisierung des Sinus coronarius — Indikationen, Technik, Ergebnisse. Thoraxchirurgie, 21, 295—301.

Pakalska E. (1977): Number of thebesian veins in the myocardium of the ventricles i. human and ome animals.: Div. of Art. Organs, University of Utah, USA (prepared for press)

Ratajczyk-Pakalska E. (1970): Cardiac veins. Folia Med. Lodz., 10, 45—72.

Ratajczyk-Pakalska E., Moll J. W., Edelman M., Chltkowska E. (1974): Studies on the venous system of ventricular myocardium following ligation of the coronary arteries. Kardiol. Pol. 17, 133—141.

Samojlowa S. V. (1970): Anatomy of the cardiac blood vessels. Medicina, Leningrad.

E. P., Depart. of Normal Anatomy IBM, Narutowicza 60, Łódź 90 131, Poland

THE INDEX OF PERMEABILITY OF CORONARY ARTERIES TO ALBUMIN

U. FUCHS, M. JOBST and G. SCHNEIDER

Department of Experimental Pathology, Institute of Pathology, and Department of Nuclear Medicine, Clinic of Radiology, Karl Marx University, Leipzig, G.D.R.

Introduction

Various types of tracers may be used to test the permeability of the arterial vascular wall (*Adams*, 1967; *Fuchs*, 1977; *Jellinek*, 1974). Labeled albumin has been used in tests conducted by the authors. The results obtained for coronary vessels are described in this paper.

Materials and methods

Human serum albumin labeled with ^{51}chromium is intravenously administered to ra·bits. After five and forty-five minutes after administration, the permeability index (*Duncan, et al.*, 1958; *Stefanovich and Core*, 1971) is determined. After fifteen minutes from the administration of albumin, 1.5 µg of bradykinin per kilogram of body weight is intracordially administered to some of the test animals. Additional tests are run to measure the blood pressure in the ascending thoracic aorta.

Results

The permeability index, after an albumin circulatory time of five minutes (P_{5min}), is higher in the coronary arteries than in the aorta, femoral artery, and pulmonary trunk, but lower than in the aortic valve. In the aorta, maximum values are measured in the aortic arch. If this result is set equal to 100 percent, then P_{5min} is 160 percent for the coronary arteries. After a circulatory time of albumin of forty-five minutes (P_{45min}), the permeability index increases to 285 percent, while the entire aorta attains only 113 percent. Intracordially administered bradykinin tends to increase the P_{45min} index in the coronary arteries by approximately 38 percent. The mean aortal pressure shows a considerable decrease (down to 60 percent) subsequent to the administration of bradykinin and thereafter levels off sinusoidally, with the initial value being temporarily exceeded (approximately 140 percent).

Discussion

The permeability to labeled albumin is different for different arteries. The results of studies on the aorta suggest that the vascular tension, the surface-to-weight ratio, the topographically different structures of intercellular junctions and the cytopempsis are of major importance in this connection. The increase in vessel wall permeability observed after the administration of bradykinin might be regarded as being due predominantly to endothelial changes (*Constantinides and Robinson*, 1969) as well as to sinusoidally reactive increases in the blood pressure. A short-time increase in the intravascular pressure is sufficient to cause an increase of the permeability of the vessel wall (Fuchs, et al., 1974). That the effect of the administration of bradykinin may still be detected after thirty minutes from the application thereof is considered to be due primarily to the "trap door" effect (*Robertson and Khairallah*, 1973). The high permeability of coronary arteries should contribute to atherogenesis in these vascular regions that are so frequently affected with serious diseases.

Conclusion

The permeability of the coronary arteries of rabbits has been studied using labelled albumin. The permeability index of these arteries was observed to be higher than that of the aorta after a relatively short circulatory time of albumin and also exhibits a greater increase after an extended circulatory time of the tracer. Bradykinin tends to increase the permeability index.

REFERENCES

Adams, C. W. M. (1967): Vascular Histochemistry. London: Lloyd-Luke.

Constantinides, P., Robinson, M. (1969): Ultrastructural injury of arterial endothelium. II. Effects of vasoactive amines. Arch. Path. 88, 106–112.

Duncan, L. E. jr., Cornfield, J., Buck, K. (1958): Circulation of iodinated albumin through aortic and other connective tissues of the rabbit. Circ. Res. 6, 244–255.

Fuchs, U. (1977): Submicroscopy of the arterial vascular wall. Exper. Path. Supp, 2, Jena: Fischer.

Fuchs, U., Gepp, G., Löbe, J., Hauffe, W., Riethling, A. K. (1974): Labelled serum albumin in the aortic wall after short-term blood pressure increase by angiotensin II. Paroi Artérielle 3, 187–199.

Jellinek, H. (1974): Arterial lesions and arteriosclerosis. AkadémiaiKiadó. Budapest.

Robertson, A. L. jr., Khairallah, P. A. (1973): Role of temporary endothelial cell contraction and circulating platelets in the initial stages of vascular disease. The "trap door" effect. Int. Res. Commun. Syst. 1–2–1.

Stefanovich, V., Core, J. (1971): Cholesterol diet and permeability of rabbit aorta. Exp. mol. Path. 14, 20–29.

U. F., Pathologisches Institut der Karl-Marx-Universität, Liebigstr. 26, 701 Leipzig, G.D.R.

PATHOLOGICAL CHANGES OF THE SMALL CORONARY ARTERIES IN POSTINFARCTION ANEURYSMS

F. KÖLBEL, V. DORAZILOVÁ, J. VANČURA,
J. LICHTENBERG and M. ASCHERMANN

3rd Medical Department, 1st Department of Surgery and the 1st Institute
for Pathological Anatomy, Faculty of General Medicine, Charles University,
Prague, Czechoslovakia

Recently, interest in the pathology of the small coronary arteries has increased (1). This category of vessels includes arterial branches with a diameter of 0.1 to 1.0 mm. Some of them can be identified as special branches supplying important structures in the heart such as the sinus node, atrioventricular junction and chemoreceptors in the left ventricular wall and some of them form the Viussens arterial ring, such as Kugel's artery (arteria anastomotica auricularis magna). The greatest number of these arteries is present in the heart as peripheral branches of the right and left coronary arteries, and as intercoronary anastomoses (2, 3). Only seldom, however, we are able to diagnose their pathological changes intravitally, as only some of them can be irregularly visualised using coronary angiography.

Pathological changes of these arteries can be detected in a number of diseases such as diabetes mellitus, amyloidosis, cardiomyopathies, and in inflammatory as well as in degenerative diseases of the heart. From the point of view of their functional significance, they are most frequently associated with rhythm disturbances and with scattered focal fibrosis of the ventricular myocardium. Microscopically, a broad spectrum of changes within these arteries can be detected, ranging from the intraluminal thrombosis over medionecrosis to fibromuscular dysplasia of the arterial wall (3).

In our present studies, we focused our attention on changes of the small coronary arteries in samples of surgically removed left ventricular postinfarction aneurysms, and we were surprised to find them in about 10 percent of the samples investigated (in 3 out of 28 aneurysms). All three patients had a history of myocardial infarction with subsequent appearance of a akinetic and/or a dyskinetic zone in coronary angiography. The most typical findings in one of the three patients were published separately (4). In a brief summary, using coronary angiography, both patient coronary arteries were found as well as both major branches of the left coronary artery. However, the left descending branch was relatively narrow and ended at about one half the distance between its origin and the apex of the heart. Using left ventriculography, an akinetic zone in the anterior wall of the left ventricle was observed. The anatomical sub-

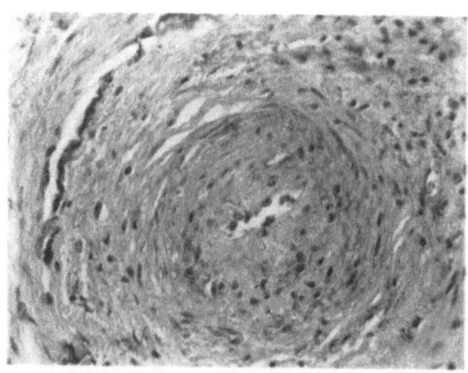

Fig. 1. Fibromuscular dysplasia of a small, coronary artey from a postinfarction aneurysm removed surgically, with a narrowing of the inner diameter of the artery. Hematoxylin-eosin-elastica stain, magn. 400 times.

strate of the akinetic zone was identified by the surgeon as a true aneurysm adhering to pericardium and filled with mural thrombus.

In microscopical investigations very similar changes were observed in all three aneurysms without any major difference. They can be summarized as follows (Fig. 1, 2):

1. fragmentation of both the internal and external elastic laminae;

2. the inner diameter of the small arteries was severely narrowed and/or obstructed by proliferating fibroblasts and muscle cells was observed;

3. the clusters of intimal cells can sometimes be observed in place of the obstructed arterial lumen;

4. necrotic and/or inflammatory changes within the arterial wall were not observed in any sample, nor was atheromatosis of these arteries found.

The condition of all three patients was improved by the aneurysmectomy performed. In one of them, new anginal attacks were observed 2 1/2 years after the aneurysmectomy, caused by stenosis of the initial part of the left descending branch.

In conclusion, we were able to observe small coronary artery disease in 10 per cent of the patients with surgically removed postinfarction aneurysms of the left ventricle. In the arterial walls, a mixture of proliferation of fibroblasts and muscle can be observed together with fragmentation of the elastic laminae. In no case was necrotic, inflammatory and/or atheromatous changes of these arteries observed.

It is not possible, however, to clarify whether the primary sites of these changes are the small coronary arteries with subsequent narrowing of the large arteries due to decreased blood flow, or vice versa. From prolonged postoperative observations it seems probable that fibromuscular dysplasia of the small coronary arteries will be combined with atheromatosis of the large arteries.

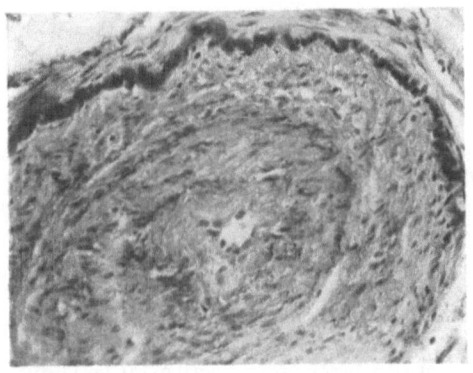

Fig. 2. Another artery with fragmentation of both internal and external elastic laminae and with intimal proliferation responsible for the narrowing of the inner diameter of the vessel. Hematoxylin-eosin-elastica stain, magn. 400 times.

REFERENCES

1. *Esente P., Gemini, G. G., Huntigton, P. P., Kelly, A. E., Black, A. (1974):* Left ventricular aneurysm without coronary arterial obstruction or occlusion. Amer. J. Cardiol. 34: 658—663.
2. *James, T. N. (1967):* Pathology of small coronary arteries. Amer. J. Cardiol. 20: 679—691.
3. *James, T. N. (1977):* Small arteries of the heart. Circulation 56: 2—14.
4. *Kölbel, F., Dorazilová, V., Vančura, J., Lichtenberg, J., Hampl, J., Aschermann, M., Petráček, J. (1977):* Left ventricular aneurysm without trunk or main coronary artery branch occlusion (Czech text). Sborník lék. 79: 231 až 236.

F. K., 3rd Medical Department, Faculty of General Medicine, Charles University, U nemocnice 1, 128 21 Prague 2, Czechoslovakia

CALCIUM ACTIVATION PROCESSES IN THE SMOOTH MUSCLE OF CORONARY ARTERIES AND THEIR SELECTIVE INHIBITION

K. GOLENHOFEN and G. NEUSER

Department of Physiology, University of Marburg, F.R.G.

Two types of calcium activation processes can be distinguished in smooth muscles by selective blockade; they have been called the P-system and the T-system. As the susceptibility of these processes to the antagonist nifedipine is the main criterion for this differentiation, the two mechanisms can alternatively be called the "nifedipine-sensitive system" (NSS) and the "nifedipine-resistant system" (NRS).

Methods

Helical strips were cut from dog, pig and human coronary arteries. Arteries of various sizes with an outer diameter 0.5–3 mm were used. Up to 8 strips were dissected from one and the same heart. They were mounted in thermostatically controlled organ baths filled with physiological salt solution of the following composition: Na^+ 137, K^+ 5.9, Ca^{2+} 2.5, Mg^{2+} 1.2, Cl^- 124, HCO_3 25, H_2PO_4 1.2, glucose 11.5 mmol/l; equilibrated with 95% O_2 and 5% CO_2; pH 7.4; 35 or 37 °C. The preparations were stretched to approximately in situ tension. The following substances were used: nifedipine, nitroprusside sodium, noradrenaline, propranolol, nitroglycerin.

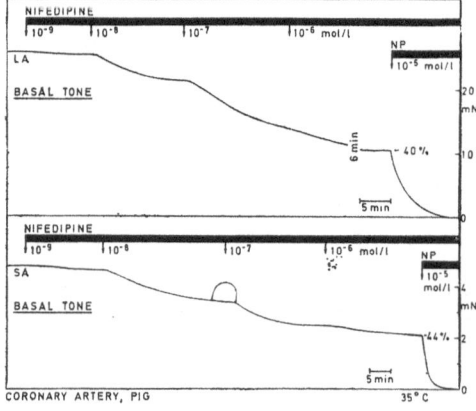

Fig. 1.

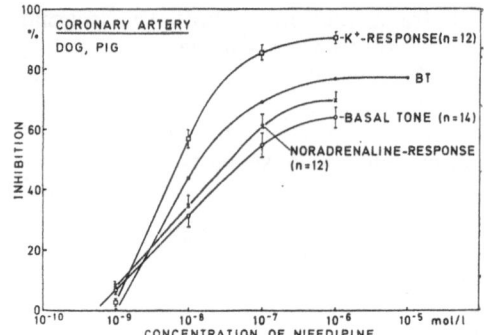

Fig. 2.

Results

Strips of coronary arteries had a great tendency to spontaneously develop an active basal tone. The effect of nifedipine on strips of a large and a small artery is shown in Fig. 1. Nifedipine was applied cumulatively with a concentration increase every 10–15 min up to 10^{-6} mol/l or, in some experiments, up to 10^{-5} mol/l. The threshold for the inhibitory effect was near 10^{-9} mol/l and the maximum inhibitory effect was reached at about 10^{-6} mol/l. A further increase of the nifedipine concentration to 10^{-5} mol/l produced negligible further inhibition (Fig. 2). The active tension persisting after nifedipine treatment (10^{-6} mol/l) for 10–20 min can therefore be interpreted as nifedipine-resistant (*Golenhofen et al.,* 1977). The nifedipine resistant component of basal tone was 35.9 ± 3.5% (mean ± SE, n = 14) of the initial basal tone (Fig. 2). The nifedipine resistant component was suppressed by nitroprusside sodium 10^{-5} mol/l (Fig. 1), and this drug was therefore used for the determination of the zero point of active tension.

686

The effect of nifedipine was also studied during α-adrenergic stimulation of the preparations, produced by application of noradrenaline ($5 . 10^{-6}$ mol/l) in combination with a blockade of the β-adrenergic receptors by propranolol (10^{-5} mol/l). The inhibitory effect of nifedipine on that type of activation was similar to that on basal tone. The nifedipine resistant component was $28.9 \pm 2.7\%$. The average effect of nifedipine on potassium-induced activation (40 mmol/l K^+) was stronger, and only $9.5 \pm 2.3\%$ (n = 12) was nifedipine resistant (Fig. 2).

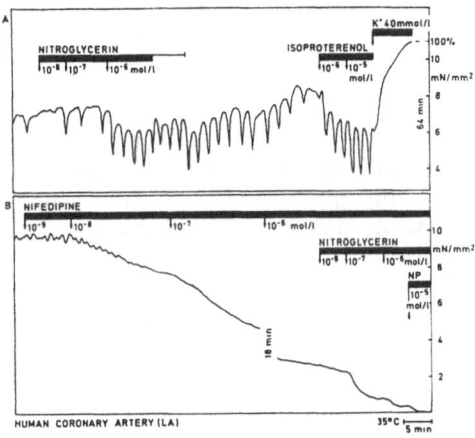

Fig. 3.

Strips of human coronary arteries, excised 3–6 hours after death, developed particularly strong spontaneous activity, often with marked fluctuations of the minute-rhythm type. Nitroglycerin had relatively little effect on such spontaneous activity. Nifedipine suppressed the greater part of this activity and all phasic components were abolished during nifedipine treatment. Nitroglycerin was very effective in suppressing the nifedipine-resistant tonic component: even 10^{-7} mol/l, which was ineffective under normal conditions, nearly completely suppressed the nifedipine-resistant component. In general, the results obtained on human coronary muscles were similar to those observed in canine and porcine preparations. (Fig. 1).

Discussion

The main result is that, in coronary smooth muscles, both activation systems exist, NSS and NRS, and that these mechanisms contribute in different proportions to the various types of activation. This indicates that the two systems are not only selectively blocked by specific antagonists but may also be separately controlled during physiological regulation. The NSS predominates in the activations studied so far. As the processes involved in the development of angina pectoris and coronary infarction are not fully understood, the possibility should be kept in mind that, in pathophysiological processes, the NRS may play a greater role. The particularly strong antianginal effect of nitroglycerin may be taken as an indication of this.

Our results are in good agreement with those of *Peiper and Schmidt* (1972) who observed only a partial relaxation of coronary arteries after application of verapamil which has a similar mode of action to that of nifedipine. *Fleckenstein and coworkers* (*1977*), however, did not observe a nifedipineresistant activation mechanism in coronary arteries. The differences in the calcium concentration used — 1 mmol/l was usually used by *Fleckenstein* and coworkers — can explain quantitative but not the qualitative differences. The differences may be mainly due to the fact that the conclusions of *Fleckenstein et al.*, are largely (*1976·1975*), based on studies of the potassium-induced activation where the nifedipine-resistant component at 1 mmol/l calcium is often negligible, and that the zero point of active tension was not directly determined by these authors (*Fleckstein*, personal communication) by a procedure such as application of nitroprusside sodium or papaverine or removal of calcium, which suppresses all active components with certainty.

K. H., Inst. of Physiology, Deutschbausstr. 2, D-3550, Mahrburg/Lahn, F.R.G.

CORONARY ARTERIES AND MYOCARDIAL METABOLISM

J. FABIÁN, V. BRODAN, J. SPÁČIL and A. BELÁN

*Cardiovascular Research Centre, Institute of Clinical
and Experimental Medicine, Prague, Czechoslovakia*

The clinical diagnosis of ischemic heart disease is based on angina pectoris or a history of myocardial infarction. In the majority of patients the clinical feature correlates with ECG signs of coronary insufficiency at rest or during exercise and angiographic evidence of coronary artery disease. However, these findings do not necessarily correlate. Occasionally, even all three findings combined cannot definitively confirm or exclude the diagnosis of ischemic heart disease. There is some evidence that in such situations a study of myocardial metabolism and a pacing test are useful (1, 3, 4, 5, 6). To evaluate the clinical significance of these investigations we studied myocardial metabolism in two different and clinically quite opposite groups of patients:

a) 41 of them had angina pectoris with corresponding ECG signs of coronary insufficiency and/or previous myocardial infarction and with angiographically proven significant coronary artery disease involving at least one, but usually two or three coronary arteries, and

b) 29 patients with no characteristic symptoms, normal or atypical ECG findings and no or minimal coronary artery disease.

Myocardial metabolism was assesed from blood samples collected from a systemic artery and the coronary sinus at rest and during right atrial, rarely right ventricular pacing. For the purposes of this study the changes of lactate and pyruvate values and their ratio were evaluated. A negative arteriovenous (= a−v) difference of lactate, or lactate: pyruvate ratio (= La: Py), or both were interpreted as metabolic signs of myocardial ischemia. Of the other parameters we studied also

the concentrations of glucose, free fatty acids, potassium, natrium, chlorides, phosphates, GOT and CPC in arterial and coronary sinus blood.

The following two figures show the metabolic values compared with the angiographic pattern of coronary arteries.

(Fig. 1) During pacing, all patients with significant coronary artery disease (right columns of the pairs) showed a significantly higher rate of negative a−v difference for lactate and a lower rate of negative a−v difference for pyruvate than those with no or minimal coronary artery disease (left columns of the pairs).

(Fig. 2) In patients with significant coronary artery disease a negative a−v difference for free fatty acids was significantly less common, as opposed to a significantly more frequent negative a−v difference for potassium.

The remaining parameters showed only minimal and statistically insignificant differences between our two groups of patients.

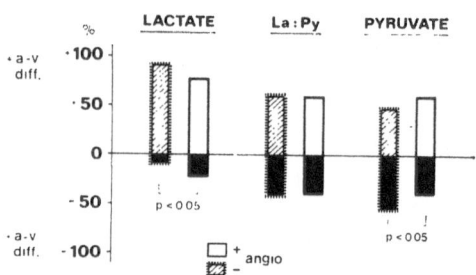

Fig. 1. Comparison of the rate of positive or negative arteriovenous (= a−v) difference of lactate, lactate/pyruvate ratio = La : Py) and pyruvate in patients with significant coronary artery disease (= angio +) and those with no or minimal coronary artery disease (= angio −). The negative a−v differences are below zero.

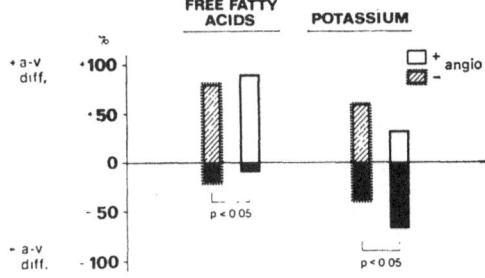

Fig. 2. Comparison of the rate of positive or negative arteriovenous differences of free fatty acids and potassium with angiographic findings. For details see fig. 1.

Higher myocardial lactate production against a lower pyruvate wash-out indicates accentuated anaerobic glycolysis. In the end-stage of anaerobic glycolysis, pyruvate-to-lactate conversion was significantly more common in patients with coronary artery disease than in those with no or minimal changes in the coronary arteries. Despite of the fact that in patient with a highly pathologic coronary artery pattern lactate increases and/or pyruvate decreases occurred more frequently, these patients did not produce a significantly higher La : Py ratio. The less common negative a–v difference of free fatty acids suggests that the latter are taken up and converted to triglycerides, which is a characteristic feature of ischemia. Just as typical is the more frequent potassium wash-out, which is related to glycogen decomposition.

A comparison between the angiographic findings and metabolic or clinical (=angina pectoris and/or S–T segment depression in V_5) signs of ischemia during the pacing test showed no close relationship between these criteria. Agreement between angiography and the metabolic signs of ischemia was found in 46.8% of patients, between angiography and the clinical signs of ischemia in 56.0% of patients, and between the metabolic and clinical signs of ischemia in 52.0% of patients. The remaining patients showed a discrepancy between each of the two compared criteria.

The distribution of all three positive criteria is shown in Figure 3, excl. 9 patients with all findings within normal limits. Note that each of the three parameters was present in about 40–50% of patients. A similar percentage of patients had only one positive criterion. Two of the evaluated criteria were found in about 10% of patients. We can pressume that myocardial lactate production is absent in normals even under stress, i. e. we cannot expect false positive results. On the other hand, myocardial ischemia can be easily undetected due to low pacing stress or poor venous blood mixing or when venous drainage of the ischemic area is below the site of blood sampling. So we cannot exclude the possibility of false negative results.

To sum up, the relationship between angiographically proven coronary artery disease and metabolic and/or clinical signs of ischemia induced by pacing is rather loose. The present techniques for evaluating myocardial metabolism in cardiology have a limited clinical value, but in some patients with inconclusive other results they can be help to prove the presence of ischemic heart disease. However, the study of myocardial metabolism is important for basic research (A).

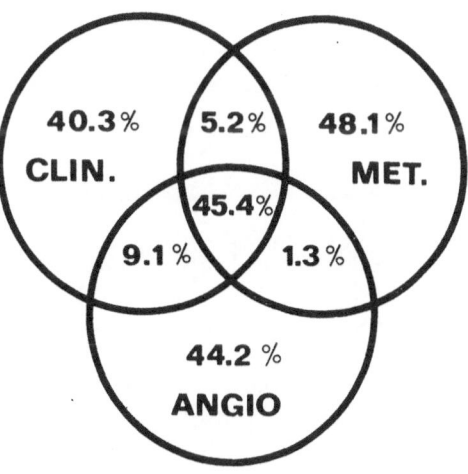

Fig. 3. Distribution of all evaluated positive results-angiographic findings (=angio), metabolic (=met) and clinical (=clin) signs of ischemia during pacing.

689

REFERENCES

1. *Boudoulas, H., et al.* (1974): Myocardial lactate production in patients with angina-like chest pain and angiographically normal coronary arteries and left ventricle. Amer. J. Cardiol. 34, 5, 501—505.
2. *Brodan, V., et al. (1978):* Myocardial amino acid metabolism in patients with chronic ischemic heart disease. Basic Res. Cardiol. 73, 160—170.
3. *Livesley, B., Oram, S. (1973):* Diagnosis of doubtful angina. Comparison of radiotelemetric exercise electrocardiogram with lactate content of coronary-sinus blood after pacing. Lancet 30, 1461—1465.
4. *Mammohansingh, P., Parker, J. O. (1975):* Angina pectoris with normal coronary arteriograms: Hemodynamic and metabolic response to atrial pacing. Amer. Heart J. 90, 5, 555 to 561.
5. *Rajasalmi, M., Takkunen, J.* (1977): Angina pectoris in young patients: Clinical appraisal and evaluation by exercise, atrial pacing, and myocardial lactate metabolism. Acta Med. Scand. 202, 341—347.
6. *Robson, R. H., Pridie, R., Fluck, D. C.* (1976): Evaluation of rapid atrial pacing in diagnosis of coronary artery disease. Evaluation of atrial pacing test. Brit. Heart J. 38, 986—989.

J. F., Inst. of Clinical and Experimental Medicine, Videňská 800, 140 00 Praha 4, Czechoslovakia

IDENTIFICATION AND MANAGEMENT OF THE CANDIDATE FOR SUDDEN CARDIAC DEATH

E. CORDAY

Clinical Professor of Medicine, University of California, School of Medicine, Los Angeles, U.S.A.

Sudden cardiac death is now recognized as the leading cause of death in the U.S.A. accounting for the loss of 300.000 to 400.000 lives each year. It is principally due to ischemia of the myocardium. Prior to the 1940's it was believed that sudden death was an unavoidable blessing if it was sudden and the patient did not suffer. New methods have been developed to prevent and treat the fearful catastrophe so that now we are beginning to look upon this as an avoidable condition.

Definition

There are many different definitions of sudden cardiac death. It may be instantaneous, or may occur at variable periods after the onset of symptoms. The definition used by the cardiac programs office of the National Heart, Lung and Blood Institute to provide the stratification of scientific data, considers it to be death due to primary cardiac causes or mechanism occurring within 24 hours of the onset of acute illness in a person thought to be free of, or with symptomatically mild heart disease, or simply prehospital death. This should not be confused with the term used to describe "instantaneous" death which refers to death within minutes, or up to 1 hour after the onset of symptoms.

Etiology

Most instances of cardiac arrest are due to ventricular fibrillation and a smaller percentage of less than 10 percent are due to ventricular standstill. Frequent premature ventricular systoles often precede the onset of ventricular fibrillation. The data derived from the Framingham Study suggest these frequent ectopic beats become a considerable risk factor when they are associated with arteriosclerotic heart disease or hypertrophy of the ventricles. Several investigations indicate that coronary artery disease accounts for 90 percent of the victims of sudden cardiac death, but there are many other cardiac causes of less frequency which include rheumatic fever, aortic valve disease, hypertensive heart disease, Wolff-Parkinson disease, cardiomyopathy, congenital heart disease, bacterial endocartitits, coronary embolism, aortic aneurysm with dissection, idiopathic myocardial hypertrophy, or idiopathic hypertrophic subaortic stenosis and prolapsed mitral valve syndrome.

Although it is well documented that coronary disease is the principal etiologic factor, it has been noted at autopsy that recent myocardial infarction or acute coronary thrombosis was causally related in only 5—10 percent of those who died. Of course, this figure might actually be on the low side because it is difficult to recognize progressive histopathologic evidence of infarction at autopsy until 24—48 hours after occlusion. It is also possible that the evidence of coronary occlusion due to an obstructive coronary thrombus might have been washed away by lytic action. The comprehensive review of data obtained of those that died in placebo groups of the cooperative drug program, noted severe chronic damage to the myocardium was a common finding in victims of sudden cardiac death. Also, many who died suddenly were taking cardiac drugs such as digitalis, diuretics, and antiarrhythmic agents that in themselves, may cause fatal arrhythmias.

Many reports reiterate the most important risk factor for sudden cardiac death was previous history of myocardial infarction of significant severity manifested by residual impairment of cardiac function. Many reports indicate the incidence of hypertension and blood lipids are not abnormally elevated so that they can be rated low as an associated condition of risk. Standard risk factors which are believed to cause arteriosclerosis do not appear to have been more evident in sudden coronary death victims and therefore they do not appear to play a prominent role in its etiology.

The significant electrocardiographic findings in those who died were residual ST segment depression and Q waves which provided evidence of previous myocardial infarction or cardiomegaly. The associated finding of congestive heart failure was often evident. Patients who succumbed had an increased incidence of ventricular tachycardia. To identify such arrhythmias, it became evident that routine 12-lead electrocardiograms which consider only a few minutes recording time had little opportunity of documenting ominous arrhythmias, but that the Holter Monitor which reviews every heartbeat for a period up to 24 hours made it possible to identify the candidate who might sustain sudden cardiac death. Holter monitoring also provides a more appropriate assessment of effectiveness and applicability of antiarrhythmic agents.

Many reports indicate a higher incidence of sudden cardiac death in those who have sustained an acute myocardial infarction within 6 months. *Moss* noted that 60% of the 42 deaths in 759 patients occurred within the first 6 months after hospital discharge for myocardial infarction. *Vismara* noted that frequent ventricular ectopic beats which occur in the first week after infarction were not of prognostic significance, but if they were noted in the second and third week, they indicate a bad prognosis of possible sudden cardiac death. This observation highlights the vulnerability of the early posthospital interval and suggests well-directed preventive programs may reduce cardiac mortality. Therefore, we recommend that every patient should have a 24-hour Holter monitor performed before discharge from a CCU to determine if he has considerable ectopic activity which indicates a need for a long term course of antiarrhythmic medication. In addition to such special 24-hour monitoring, nuclear scans should be performed in all such patients before discharge, particularly if they continue to have anginal pain, to learn whether they still have residual areas of ischemia, which might result in devastating electrical instability. *Harrison et al* report that patients admitted to the coronary care unit suspected of having had a myocardial infarct and sent home after 2 days of observation as ruled out infarction, should be considered to be at high risk of sudden death. They should have further investigative study because 10% died and an equal number sustained a non-fatal infarction within a 6-month period.

We noted the magnitude of ST segment depression or elevation immediately following acute myocardial infarction is also an important finding because those animals and humans that developed fatal ventricular fibrillation within 1 hour after coronary occlusion had the tallest ST segment elevations that persisted during the acute phase. They also had higher resting heart rates after coronary occlusion, suggesting they might be experiencing a stronger sympathetic autonomic tone than the survivors. In our attempt to determine the causation of sudden cardiac death, we noted that those that subsequently developed ventricular fibrillation suffered the severe abnormalities of metabolic function in the ischemic zone which was demonstrated by lactate production, potassium loss, and reduced pH. Just a few minutes before the onset of ventricular fibrillation, a sudden explosive deterioration in metabolism in the regionally ischemic zone supervened. We noted that in the first 2 hours after coronary occlusion gross ST segment elevations were usually associated with the most severe regional loss in potassium. Such severe metabolic derangements in the ischemic zone produces abnormal electromotive forces which trigger a regional electrocution mechanism.

Premonitory symptoms of sudden cardiac death

Fifty percent of sudden cardiac death victims die within one hour of the onset of their acute illness. On retrospective questioning of the family of sudden cardiac death victims about any new or modified symptomotology preceding death, we learned that two-thirds of sudden cardiac death victims experienced symptoms for a few minutes to many days preceding the fatal event. These included (1) chest discomfort, (2) an increase in anginal pattern, (3) breathlessness for no apparent reason, (4) symptoms referable to the musculoskeletal and gastrointestinal tract, (5) overwhelming fatigue and (6) depression.

Techniques used to identify the candidate for sudden cardiac death

Of the above noted markers it appears the clinical history, the ECG and radionuclear stress tests are of greatest value to identify those individuals at greater risk. The ECG changes during stress testing are not as significant as other measurements of physiologic function. The studies by *Bruce* on the effect of exertional hypotension that supervened during exercise testing, noted that 6 men that became hypotensive later sustained fatal ventricular fibrillation. They consider such blood pressure responses to exercise superior to the occurrence of ST segment depression and the presence of arrhythmias, the traditional predictors used in stress testing. This suggests that the blood pressure should be taken on all individuals during stress testing because it might delineate those who are at great risk of sudden cardiac death. *Richtie et al.* using radionuclide Thallium for myocardial imaging in 21 long term survivors who were previously resuscitated, revealed that 11 had an unstable area of myocardial tissue. A new unstable nuclear defect was also evident in 10—13 of these patients submitted to exercise testing. Detection of such trigger areas are of prognostic importance for identifying the candidate for sudden cardiac death.

*Why is it important to identify
the individual candidate for sudden
cardiac death?*

Our studies which demonstrated a 60 percent mortality within the first 30 minutes after experimental coronary occlusion, suggest that antiarrhythmic therapy must be applied either prophylactically or immediately after the onset of ischemic symptoms. Individuals at great risk of sudden cardiac death should receive prophylactic antiarrhythmic therapy either in the form of beta blocking drugs, quinidine, or procaine amide, to prevent the occurrence of cardiac arrest. Several studies postulated that propranolol, a beta blockade, may prevent cardiac arrest, but certain pitfalls were noted in the design of such studies. To prove the point, the NHLBI has set up a program which will try to better identify and prove whether propranolol should be used in all patients labeled as likely candidates for sudden cardiac death.

Lown has demonstrated that many fatal arrhythmias have a neuro or psychological mechanism and postulates that the sympathetic pathway eminating from the hypothalamus can lower the ventricular vulnerability threshold and thus provoke a variety of arrhythmias. He noted that any agents which will reduce norepinephrine release in the localized myocardial sites, such as beta blocking agents, may afford nearly complete protection against ventricular fibrillation after coronary occlusion. They remphasize that environ-mental stress of diverse types can affect the hear¹ and lower the vulnerability threshold to ventricular fibrillation which provokes potentially malignant ventricular arrhythmias. These studies would suggest a need to find drugs which have a more favorable effect on the neurochemistry. Psychotrophic drugs and psychiatric care might be of benefit to prevent fatal arrhythmias in many patients.

Principles of treatment

Our studies, which demonstrated a 67 percent mortality rate in the first 30 minutes after experimental coronary occlusion, suggest that therapy must be applied prophylactically or soon after symptoms appear. Therefore, because of the early onset of fatal ventricular fibrillation, the measures to reduce the mortality of patients identified at high risk must (1) encompass prophylactic antiarrhythmic therapy of proved efficacy in the presence of regional ischemia, (2) prompt treatment of arrhythmias occurring during acute myocardial ischemia, and (3) prompt and effective cardiac resuscitation from ventricular fibrillation. So far, the search for better antiarrhythmic agents that will work in the presence of ischemia has been disappointing. At present there are so few drugs that have proved ability as antiarrhythmic agents for the prevention of sudden cardiac death that the national need commands an increased priority of effort directed to this major health problem.

E. C., Institute of Med. Research, Fountain ave. 4751, Los Angeles, Cal. 90020, U.S.A.

693

CORONARY HEART DISEASE IN PATIENTS WITH PERIPHERAL ARTERIAL OCCLUSION

M. KORNOTZKI and H. HEINE

Governmental Hospital and Central Institute of Cardiovascular Regulation Research, Academy of Sciences, Berlin, G.D.R.

The prognosis of patients suffering from peripheral vascular disease is determined to a considerable extent by the coincidence of arteriosclerotic changes in the coronary arteries. Coronary heart disease (CHD) in this group of patients is to be expected earlier than in the corresponding normal population. In our experience, however, the case-history is insufficient for the diagnosis of CHD in 35% of these patients. But early diagnosis of CHD is essential for all preventive and therapeutic measures.

In the Angiological Unit of the IInd Medical Department of Charité Hospital, Humboldt-University Berlin, 200 unselected male patients with the angiographic diagnosis of arterial occlusion in the legs were examined by experienced cardiologists to detect the presence of CHD. The diagnosis was based on the case-history, clinical findings, ECG and ECG after exercise. On admission three fourth of our patients were in stage II according to *Fontaine*. Intermittent claudication developed on the average 8.5 years ago. The rate of risk factors of arteriosclerosis was as follows. On the top of the list is cigarette smokings followed by overweight and hypertension. Underweight, however, was recorded in 38% of the males suffering from peripheral arterial disease. Only 28% of the patients had X − ray findings typical of left ventricular hypertrophy. 22% of

Tab. I. Risk factors in 200 patients suffering from peripheral arterial occlusion

smoking	198	99%
obesity	116	58%
hypertension	82	41%
hyperlipidemia	73	36.5%
diabetes mell.	32	16%

the patients had signs of manifest myocardial insufficiency.

In our study special importance was ascribed to ECG after exercise which is considered a sufficiently sensitive and specific method to recognize CHD. Therefore we have deliberately omitted correlation of ECG after exercise and coronarography.

Results

In 63.5% of all cases we found signs of coronary insufficiency. In 11% the ECG was normal, but the ECG after exercise was pathological. ECG after exercise was performed in principle only after the necessary elimination time for glycosides. In

Tab. II. Signs of CHD in 200 patients suffering from peripheral arterial occlusion

Symptom	n	%	
angina pectoris	101	50.5	
state after heart infarction	37	18.5	
path. ECG	105	52.5	
path. ergometry by normal ECG	22	11.0	63.5%
ergometry impracticable	27	13.5	

29% the ECG and exercise ECG were normal. Arm crank ergometry was used in cases of coxarthrosis, kneejoint stiffness, amputation or severe claudication.

In 13.5% of all patients ECG after exercise was contraindicated for different reasons. If we assume that CHD exists in all these cases with general advanced vascular disease at least as frequently, as in the others, we can state, that approximately

70% of all patients with peripheral arterial disorders of the legs suffered from ischemic heart disease.

50.5% of the patients had angina pectoris.

17.5% survived after one or more myocardial infarctions.

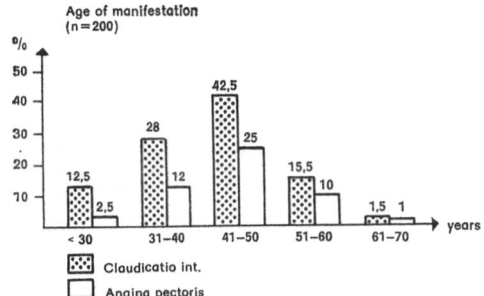

Manifestation of intermittent claudication before the age of 50 years in 83% of the cases is remarkable (first three columns). In 76% of all patients manifestation of claudication precedes angina pectoris. 16% of the patients reported previously angina pectoris. In 8% angina and claudication occurred at the same time. Smoking habits were of special interest to us, because only two patients did not smoke.

The average number of cigarettes smoked per day was 16. But 87 patients admitted smoking 30—40 cigarettes daily most of them for a period of about 20 years. Peripheral arterial disease developed in 82% within 20 years of smoking.

Irrespective of the localization of the occlusion in the leg (distal or proximal), the incidence of angina pectoris was the same.

In stage III according to *Fountaine* angina pectoris is significantly more frequent than in all other stages. This corresponds with the ECG results. Most of the pathological ECG were found in stage III and in cases with polytopic arteriosclerosis, that means ileofemoro-popliteal types.

Our results agree with the coronarographic studies of *Kiefer* (1969) in patients with peripheral arterial disorders, who revealed the coincidence of coronary sclerosis in up to 70%.

Conclusions

1. It is to be expected that CHD is present in about 70% of all patients suffering from arteriosclerotic disorders of the legs.
2. Approximately half of these patients complain of angina pectoris.
3. There are pathological ECG's in more than 50% of the cases. ECG after exercise increases the rate of pathological ECG findings by 11%
4. Peripheral arteriosclerosis precedes coronary sclerosis in 76% by 2.4 years on the average (between 1 and 17 years).
5. Cigarette smoking is the most frequent risk factor of CHD as well as of peripheral vascular disease. Claudication develops on the average after 24 years of smoking.
6. Early recognition of peripheral arteriosclerosis is of great importance for detection of accompanying changes in the coronary arteries and should be included in every screening and preventive programme of CHD.

REFERENCE

Kiefer, H. (1969): Die klinische Bedeutung der Koronararteriographie. Med. Welt 13, 710—714.

M. K., Governmental Hospital 104 Berlin. Scharnhorststraße 37, G.D.R.

CHANGES IN MYOCARDIAL TRACE ELEMENT LEVEL IN EXPERIMENTAL CORONARY OCCLUSION AND MYOCARDIAL INFARCTION

J. DANYS, M. KUŠLEIKAITÉ and P. SIMAŠKA

Institute of Cardiovascular Research, Kaunas, Lithuanian S.S.R., U.S.S.R.

We studied the content of manganese, nickel, copper and zinc in the myocardium during experimental coronary occlusion of various duration, and the level of manganese, nickel, copper, zinc, chromium, calcium and magnesium in the cardiac muscle of patients who have died of myocardial infarction.

Materials and methods

The experiments were carried out on 45 rabbits of 2—3 kg body weight. After thoracotomy the descending branch of the anterior coronary artery was ligated and thus an occlusion was made which was of 30, 40, 50, 60 minutes and 3, 6, 12, 24 hours duration. The content of Mn, Ni, Cu and Zn was estimated in the intact myocardium of the left ventricle and in the ischemic zone. For control, the same trace elements were estimated in the left ventricle of intact rabbits. The trace elements were estimated with a Perkin Elmer atomic absorption spectrophotometer 503.

Results

The curves, showing changes in the content of the trace elements in 1 g od dry substance of the myocardium, revealed a more pronounced increase in the content of the trace elements in an occlusion of 30—60 minutes and 12—24 hours duration. The statistically significant increase (in comparison with controls) in the content of Ni in the intact myocardium in cases of an occlusion of 30-minutes duration, the content of Mn in the ischemic zone of the cardiac muscle after an occlusion of 50 minutes, and the level of Zn in both zones after 30-60-minute-occlusion was connected not only with a lesion of muscle fibres but also with some phenomena of adaptation. The presented point becomes clearer if data obtained by *I. A.*

Shevtchuk (1972), that Zn of musclar fibers of the heart plays an important role in the activation of ATP-ase and enzymatic systems of the cell necessary for utilization of glucose, are taken into account.

After a 3—5 hours occlusion of the coronary artery the content of Zn in both zones increased insignificantly. This may be explained by a progressive destruction of myocardial cells. The degenerative character of the processes developing in the tissues of the heart during this period of occlusion is also confirmed by the manner of changes in the content of Ni in relation to the changes in the level of Mn. The character of the changes in the content of Ni in relation to the level of Mn was the same in the intact myocardium and in the ischemic zone. As ions of Ni activate slow sodium-calcium current, blocked by ions of Mn (*Donskikh*, 1971), it may be supposed that the antagonism between these ions does not manifest itself during an occlusion of 3—6—12 hours duration. During an occlusion of 30, 40, 50, 60-minutes, and 12-24 hours duration the changes in the content of Mn and Ni (as they are shown by the curves) had an opposite character in the ischemic zone as well as in the intact myocardium. It may be supposed that during this period of occlusion ions of Mn and Ni behave like antagonists in respect of their influence on the conduction in the slow sodium-calcium channel in membranes of myocardial fibers. In a 12—24-hours-occlusion, the concentration of zinc in both zones of the myocardium and the content of copper in the intact heart muscle increase statistically significantly (in comparison with con-

Table I. Changes in the content of trace elements in cardiac tissue of patients who have died of myocardial infarction (µg/g)

Investigated material	n	Mn $\bar{x} \pm S\bar{x}$	Ni $\bar{x} \pm S\bar{x}$	Cu $\bar{x} \pm S\bar{x}$	Zn $\bar{x} \pm S\bar{x}$	Cr $\bar{x} \pm S\bar{x}$	Ca $\bar{x} \pm S\bar{x}$	Mg $\bar{x} \pm S\bar{x}$
Acute myocardial infarction	Isch zone 16	0.89 ± 0.48	1.62 ± 0.55	22.58 ± 16.27	67.98 ± 27.89	14.13 ± 8.66	454.20 ± 343.40	173.80 ± 68.24
	Int area 16	0.77 ± 0.44	1.32 ± 0.71	10.00 ± 6.33	55.34 ± 34.13	4.80 ± 2.60	174.63 ± 111.34	190.94 ± 161.66
	t	1.0710	0.2790	2.472	0.9793	3.5742	2.4740	0.3322
	p	<0.05	<0.05	<0.05	<0.05	<0.01	<0.05	<0.05
Myocardial infarction in the stage of resorption and organization	Isch zone 13	0.67 ± 0.46	1.78 ± 1.10	3.32 ± 1.14	27.47 ± 14.43	4.91 ± 2.25	156.83 ± 110.62	97.61 ± 81.72
	Int area 13	0.66 ± 0.31	1.98 ± 1.21	4.44 ± 0.91	44.03 ± 21.62	6.75 ± 5.20	202.30 ± 102.23	156.30 ± 28.03
	t	0.5260	0.3032	2.2431	1.8213	0.9231	0.8570	1.9381
	p	<0.05	<0.05	<0.05	<0.05	<0.05	<0.05	<0.05

trols), the level of copper in the ischemic zone lowers. This permits us to suppose that in this period of occlusion intracellular compensatory processes manifest themselves, especially in the zone of the intact myocardium, together with progressing destructive changes. Changes in the concentration of trace elements in the heart during occlusion of the coronary artery may help us to understand some aspects of acute ischemia of the heart.

Having all this in mind we decided to investigate changes in the content of the trace elements (Mn, Ni, Cu, Zn, Cr, Ca, Mg) in tissues of the heart of persons who have died of myocardial infarction. The data obtained have shown that in most cases of acute myocardial infarction the level of the investigated trace elements was higher than in the intact zone (Table I). Apparently, adaptation of metabolic processes to the new conditions had not enough time to develop in the intact zone.

During the stage of resorption and organization, the ratio of the content of the trace elements in the focus of necrosis and in the prenecrotic area had a different character, i. e. the concentration of the investigated trace elements in the intact zone was higher than in the area of necrosis. The augmentation of concentration of the trace elements in the intact zone is evidence of compensatory-adaptive processes occurring in this area of the myocardium.

REFERENCES

Donskikh, E. A. (1971): Influence of nickel on the myocardium. Moscow.
Shevchuk, I. A. (1972): The content and distribution of zinc in the heart. In Metabolism and Structure of the Normal and Pathologic Heart. Novosibirsk, 511—512.

J. D., Institute of Cardiovascular Research, Eiveniu 4, Kaunas, Lithuanian SSR, U.S.S.R.

AUTONOMIC CONTROL OF CONDUIT CORONARY ARTERY DIAMETER

MÁRIA GEROVÁ, E. BARTA and J. GERO

Institute of Normal and Pathological Physiology, Slovak Academy of Sciences and II. Dept. of Surgery, Faculty of Medicine, Comenius University, Bratislava, Czechoslovakia

The pattern of adrenergic innervation of major coronary arteries corresponds to the general innervation pattern of large and middle sized arteries: the nerve terminals are located on the adventitia — media border, remote from the effector smooth muscle cells (*Denn and Stone*, 1976, *Doležel et al.* 1973, 1978). It became of interest to determine the functional consequence of this structural pattern. The urgency of this problem was underlined by the fact that no data dealing with sympathetic control of major coronary arteries is available. On the other hand, there are reports on temporary and segmental spasms of major coronary artery, whose nature is unknown (*Rose et al.*, 1974).

To study the sympathetic control of the major coronary artery and underlying mechanism, the following model was designed. The heart was arrested by a mercury tamponade of its microcirculation and the anterior half of the body including a 5 cm long segment of ramus interventricularis ventralis (RIV) — a branch of the left coronary artery was perfused at a constant pressure by cardiopulmonary bypass. BP (Stattham electromanometer) and diameter of RIV (inductive transformer) were directly and continuously monitored. The respective postganglionic sympathetic fibers were stimulated by bipolar platinum electrodes.

Bilateral stimulation of stellate ganglion (SG) ellicits a diameter reduction of RIV (Figure 1) peculiar from two points of view.

(1) Maximum diameter reduction of RIV represents 4% of the resting outer diameter; taking into account the wall thickness (*Boucek et al.*, 1963) this value corresponds to 8% of the inner diameter reduction.

Because of uncertainty concerning the coronary sympathetic pathways, additional sympathetic fibres were stimulated. The diameter reduction induced by bilateral stimulation of fibres leaving thoracic sympathetic ganglia (Th_{2-3-4}) was only 1.2%; stimulation of caudal cerv. ggl. did not effect the RIV diameter.

One possible explanation of the relatively small range of sympathetic control could be the long neuro-effector distance. Transmitter released during stimulation, after having been reuptaked partly by the nerve terminal, diffuses radially and thus a considerable fraction is directed to the adventitia. This part is lost for effective contraction and only the remainder can

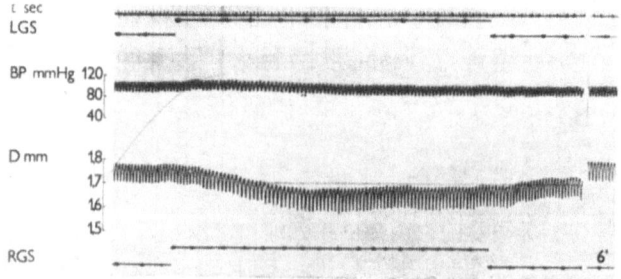

Fig. 1. Blood pressure and diameter of RIV during bilateral stellate ganglia stimulation (LGS, RGS); time in sec.

associate with smooth muscle receptors and is relevant for constriction.

Bearing in mind that a majority of large and middle sized vessels have a similar localization of adrenergic terminals in vessel wall, we compared the extent of maximum sympathetic constriction of several segments in the arterial tree. It can be seen in Figure 2 that RIV and the carotid artery have the smallest extent of maximum sympathetic contraction.

Moreover, in spite of the fact that innervation density of RIV is far higher (60 – 100 terminals/cross section) than the density of femoral artery (5 terminals/cross section), the constriction of the femoral artery is 3 times larger than that of RIV.

Since neither the localization nor the density of innervation seem to be responsible for the small extent of RIV constriction, attention was focused to the coronary smooth muscle itself.

In coronary arteries beta-receptors were described and hence it can be suggested that the small extent of contraction might reflect simultaneous activation of both alpha-and beta-receptors; the effective constriction might be determined by the inter-

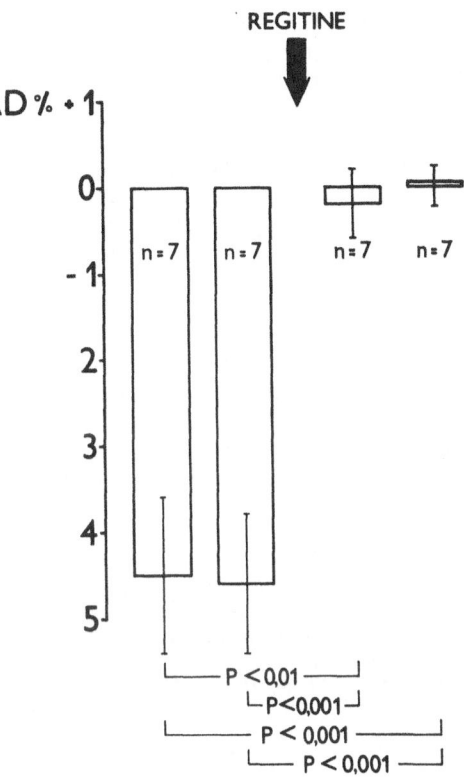

Fig. 3. The RIV diameter changes (mean values ± SEM) in response to bilateral SG stimulation before (10 – 5 min) and after (5 – 10 min) blocking of alpha-receptors by phentolamine (2 mg/kg i. v.).

action of simultaneous alpha- and beta-response.

To interfere in the system of receptors, phentolamine 2 mg/kg was administered. Although, before alpha-receptor blockade, SG stimulation induced appropriate diameter reduction, 5 minutes after administration phentolamine, the same stimulation does not evoke any constriction; however, no dilation was found either (Figure 3). These results indicate that, during sympathetic stimulation in the major coronary artery, only alpha-receptors are activated, whereas beta-receptors are not involved. Thus, a small reactivity of the major coronary artery to released noradrenaline can be deduced from all these experiments. The experiments *in vitro* with coronary

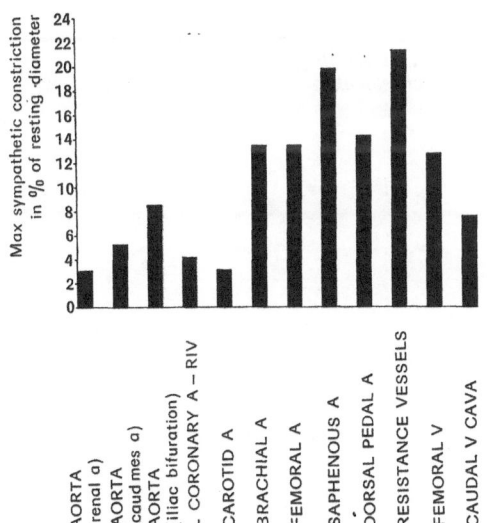

Fig. 2. The extent of maximal sympathetic constriction in percentage of resting diameter in individual segments of the vessel tree.

strips cut from the same part of RIV where the diameter was registered, extend the low sensitivity of major coronaries to exogenous noradrenaline. The response of a strip cut from coronary artery was 7 times smaller than that of femoral artery and 10 times lower than that from rabbit aorta.

(2) The second peculiarity was the low rate of sympathetic constriction of major coronary artery. Steady-state diameter reduction during sympathetic stimulation is attained between 60—90 sec, i. e. in a time which is 4—6 times longer than that of the portal vein or arterioles. The slow velocity points to successive recruitment into contraction of smooth muscle layers remote from nerve endings very probably due to diffusion of the transmitter, in a way similar to that which was shown in the dorsal pedal or saphenous artery (*Gerová et al.*, 1967, *Doležel et al.*, 1975).

The results of the experiments can be summarized: sympathetic nervous system induces a constriction of major coronary arteries via association of released-noradrenaline to alpha-receptors. The constriction is moderate and slow. The small extent of constriction can be ascribed to both a long neuro-effector distance and low sensitivity to noradrenaline; the low rate is very probably due to the diffusion of released noradrenaline across the vessel wall.

REFERENCES

Boucek, R. J., Takashita, R., Foiaco R. (1963): Relation between microanatomy and functional properties of the coronary arteries. Anat. Rec. 147: 199—207.

Denn, M. J., Stone, H. L. (1976): Autonomic innervation of dog coronary arteries. J. Appl. Physiol. 41: 30—35.

Doležel, S., Gerová, M., Gero, J., Feit, J. (1975): Diffusion through the vessel wall of transmitter released by sympathetic stimulation. Blood Vessels 12: 108—121.

Doležel, S., Gerová, M., Gero, J., Sládek, T., Vašku, J. (1978): Adrenergic innervation of the coronary arteries and the myocardium. Acta anat. 100: 306—316.

Gerová, M., Gero, J., Doležel, S. (1967): Mechanism of sympathetic regulation of arterial smooth muscle. Experientia 23: 639—640.

Rose, F. J., Johnson, A. D., Carleton, R. A. (1974): Spasm of the left anterior descending coronary artery. Chest 66: 719—721.

M. G., Institut of Normal and Pathological Physiology, S. A. S., Sienkiewiczova 1, 884 23 Bratislava, Czechoslovakia

SYSTOLIC TIME INTERVALS UNDER CONDITIONS OF PHYSICAL EXERCISE IN INVESTIGATION OF THE 40—59 YEAR OLD MALE POPULATION

S. I. PLAVINSKAYA

The Anitchkov Department of Biochemistry of Lipids and Atherosclerosis, Institute of Experimental Medicine, Leningrad, U.S.S.R.

This investigation was carried out to determine the potentialities of the polycardiographic (PCG) method under conditions of physical exercise on a treadmill for revealing insidious coronary insufficiency.

In an epidemiological investigation of the population in one of the districts of the city of Leningrad 468 men of the age of 40—59 were picked by the method of random selection. Persons with arterial hypertension (AP $\leq$ 160/95) were excluded. All the studied persons performed a standard physical exercise on a treadmill according to the *Bruce* scheme. The exercise period was determined according to the number of heart contractions, taking into account the age and degree of training condition. PCG was recorded three times on an "Elema" mingograph — prior to exercise and 1 minute and 6 minutes after the exercise. Analysis of the left ventricle phase structure was carried out by the *Blumberger* method using the modification of *Carpman*. Pulse rate, arterial pressure and ECG were registered periodically throughout the whole exercise and 6 minutes after it ended.

366 of the investigated persons (78%) performed the set submaximal exercise completely; in these cases neither electrocardiographic nor clinical symptoms of coronary insufficiency were noted. The latter made up group 1 (control). In 61 cases (13%) the exercise was stopped due to fatigue or the appearance of labored breathing (dyspnea) — group 2; in 41 cases (9%) the cause for terminating the exercise was an ischemic reaction (a drop of the horizontal or concave ST segment by not less than 1 mm; the onset of attacks of stenocardia, a drop in the systolic arterial pressure) — group 3.

The exercise duration in group 1 and 2 were approximately the same: 10.3 ± 0.14 and 10.2 ± 0.28 min., while as the heart rate attained in these two groups proved to be statistically different; in the 1st group it was 167 ± 0.4 beats per min. and 150 beats per min. ($p < 0.001$) in the 2nd group. In the 3rd group the maximum heart rate attained was on an average only 135 ± 2.5 beats per min., at a mean exercise duration of 7.2 ± 0.45 min. The low chronotropic heart reserve in the 3rd group investigated is connected with the fact that continuation of the exercise was impossible due to development of an ischemic reaction. The drop of the chronotropic reserve in the 2nd group to 89.7 ± 1.2 against 107.3 ± 1.1 in the control group ($p < 0.001$) cannot be explained by a typical manifestation of coronary insufficiency. The tolerance decrease to the exercise may be connected with latent heart insufficiency, which is reflected as changes in the PCG-picture. When studying the systolic time intervals (to PCG data) in a state of rest there were no significant differences among the above three groups. Significant differences appear in the 2nd and 3rd groups, compared with the control (see Table I), during the period of early restitution after physical exercise.

As seen from the above data, the left ventricular ejection time (LVET) and preejection period (PEP) are extended, the mean acceleration of intraventricular pressure is decreased, i. e. the physical exercise revealed cardiodynamic distrubances ac-

Table I. Some indices of systolic time intervals in the 40—59 year old male population in a state of rest and after a treadmill-test (M ± m)

Group investigator	PEP		LVET		Mean acceleration of intraventrilucar pressure (mm Hg/sec)	
	prior to exercise	1.5 min. after test	prior to exercise	1.5 min. after test	prior to exercise	1.5 min. after test
Group No. 1 Control	0.98± 0.01	0.63± 0.02	0.305± 0.02	0.215± 0.02	1N94± 108	10396± 1070
Group No. 2 with reduced tolerance to exercise	1.01± 0.02	0.68± 0.02	0.305± 0.03	0.233± 0.03	1807± 131	5673± 1053
Group No. 3 with ischemic reaction to exercise	1.02± 0.03	0.72± 0.03	0.308± 0.04	0.271 ± 0.05	1517± 73	5300± 1458

cording to the type of hypodynamia phase syndrome. There is evident ECG proof or clinical manifestations of coronary insufficiency, which explain the cardiodynamic disturbances in the 3rd group investigated.

The shift similarity of systolic time intervals in the 2nd and 3rd groups, the absence of other reasons in addition to coronary insufficiency, which could explain the PCG changes and decreased tolerance to exercise, suggest that insuf-

ficiency of coronary circulation underlies the inadequate reaction to exercise in the 2nd group. A number of other authors hold to the same opinion (*Kavtaradze et al.*, 1975, *Cooper*, 1975).

The data support use of the PCG method under conditions of physical exercise for diagnosing insidious disturbance of the myocardium contractile function connected. in particular, with ischemic heart disease.

REFERENCES

Kavtaradze V. G., Didebuladze T. G., Bregvadze G. I. (1975): Chronotropic heart reserve and indices of physical working capacity in persons with coronary atherosclerosis and hypertension. Ther. Arch., 7, 77—82 (Russian).

Carpman V. L. (1965): Phase analysis of heart activity. Moscow, Medizina (Russian).

Blumberger K. (1940): Die Auspannungszeit und Austreibungzeit beim Menschen. Arch. Kreislaufforsch., 6, 203—292.

Bruce R. (1973): Principles of Exercise Testing in: "Exercise Testing and Exercise Training in Coronary Heart disease". N.-Y., Ed. by Naughton, Hellerstein, 45—61.

Cooper M. (1975): The Symptom-Limited Exercise Tolerance Test in the Diagnosis of Coronary Artery Disease. Cardiol. Dig., 10, 7, 11—20.

S. I. P., The Anitchkov Dept. of Biochemistry of Lipids and Atherosclerosis, Inst. of Experim. Med., 12 Pavlov St., Leningrad 197022, U.S.S.R.

ANGIOCARDIOGRAPHIC AND ECHOCARDIOGRAPHIC EVALUATION OF LEFT VENTRICULAR FUNCTION

M. ŠIMO, I. RIEČANSKÝ, E. BÁRTA, J. ZELENAY,
O. KUNA, and L. KUŽELA,

Second Medical and Surgical Clinic, Comenius University Bratislava, Czechoslovakia

Measurement of the left ventricular systolic performance, expressed mostly in terms of the ejection fraction, has proved to be an important indicator of prognosis in patients with heart disease. Preoperatively measured, it has been a good predictor of the risks and results of surgery in patients undergoing coronary arterial revascularization or valve replacement. Thus, efforts have been made to obtain this value not only by invasive but also by noninvasive methods. One of the most promising noninvasive methods from this point of view seems to be echocardiography. This method enables registration not only of the motion of valves but also of the internal left ventricular dimensions, volumes, ejection fraction and mean velocity of circumferential shortening of fibers. Several authors have found good correlations between echocardiographically and

angiographically determined values of ejection fraction and other measures of contractile function (*Pombo*, 1971; *Fortuin*, 1971). On the other hand it should be emphasized that echocardiographic indexes of the ventricular function are unreliable in patients with segmental asynergy resulting from coronary artery disease or fibrosis of the ,papillary muscles (*Feigenbaum*, 1976; *Horwitz*, 1973).

In 1977 *Massie et al.* proposed a new echocardiographic index of left ventricular function. These authors observed that, in normal subjects, the anterior mitral valve leaflet closely approaches the interventricular septum in early diastole, at the E point in its cycle. In patients with depressed ventricular function they noted increased mitral E point-septal separation. The purpose of the present study was to determine whether measurements of the

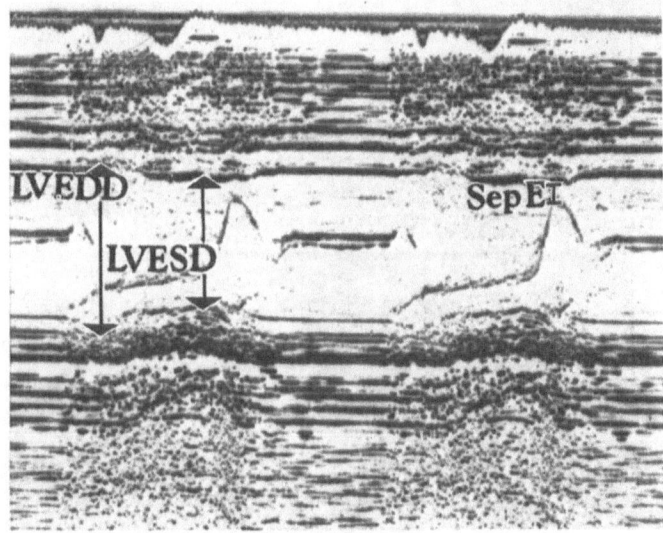

Fig. 1. Left ventricular echocardiogram showing some of the measurements that can be obtained from such an examination.
LVEDD = Left ventricular internal diameter in diastole
LVESD = Left ventricular internal diameter in systole
Sep E = Mitra-septal separation (E point separation).

mitral-septal separation also provide a useful measure of the ventricular function in patients with coronary artery disease and segmental asynergy of the left ventricle resulting from it.

A total of 50 patients with coronary artery disease underwent echocardiographic left ventriculography and coronarography within an interval of 2 days over a 12 month period at our laboratory. 10 patients were excluded because angiographic or echocardiographic studies were technically inadequate for analysis. Echocardiograms were performed using a 1.3 cm, 2.25 megahertz focused transducer and Picker Echoview 10 ultrasonoscopes with a Honeywell recorder. The left ventricular dimensions were measured at a level just below the anterior mitral valve leaflet.

An echocardiographically measured ejection fraction (EF) was computed using the formula for end-systolic volume (ESV) and end-diastolic volume (EDV) developed by *Teichholz et al.* (1975). The amount of mitral-septal separation was defined as the distance between the E point of the anterior mitral leaflet and a tangent drawn to the most posterior point reached by the interventricular septum within the same cycle.

Selective coronary arteriograms were

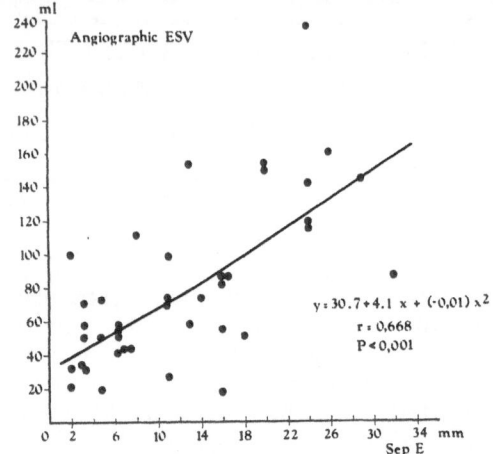

Fig. 3. Correlation between E point separation (Sep E) and angiographic end-systolic volume of the left ventricle (ESV).

performed by the *Judkin* method. Left ventricular cineangiograms were taken in the 30° right anterior oblique projection after an injection of 42 ml of 76 percent Verographin. Left ventricular volumes at end-diastole and end-systole were obtained by the method of *Greene and Snow* (1961; 1969). All patients had pathologic changes on arteriograms and various types of asynergy on ventriculograms. A statistically significant difference was found between the value of the ejection fraction measured angiographically ($P < 0.005$). The relationship between mitral-septal separation and the angiographically measured ejection fraction is shown in Figure 2. There exists a highly significant negative correlation between the value of the E point separation and ejection fraction ($r = -0.807$, $P < 0.001$). The correlations between the E point separation and angiographically measured end-diastolic volume as well as the stroke volume ($r = 0.438$, $P < 0.01$ and $r = -0.352$, $P < 0.05$ respectively) were statistically significant.

Figure 3 demonstrates the relationship between mitral-septal separation and angiographically estimated end-systolic volume.

A highly significant positive correlation was found ($r = 0.668$, $P < 0.001$).

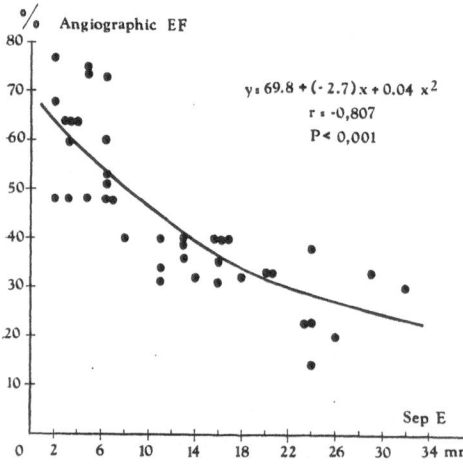

Fig. 2. Correlation between E point separation (Sep E) and angiographic ejection fraction (EF).

Our results thus indicate that the amount of mitral-septal separation in early diastole correlates well with the ventriculographically measured ejection fraction in patients with coronary artery disease. The reliability of this index in these patients is noteworthy. The utility of this variable is enhanced by the relative simplicity of obtaining simultaneous echoes from the anterior mitral leaflet and the interventricular septum. In addition, E point separation can be measured rapidly and no further computation is required, thus allowing a rapid estimation of ventricular function.

REFERENCES

Feigenbaum, H., (1976): Echocardiography. Philadelphia, Lea and Febiger 298—380.

Fortuin, N. J., Hood, Jr. W. P., Sherman, E., Craige, E., (1971): Determination of left ventricular volumes by ultrasound. Circulation 44, 575—584.

Horwitz, L. D., Mullins, Ch. B., Payne, R. M., Curry, G. C., (1973): Left ventricular function in mitral stenosis. Chest 64, 609—914.

Massie, B. M., Schiller, N. B., Ratshin, R. A., Parmley, W. W., (1977): Mitra-septal separation: New echocardiographic index of left ventricular function. Amer. J. Cardiol. 39, 1008—1016.

Pombo, J. F., Troy, B. L., Russell, R. O., (1971): Left ventricular volumes and ejection fraction by echocardiography. Circulation 43, 480 to 490.

Teichholz, L. E., Kreulen, T. H., Heman, M. V., Gorlin, R., (1975): Problems in echocardiographic volume determinations: Echocardiographic-angiographic correlations in the presence or absence of asynergy. Amer. J. Cardiol. 37. 7—11.

M. Š., II-nd Medical Clinic, KU, Partizánska 2., 88326 Bratislava, Czechoslovakia

A REAL-TIME ECHOCARDIOGRAPHIC TRACKING SYSTEM FOR ANTERIOR VENTRICULAR WALL MOTION

G. S. MALINDZAK, JR., M. S. HOSTETLER, L. E. ROEMER, M. L. PETROVICK and E. J. CAUFFIELD

Northeastern Ohio Universities, College of Medicine, Rootstown, Ohio, U.S.A.

The non-invasive echocardiographic assessment of ventricular volume, ejection fraction and myocardial contractility has been shown to provide valuable information regarding the cardiovascular status of patients, particularly those with cardiac disease (*Fortuin, et al.*, 1971). Additional studies have shown that the dynamic motion of the heart and cardiac structures can be tracked and ventricular function evaluated utilizing modifications of conventional echocardiographic techniques (*Petrovick, et al.*, 1974; *Petrovick, et al.*, 1976; *Emerson, et al.*, 1977). The major purpose of this paper is to present a working model of a real-time digital echocardiographic tracking system designed to detect the motion and evaluate the function of the anterior and posterior ventricular wall simultaneously.

An echocardiographic tracking system has been designed which utilizes an IREX to furnish an analog signal for the simultaneous tracking of the proximal and distal boundaries of the left ventricle of man in real time. The entire tracking system is digital and controlled by a microprocessor (Intel 8080). Each ultrasonic echocardiographic pattern from the transducer burst (1500 Hz repetition rate) is digitized for the first 500 microseconds (at a rate of slightly greater than 1 MHz — 0.977 μsec/sample) following the pulse transmission and stored in a buffer memory as a data set representing that time period. Each data set is processed using the criteria described in this paper prior to the sampling and digitization of the echo patterns from subsequent transducer bursts. The tracking function is accomplished by identifying the anterior and posterior wall boundaries (using the microprocessor based system) within each data set continuously and in real-time.

Initially the composite echo pattern from the heart is viewed in the A-mode. In this mode, range gates are positioned around the echo pattern corresponding to the anterior left ventricular wall and posterior left ventricular wall. The position (depth), width and threshold of each range gate are independently adjustable and are initially set manually from potentiometers mounted on the front of the tracking control module. The effect of these adjustments are superimposed on the A-mode display and are monitored visually during the initialization procedure. The criterion for computer detection of each echo within each range gate may be the peak, the leading slope or the trailing slope of the echo pattern (Figure 1).

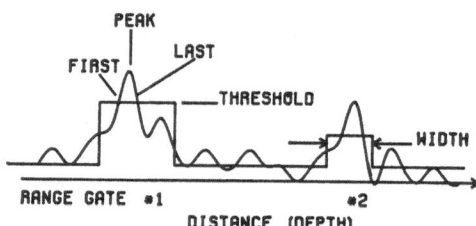

Fig. 1. A-mode display (simulated) showing the superposition of the two range gates and the envelope of the echo pattern from the ventricle.

Once these selection criteria are established, the system is switched into the automatic tracking mode during which the microprocessor takes over the function of echo selection and tracking. In the automatic tracking mode, the microprocessor processes only the data set information that falls within the range gates for positional and velocity information on each moving boundary. The position of the range gate for each data set subsequent to that selected during the initialization period is updated to center the range gate around the future predicted boundary position.

Several algorithms have been evaluated to compute the probable future position of the echo (S_{n+1}); they were all of the general form

$$S_{n+1} = K_0 \cdot S_n + K \cdot S_{n-1} + \\ + K_2 \cdot S_{n-2} + K_3 \cdot S_{n-3} + \cdots +$$

where K's are specified constants and S's are past detected echo positions.

The width of the range gate is designed to be a function of the boundary velocity (Figure 2). At low velocities, the range gate is set to a minimum width; at rapid velocities, the range gate width is increased above the minimum width to increase the probability that the echo boundary being tracked does not fall outside the range gate and fails to be detected. In the automatic tracking mode, the range gate width is increased or decreased according to the boundary velocity, but never less than the minimum width.

In the event an echo is lost or the detection criteria are not met, the range gate width is increased incrementally and symetrically around the last detected position

until an echo is found or a maximum width is reached. Until a valid signal is reacquired, no tracking signal is available and the oscillographic traces are blanked.

SIMULATED ECHO TRACKING

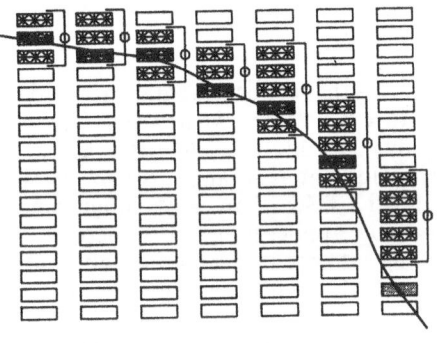

→ TIME

Fig. 2. An illustration of the changing range gate width as a function of velocity according to a specific algorithm.

REFERENCES

Emerson, R., Donnerstein, R., Kronzon, I., Schloss, M., and Glassman, E. (1977): Maximal instantaneous mitral valve velocities measured with a digital echocardiographic tracking system. IEEE Trans. Biomed. Eng. Vol. BME-24: 71—73.

Fortuin, N. J., Hood, W. P., Sherman, M. E. & Craige, E. (1971): Determination of left ventricular volumes by ultrasound. Circ. 54: 575—584.

Petrovick, M. L., Malindzak, G. S., Jr. & Knelson, J. H. (1974): A non-invasive cardiac output processor for clinical echocardiography. 27th Ann. Conf. Eng. Med. Biol., p. 267.

Petrovick, M. L., Malindzak, G. S., Jr. & Haak, E. D., Jr. (1976): An analog echocardiogram for estimating ventricular stroke volume. Ultrasound in Medicine, Edited by D. White and R. Barnes, Vol. 2: 351—361.

G. S. M., Program in Physiology, Northeastern Ohio Universities, College of Medicine Rootstown, Ohio 44272, U.S.A.

ECHOCARDIOGRAPHIC ASSESSMENT OF LEFT VENTRICULAR PERFORMANCE IN PATIENTS WITH ARTERIAL HYPERTENSION

L. PAHL

Central Institute of Cardiovascular Regulation Research, Academy of Sciences, Berlin, G.D.R.

Reports that echocardiography could be used to evaluate left ventricular function probably had more to do with the rapid world-wide interest and growth in this diagnostic field than any other single diagnostic application. Also there is increasing interest in evaluating left ventricular function with this noninvasive technique in patients with arterial hypertension. The echocardiographic method can be of special diagnostic value when it is possible to evaluate the characteristic parameters of the left ventricle (LV). Therefore accurate evaluation of the contractility and the pump function of the LV is necessary.

Our study examined the influence of the actual level of blood pressure (i. e. mean arterial blood pressure = MABp) and the effect of the duration of hypertension on the heart with regard to age and sex differences. The studies were performed with the Organon teknika ultrasonic cardiograph Echocardiovisor. We used the conventional one-dimensional single beam technique with time-motion-registration for the qualitative and quantitative evaluation. The configuration of the heart, the geometry of the ventricles and the motion pattern of the heart valves were examined with two-dimensional images with the multielement-system. In each patient we scanned the heart from the base to the apex and the echo from the LV was registered in standard position according to *Popp and Harrison* (1969). (Figure 1).

We measured the thickness of the walls, the internal diameters and the amplitude and velocity of the posterior wall movement. Therefore we can calculate fractional shortening, the mean velocity of circumferential fibre shortening (Vcf) and, assuming an idealized geometrical model of the LV, also the stroke volume, the ejection fraction and the myocardial mass of the LV (*Teichholz et al.*, 1976, *Feigenbaum*, 1972). The Vcf is a sensitive criterion of left ventricular performance and makes possible representative evaluation of the basic contractility of the ventricle (*Yonoussi*, 1976). This conclusion was also reached by other authors (*Feigenbaum*, 1972, *Karliner*, 1971).

Ejection fraction (EF) and fractional shortening can be used as an index of the pump function of the LV (*Krayenbühl*, 1977, *Karliner* 1971). We investigated 295 of our hospital patients without therapy. In 205 patients we could make an adequate

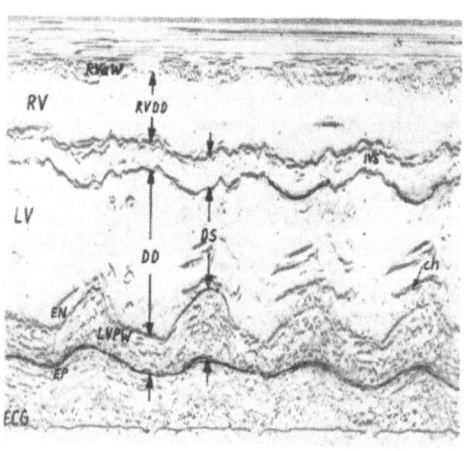

Fig. 1. Echocardiogram of the left ventricle in standard position. RV = right ventricle, LV = left ventricle, IVS = interventricular septum, EN = endocard, EP = epicard, Ch = chordae mitralis, LVPW = left ventricular posterior wall, DD = enddiastolic diameter, DS = endsystolic diameter.

echo from the LV, i. e. 62.9% of the cases. This shows the difficulties and limits of this method. 185 of the 205 patients had arterial hypertension, 20 of the patients were normotensives, all aged 18 to 60. 105 of the hypertensives were men and 80 were women. We formed 4 groups according to the level of MABp and 3 groups to the duration of hypertension.

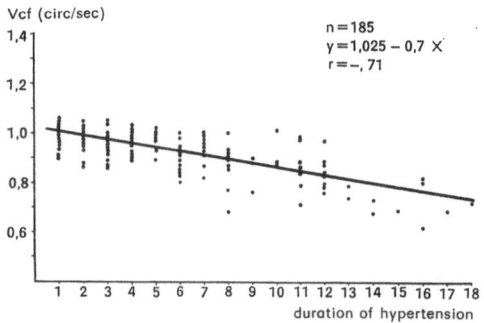

Vcf (circ/sec)

$n = 185$
$y = 1,025 - 0,7 \times$
$r = -,71$

duration of hypertension (years)

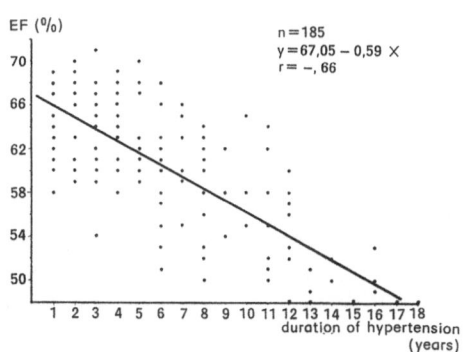

EF (%)

$n = 185$
$y = 67,05 - 0,59 \times$
$r = -,66$

duration of hypertension (years)

Fig. 2. Correlation of Vcf and EF to the duration of hypertension (years)

The correlation of Vcf to the duration of hypertension shows a linear relationship between the decrease in Vcf with increased lengh of hypertension. Also the EF shows a linear relationship its decrease with increased duration of hypertension. In women older than 41 years we registered higher values of myocardial mass, but we cannot explain this fact; indeed influences like body weight were not taken in consideration. With regard to the level of MABp with a general decreasing tendency

of Vcf with increased blood pressure we could see that the largest differences exist between the control group and group I of hypertensives. (Figure 3). In consideration of the fact that group I consists of patients in the early stages of hypertension, we can conclude that a restriction of contractility already exists in this stage of the disease.

The EF also shows a significant difference in the relationship of the control group to group I, but within the hypertensive groups I to III differences are not as important. Thus, in contrast to contractility, the pump function in hypertensives is not greatly decreased with exception of group IV.

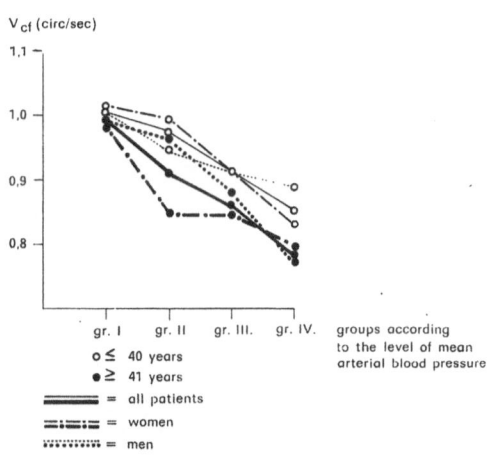

V_{cf} (circ/sec)

| gr. I | gr. II | gr. III. | gr. IV. | groups according to the level of mean arterial blood pressure |

o ≤ 40 years
● ≥ 41 years
= all patients
= women
= men

Fig. 3. Relationship between Vcf and the level of mean arterial blood pressure (MABp). Group I ≤ 110 mm Hg, Group II = 111 to 130 mm Hg, Group III = 131 to 140 mm Hg, Group IV ≥ 141 mm Hg.

Our results show that the echocardiographic parameters Vcf and EF are suited to judge an early beginning of restriction of the myocardial function in patients with arterial hypertension.

In 54 of our patients angiographic examinations with evaluation of Vcf showed good correlation with our results with an correlation index of $r = 0.87$. As we know from experience, there is a good correlation between angiographic and echocardiographic methods, when − the standardized echographic left ventricular internal dimensions approximates the left ventricular minor axis.

— there are no segmental changes in heart function.
— the measurement error is less or the same for echo, when properly performed.

But it should also be considered that there are various possible errors in obtaining echo information and in the calculation of derived indices using geometrical models. The latter fact however is true for both the echo and angiocardiographic method. Despite all these limitations, left ventricular echographic parameters are very important in the assessment of left ventricular function.

REFERENCES

Popp, R. L., Harrison, D. C. (1969): Circulation 40, 905.

Teichholz, H., Kruelen, T., Herman, M. V. et al. (1976): Amer. J. Cardiol. 37, 7.

Feigenbaum, H. (1972): Prog. Cardiovasc. Dis. 14, 531.

Yonoussi, K. (1976): Z. Kardiol. 65, 143.

Karliner, J. S. et al. (1971): Circulation 44, 323.

L. P., Central Inst. of Cardiovasc. Regulation Research, Academy of Sciences, 1115 Berlin, Wiltbergstr. 50. G.D.R.

FIRST PASS NITROGLYCERIN RAO RADIONUCLIDE ANGIOGRAPHY: NONINVASIVE EVALUATION OF MYOCARDIAL VIABILITY

CH. HELLMAN, F. BLAU, W. D. JOHNSON and D. SCHMIDT

University of Wisconsin, Mount Sinai Medical Center, Milwaukee, Wisconsin, U.S.A.

At present there are few diagnostic tests to screen for reversible as opposed to non-reversible depression of myocardial function due to coronary artery disease. Those tests that have been devised to test this aspect of left ventricular function — namely, postextra systolic potentiation (*Popio et al.*, 1977) and nitroglycerin potentiation (*Helfant et al.*, 1974) — have required cardiac catheterization and contrast ventriculography, both of which involve a small but significant risk to the patient. In order to provide an alternative noninvasive technique to evaluate the risk and the potential benefit of myocardial revascularization surgery in patients with left ventricular dysfunction, this study was designed to differentiate scar tissue from viable muscle utilizing first pass RAO radionuclide angiography. For this purpose, ejection fraction and regional wall motion were examined preoperatively by contrast ventriculography and radionuclide angiography and compared. The radionuclide studies were then repeated after nitroglycerin and the changes produced in ejection fraction and regional wall motion compared to those seen following surgery.

Fourteen consecutive patients with abnormal regional wall motion demonstrated by routine contrast left ventriculography who subsequently underwent myocardial revascularization formed the basis of this study (Table I). The average age was 56.4 years with a range of 37 to 77 years. There were three females and 11 males. Preoperative ejection fraction ranged from 15% to 50% with a mean ejection fraction of 31%, and the average number of bypass grafts placed at the time of surgery was 3.6.

All patients had 30° contrast ventriculography after coronary angiography by either the Sones or a modified Judkins technique. One to four days preoperatively, all patients had 30° nuclear cardiac dynamic studies for the determination of baseline ejection fraction and wall motion; this test was immediately followed by a repeat determination four minutes after administering 0.4 mg. of sublingual nitroglycerin while monitoring blood pressure and heart rate. A third radionuclide examination was done seven to 10 days postoperatively to assess the same parameters. All studied were done with the patient not having received any nitroglycerin preparation for the previous four hours.

Nuclear cardiac dynamic studies in our laboratory are performed with a Baird-Atomic System 77 multicrystal camera using the first pass technique as previously reported with a modified background correction for the RAO view (*Hellman and Schmidt*, 1978). For this study, the left ventricle and surrounding background were flagged. Total counts over the left ventricle averaged 15.000 – 20.000 per second; only beats that had 50% or greater of the maximum count were used for calculation. By summing the peak and valley

Table I. Study Group

STUDY GROUP	N = 14	
11 MALES		
3 FEMALES		
AGE	$\overline{56.4}$	(37-77)
EJECTION FRACTION	$\overline{31\%}$	(15-30)
# GRAFTS	$\overline{3.6}$	(1-6)

(end-diastole and end-systole) counts of those beats used, ejection fraction was calculated in the standard manner. Using the summed beats, a representative cycle or superbeat image was formed. Using this representative cycle which was the higher summed number of counts and, therefore, better statistics, and end-diastolic perimeter is produced along with an end-systolic image (Figure 1). Measuring the distance between the end-diastolic perimeter and the border of the end-systolic image, estimates wall motion.

The images of the RAO radionuclide angiogram were divided into six segments for analysis of wall motion by trisecting the long axis of the left ventricle.

An example of a typical study is shown in Figure 1. This was a 57 year old woman admitted for chest pain who at cardiac catheterization showed significant disease in two coronary arteries and akinetic apical wall motion and an ejection fraction of 33%. Radioisotope studies showed an ejection fraction of 29% and similar wall motion. After nitroglycerin, there was marked improvement in wall motion and the ejection fraction rose to 46%. After surgery,

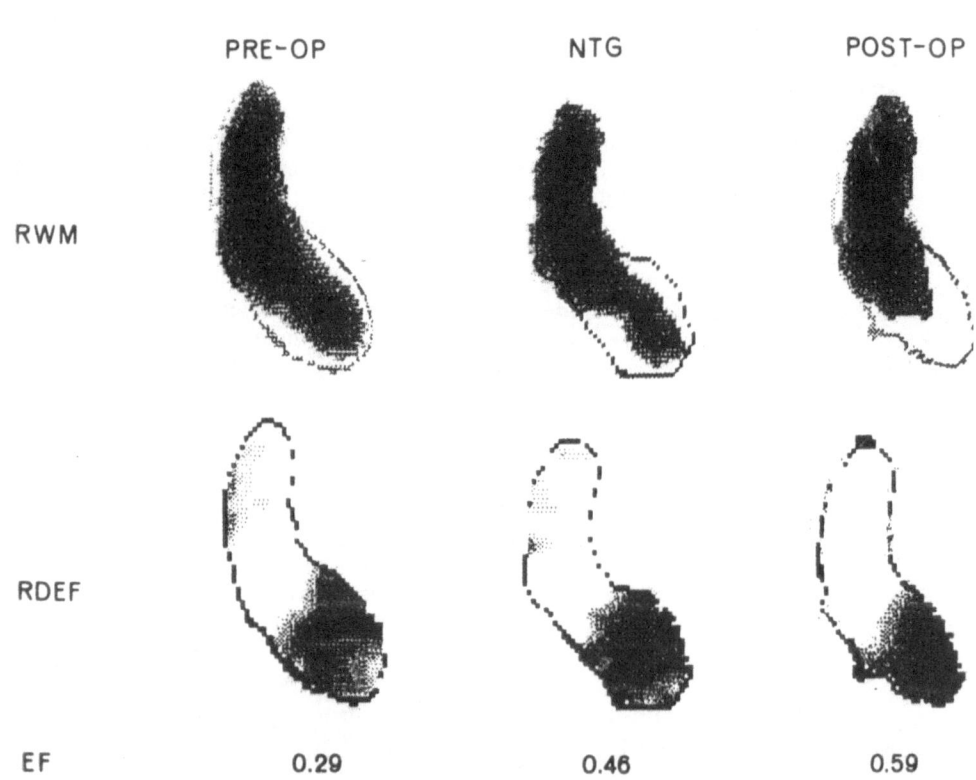

E.D. 42470 AGE 57

PRE-OP NTG POST-OP

RWM

RDEF

EF 0.29 0.46 0.59

Fig. 1. A typical study. RAO radionuclide angiography reveals an ejection fraction of 29% preoperatively with poor apical wall motion. Following nitroglycerin intervention in the center panel, the wall motion improves as does the regional distribution of ejection fraction and the global ejection fraction goes up to 46%. After surgery there was normalization of wall motion and the ejection fraction rose to 59%. NTG = nitroglycerin, EF − ejection fraction, RWM − regional wall motion, RDEF = regional distribution of ejection fraction image (a functional image of the part of the ventricle which is ejecting blood).

there was normalization of wall motion and an ejection fraction of 59%.

Analyzing the entire group of patients, 30° RAO preoperative nuclear cardiology ejection fraction correlated well with preoperative 30° RAO contrast angiography; the correlation coefficient being 0.96 with a standard error of the estimate of ±2%. Then, comparing the preoperative ejection fraction to that after nitroglycerin demonstrated the ejection fraction rose by more than 10% in 10 of 14 patients (Figure 2).

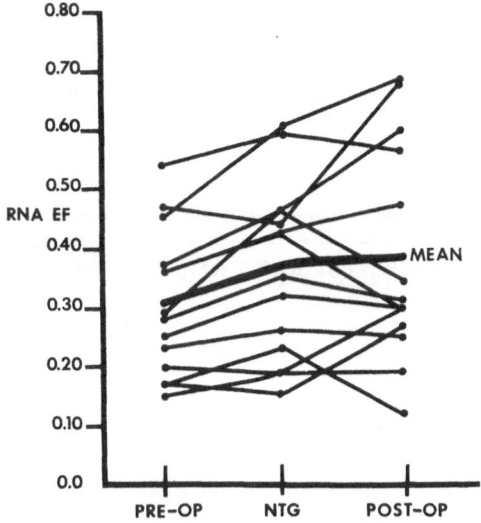

Fig. 2. Four minutes after nitroglycerin administration the ejection fraction rose from 31% to 37%. Postoperatively the ejection fraction rose to 38%.
RNA EF = radionuclide angiography ejection fraction, Pre-op = preoperative control studies, NTG = nitroglycerin intervention, Post-op = postoperative study.

Mean ejection fraction rose from 30.6% to 36.6% (p < .01). Postoperatively, ejection fraction rose in 9 of these 10 patients with the mean ejection fraction rising to 38.1% (p < .02). Regional wall motion analysis showed similar changes. Of 84 total segments analyzed, 20 were normal, 45 were hypokinetic (decreased wall motion), 12 were akinetic (no motion) and 7 were dyskinetic (paradoxical motion). Of 7 total dyskinetic segments, none improved either after nitroglycerin nor after bypass graft surgery. Of 12 total akinetic segments, five improved after nitroglycerin; four of these five akinetic segments were the only akinetic segments to improve after surgery. Of 45 hypokinetic segments, 26 improved with nitroglycerin. Of these 26, 12 normalized after nitroglycerin and of these, 9 also improved after surgery. Fourteen additional hypokinetic segments also showed improvement after nitroglycerin but did not normalize. Of these 14 segments, 9 improved after surgery including 5 which normalized. Of all segments analyzed to move abnormally preoperatively, only 6 showed improvement after surgery that was not predicted by nitroglycerin.

In summary, in patients with ischemic cardiomyopathy, first pass RAO nuclear angiography after sublingual nitroglycerin is a sensitive and specific predictor of potential improvement of left ventricular ejection fraction and regional wall motion after successful coronary bypass surgery. Therefore, this ninonvasive test can be used to distinguish viable muscle from scar tissue and thus contribute to therapeutic decisions in patients with left ventricular dysfunction.

REFERENCES

Helfant, R. H., Pine, R., Meister, S. G., Feldman, M. S., Trout, R. G., Banka, V. S. (1974): Nitroglycerin to unmask reversible asynergy: Correlation with post coronary artery bypass ventriculography. Circulation 50: 108—113.
Hellman, C., Schmidt, D. H. (1978): First pass RAO radionuclide angiography after nitroglycerin to assess myocardial viability. Clin. Res. 26: 239A.
Popio, K. A., Gorlin, R. H., Bechtel, D., Levine, J. A. (1977): Post extrasystolic potentiation as a predictor of potential myocardial viability: Preoperative analysis compared with studies after coronary bypass surgery. Am. J. Cardiol. 39: 945—953.

C. H., Mount Sinai Med. Center, 950 North 12th Street, Milwaukee, Wisconsin 53201, U.S.A.

STUDIES OF VASOACTIVE SUBSTANCES IN ISOLATED CORONARY ARTERIES USING A MODIFIED PERFUSION TECHNIQUE

M. F. CRASS, III, P. L. CHAN, R. L. ROSETT and D. J. PAULSON

Dept. of Physiology, Texas Tech. University School of Medicine, Lubbock, Texas, U.S.A.

Introduction

Most studies of coronary artery physiology and pharmacology have employed the intact *in situ* vascular bed or isometrically-contracting helical strips *in vivo*. Relatively few studies have been reported using coronary segment perfusion (*Zuberbuhler and Bohr*, 1965; *Kupke*, 1972; *Trinker*, 1973; *Cornish et al.*, 1974; *Sarma et al.*, 1975); an approach which avoids the effects of myocardial vasodilator substances and extrinsic neural factors. The present technique (*Crass et al.*, 1977) employs longer (6–10 cm) perfused segments and direct monitoring of flow changes using electromagnetic flow probes. This report describes the responses of this isolated perfused canine left circumflex artery preparation to certain known vasoactive agents.

Materials and methods

Adult mongrel dogs (15–30 kg) were anesthetized with sodium pentobarbital (30 mg/kg i.v.), ventilated with room air, and thoracotomized. The left circumflex artery was dissected free of surrounding tissue, the small branches ligated with a distal branch left patent, cannulated through the left coronary ostium and mounted for perfusion. The perfusion medium (Krebs bicarbonate buffer) was maintained at 37 °C and consisted of (mM): NaCl, 119.8; KCl, 4.8; $MgSO_4$, 1.2; KH_2PO_4, 1.2; $CaCl_2$, 1.3; and glucose, 11.0. The medium also contained whole dog serum, 5% v/v and was equilibrated with humidified 95% O_2 – 5% CO_2. A hydrostatic perfusion pressure of 70 mm Hg was maintained constant. An electromagnetic flow probe (7 or 9 mm) was placed on the vessel and flow was monitored with a Model 501D square-wave electromagnetic flowmeter (Carolina Medical Electronics, King, N. C.). Flow rates and pressures were recorded on a Model 78 Grass recorder. Angiotensin II (A–II) (Hypertensin, Ciba) or norepinephrine (NE) (Levophed bitartrate, Winthrop) were dissolved in 0.9% NaCl and administered in 0.2 ml bolus injections. Isotonic saline was similarly administered in control vessels.

Results

The response to varying doses of A-II by the isolated perfused left circumflex coronary artery can be seen in Table 1.

Table I. Effects of A-II and NE on Flow Rate ($\dot{Q}$)

Angiotensin II (µg)*	$\varDelta\dot{Q}$ (ml/min ± SEM)†
Control	0
0.2	0
0.5	(−) 4.66 ± 1.20
1.0	(−) 13.00 ± 3.46
10.0	(−) 35.28 ± 6.73
Norepinephrine (µg)*	
Control	0
1.0	(+) 2.25 ± 0.25
20.0	(+) 6.25 ± 1.88
57.0	(+) 10.60 ± 2.13

* Injected into perfusion system dissolved in 0.2 ml 0.9% NaCl. Control = 0.2 ml 0.9% NaCl.
† $\varDelta\dot{Q}$ = maximum quantitative difference in $\dot{Q}$ relative to pre-injection or baseline $\dot{Q}$. (−) & (+) = decrease and increase in $\dot{Q}$, respectively.

The vessels were highly responsive to A-II. The threshold dose was approximately 0.5 µg, which elicited a slight vasoconstrictor response. Increased vasoconstriction occurred in dose-dependent fashion commensurate with increased A-II concentrations. Times of onset, peak and duration of the vasoconstrictor effect varied with the dose administered. Tachyphylaxis to A-II was consistently observed for periods approximating 45 min. The

714

presence of serum in the perfusion medium (see Materials and methods) markedly enhanced the vasoconstrictor response to A-II. As shown in Table II, vessels perfused with buffer containing 1.0 µg A-II in the presence of serum exhibited a ninefold increase in the vasoconstrictor response vis-a-vis vessels perfused without serum. Serum potentiation was less marked at a dose of 10.0 µg A-II, albeit still amounting to a twofold increase in the response. Table I also shows the response of the perfused vessel to NE. Over the concentration range shown, NE produced a dose-dependent vasodilation. In the recirculated system employed, NE-induced vasodilation persisted indefinitely, or until the perfusate was changed.

Table II. Potentiation of the Vasopressor Activity of Angiotensin II by Serum

Angiotensin II (µg)*	Serum (5% v/v)	$\Delta\dot{Q}$ (ml/min $\pm$ $\pm$ SEM)†
1.0	— —	(−) 1.20 $\pm$ 0.37
	+	(−) 10.50 $\pm$ 3.50
10.0	— —	(−) 16.60 $\pm$ 3.50
10.0	— —	(−) 16.60 $\pm$ 2.68
	+	(−) 35.28 $\pm$ 6.73

*† as in legend to Table I.

Discussion

The perfusion system employed in the present studies was developed to investigate vessel wall function in the intact isolated coronary artery. The advantages of this approach include a) considerably greater segment length (6 – 10 cm) relative to previous methods and b) direct monitoring of flow using an electromagnetic flowmeter. Flow and perfusion pressures were stable for up to 8 hours. It is clear from our data shown that the perfused vessel preparation is highly responsive to vasoactive substances of major physiological importance, i. e., A-II and NE. Vessel integrity, geometry and length can be kept reasonably normal by tethering. As opposed to an isometrically-contracting helical strip preparation, the isolated coronary perfusion approach enabled a greater reactive surface area for evaluation of hormone responsiveness and amplification of metabolic events. The role of serum in potentiating the A-II response is not clear at the present time. Facilitation of hormone responsiveness in vascular smooth muscle by plasma or serum is not a new finding as evidenced by other published reports (*Wurzel*, 1963; *Bohr and Sobieski*, 1968). The complexity of the hormone and kinin composition of serum precludes a simple explanation for the effects observed in the present study.

REFERENCES

Bohr, D. F., Sobieski, J. (1968): A vasoactive factor in plasma. Federation Proc. 27, 1396.
Cornish, E. J., Miller, R. C., Tolmer, P. R. (1974): An isolated perfused coronary artery preparation from the kitten. J. Pharm. Pharmac. 26, 733.
Crass, M. F., III, Chan, P. L., Paulson, D. J., Rosett, R. L., Song, W. (1977): An isolated perfused canine left circumflex coronary artery preparation for studies of vascular smooth muscle function. Federation Proc. 36, 520.
Kupke, I. R. (1972): Biosynthesis of lipids in perfused dog aorta and coronary artery. J. Mol. Cell. Cardiol. 4, 11.

Sarma, J. S. M., Tillmann, H., Ikeda, S., Bing, R. J. (1975): The effect of carbon monoxide on lipid metabolism of human coronary arteries. Atherosclerosis, 22, 193.
Trinker, F. R. (1973): The effects of catecholamines on isolated perfused coronary arteries in the dog. Arch. int. Pharmacodyn. 205, 218.
Wurzel, M. (1963): On a vasoactive peptide (?) in rabbit serum. Arch. int. Pharmacodyn. 143, 550.
Zuberbuhler, R. C., Bohr, D. F. (1965): Responses of coronary smooth muscle to catecholamines. Circulation Res. 16, 431.

M. F. C. III, Dept. of Physiology Texas Tech. University School of Medicine Lubbock, Texas 79409, U.S.A.

FREE AMINO ACIDS AS INDICATORS OF ACUTE MYOCARDIAL ISCHAEMIA

V. BRODAN, J. FABIÁN and M. ANDĚL

Institute for Clinical and Experimental Medicine, Prague, Czechoslovakia

The main diagnostic problem during pacing is sufficiently sensitive proof of acute induced myocardial ischaemia. In addition to clinical signs, i. e. angina pectoris and depression of ST segment on ECG, the diagnosis of acute ischaemia depends especially on differences in the concentrations of some metabolic parameters between arterial blood and the blood in coronary sinus (a-cs diff). One of the most important metabolic signs of myocardial ischaemia is the lactate (La) production in the heart (i. e. negative a-cs diff for La). Another valuable parameter is the increase in the lactate: pyruvate ratio (La : Py) across the myocardium (i. e. negative a-cs diff for La : Py) (*Opie and Mansford*, 1971). The investigation of many other metabolic parameters as a-cs differences of kalium, some enzymes (transaminases and creatinphosphokinase), phosphates, pyruvate, pO_2 and oxygen saturation, pCO_2 and pH is much more contradictory and the results are very poorly correlated with both basic clinical (angina pectoris and ST-segment depression) and metabolic (negative a-cs diff for La and La : Py) signs of myocardial ischaemia. In this paper we are concerned with the diagnostic value of a-cs differences of free amino acids at rest and during pacing and also with some theoretical aspects connected with their changes.

Nine men aged 37 — 55 years with angina pectoris were examined. All had a myocardial infarction case history. At rest and during pacing blood specimens were simultaneously collected from arteria and from the central portion of the coronary sinus. Lactate and pyruvate vere estimated enzymatically, amino acids were analysed on an amino acid analyzer (Beckmann 119 Automatic).

Table I.

Arterio-coronary sinus differences	Alanine	Glutamine	Alanine + glutamine
Lactate	−0.6309 p < 0.01	−0.5400 p < 0.05	−0.6414 p < 0.01
Lactate: Pyruvate	−0.4921 p < 0.05	−0.4832 p < 0.05	−0.4715 p < 0.05

During pacing were found significant positive a-cs diff in glutamate, leucine, isoleucine and aspartate (which has significantly positive a-cs diff also at rest). Negative significant differences were found in cystine-cysteine, glutamine, asparagine and alanine.

Table I shows that a-cs differences in alanine glutamine and in sum of both amino acids are significantly negatively correlated both with lactate and (less closely) with the La : Py ratio. A-cs differences in other amino acids are not correlated with basic metabolic indicators of ischaemia. In Table II are shown the relation-

Table II.

Less negative (or positive) a-cs diff during pacing		Metabolic ischaemia (neg a-cs diff La and La: Py)		Clinical ischaemia (angina pectoris, ↓ ST segm. ECG)	
		NO	YES	NO	YES
Alanine	NO	6	1	5	2
	YES	1	1	1	1
Glutamine	NO	4	1	4	2
	YES	3	1	2	1

ships between less negative a-cs differences (or even positive a-cs diff) in alanine and glutamine during pacing and metabolic and or clinical signs of ischaemia. Changes in alanine are in keeping with metabolic signs in 77.7% and with clinical signs in 66.7%. Changes in glutamine agree with both groups of ischaemia signs in 55.6%.

During cardiac revolution in the myocardium, ATP is utilised and ADP is formed. The minor portion of ADP is degradated via AMP, IMP, adenosine, inosine, hypoxanthine, xanthine and uric acid. Most of adenosine or IMP is transformed back to AMP (*Lowenstein*, 1972). In these reactions ammonia is formed, a small portion of which is released from the myocardium or transformed on the spot into urea (*Smirnov et al.*, 1974). Most of the ammonia, however, is detoxicated by combination with alpha-ketoglutarate and glutamate, whereby glutamate and glutamine are formed (*Kato*, 1968). Glutamate participates simultaneously in the transamination where it is transformed back to alpha-ketoglutarate and pyruvate is at the same time transformed to alanine. Alanine and glutamine production thus run parallel to a-cs diff in both metabolites and is highly significantly positi-

vely correlated. The release of alanine may be considered as a part of Felig's glucose-alanine cycle in which alanine is transported from the muscle into the liver where it is desaminated and transformed back into glucose (*Felig et al.*, 1970).

Pyruvate is formed in the myocardium by the glycolysis and under aerobic conditions from lactate which is one of the most important substrates. During ischaemia the sequence of reactions is reversed and from pyruvate lactate is formed as the final product of the anaerobic glycolysis (*Opie*, 1968). When the lactate production from pyruvate increases, the pyruvate transformation into the alanine decreases and vice versa.

The decrease of alanine production in myocardium, i. e. its less negative or even positive a-cs diff may be thus used as an indicator of the acute induced myocardial ischaemia. Glutamine changes parallel those of alanine. During ischaemia the ammonia production from ATP probably decreases simultaneously. Thus also changes in a-cs diff in glutamine are useful in evaluation of the degree of ischaemia although their relationship to the main metabolic indicators of ischaemia is less close and reliable.

REFERENCES

Kato, T. (1968): Myocardial amino-nitrogen metabolism with special reference to ammonia metabolism. Jap. Circulat. J. 32, 1401—1416.

Lowenstein, J. M. (1972): Ammonia production in the muscle and in other tissues: Purine nucleotide cycle. Physiol. Rev., 52, 382—414.

Opie, L. H. (1968): Metabolism of the heart in health and disease. Part I., Amer. Heart. J. 76, 685—698.

Opie, L. H., Mansford, K. R. L. (1971): Value of lactate and pyruvate measurements in the assesment of the redox state of free nicotinamideadenine dinucleotide in the cytoplasma of the perfused rat heart. Eur. J. Clin. Invest. 1, 295—306.

Smirnov, V. N., Asafov, G. F. et al. (1974): Ammonia neutralisation and urea synthesis in cardiac muscle. Circulat. Res. 35, Suppl. III, 58—69.

V. B., IKEM, Vídeňská 800, 146 22 Prague 4, Czechoslovakia

ISCHAEMIC HEART DISEASE IN YOUNG WOMEN AND THEIR OVARIAN FUNCTION

KVĚTA SOUKUPOVÁ and JITKA KOBILKOVÁ

*4th Medical Department and 1st Gynecological Department,
University Hospital, Charles University, Prague, Czechoslovakia*

The problem of IHD in women of reproductive age has lately aroused great interest. Most papers published on this subject (*Wink*, 1972, *Bengtosson*, 1973, *Oliver*, 1970, 1974, *Mann*, 1975, *Morris*, 1976) mention the relationship between this disease and the known risk factors of IHD and/or hormonal contraceptives. But there is a small number of women with IHD who do not have any of the known risk factors. For this reason we focussed our attention on the activity of oestrogens.

Our hypothesis is that normal levels of oestrogens have a protective influence against IHD in women of reproductive age. If their protective role stops, an increasing number of cases of IHD may occur.

In order to exclude the influence of an early climactery, we investigated those women with IHD who were younger than 40 years of age and had normal menstruation.

Subjects

Eighteen women with a mean age of 35.2 years (23 — 40 years) were investigated. Five had myocardial infarction, seven unstable angina and six had angina pectoris with ECG evidence at rest or after exercise and with positive nitroglycerin test.

Methods

We searched for a positive family history of myocardial infarction in those near relatives who were younger than 60 years of age. In addition to this, the following parameters were taken into account: smoking of 10 cigarettes or more, oral contraceptives, obesity more than 15% above ideal weight according to Broca, hypertension actual or treated, hypercholesterolaemia 260 mg% or more, pathological glucose tolerance test, plasma uric acid level of 5 mg% or more (using enzymic spectrophotometric method).

Functions of the ovaries were estimated by means of vaginal cytology: karyopycnotic and eosinophilic indices were estimated every third day in the course of the cycle. To determine the gestagen activity, the basal temperature and urine pregnandiol were measured (*Kobilková*, 1967).

Results

Of 18 patients, 10 had positive family history, 3 were smokers, one took oral contraceptives, obesity was found in 7 women, hypertension in 6, hypercholesterolaemia in 6, pathological glucose tolerance test (but no manifest diabetes) in 6 and elevated uricaemia in 9 patients.

As for as the hypo-oestrinism is concerned, 12 of 18 women with normal menstruation had low oestrogen indices, i. e. either at the lower level of the normal range or lower still, at least in one phase of the cycle.

The patients mostly had several risk factors, only one female had smoking as the only risk factor and another had only hypercholesterolaemia. Three patients had none of the known risk factors but had hypo-oestrinism.

RESULTS

	55,55 % FAMILY HISTORY
	16,67 % SMOKING
	5,56 % HORMONAL CONTRACEPTIVES
	38,89 % OBESITY
	33,34 % HYPERTENSION
	33,34 % HYPERCHOLESTEROLAEMIA
	33,34 % GLUCOSE TOLERANCE
	50,00 % URICAEMIA
	66,67 % HYPOOESTRINISM
	100,00 % TOTAL NUMBER OBSERVED

Conclusion

From our results we can conclude that a change in the level of oestrogens to which women in their reproductive age are adapted could be a risk factor or could have an auxilliary influence for the development of IHD.

REFERENCES

Bengtsson, C. (1973): Ischaemic heart disease in women. Acta Med. Scand. Suppl. 549.

Kobilková, J. (1967): Cytologic study of the level of oestrogen during productive age. Acta cytologica 11, 497.

Mann, J. J., W. H. W. Inman (1975): Oral contraceptives and death from myocardial infarction. Brit. Med. J. 2, 245.

Morris, D. C., J. W. Hurst, R. B. Logue (1976): Myocardial infarction in young women. Am. J. Cardiol. 7, 38, 299.

Oliver, M. F. (1970): Oral contraceptives and myocardial infarction. Brit. Med. J. 2, 110.

Oliver, M. F. (1974): Ischaemic heart disease in young women. Brit. Med. J. 4, 253.

K. S., IVth Internal Clinic, FVL UK, U nemocnice 2, 128 08 Prague 2, Czechoslovakia

THE INFLUENCE OF MECHANICAL HEART ASSIST (MHA) UPON SOME FEATURES OF THE MYOCARDIAL METABOLISM IN EXPERIMENTAL INFARCTION

J. VAŠKŮ, E. URBÁNEK, S. DOLEŽEL, T. SLÁDEK, M. DOSTÁL, B. HARTMANOVÁ and P. URBÁNEK

Institute of Pathophysiology, Faculty of Medicine, UJEP Brno, Czechoslovakia

Our articles contributing to the problem of haemodynamics using mechanical heart assist (MHA) are published elsewhere. This communication is dedicated to the integration of some findings gained during the study of different features of the cardiac metabolism of the infarcted myocardium after the action of MHA.

Electrolyte changes in the myocardial tissue

We could prove that during short (3 hours) action of MHA as marked increase in the calcium level in the acutely infarcted myocardium can be prevented. Also other electrolytes in the myocardium are greatly normalised. Most effective is especially the combination of bypass and counterpulsation in one device. used for MHA.

The stabilization of the heart electrolytes is very similar to the stabilization achieved using polarising solutions (K—Mg—Aspartate). (Figure 1, see p. 721.)

Changes in the monoaminergic innervation of the myocardium

In explaining of the effect of MHA the monoaminergic nerve terminals in myo-

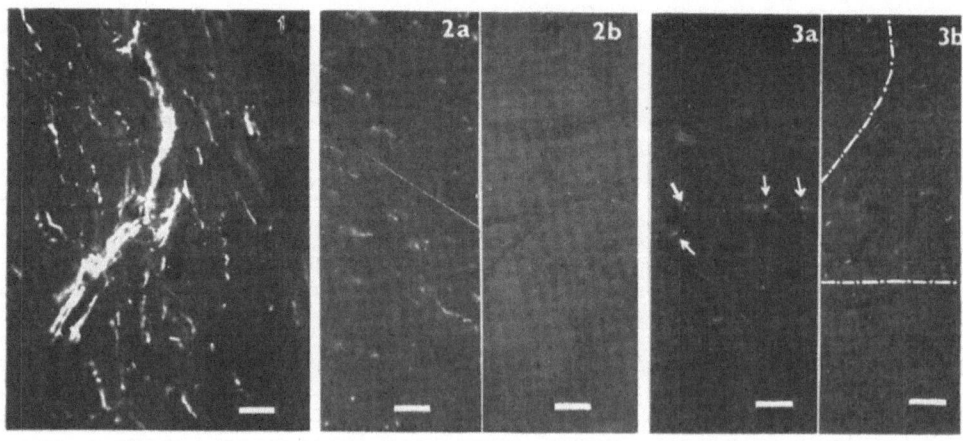

Fig. 2. 1 — Myocardium in dogs, normal innervation of vessels (thick nerves) and direct myocardial innervation (thin, irregular nerve fibers) 2a) — Rat myocardium — 2 hours lasting experimental infarction. Regeneration of fluorescence in Krebs-Ringer-O_2 solution. 2b) — Rat myocardium — 2 hours lasting experimental infarction. Krebs-Ringer-N_2 solution prevents the regeneration. 3a) — Dog myocardium — experimental infarction lasting 25 hours. Regeneration of fluorescence after 2 hours of IABC in perivascular nerves (arrows). 3b) — Dog myocardium — experimental infarction lasting 25 hours. Center of infarction (down and upper left) demarcated with the interrupted line from the peripheral transition zone (middle and upper right). Without IABC. No signs of regeneration. Calibration = 50 μm.

cardium are very important. In experiments on dogs with acute ligation of the ramus intraventricularis ventralis for two hours, using the method of *Falck*, we could observe that the varicosities of the sympathetic ground plexus were depleted of noradrenaline within the infarcted area during the second hour after ligation. The method is described elsewhere. (Figure 2.)

The depletion of catecholamines is expressed by disappearance of fluorescence. The fluorescence could be regenerated

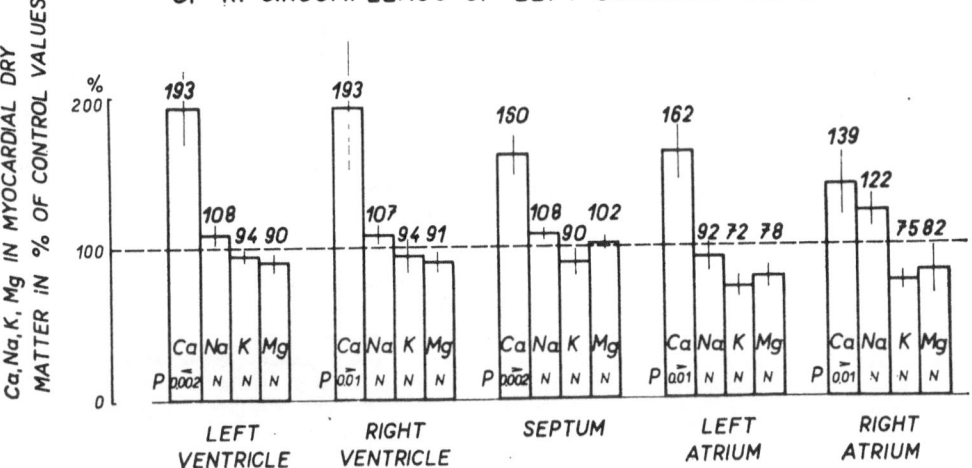

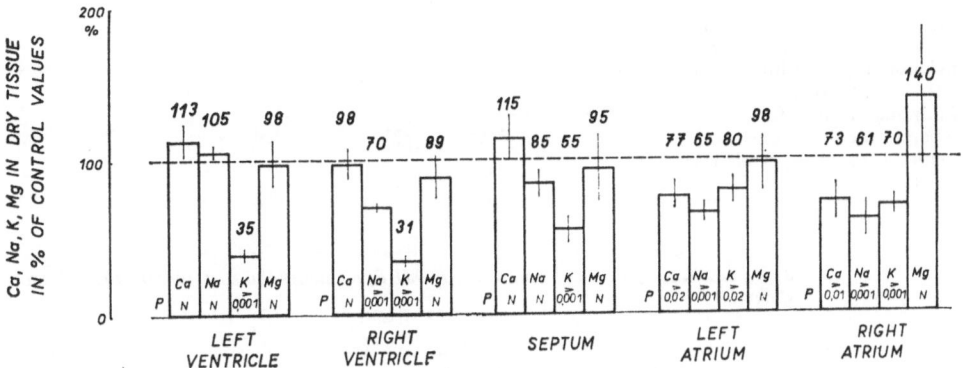

Fig. 1. The electrolyte changes in the myocardium with experimentally induced infarction and after 3 hour action of combined heart pump for simultaneous bypass and counterpulsation regimen. Experiments in dogs. Normalization of electrolyte pattern in treated dogs.

either by aeration by pneumoxyd of the tissue specimen *in vitro*, or *in vivo* after 2 hour intraaortic balloon counterpulsation. The striking increase in the fluorescence after IABC is explained by the regeneration of the release — reuptake activity of the sympathetic nerve terminals. This mechanism of normalization of noradrenaline depletion by short IABC can be useful in the elucidation of the well known prolonged effect, even if IABC was used only for a few hours.

Attempts for precise estimation of the area of infarction and its possible reduction

In experiments on 20 dogs, in which 150 min infarction by ligation of ramus intraventricularis ventralis was induced, the area of infarction was visualised by means of PAS stain for glycogen, by pH changes and by spreading of fluorescein into the infarcted area. (Figure 3.)

The area of decreased perfusion with accumulation of fluorescein agrees with the area of glycogen depletion. The area of acidosis is always smaller. Peripheral alcaline borderline of ischemic lesion plus the central acidotic area agrees with the area of decreased oxygen perfusion, demarcated by means of glycogen estimation and fluorescein accumulation. Administration of IABC especially in combination with thiamin, both studied immediately after occlusion effectively decreases the ischemic area.

THE AMOUNT OF THE ISCHEMIC TISSUE IN TREATED AND CONTROL DOGS

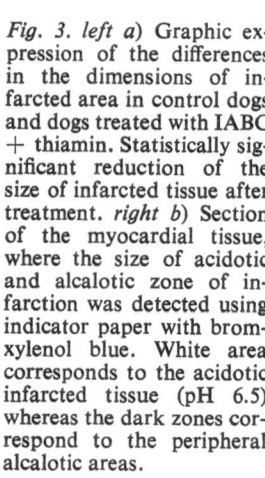
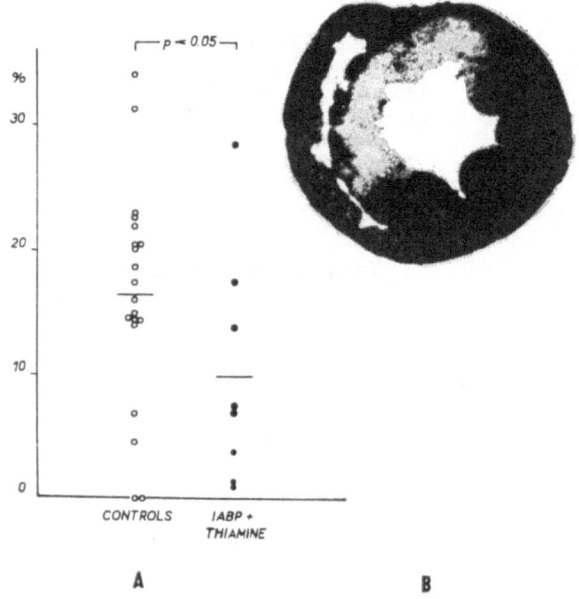

Fig. 3. left a) Graphic expression of the differences in the dimensions of infarcted area in control dogs and dogs treated with IABC + thiamin. Statistically significant reduction of the size of infarcted tissue after treatment. *right b*) Section of the myocardial tissue, where the size of acidotic and alcalotic zone of infarction was detected using indicator paper with bromxylenol blue. White area corresponds to the acidotic infarcted tissue (pH 6.5) whereas the dark zones correspond to the peripheral alcalotic areas.

J. V., Institute of Pathophysiology, LF UJEP, Komenského n. 2, 600 00 Brno, Czechoslovakia

ASSISTANT CIRCULATION WITH AN INTRAAORTAL BALLOON PULSATION (IABP) — SYSTEM IN MYOCARDIAL INFARCTION: CHANGES IN BLOOD COAGULATION

M. FISCHER, P. HOPMEIER, M. LURF, W. ENENKEL and N. NOBIS

Central Laboratory. 4th Medical Department for Cardiac Diseases, Municipal Hospital, Lainz, Vienna, Austria

From November 1976 to May 1978, a study was carried out by the Central Laboratory, together with the 4th Medical Department of the Vienna Municipal Hospital, Lainz, on 20 patients of the Cardiac Care Unit (CCU) who had to undergo treatment with an IABP-system. After adequate preparation, 16 patients were treated with an assistant circulation of the type of AVCO-IABP-Systems/Medical Instruments — USA. This is an automatically controlled system with a specially developed three-chamber-balloon with antithrombotic qualities.

All patients suffering from acute myocardial infarction, who were admitted to the CCU, underwent anticoagulant therapy with heparin (22.500 I.U./d). If, however, therapy with an IABP-system proved necessary, 5.000 I.U. of heparin were additionally applied before the balloon-catheter was inserted. Later on, during assistant circulation, the heparin dosis given was 12.000 — 20.000 I.U. in 24 hours.

As possible changes in the coagulation system during the assistant circulation time had been taken into consideration, coagulation tests were carried out on all the patients during and after treatment with the IABP-system. It was considered important to discover a possible consumption reaction in an early stage, which may be caused by activation of the blood due to contact with non-physiological surfaces.

The diagnosis of a consumption reaction was based on the finding of a thrombocytopenia and hypofibrinogenemia, of circulating fibrinogen monomers and a decrease in antithrombin III. Moreover, diagnostic importance was given to a progressive increase of the coagulation disorder.

Results

16 patients underwent an assistant circulation therapy of the AVCO-IABP type under heparin. The duration of the assistant circulation therapy varied with different patients.

a) Control of heparin therapy: Thrombin time and PTT. After an intravenous injection of 5.000 I.U. heparin, an infusion of, on the average, 15.000 I.U. heparin (12.000 — 20.000 I.U.) per day was given during IABP-therapy. Under heparin medication, the thrombin time of all treatment groups became more than 3 times longer than before and also the activated PTT became double as long and even longer.

b) Platelets: Before assistant circulation was started, the mean value of the platelet count was 224.000 $\pm$ 32.000. The group of patients undergoing IABP — therapy for approximately 15.5 hours showed a reduction of about 30%, in case of 108.6 hours, the reduction was more than 60%. After the end of IABP — therapy, the platelet count increased slowly but exceedingly. The normal count values were reached 4 days after operation, the maximum value after 7 days.

c) Fibrinogen: Controls of fibrinogen showed an increase. Only in group 4 there was a small decrease in accordance with the duration of IABP — therapy. Several determinations showed that the half-life period of fibrinogen had decreased.

d) Thrombin coagulase, Ethanol test, Fibrin degradation products, Plasminogen: According to the duration of the IABP — therapy, the thrombin coagulase time showed a clear increase. During IABP — therapy, the ethanol test was positive in about 75% of the cases. 2 out of 3 patients undegoing IABP — therapy for more than 92 hours showed a reactive fibrinolysis with a decrease of plasminogen, an increase of plasmin and FDP in the serum.

e) Antithrombin III: Before therapy, the average plasma antithrombin III level was 27.3 ± 6.1. This is in the upper range of normal values. With increasing duration of IABP — therapy a reduction of antihrombin II could be noticed. At the end of the IABP — treatment a fast and exceeding increase was noted.

Hemorrhagic and Thromboembolic complications

With 4 out of 16 patients, hemorrhagic complications (hematuria (2 cases), multiple large hematoma (1 case), metrorrhagia (1 case)) occurred during IABP — treatment in spite of the fact that there was a strong heparin response (thrombin time >90 seconds). With all these patients, the duration of the IABP — therapy was more than 60 hours and they suffered from severe thrombocytopenia (platelet count <90.000).

With 3 patients, a thrombosis occurred in the region of the femoral or iliac artery. Twice this happened at the end of the IABP-therapy, once shortly after the catheter was removed.

After surgery, circulation was normal again.

Towards the end of the IABP-therapy, all patients had elevated temperatures.

Conclusion

In connection with the IABP-treatment for patients suffering from myocardial infarction, signs of a consumption reaction occurred in spite of a specially developed balloon-catheter with anti-thrombotic qualities and a closely observed heparin therapy. Thrombocytopenia, an increased turnover of fibrinogen, formation of fibrin monomer complexes, a decrease in antithrombin III and reactive fibrinolysis were noted. The degree of changes is in direct connec:ion to the duration of the assistant circulation. After IABP-therapy, an exceeding normalization could be noticed.

The dosage of heparin must be chosen in such a way that on the one hand the consumption reaction must not be too distinct and on the other hand, as has been learned by former experience, hemorrhagic complications should not additionally endanger the patient, whose circulation has already been affected.

REFERENCES

Bregmann D.: Assessment of IABP in cardiogenic shock. Critical Care Medicine 3, 90, 1975.

Enenkel W., E. Wolner, M. Deutsch, W. Fasching, S. Leodolter, H. Thoma: Klinische Erfahrungen mit der assistierten Zirkulation. Intensivmed. 9. 363, 1972.

Fekete L. F., R. L. Bick: Laboratory Modalities for Assessing Hemostasis During Cardiopulmonary Bypass. Sem. Thrombosis & Diathesis Vol. III, 90, 1976.

Fischer M.: Diagnose der Verbrauchskoagulopathie Wien Klin. Wschr. 85, 319, 1973.

McCabe J. C., R. M. Abel, V. A. Subramanian, W. A. Gay: Complications of Intraaortic Balloon Insertion and Counterpulsation. 1st

Europ. Aortic Balloon Pump Congress, Rotterdam, March 1978. Abstr.

McEnany M. T., W. G. Austen: Surgical Intervention for the Mechanical Complications of acute myocardial Infarction, in "Current Cardiovascular Topics", Vol. IV, S. 207, Thieme 1978.

Mueller H. S.: Role of Cardiac Assistance in the Treatment of Cardiogenic Shock. In Intensivmedizin, Notfallmedizin, Anästhesiologie Bd. 6. S. 80—91. Thieme, 1977.

Wolner E.: Diskussionbemerkung zu "AC-Therapie während IABP-behandlung" in Intensivmedizin, Notfallmedizin, Anästhesiologie, Band 6, S. 206, Thieme, 1977.

M. F., Centrallaboratory, Municipal Hospital Vienna-Lainz, Wolkersbergenstr. 1, A-1130, Vienna, Austria

INTERACTION OF VENOUS ENDOTHELIUM AND RIGHT VENTRICLE ENDOCARDIUM TO LONG-TERM CARDIAC PACING LEADS

Z. NÁPRSTEK, A. LYSENKOVÁ, M. KRAJÍČEK, Č. ŠVORČÍK,
J. NÁPRSTKOVÁ, B. DOLEŽEL and M. HACO

Institute for Clinical and Experimental Medicine, Prague
Institute of Law-Medicine, Dept. of Pathology, Med. Hyg. Faculty
Charles University, Prague, Czechoslovakia

The implanted electrode for long-term cardiac pacing creates an important integrate part of the pacemaker complex. Its endovasal implantation performs the most common approach concerning about 92% of all operations.

Figure 1. summarizes our increasing clinical survey started in 1962, now with 4206 operations, endovasal approach in 1442 out of 1524 patients, still living 1043.

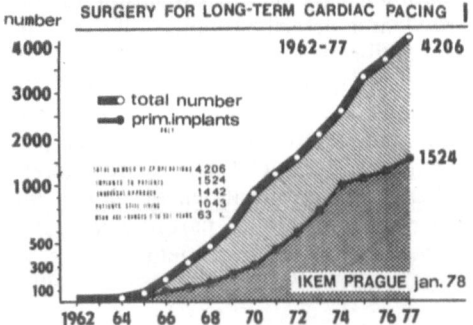

Fig. 1.

It is very difficult to establish some specific mortality rate in relation to pacing of myocardium because of prevailing older age groups of patients suffering from cardiovascular diseases, mean age 63 years. However, the surviving pattern-group in a 5 years period shows very good results (69 – 78% of survivors) in middle aged patients, still good over 70, with poor effect at 80 years.

For longitudinal phlebologic studies the endovasal electrode leading the signals from the subcutaneous pacemaker through the peripheral venous tree into the right ventricle seems to be a unique reasonable model of polymere interaction to venous endothelium and healing resistance as well.

Three main vector-moving forces influence the stability of the endovasal lead in different directions and repeated little injuries to the intimal layer (Figure 2). 1. undulating longitudinal movements corresponding with heart beats, 2. tangential flexibility – wrapping insulation layer and 3. irregular side-tractions by differently fixing fibrous bridges to the venous wall (VW, FR in picture). These bridges start originally from bland organized thrombi on the electrode. The obvious apprehension of high-risk thrombo-embolic complications – particularly on the damaged surface did not correspond with proved long-term experience of low rate embolism (comparing published data of *Furman, Groegler* and *Calderoli* – 1974 – 76 – all 0.5 – 1.2%, with our 1% we see the incidence increasing to 6% (our to 4%)) if the area is infected. From our previous group of autopsies there is a high

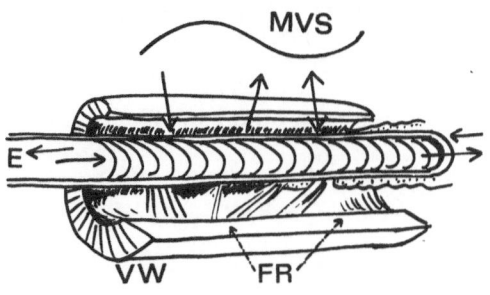

Fig. 2.

725

incidence of ischemic heart disease with proved infarction zone in almost 19%, angina 2.7%. Different types of gradually changing intensity of intimal reactions have been studied, with fibroproduction often beginning in vena cava location, later with organized adhesions by encapsulating tubes and tunnels in the right ventricle. From a randomized group of 63 postmortem (Figure 3) we established typical standard reactions: No. 1. (17%) very poor fibrous reaction, little bridges in v. cava, No. 2. (28%) with electrode mostly uncovered, divided fibrous bridges in the right atrium and ventricle, No. 3. (42%) often with rich but irregular adhesions to the wall, sometimes with fibrous tube on

free moving lead, and No. 4. (11%), smooth but incompleted endothelization of almost the whole surface of this foreign body. The quality of these reactions is important for the expectancy of complications as displacement, broken wire and other. To improve this endothelization to a programmed degree we developed a special electrode with colagen-antibiotics layer for better biological fixation and we used this approach in 34 high-risk patients without complications. This type of electrode allows total endothelization Complex study has been completed by investigation of movements and fixation of different electrodes to the cardiac wall in living patients by the use of X-ray right-ventriculography, biprojectional technique, taken on movie film. The frames show a cylindrically formed channel as shown on anatomic study, deep penetration of the tip, intensive fibrous encapsulation at colagen lead and other formation.

MEAN TYPES OF FIBROUS REACTION

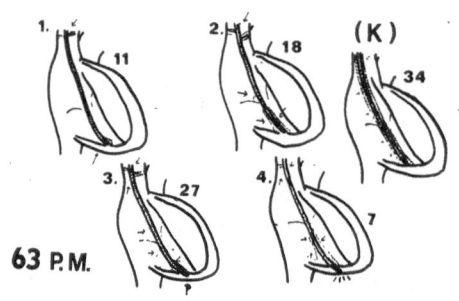

63 P.M.

Fig. 3.

Summarizing this investigation we observed and described some different and diverse fibrous reactions in long-term cardiac pacing, in interaction between the venous, atrial and ventricular wall and implanted electrode. We suppose the permanent electrode-lead must be recognized and treated as not only encapsulated, but healed-in foreign body, partially occluding the venous tree of the patient.

REFERENCES

1. *Bredikis J. I.* (1972): Električeskaja stimulacija serdca. Proc. Kaunas Med. Publ.
2. *Furman S., D. J. Escher,* Principles and techniques of cardiac pacing. Harper & Row, N. Y. 1971.
3. *Groegler F. M. et al.* (1975): J. Thor. cardiovasc. Surg. 69/1975/895—900 (Edit.).

4. *Náprstek Z.* in Cardiac Pacing, Proceedings Tokyo, Excerpta Medica, Amsterdam 1977, 499—500.
4. *Parsonnet V., L. Gilbert* (1973): The natural history of pacemaker wires, J. Thor. cardiovasc. Surg. 65, 315—322.

Z. N., IKEM, Vídeňská 800, 146 22, Prague 4 Krč, Czechoslovakia

VIDEODENSIMETRIC MEASUREMENT OF PHASIC BLOOD FLOW IN AORTOCORONARY BYPASS GRAFTS

P. SPILLER, U. FERMOR, K. L. NEUHAUS, H. PANNEK and F. K. SCHMIEL

Medical Clinic and Policlinic B, Düsseldorf University, Düsseldorf, F.R.G.

Aortocoronary bypass surgery is now widely applied for the treatment of coronary artery disease. Although numerous reports have appeared describing the surgical technique, mortality, graft patency, changes in ventricular performance and relief of anginal symptoms, little is known about the function of aortocoronary vein grafts. Currently, estimation of flow in bypass grafts primarily depends on subjective evaluations of the vessel structure and the "run off" of contrast media, visualized by angiography.

The purpose of this paper was to present the results of videodensimetric measurements of phasic blood flow in aortocoronary bypass grafts, thereby providing a quantitative analysis of vein graft function.

The densimetric flow measurements were based on the determination of the mean transit times of contrast media in the bypass grafts. The transit times were evaluated from the leading slopes of the densograms at two measuring points. Due to the short spatial distance between these points, flow was measured as an average of relatively short periods of the cardiac cycle. To obtain representative values of blood flow, at least three measurements were taken at different times during the cycle, using a sampling technique. This was achieved by ECG-controlled injections of contrast boli (Amidotrizoate, 1 ml at a flow rate of 4 ml s^{-1}).

Figure 1 shows a typical example of the flow measurements in a bypass graft to the descending branch of the left coronary artery. The horizontal bars in the upper part indicate the flow, the length of the bars representing the average interval between the leading slopes of the two densograms. As reference signals the aortic pressure and the ECG are shown in the lower part. Five contrast boli were injected at different phases of different cardiac cycles. During the systole, the flow amounted to 85 ml min^{-1}. During the early diastole, the flow was higher (175 ml min^{-1}) than during the late diastole (140 ml min^{-1}).

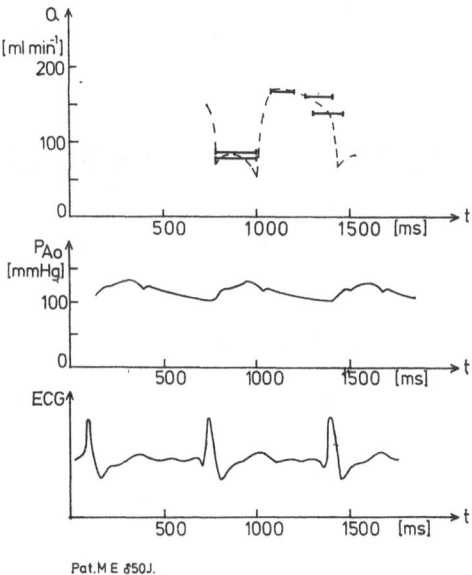

Pat.M E ∂50J.

Fig. 1. Systolic, early and late diastolic flow in a vein graft to the left anterior descending coronary artery in a patient with coronary artery disease.

P_{Ao}: aortic pressure, ECG: electrocardiogram. Diastolic flow is considerably higher than systolic flow.

Repetitions of measurements (as shown in Fig. 1 at systole) revealed a good reproducibility. The correlation coefficient was $r = 0.98$, the standard deviation was 8.5 ml min^{-1}.

Figure 2 summarizes the results of flow measurements in 15 aortocoronary bypass vein grafts. The mean of systolic flow was 77 ± 33 ml min^{-1}. During the early diastole, mean flow was 132 ± 73 ml min^{-1}, during the late diastole 122 ± 57 ml min^{-1}. The differences between systolic, early and diastolic flow were highly significant. The results show that phasic flow in aortocoronary bypass grafts can be measured videodensimetrically with a good reproducibility. The *in vivo* flow measurements in individual vessels provide a quantitative evaluation of coronary artery function.

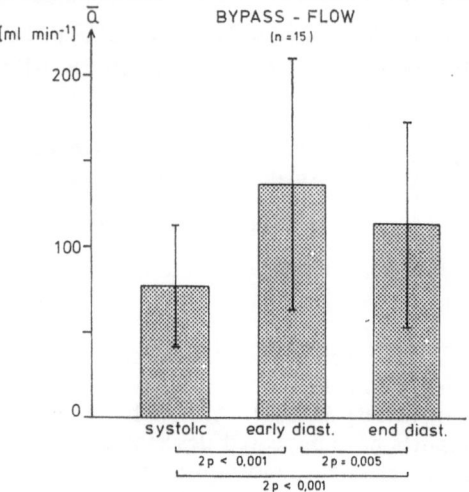

Fig. 2. Mean values $\pm$ S.D. of systolic, early and enddiastolic flow in 15 aortocoronary vein bypass grafts. The differences between the mean values are highly significant.

REFERENCES

Rutishauser, W., Bussmann, W.-D., Noseda, G., Meier, W., Wellauer, J. (1970): Blood flow measurements through single coronary arteries by roentgen densitometry, Part I. Amer. J. Roentgenol. Rad. Therapy & Nuclear Med. 109, 12.

Smith, H. C., Frye, R. L., Donald, D. E., Davis, G. D., Pluth, J. R., Sturm, R. E., Wood, E. H. (1971): Roentgen videodensitometric measure of coronary blood flow. Mayo Clin. Proc. 46, 800.

Schmiel, F. K., Huber, H., Neuhaus, K. L., Spiller, P. (1978): Densitometric measurement of coronary blood flow. Methodical improvements. in: Heintzen, P. H., Bürsch, J. H.: Roentgen-Video-Techniques Stuttgart, Thieme.

P. S., Med. Klinik und Poliklinik B der Univ., Moorenstrasse 5, 4000 Düsseldorf, F.R.G.

MICROCIRCULATORY CHANGES AND EARLY MYOCARDIAL REVASCULARIZATION

J. P. CAMILLERI, D. JOSEPH and J. N. FABIANI

Laboratory of Pathologic Anatomy, Center of University of Cordeliers, Paris, France

Several experimental studies have established that early reperfusion following temporary ischemia could reduce the extent of tissue necrosis (*Maroko et al.* 1971, 1972; *Ginks et al.* 1972). However, tests by various groups showed contradictory results. In a study using the rat as an experimental animal, we obtained heterogeneous results and demonstrated the possibility of localized infarcts following brief periods of ischemia. (*Deloche et al.* 1972; *Fontaliran et al.* 1972; *Camilleri et al.* 1975). To investigate the factors at work, the following study was undertaken to determine microcirculatory changes after varying duration of ischemia.

Materials and methods

The rat was chosen because of the possibility of working with large series and the reproducibility of the lesions obtained. Two hundred rats were used for this study.

Briefly, infarction of the left ventricle was created by ligation of the left coronary artery at its origin using the technique of Johns and Olson (1954) as modified by *Selye et al.* (1960). Reperfusion of the coronary bed was obtained by an original method of temporary ligature. The animals were divided into two groups: permanent ischemia (15—30—45—60—120 minutes), transient ischemia (the ligature was released at different time intervals and the heart removed after 15—30 minutes of reperfusion).

At the end of each experiment, fixation-perfusion was performed in all animals. Under ether anesthesia, the aorta was catheterized and the catheter attached to a constant perfusion pump with a flow rate of 50 ml per minute. Following injection of heparin and 1% potassium chloride (KCl), into the vena cava cardiac arrest occurred in diastole and the hearts were then perfused for 5 minutes with 2% glutaraldehyde made in 0.15 M cacodylate buffer pH 7.3.

In order to visualize the capillary network, a suspension of 20% colloidal carbon in gelatin (China Ink Pelikan Werke) was injected after fixation via the same aortic catheter. Transverse sections were made (50 to 100 μ in thickness) and examined with a binocular loup. For each myocardial section, the surface of injected and non-injected areas were measured by projection

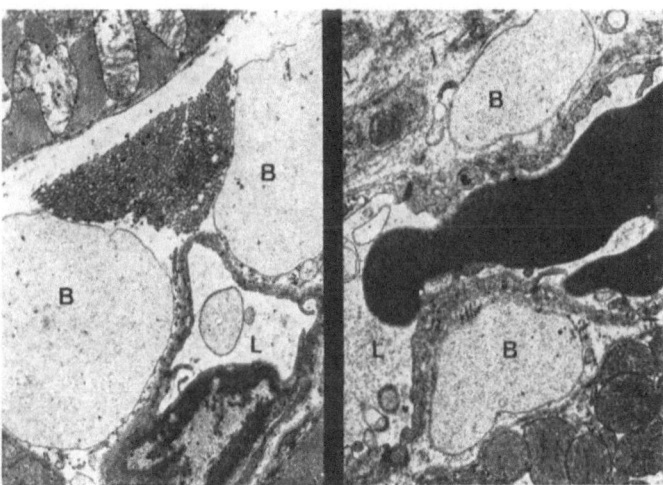

Fig. 1. Myocardium made ischemic for 30 minutes and reperfused 15 minutes. Electron micrograph of a capillary showing the lumen (L) compressed by interstitial oedematous blebs (B) on transverse (left) and longitudinal (right) sections. G = ×14.000.

on a grid using a simple planimetric method.

For electron microscopy, blocks of selected myocardial areas were dropped into 1 mm square fragments. Following fixation in 3% glutaraldehyde these samples were washed in cold buffer, post-fixed in 1% osmium tetraoxide, dehydrated and embedded in epon.

The sarcolemmal and endothelial permeability was investigated in the early phase of ischemic injury by using the diffusion tracer, horse radish peroxidase (HRP). The tracer HRP (Sigma type II) was injected through a femoral vein in dose of 10 mg/100 g body weight. Animals were sacrified following 6 minutes HRP circulation time by perfusion of the fixative.

Results

Colloidal carbon black injection

After permanent ligation, no injection was seen in the ischemic myocardial area. In the reperfused group restoration of blood flow was accompanied by the absence of capillary injection in varying areas. This no-reflow phenomenon was observed for periods of ischemia of short duration, i.e. 15 minutes. The severity of this phenomenon was in direct proportion to the length of ischemia time.

Electron microscopy

After 15 to 45 minutes of blood flow interruption, a few endothelial cells showed margination of chromatin, dilatation of endoplasmic reticulum and cellular swelling. At this phase, the collapse of the capillary bed appeared to be due chiefly to interstitial and myocardial cell edema (Fig. 1, 2),

After the first hour, almost all the sections of the vessels showed pale, empty endothelial cells with protrusion of cytoplasmic blebs and obstruction of capillary lumen.

In cases of temporary ischemia followed by reperfusion, cellular swelling was increased. Reperfusion after 60 minutes of ischemia led to a dramatic deterioration of the myocardial cell with capillary rupture, interstitial hemorrhages and fibrin deposits.

Protein tracer study (HRP)

In ischemic myocardium, the enzymatic reaction product visualized the irregularly widened interstitial spaces. After 15 minutes of blood flow interruption and 6 minutes of HRP circulation time, the tracer did not appear in the muscle cells. After 15 minutes of ischemia followed by 15 minutes of reperfusion, the reaction product was detected in some muscle cells randomly distributed throughout the myocardium. After 30 minutes of ischemia followed by 15 minutes of reperfusion, the tracer appeared in groups of neighbouring muscle cells. Electron microscopy identified intracytoplasmic localization of HRP (Figure 3).

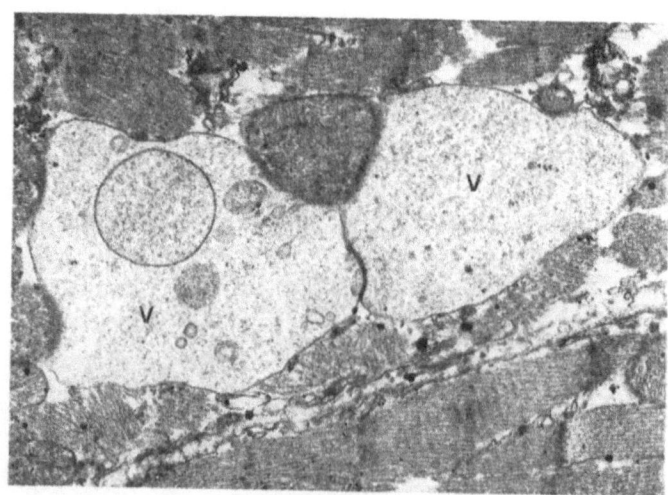

Fig. 2. Intracytoplasmic vacuoles (V) in myocardium made ischemic for 30 minutes. G = ×40.000.

Fig. 3. 30 minutes tempo-
rary ischemia followed by
15 minutes of reperfusion
including 6 minutes of HRP
circulation time. a) HRP
reaction products are seen
in the pericapillary space
and in the sarcoplasm of
a myocardial cell (arrows =
sarcolemma; L = lumen;
M = mitochondria). b)
Heavy deposit of HRP re-
action is evident in the
sarcoplasm and around the
mitochondria (M).

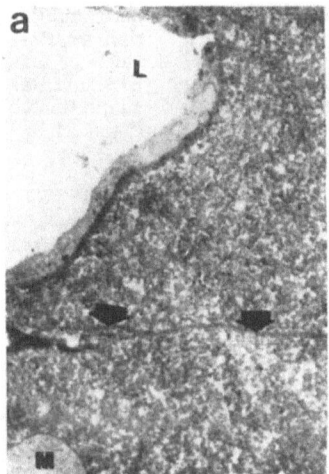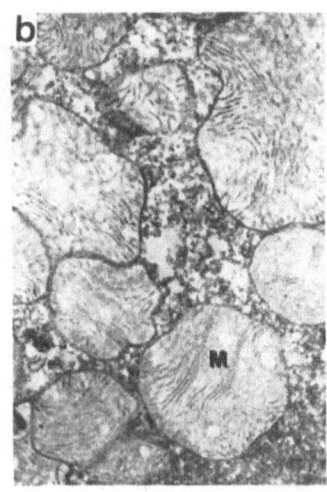

Comments

It appears that restoration of blood flow
following temporary ischemia may result
in removal of large areas from the effects
of reperfusion (*Kloner et al.* 1974; *Camilleri et al.* 1976). This so-called "no-reflow"
phenomenon has already been observed
in the kidney (*Flores et al.* 1972) and brain
(*Majno et al.* 1967). The localized reduced
perfusion may be explained on the basis
of hypoxic cellular swelling (*Ganote et al.*
1977). The myocardial cell membrane loses
its selective permeability and, on restoration of blood flow, allows leakage of intra-

cellular enzymes from the cell and the influx of ions, water and extracellular macromolecular tracer into the cell as HRP
(*Rona et al.* 1977). Our fine structural
findings in the first 40 minutes of ischemia
suggest that a definite relationship exists
between capillary block and sarcolemmal
permeability.

More changes can be seen in the blood
vessels after ischemias lasting one hour or
more. The degree of damage is dependent
on the duration of the ischemia. In late
reperfusions partial disruption of the capillary wall may explain the deleterious effect
of the restoration of blood flow.

REFERENCES

*Camilleri J. P., Fabiani J. N., Deloche A., Gurd-
jian C.:* Etude histochimique et histoenzymo-
logique de l'infarctus expérimental du rat
après ligature permanente ou temporaire de la
coronaire gauche. Virch. Arch. A Path. Anat.
366, 149—175, 1975.

*Camilleri J. P., Joseph D., Fabiani J. N., Deloche
A., Schlumberger M., Relland J., Carpentier A.:*
Microcirculatory changes following early reperfusion in experimental myocardial infarction. Virch. Arch. A Path. Anat. 369, 315—
333, 1976.

*Deloche A., Fontaliran F., Fabiani J. N., Pennecot
G., Carpentier A., Dubost Ch.:* Etude expérimentale de la revascularisation chirurgicale
précoce de l'infarctus du myocarde. Ann.
Chir. Thor. Cardiovasc. 11, 89—105, 1972.

*Fontaliran F., Deloche A., Camilleri J. P., Car-
pentier A., Diebolo J.:* Effets de la revascularisation sur l'évolution histopathologique de
l'infarctus expérimental du Rat. Path. Biol.
20, 393—400, 1972.

*Ginks W. R., Sybers H. D., Maroko P. R., Covell
J. W., Sobel B. E., Ross J.:* Coronary artery
reperfusion: II-Reduction of myocardial infarct size at 1 week after the coronary occlusion. J. Clin. Invest. 51, 2717—2733, 1972.

Flores J., Dibona D. R.. Beck C. H., Leaf A.:
The role of cell swelling in ischemic renal
damage and the protective effect of hypertonic
solute. J. Clin. Invest. 51, 118—126, 1972.

Kloner R. A., Gandte C. E., Jennings R. B.: The
"no-reflow" phenomenon after temporary
coronary occlusion in the dog. J. Clin. Invest.
54, 1496—1508, 1974.

Majno G., Ames A., Chaing J., Wright R. L.: No reflow cerebral ischemia. Lancet, 2, 569 to 570, 1967.

Maroko P. R., Kjeskhus J. K., Sobel B. E., Watanabe T., Covell J. W., Ross J., Braunwald E.: Factors influencing infarct size following experimental coronary artery occlusion. Circulation, 43, 67—82, 1971.

Rona G., Huttner I., Dusek J., Badonne M. C.: Experimental studies on cardiac muscle cell adaptation to insult. Basic Res. Cardiol. 72, 214—221, 1977.

J. P. C., Centre Universitaire des Cordeliers, 15—21, rue de l'Ecole-de-Médecine 75270 Paris Cedex, France

ROLE OF NUCLEAR CARDIOLOGY IN THE PRESENT PRACTICE OF CORONARY SURGERY

W. D. JOHNSON, R. T. SHORE and D. H. SCHMIDT

University of Wisconsin, Mount Sinai Medical Center, Milwaukee, Wisconsin U.S.A.

Recent advances in nuclear cardiology have made these techniques particularly suited for the evaluation of patients prior to and following coronary surgery. The techniques available are listed in Table I. The studies applicable to surgery include technetium pyrophosphate scans, of which we have done 1.025 studies, rest and stress thallium[201] scans to measure regional myocardial perfusion, of which we have done 525, and first pass dynamic studies either at rest, with nitroglycerin intervention, or with exercise, of which we have done 1.250. Additional studies done at the time of catheterization include Xenon[133] quantitative regional myocardial blood flow and microsphere perfusion tests.

We consider pre and postoperative technetium pyrophosphate scans as the most accurate means to evaluate perioperative infarcts. In a study which we have recently completed (*Wadhwa et al.*, 1977), 178 patients had preoperative MI scans and had these studies repeated three to five days following surgery. In this group of patients, there was an overall 9% incidence of perioperative infarction. In the same group of patients, 4% developed new electrocardiographic evidence of infarction namely developed a new Q wave. In one patient, Q waves were noted in the inferior leads following surgery in the presence of a negative MI scan. Of more importance though, this technique closely defines the area and extent of damage to the ventricle and can be correlated with the specific bypass performed. Our data, therefore, show it to be more specific than enzymes or the electrocardiogram, hence it has largely supplemented these studies on our service.

It has been well shown that stress thallium scintigrams done in conjunction with conventional stress testing is more sensitive in defining coronary insufficiency than conventional stress tests alone. Microsphere perfusion studies done at the time of catheterization provide virtually the same information as a resting thallium study. Neither procedure unequivocally differentiates severely ischemic muscle from scar and cannot be used, in our opinion, to reject patients for surgery. Postoperative thallium[201] studies are useful to assess the results of revascularization and to follow graft patency. In a recent study, comparing the pre and postoperative thallium scintigrams in 75 patients, an analysis was made of defects pre and postoperatively. Sixty-three percent or 201 out of 319 were better, 31% or 91 out of 319 remained the same, and 6% or 20 out of 319 became larger and more clearly

Table 1. Techniques available.

NUCLEAR CARDIOLOGY

TECHNIQUES AVAILABLE

I. NONINVASIVE

    A. STATIC IMAGING

        1) TECHNETIUM PYROPHOSPHATE

          (MI SCANS)

        2) THALLIUM [201] SCANS

          (REGIONAL MYOCARDIAL PERFUSION)

    B. DYNAMIC STUDIES

        (FIRST TRANSIT)

        1) REST (RAO AND LAO)

        2) INTERVENTION (NITROGLYCERIN)

        3) EXERCISE

II. INVASIVE

    A. PARTICLE PERFUSION STUDIES

        (MACROAGGREGATES AND MICROSPHERES)

    B. QUANTITATIVE REGIONAL MYOCARDIAL BLOOD FLOW

        (XENON [133])

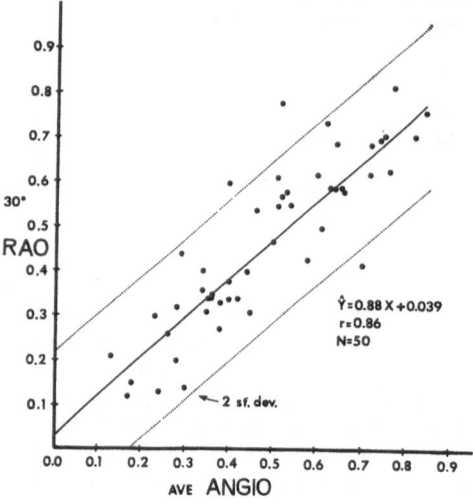

EJECTION FRACTION

Fig. 1. Regression analysis of 50 patients comparing RAO radionuclide angiography to biplane contrast angiography. The ejection fractions range from .12 to .80. There is good correlation with r = 0.86. RAO = right anterior oblique radionuclide angiography, Average Angio = biplane contrast ventriculography.

defined. If one of these defects which improved with surgery documenting successful revascularization again reappeared in follow-up at a later date, we would feel that this represented a graft closure. Perfusion studies have been most valuable in selecting borderline patients for surgery. A number of patients have negative stress tests and equivocal lesions on coronary arteriography. A positive thallium scintigram in this situation signifies to us a functionally significant lesion and we would recommend surgery.

Recent studies in our laboratory using Xenon[133] at rest and following isuprel infusions would suggest that internal mammary bypass grafts respond to increased demand equally as well as vein bypass grafts and very similar to the normal coronary circulation.

Dynamic studies, that is, studies to evaluate ventricular function, utilizing radionuclide techniques are done by the first transit method which has been adequately

described in the literature (*Marshall et al.,* 1977; *Bodenheimer et al.,* 1978; *Schad et al.,* 1978). We routinely perform these tests in both the right anterior oblique and left anterior oblique projections, thereby enabling us to look at the overall wall motion. They accurately correlate with contrast ventriculography in our laboratory as shown in Figure 2. Not only can these

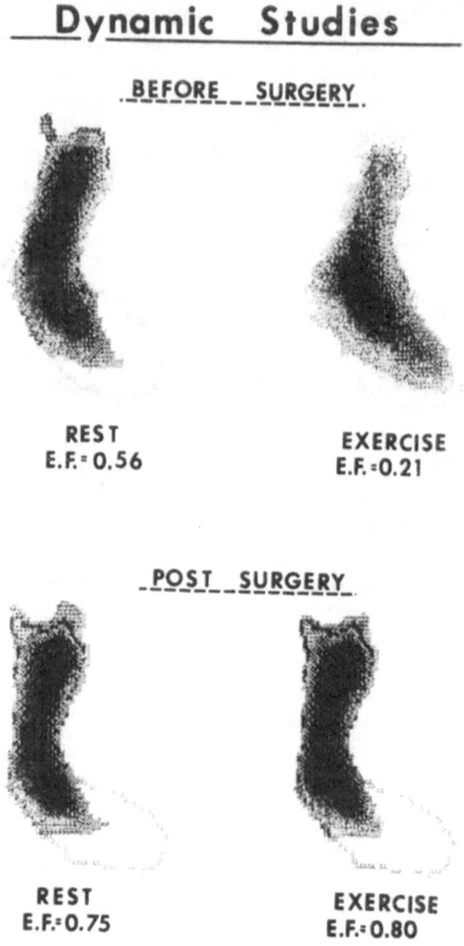

Dynamic Studies

BEFORE SURGERY

REST
E.F. = 0.56

EXERCISE
E.F. = 0.21

POST SURGERY

REST
E.F. = 0.75

EXERCISE
E.F. = 0.80

Fig. 2. Radionuclide angiography in the RAO position at rest and during exercise before surgery in a patient with a left main coronary artery stenosis and after myocardial revascularization. Before surgery the resting ejection fraction was .56 and fell to .21 with exercise. Following bypass surgery the resting ejection fraction was .75 and rose to .80 with exercise.
EF = ejection fraction.

734

studies be done at rest, but of equal importance are intervention studies where the test can be performed after nitroglycerin. Improved function and wall motion following the administration of nitroglycerin helps to differentiate between viable muscle and scar tissue.

An exciting new area of evaluation consists of doing exercise dynamics. For this purpose, the patient is positioned on a bicycle ergometer and exercise. Initially, a rest study is done in this same position and then the patient is exercised and while performing a given level of exercise, a second dynamic study is performed. Most hearts perform normally at rest but in the patient with significant coronary artery disease with exercise and the ventricle becoming ischemic, the ejection fraction will stay the same or will fall rather than going up as it normally does with exercise (*Rerych et al.*, 1978). In Figure 3 we have shown the results of a rest and exercise study in a patient preoperatively, where the ejection fraction fell from 56% to 21% with mild exercise. Postoperatively, following successful revascularization, the resting ejection fraction was 75% which went up to 80% with exercise.

In summary, the dynamic studies can be done safely, repeatedly and cost-effectively to evaluate the effect of drugs, surgery and exercise. In combination with the technetium pyrophosphate MI scan, they accurately define the area and the effect of any infarct on performance. In summary, our data demonstrates that nuclear cardiology is very helpful in the practice of coronary artery surgery. These studies quantitate perioperative infarcts, screen and eliminate the need for catheterization, influence the selection of a patient for surgery and serially measure ventricular function to guide the rehabilitation of postoperative patients.

REFERENCES

Bodenheimer M. M., Banka V. S., Fooshee C. M., Hermann G. A., Helfant R. H. (1978): Quantitative radionuclide angiography in the right anterior oblique view: Comparison with contrast ventriculography Am. J. Card. 41: 718.

Marshall R. C., Berger H. J., Costin J. C., Freedman, G. S., Wolberg J., Cohen L. S., Gottschalk A., Zaret B. L. (1977): Assessment of cardiac performance with quantitative radionuclide angiography: Sequential left ventricular ejection fraction, normalized left ventricular ejection rate, and regional wall motion. Circulation 56: 820—829.

Rerych S. K., Scholz P. M., Newman G. E., Sa-
biston D. C., Jones R. H. (1978): Cardiac function at rest and during exercise in normals and in patients with coronary heart disease: Evaluation by radionuclide angiocardiography. Ann. Surg. 187: 449—464.

Schad N., Nickel O. (1978): Radionuclide angiography of the heart in coronary heart disease Where do we stand? Cardiovasc. Radiol. 1: 27—35.

Wadhwa S. K., Schmidt D. H., Johnson W. D. (1977): Myocardial infarction in coronary artery surgery: Correlation of scintigrams, enzymes, electrocardiograms and vectorcardiograms. Clin. Res. 25: 261A.

W. D. J., Mont Sinai Med. Center, 950 N. 12th Street, Milwaukee, Wisconsin 52301, U.S.A.

CURRENT STATUS AND PROSPECTS OF CORONARY SURGERY

L. HEJHAL, J. FABIÁN, P. FIRT and A. BELÁN

Institute for Clinical and Experimental Medicine, Prague, Czechoslovakia

Up to the end of the sixties, the unprecedented progress in cardiac surgery had little effect on the management of ischaemic heart disease. In the past decade, the development of cardiovascular surgery for acquired or congenital diseases has slowed down. In contrast, surgical management of ischaemic heart disease is making progress which, because of its rate and social impact surpasses all other spheres of cardiovascular surgery. At present, patients with ischaemic heart disease make up 60% of all candidates for cardiac surgery.

ACBG IN THE USA

Year	No.
1968-1974	100 000
1975	54 000
1976	60 000
1977	80 000

Over the past seven years — 1968—1974 — more than 100 000 by-pass procedures have been performed in the United States — and in 1977 alone the number rose to over 80 000.

The high and steadily growing number of operations can be attributed to the high incidence of ischaemic heart disease. Another reason is low operative mortality, along with a significant improvement of symptoms and the quality of life in the majority of the operated patients.

Ischaemic heart disease is the main cause of death in industrial countries. In addition, millions of people all over the world suffer from and are incapacitated by this disease. An allout use of all possibilities offered by surgery of ischaemic heart disease is becoming an extraordinarily important problem medically, scientifically and socially. A more accurate evaluation of the experience gathered would help to further improve the results, define the indication and improve organizational measures.

The effect of this procedure on life expectancy is still being discussed. So far, an unequivocal and generally accepted proof of the benefits of this operation for longer life expectancy is available only for symptomatic narrowing of the main left coronary artery. The results of studies on the effect of surgical management of other patients are still ambiguous. However, the nature of the operation promises a far greater effect on life expectancy than has been hitherto realized. This realization will grow with increasing improvement of diagnosis, surgical techniques and postoperative care.

In the light of the high rate of immediate death from myocardial infarction, preventive operation of not too symptomatic and even asymptomatic patients seems to be fully justified in the near future. At the same time, the patients with severe left ventricular dysfunction can be operated and their prognosis may be better than without surgery.

Closer attention should be paid to more effective utilisation of the current knowledge and techniques in the management of acute coronary attacks. Modern coronary units should be equipped with facilities for urgent coronary arteriography and surgical intervention and should make full use of all facilities for postoperative care including intra-aortic balloon counterpulsation. The possibilities of therapeutic management of acute coronary heart attacks and the facilities employed to control them will shortly be the main criterion for the assessment of the professional and organisational standards of cardiovascular centres.

Perfect organization and economy of work are of utmost importance in the surgical management of ischaemic heart disease. Full-scale medical care for all who

736

need it represents a great financial burden even for wealthy societies, due to the high costs of diagnostic and surgical procedures and the high incidence of this disease. Yet, the number of operations will necessarily grow in most countries. For reasons of economy and professional standards, it is desirable to expand the capacity of the existing centres rather than to build new, poor-quality ones. The lowest admissible number of surgical procedures for ischaemic heart disease should be about 200 annually. Only such or a higher case-load assures economic utilisation of expensive equipment, which is also essential for the attainment and maintenance of high professional standards of the team and for optimum patient care.

At this point, the total required capacity cannot be predicted with absolute accuracy. A reasonable lower but appropriate limit for most European countries seems to be 200 procedures annually per 1 million population. So far, the facilities available in a great majority of European countries lag behind this requirement. Inadequate application of our present knowledge to the treatment and prevention of cardiovascular disease is a problem of growing importance and is true not only for surgical management of ischaemic heart disease.

Therefore a general application of new and effective medical and surgical techniques and procedures is the major task of medical care. Organisation of diagnostic and medical care should rely on realistic prognosis and possibilities of the societies, rather than on unrealistic ideas and hypothesis.

L. H., IKEM, Vídeňská 800, 146 22 Prague 4, Czechoslovakia

MYOCARDIAL REVASCULARIZATION IN MARKED LEFT VENTRICULAR DYSFUNCTION

D. H. SCHMIDT, CH. K. HELLMAN and W. D. JOHNSON

University of Wisconsin, Mount Sinai Medical Center, Milwaukee, Wisconsin, U.S.A.

Coronary artery bypass graft surgery in patients with marked left ventricular dysfunction remains a controversial subject. It has been stated frequently in the recent literature that coronary artery surgery in patients with marked left ventricular dysfunction carries a prohibitively high perioperative mortality and provides little evidence to show improvement in left ventricular function (*Spencer, et al.* 1971; *Solignac, et al.* 1974; *Hammermeister, et al.* 1974). In many medical centers the finding of marked left ventricular dysfunction is considered enough to rule out myocardial revascularization. To evaluate this frequently encountered problem, 43 consecutive patients with an ejection fraction of less than 0.40 by both conventional contrast left ventriculography and first pass radionuclide angiography were prospectively studied. All patients had coronary arteriography and left ventricular angiography by either the *Sones* or a modified *Judkins* technique, and pre and postoperative first pass right anterior oblique and left anterior oblique nuclear cardiac dynamics studies using a multiple crystal camera.

Radionuclide dynamic studies were analyzed for overall ejection fraction and regional wall motion by the method previously reported by our own as well as other institutions (*Hellman and Schmidt,* 1978). Summing the end-diastolic and end-systolic counts of the beats as the radioactive bolus passes through the left ventricle, ejection fraction is calculated in the standard manner. Using the summed beats, a representative cycle is formed. With its higher number of counts an end-diastolic perimeter is produced along with an end-systolic image.

In addition, in 41 of 43 followed patients, pre and postoperative technetium – 99 m pyrophosphate myocardial infarction scans were performed by the multicrystal camera in the anterior LAO and left lateral views. Following surgery, all patients were followed periodically by our own staff with follow-up visits as well as by telephone.

The patient population is summarized in Table I. There were 43 patients with a defined ejection fraction of less than 40 operated on from January 14, 1976 to February 28, 1978, with 15 having coronary artery bypass graft surgery alone, 28 having resection of an akinetic or dyskinetic area in addition to grafting. The average age of the population was 56.5 years. There was essentially three-vessel disease in each patient and the number of grafts placed per patient averaged 3.5. The patients were further subdivided on the basis of specific surgical procedure with 15 having myocardial revascularization alone (Group 1), 12 having bypass graft surgery and resection of an angiographically demonstrated akinetic area (Group

TABLE I: POPULATION PROFILE

	(T) TOTAL POPULATION	(I) CABGS ALONE	(II) CABGS & RAA	(III) CABGS & RDA
1. TOTAL NUMBER	43	15	12	16
2. AGE	57.6	56.5	57.1	58.1
3. DISEASED VESSELS	2.8	2.7	3.0	2.7
4. GRAFTS	3.6	4.1	3.8	2.3
5. PRE-OP EJECTION FRACTION	0.26	0.30	0.26	0.20

CABGS = CORONARY ARTERY BYPASS GRAFT SURGERY
RAA = RESECTION OF AN AKINETIC AREA
RDA = RESECTION OF A DYSKINETIC AREA

2), and 16 patients who had bypass graft surgery and aneurysmectomy of a dyskinetic area.

When the radionuclide angiogram fractions were compared to conventional contrast ventriculography, there was good correlation using linear regression analysis with an r value of .82. The effect of surgery on ventricular performance as measured by radionuclide angiography is shown in Figure 1. Examining the total population, there is a very significant overall increase in ejection fraction after surgery, with a mean increase in the radionuclide ejection fraction from .25 to .34 (p < .001).

Closer analysis of ventricular performance following surgery revealed the following: patients who had coronary artery bypass graft surgery alone had a significant increase in the mean nuclear cardiac dynamic ejection fraction from .30 to .38; patients who had coronary artery bypass graft surgery combined with resection of an akinetic area also had a significant increase in the ejection fraction from .26 to 0.32; patients who had a coronary artery bypass graft surgery combined with resection of a dyskinetic area had a more significant increase in the radionuclide ejection fraction from 0.20 to 0.33. Therefore, all subsets showed significant improvement in left ventricular function with the patients having both coronary artery bypass graft surgery and resection of a dyskinetic area showing the greatest postoperative to preoperative change, namely 65%.

Follow-up of the patient population also yields interesting information. Of 43 patients followed up to 114 weeks post surgery − a mean of 52 weeks − shows no operative deaths, one death before patient discharge from the hospital and six patient deaths post discharge from the hospital. In the seven deaths, the average patient was similar to that of the total population, the average time of surgery to death interval was 20.6 weeks, there was a nonsignificant increase in mean ejection fractions in these patients from 0.25 to 0.28 and in all five patients in whom a postoperative myocardial infarction scan was done, it was positive.

The positive myocardial infarction scans are all the more significant when considering the postoperative myocardial infarction scans as a whole. The overall perioperative infarction rate at our institution is 9% by the positive myocardial infarction scan criteria (3% by ECG criteria). To reiterate, all of the five studied patients who died had a new positive MI scan after surgery. This is despite the fact that all five had some increase in ejection fraction postoperatively and only two of seven had new ECG changes.

In summary, coronary artery bypass graft surgery in patients with marked left ventricular dysfunction generally does

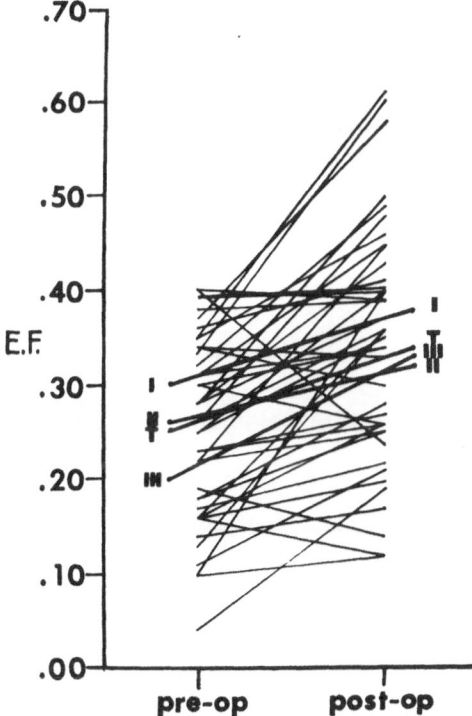

Fig. 1. The effect of surgery on ventricular performance as measured by radionuclide angiography.
EF = ejection fraction, Pre-op = preoperative, Post-op = postoperative, T = mean value of total population, I = mean value of Group 1, II = mean value of Group 2, III = mean value of Group 3.

significantly improve left ventricular ejection fraction. In patients with an angiographically demonstrated dyskinetic area, myocardial revascularization combined with aneurysmectomy offers marked potential improvement in left ventricular ejection fraction over graft surgery alone. Furthermore, patients dying in the first year following surgery appear to be identified by a positive myocardial infarction scan in this series and finally, noninvasive nuclear cardiac dynamic studies are a quantitative method to assess the results of coronary artery bypass graft surgery, and potentially help in the planning of post-surgical therapy.

REFERENCES

Hammermeister K. E., Kennedy K. W., Hamilton J. E., Steward D. K., Gould K. L., Lipscomb, F., Murray J. A. (1974): Aortocoronary saphenous vein bypass: failure of successful grafting to improve resting left ventricular function in chronic angina. N. Engl. J. Med. 290: 186 to 192.

Hellman C., Schmidt D. H. (1978): First pass RAO radionuclide angiography after nitroglycerin to assess myocardial viability. Clin. Res. 26: 239A.

Solignac A., Lespviance J., Gronden P., Campeace L. (1974): Aorta-to-coronary bypass operation for chronic intractible heart failure. Can. J. Surg. 17: 76—84.

Spencer F. C., Green G. E., Tice G. A., Wallsch E., Mills N. L., Glassman E. (1971): Coronary artery bypass grafts for congestive heart failure: a report of experiences with 43 patients. J. Thorac. Cardiovasc. Surg. 62: 529—538.

D. H. S., Mount Sinai Med. Center, 950 N. 12th Street, Milwaukee, Wisconsin 53201, U.S.A.

VALIDITY OF AORTO-CORONARY BYPASS SURGERY IN IMPENDING MYOCARDIAL INFARCTION

K. TAMURA, N. HIGUMA, S. BANNAI and T. OZAWA

Niigata University School of Medicine, Niigata, Japan

Introduction

The efficacy of aorto-coronary bypass surgery in impending myocardial infarction has not yet been established in spite of much research in this field. The main reason for this problem is the lack of good evaluation of the surgical results (*Chatter-* *jee, 1973*). Therefore, this study was carried out to evaluate the efficacy of this surgery in impending myocardial infarction comparing the pre- and the post-surgical data as follows: (i) symptoms, (ii) electrocardiogram, (iii) coronary circulation, (iv) myocardial metabolism and (v) systemic hemodynamics.

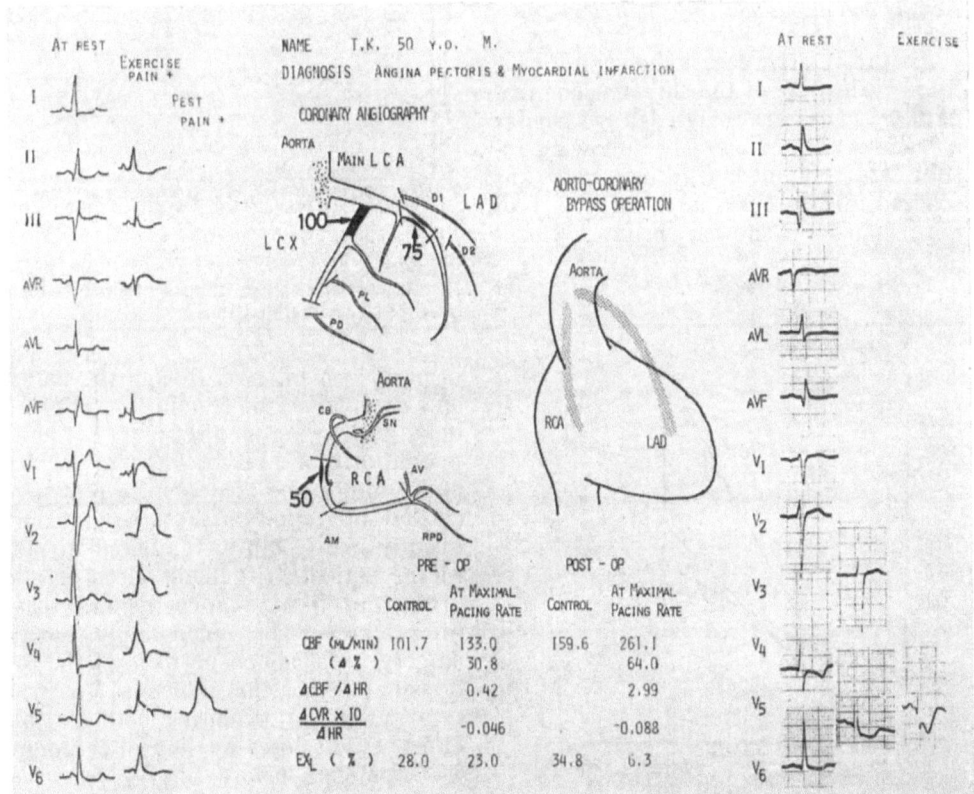

Fig. 1. A representative case of polyparametric evaluation of a−c bypass surgery. CBF = coronary sinus blood flow, HR = heart rate, CVR = coronary vascular resistance, EX_1 = myocardial extraction ratio of lactate.

Materials and methods

The patients underwent this surgery were as follows: (i) patients who were resistant to the usual medical therapy, (ii) patients with a critical stenotic lesion in the coronary artery disclosed by coronary angiogram and (iii) patients with social indications. 11 cases all male, with age ranging from 39 to 63 years were selected for this study.

Methods were as follows, taking the poly-parametric approach for the evaluation: (i) symptoms, (ii) electrocardiogram by Holter monitor system, bed-side telemetry and "near maximal" exercise stress test by treadmill using the Ellestad protocol, (iii) coronary sinus blood flow by the continuous local thermodilution method with pacing stress test (*Sowton, 1967*), (iv) myocardial oxygen consumption and myocardial lactate extraction ratio, (v) cardiac output with left ventricular filling pressure by Swan-Ganz catheter and (vi) selective coronary angiogram.

Results and discussion

A representative case is shown in Figure 1 for evaluation of the surgery. The rest of the patients were analysed in as a similar a manner as possible. The following results were obtained. (i) Chest pain was relieved in 8/11 cases after surgery. 1 of the remaining 3 showed an improvement

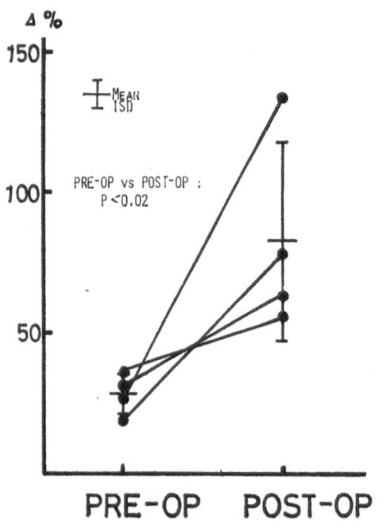

Fig. 2. Increment of coronary sinus blood flow during the pacing stress test; with postoperative data compared preoperative data.

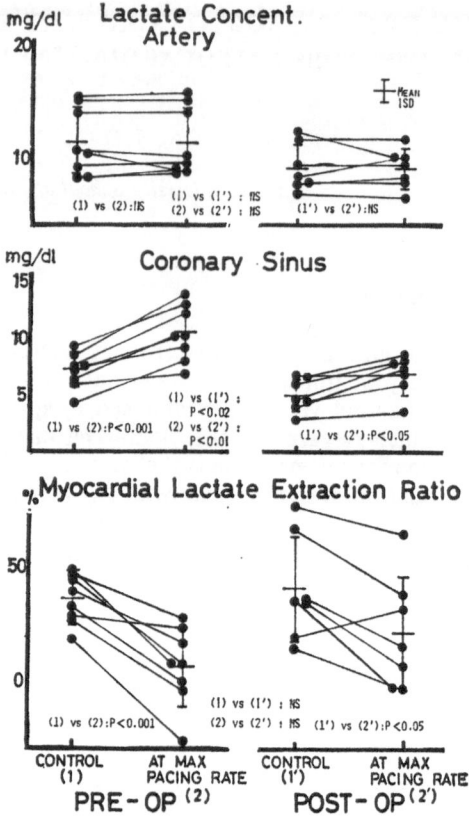

Fig. 3. Lactate changes in both preoperative and postoperative examinations.

in cardiac pain, even though the patient still complained of certain limitations in daily activities after the surgery. 1 other patient died of a cerebrovascular accident and another one died of recurrent myocardial infarction after surgery. Consequently chest pain was relieved in most of the patients. (ii) In the electrocardiogram, the Q wave appeared in 2 cases after surgery. This might imply that the surgery itself caused necrosis of the pre-exsistant myocardial ischemia. The transient ST elevation during both rest and effort was disclosed by the Holter monitor in 7 patients before surgery. However, 5/7 cases did not show this alteration after surgery. ST depression also disappeared in 2 cases with markedly improved tolerance in the treadmill stress test. The treadmill stress test showed improved exercise tolerance in 6/8 cases after the surgery. Again the electrocardiographic changes were mostly improved in these patients. (iii) The increment in the magnitude of the coronary sinus blood flow under the pacing stress test was examined. By this stress test, 7/8 cases were proved angina before surgery. However, after surgery only 1 of these patients developed anginal pain during stress. This increment in the coronary sinus blood flow during pacing stress was markedly improved in every case (Figure 2). Furthermore, the coronary vascular resistance per 10 cardiac beats was significantly decreased ($P < 0.05$). In some cases, the patency of the graft was also examined during the surgery by occluding this graft temporarily. Then the flow was calculated. By this procedure, not only the patency of the graft but also the coronary vascular reserve was quantitatively measured. From these data it follows that the flow was definitely increased after surgery. (iv) Myocardial oxygen consumption was also improved after surgery as the coronary sinus blood flow itself increased.

These data would indicate improvement of the coronary perfusion, as our previous data disclosed that the coronary sinus blood flow increment was dependent on the existence of the coronary stenosis. In the coronary ischemia this increment in the flow was less than that of the control. The change in the lactate extraction ratio was also examined as the metabolic marker of the existance of the myocardial ischemia during pacing stress (Figure 3). Before the surgery, even myocardial lactate production was observed as shown in Figure 3. However, this lactate extraction ratio was also significantly improved after surgery. However, in 2 cases this ratio to lactate production remained even after surgery. One of these two cases showed no improvement of ST depression in the exercise test. Furthermore, the remaining case also showed no improvement in symptoms and the exercise tolerance test. (V) The cardiac output remained the same. The left ventricular filling pressure and the mean arterial pressure remained almost the same.

REFERENCES

1. *Tamura K., Higuma N., Bannai S., Aoyagi R., Izumi T., Matsuoka M., Eguchi S. (1978):* Coronary circulation, myocardial metabolism and hemodynamics of pacing-induced angina. Recent Advances in Studies on Cardiac Structure and Metabolism 12: 265.
2. *Sowton G. E., Balcon R., Cross D., Frick M. H. (1967):* Measurement of the anginal threshold using atrial pacing. Cardiovasc. Res. 1: 301.
3. *Chatterjee K., Swan H. F. C., Parmley W. W., Sustaita H., Marcus H. S., Matloff J. (1973):* Influence of direct myocardial revascularization on left ventricular asynergy and function in patients with coronary heart disease. Circulation XLVII: 276.

K. T., Niigata Univ. School Med., Osaka Univ. Fukushima, 1 Chome, Fukushima-ku, Osaka 553, Japan

FUNCTIONAL CONSEQUENCES OF CORONARY RECONSTRUCTION

Chairman: J. J. Collins, Jr. (U.S.A.)

Co-Chairman: J. Fabian (Czechoslovakia)

Participants: V. Brodan (Czechoslovakia)
               P.-T. Harjola (Finland)
               W. D. Johnson (U.S.A.)

The members of the panel expressed the opinion that a successful reconstruction of coronary arteries results not only in amelioration of the patient's symptoms, but also in better physical performance due to correction of the mechanical function of the left ventricle. Direct coronary surgery is at present the only therapeutical method with a clear-cut effect on the mechanical function of the left ventricle in patients with ischemic heart disease. This has been demonstrated by direct techniques as well as by less invasive methods such as radio-isotopes etc. A successful reconstruction of the coronary arteries also helps to correct the heart muscle metabolism. More recently, the operation has been carried out in some centres even on patients with a seriously damaged function of the left ventricle. In spite of a higher mortality in this particular group of patients, it would appear that the prognosis is more favourable than with conservative treatment. However, many aspects of the problem have not yet been unanimously solved and obviously require concentrated attention.

ROUND-TABLE DISCUSSION

COUNTERPULSATION

Chairman: J. Vašků (Czechoslovakia)

Co-Chairman: M. Deutsch (Austria)

Participants: M. Kučera (Czechoslovakia)
             Z. Náprstek (Czechoslovakia)
             E. Wullner (Austria)

Vašků reviewed the present position of intraaortic baloon counterpulsation and discussed the pathophysiological basis and clinical aspects. Using own experiments, he demonstrated the effectiveness in the model of failure of the left ventricle and described the counterpulsation systems developed in the Institute of Pathological Physiology in Brno. Wullner pointed out the importance of pre-and post-operative care in cardiac surgery, particularly in patients after myocardial infarction with a low-output syndrome. Patients with impending myocardial infarction and acute coronary angiography may also be considered as candidates for IABC. The most frequent complication is aortic dissection (5%). — Náprstek pointed out that indications for the IABC at the Institute for Clinical and Experimental Medicine in Prague are similar to those of Bergman.

Care must be taken to prevent ischemia of the extremities. A frequent fault is the delayed onset of IABC. The augmentation capacity is limited by the functional condition of the myocardium. Bifocal synchronous cardiac stimulation may be an important measure in patients with serious ventricular tachyarrhythmias before IABC. — Kučera recommended more frequent application of IABC. Ideally, fully automatic equipments would be the technique of choice, but they are not available so far. The problems of IABC are closely connected to those of short-term mechanical assistance to the left ventricle.

Generally, the systems of mechanical assistance to the failing left ventricle have been considered as highly important procedures in modern cardiac surgery which may be of considerable value in improving therapeutical results.

INDEX OF SUBJECTS

AUTHOR INDEX*

---

* Numbers in bold types refer to the first page of the authors communication

753

754